OXFORD MEDICAL PUBLICATIONS

Commission of the European Communities
Health Services Research Series
No. 9

This book is one of a series concerned with health services research. It is and outcome of coordinated work by COMAC-HSR (Comité d'Action Concertée) which reports to the CGC Medical and Health Research (Comité de Gestion et de Coordination) of the Commission of the European Communities, Directorate-General Science, Research Development (DG XII).

The research is carried out by 'concerted action' method. The Commission of the European Communities pays the costs of coordination and of bringing together researchers from various countries, while the actual research is paid executed by each country. The aim is to accelerate joint research activities by Member States in selected fields, such as health services research.

1. *Perinatal Care Delivery Systems: Description and Evaluation in European Community Countries* Edited by Monique Kaminski, Gérard Bréart, Pierre Buekens, Hank J. Huisjes, Gillian McIlwaine, and Hans-Konrad Selbmann.

2. *Economic Appraisal of Health Technology in the European Community* Edited by M.F. Drummond.

3. *Technology Assessment and New Kidney Stone Treatment Methods* Edited by F. Kamper-Jørgensen, S. Challah, and T. Folmer Andersen.

4. *Expensive Health Technologies: regulatory and administrative mechanisms in Europe* Edited by Barbara Stocking.

5. *European Community Atlas of Avoidable Death* Volume One, Second edition, Edited by W.W. Holland.

6. *Home Care for Older People in Europe: A Comparison of Policies and Practices* Edited by Anne Jamieson.

7. *Equity in the Finance and Delivery of Health Care* Edited by Eddy Van Doorslaer, Adam Wagstaff, and Frans Rutten.

8. *European Community Atlas of Avoidable Death,* Volume Two, Second edition, Edited by W. W. Holland.

9. *European Community Atlas of Avoidable Death 1985–89,* Edited by W. W. Holland.

EUROPEAN COMMUNITY ATLAS OF 'AVOIDABLE DEATH' 1985–89

W. W. Holland
Project Director

EC Working Group on
Health Services and 'Avoidable Deaths'

A. Fitzgerald (Project Co-ordinator)

S. Phillips (Computer Analyst)

R. Wood (Editorial Assistant)

J. Barry, M. H. Bouvier-Colle, V. Carstairs, L. Cayolla da Motta, A. Dias, G. Feola, D. Hansen-Koenig, F. Hatton, B. Häussler, P. Hooft, E. Jougla, K. Juel, K. Kern, R. Lagasse, P. Lauriola, J. P. Mackenbach, E. Magliola, M. J. Medrano, P. L. Morosini, G. Papaevangelou, M. L. Sequeira, C. Tsimbos,

Oxford New York Tokyo
OXFORD UNIVERSITY PRESS
1997

Oxford University Press, Great Clarendon Street, Oxford OX2 6DP
Oxford New York
Athens Auckland Bangkok Bogota Bombay Buenos Aires
Calcutta Cape Town Dar es Salaam Delhi Florence Hong Kong
Istanbul Karachi Kuala Lumpur Madras Madrid Melbourne
Mexico City Nairobi Paris Singapore Taipei Tokyo Toronto
and associated companies in
Berlin Ibadan

Oxford is a trade mark of Oxford University Press

Volume Two, Second edition 1993

Publication No. EUR 11157 EN of the Commission of the European Communities, Dissemination of Scientific and Technical Knowledge Unit, Directorate-General Information Technologies and Industries, and Telecommunications, Luxembourg

Commission of the European Communities, Directorate-General Communications, Information Industries and Innovation, Luxembourg.

Library of Congress Cataloging-in-Publication Data
ISBN 0 19 262844 5

Typeset by Focal Image, London
Printed in Hong Kong

PREFACE

This edition of the European Community Atlas of 'Avoidable Death', which examines a selection of potentially unnecessary and untimely deaths, is the third to be published following the EC Concerted Action Project on Health Services and 'Avoidable Deaths'. The first edition of the atlas (published in 1988) described avoidable mortality from 17 conditions in ten countries of the European Community for the years 1974–78. The second edition (Volumes I and II) described mortality in the twelve EC countries for the years 1980–84, and changes in mortality between 1974–78 and 1980–84. This third edition also covers twelve EC countries; it describes mortality for the years 1985–89, and contains a detailed look at time-trends between this period and the 1980–84 period.

These changes are examined as annual percentage changes in age-standardized mortality rates, which is considered to be an improvement on the method used for the changes in the second edition, Volume I. Eight additional conditions were looked at in the second edition, Volume II, and three have been retained in this third edition—cancer of the breast, ischaemic heart disease and peptic ulcers—together with all 17 from the earlier editions. All whole-EC maps are presented in colour. The 1985–89 EC maps are in a yellow/brown colour scheme, and the changes maps are in a blue/red scheme. For the first time some indication of the statistical 'safety' of the data has been indicated on the whole-EC maps by the use of a striped effect. Tables have been improved to bring side-by-side data which were previously separate tables.

Also for the first time, the atlas includes essays written by the representatives in each country describing recent and ongoing work relevant to the Avoidable Deaths study. The study has now stimulated other countries, both from within the EC and non-EC members such as Greenland, Canada, USA, Japan and New Zealand, to analyse and publish papers concerning aspects of avoidable death. Some countries have published atlases for their own country, such as Belgium and Portugal, and an atlas is expected for Eastern European countries.

There is growing interest in evaluating and monitoring the performance of health services. Much effort has centred on rationalizing the enormous volume of data collected in order to produce a manageable series of measures that truly reflect the various facets of a health care system. Progress in the development of indicators of the quality and outcome of health care services has lagged behind that of measures of process and efficiency. The atlas represents an important step towards establishing outcome indicators to monitor health service performance that are applicable nationally and internationally. What is essential is that the situation across the Member States as a whole becomes known and is made publicly available as accurately and as clearly as possible, so that improvements may continue to be made in the health standards of all European citizens. Avoidable death has gained recognition and usage as a reliable and valuable performance indicator of health care provision.

Historically, maternal and infant mortality have gained wide acceptance as monitors for the quality of obstetric and infant care. This atlas extends the concept to other conditions from which most deaths should be avoidable, given timely and appropriate medical intervention or public health action. The study has led to EC funding of other projects based on conditions considered avoidable, such as a study of the variation in asthma and asthma-like symptoms and risk-factors for asthma throughout Europe and other parts of the world, a study to evaluate various measures of stroke care in eight countries, and a study to examine the frequency of risk factors of maternal morbidity and mortality and evaluation of care.

The choice of diseases covered in the atlas has reflected the conclusion of much discussion among all those who have worked so hard on its compilation, but the main criterion has been the relevance of a disease to all EC Member States, with the resulting highlighting of major aspects of national health care provision. The comparison of death rates in the regions and in the entireties of Member States has a scientific interest in its own right and it could only have been achieved by a coordinated and continuing trans-European effort. Our thanks and congratulations are due to all those whose collaborative research has resulted in this informative and thought-provoking series of publications. The series has been a valuable product of the EC Biomedical and Health Research Programme and provides an excellent example of what can be achieved though transnational use of the available and extensive data sources within EC Member States. I hope that it will stimulate further research into the organization and improvement of health services in the EC, and continue to encourage productive partnerships between our health services researchers.

December 1995
Paolo Fasella
Director-General for Science, Research and Development

PREFACE

Cette édition de l'Atlas de la *Communauté Européenne sur les 'morts évitables'* qui concerne un certain nombre de décès inutiles et prématurés, est la troisième à être publiée dans le cadre d'un projet Européen d'Action Concertée sur les services de santé et les 'morts évitables'. La première édition de l'Atlas (publiée en 1988) décrit la mortalité évitable due à dix-sept affections dans dix pays de la Communauté Européenne sur la période 1974–78. La deuxiéme édition (volume I et II) décrit la mortalité dans les douze pays communautaires sur la période 1980–84 et les modifications de la mortalité entre 1974–78 et 1980–84. Cette troisième édition couvre aussi douze pays communautaires, elle décrit la mortalité sur la période 1985–89 et comprend une vue détaillée de la tendance évolutive entre cette période et la période 1980–84.

Ces modifications sont examinées en terme de modification du pourcentage annuel du taux de mortalité standardisé en fonction de l'âge, ce qui constitue une amélioration de la méthode utilisée pour les modifications dans la deuxieme édition, volume I. Huit affections supplémentaires étaient considérées dans la deuxième édition, volume II, et trois ont été reprises dans cette troisième édition—cancer du sein, maladie ischémique cardiaque et ulcères peptiques—avec les dix-sept affections des précédentes éditions. Toutes les cartes de la Communauté sont représentées en couleur. Les cartes communautaires de la période 1985–89 sont en jaune/brun et les cartes des modifications sont en bleu/rouge. Pour la première fois, une indication de la fiabilité statistique des données a été portée sur les cartes à l'aide de stries. Les tables ont été améliorées afin de mettre côte à côte des données qui figuraient auparavant sur des tables séparées.

Pour la première fois également, l'atlas comprend des textes présentés par des représentants de chaque pays, décrivant les travaux récents ou en cours relatifs à l'étude des 'morts évitables'. Cette étude a stimulé aussi d'autres pays, communautaires mais aussi non-communautaires comme le Groenland, le Canada, les USA, le Japon et la Nouvelle-Zélande, à analyser et publier des articles concernant des aspects de la 'mort évitable'. Certains pays ont publié un atlas national spécifique, comme la Belgique et la Portugal, et un atlas pour les pays d'Europe de l'Est est prévu.

L'intérêt porté à l'évaluation et au contrôle du fonctionnement des services de santé va croissant. L'effort a été concentré sur la rationalisation de l'importante quantité de données collectées afin de produire des séries de mesures qui reflètent les différentes facettes du système de soins. Le développement des indicateurs de qualité et de rendement des services de santé est resté en retard par rapport à celui des mesures de technique et d'efficacité. L'atlas représente une étape importante vers la mise au point d'indices d'évaulation des services de santé qui soient applicables nationalement et internationalement.

Ce qui est essentiel, c'est que la situation globale à travers les Etats Membres devient connue et disponible pour le public aussi précisément et clairement que possible, se sorte que des améliorations des standards de santé peuvent continuer à être apportés pour tous les citoyens Européens. La 'mort évitable' est maintenant reconnue et utilisée comme un indicateur de performance valable en matière de soins de santé.

Historiquement, les mortalitiés infantile et maternelle ont finalement été largement considérées comme des contrôles efficaces des soins obstétricaux et pédiatriques. Cet atlas étend le concept à d'autres états pathologiques qui ne devraient pas conduire au décès si une intervention médicale ou une action de santé publique appropriée était donnée à temps.

Cette étude à conduit à financer d'autres projets relatifs à des affections considerérées comme évitables, comme par exemple une étude sur les variations de l'asthme et des symptomes asthmatiformes et les facteurs de risque de l'asthme à travers l'Europe et d'autres parties du monde, une étude pour évaluer diverses mesures de traitement des accidents vasculaires dans huit pays, et une étude relative à la fréquence de facteurs de risque morbidité et mortalité maternelles et l'évaluation des sions.

Le choix des affections prises en compte dans l'atlas reflète les conclusions de discussions parmi ceux qui ont si bien collaboré à sa compilation, mais le principal critère a été l'intérêt de l'affection pour tous les pays Européens, avec en résultat la mise en lumiére des aspects majeurs des sions de santé donnés au niveau national.

La comparaison des taux de décès dans les régions et les Etats Membres en leur entier a un intérêt scientifique en soi et n'a pu être effectuée que par un effort trans-Européen continu et coordonné.

Nos remerciements et félicitations s'adressent à tous ceux dont le recherche collaborative a conduit à cette série de publications informatives et prêtant à réflexion. Cette série est un produit appréciable issu du Programme Communautaire de Recherche en Biomédecine et Santé et constitue un excellent exemple de ce qui peut être réalisé par l'utilisation transnationale de sources de données disponibles et abondantes au sein des Etats Membres. J'espère que ceci stimulera d'autres recherches dans l'organisation et l'amélioration des services de santé dans la Communauté Européenne et continuera d'encourager des partenariats fructueux entre nos chercheurs dans le domaine des services de santé.

Decembre 1995
Paolo Fasella
Directeur Général de la Science, Recherche, et le Développement

VORWORT

Diese Ausgabe des Atlas der Europäischen Gemeinschaft über 'vermeidbare Sterbefälle', die eine Auswahl von potentiell unnötigen und vorzeitigen Sterbefällen untersucht, ist die dritte, die aus der konzertierten Aktion de EG über Gesundheitsdienste und 'vermeidbare Sterbefälle' hervorgeht. Die erste Ausgabe des Atlas (veröffentlicht 1988), beschrieb die vermeidbare Mortalität bei 17 Krankheitszustände in zehn Ländern der Europäischen Gemeinschaft für die Jahre 1974–78. Die zweite Ausgabe (Bände I und II) beschrieb die Mortalität in zwölf EG-Ländern für die Jahre 1980–84 und Ändcrungen der Mortalität zwischen 1974–78 und 1980–84. Diese dritte Ausgabe behandelt ebenfalls zwölf EG-Länder, sie beschreibt die Mortalität für die Jahre 1985–89 und en-hält eine genaue Betrachtung des zeitlichen Trends zwischen diesem Zeitraum und 1980–84.

Diese Änderungen werden untersucht in jährlichen prozentualen Veränderungen der altersstandardisierten Mortalitätsraten, eine deutliche Verbesserung gegenüber der Methode, die bei Veränderungen in der zweiten Ausgabe, Band I, angewandt wurde. Acht weitere Krankheitszustände wurden in der zweiten Ausgabe, Band II, untersucht, und drei weitere werden, zusammen mit den 17 Ursachen aus den vorhergehenden Ausgaben, in dieser dritten Ausgabe berücksichtigt: Brustkrebs, ischämische Herzkrankheit und peptisches Ulkus. Alle die gesamte EG betreffenden Karten sind in Farbe abgebildet. Die EG-Karten von 1985–89 sind gelb-braun und die Karten zu Änderungen blau-rot. Zum ersten Mal wurden in den die gesamte EG darstellenden Karten mittels eines Streifeneffekts Angaben über die statistische 'Sicherheit' der Daten gemacht. Tabellen wurden dahingehend verbessert, daß Daten, die vorher in getrennten Tabellen aufgeführt waren, jetzt nebeneinander dargestellt sind.

Ebenfalls zum ersten Mal bringt der Atlas Artikel von Vertretern der jeweiligen Länder zu neuesten und noch laufenden Arbeiten zur Studie über Vermeidbare Sterbefälle. Die Studie hat mittlerweile andere Länder sowohl innerhalb als außerhalb der EG, wie Grönland, Kanada, USA, Japan und Neuseeland, dazu bewogen, Arbeiten über vermeidbare Sterbefälle zu analysieren und zu veröffentlichen. Einige Länder wie Belgien und Portugal haben Atlanten zu ihrem eigenen Land veröffentlicht, und für die osteuropäischen Länder wird ebenfalls ein Atlas erwartet.

Es besteht ein wachsendes Interesse an der Begutachtung und Überwachung der Leistungen der Gesundheitsdienste. Besondere Anstrengung ist auf die Rationalisierung der gewaltigen Datenmenge gerichtet worden mit dem Ziel, eine handhabbare Anzahl von Maßnahmen zu entwicheln, die die verschiedenen Facetten eines Gesundheitsversorgungssystems wahrheitsgemäß widerspiegeln Fortschritte in der Weiterentwicklung von Qualitäts- und Ergebnisindikatoren in der Gesundheitsversorgung sind hinter denen von Verfahrens- und Effizienzmaßnahmen zurückgeblieben. Der Atlas stellt einen bedeutenden Schritt auf dem Weg zur Erstellung von national und international anwendbarcn Ergebnisindikatoren zur Überwachung der Leistungsfähigkeit von Gesundheitsdiensten dar. Wesentlich ist, daß die Gesamtsituation über sämtliche Mitgliedstaaten hinweg aufgezeigt wird und möglichst genau und deutlich der Öffentlichkeit zugänglich gemacht wird, um so den Gesundheitszustand der Bürger in Europa verbessern können. Der Begriff vermeidbarer Sterbefall hat Anerkennung und Verwendung gefunden als verläßlicher und wertvoller Leistungsindikator in der Gesundheitsversorgung.

Historisch gesehen sind Mütter- und Säuglingssterblichkeit weithin anerkannt zur Qualitätskontrolle in der Geburtshilfe und Säuglingsversorgung. Dieser Atlas dehnt dieses Konzept ouf andere Krankheitszustände aus, bei denen die Mehrzahl der Sterbefälle vermeidbar sein sollten bei rechzeitiger und angemessener medizinischer Behandlung oder entsprechenden Maßnahmen der öffentlichen Gesundheitdienste. Die Studie hat dazu geführt, daß EG-Finanzmittel für andere Projekte zu als vermeidbar angesehenen Krankheitszuständen bereitgestellt wurden, wie zum Beispiel eine Studie über unterschiedliche Zustände bei Asthma und asthma-ähnlichen Symptomen in Europa und anderen Teilen der Welt, eine Studie zur Auswertung unterschiedlicher Behandlungsmaßnahmen bei Schlaganfällen in acht Ländern, und eine Studie zur Untersuchung der Häufigkeit von Risikofaktoren zu Morbidität und Mortalität bei Müttern sowie Bewertung der Versorgung.

Die Auswahl der in diesem Atlas abgehandelten Krankheitszustände spiegelt das Ergebnis aus eingehenden Beratungen all derer wider, die unter großen Anstrengungen zu seiner Verwirklichung beitragen haben. Das Hauptkriterium wat jedoch die Relevanz ciner Krankheir für alle EG-Mitgliedstaaten mit der sich daraus ergebenden Hervorhebung von Besonderheiten in der nationalen Gesundheitsversorgung. Der Vergleich von Sterberaten in Regionen und jeweils gesamten Mitgliedstaaten der EG ist in sich selbst von wissenschaftlicher Bedeutung und war nur durch koordinierte und kontinuierliche transeuropäische Anstrengungen zu erreichen. Unser Dank und Glückwunsch gilt all denen, deren gemrinsame Forschungsarbeit zu dieser aufschlußreichen und zum Nachdenken anregenden Reihe von Veröffenlichungen beigetragen hat. Diese Reihe ist ein wertvolles Ergebnis des EG-Programms Biomedizinische und Gesundheitsforschung und ein hervorragendes Beispiel dafür, was durch transnationale Nutzung der in den EG-Mitgliedstaaten umfangreich vorhandenen Datenquellen erreicht werden kann. Ich hoffe, daß der Atlas anregt zu weiteren Untersuchungen zu Aufbau und Verbesserung der Gesundheitsdienste in der EG und weitere ergebnisreiche Partnerschaften zwischen unseren Forschern in Gesundheitsdiensten fördert.

Dezember 1995
Paolo Fasella
Generaldirektor für Wissenschaft, Forschung und Entwicklung

CONTENTS

LIST OF PARTICIPANTS

Belgium

Dr R. Lagasse, Laboratoire d'Epidémiologie, Université Libre de Bruxelles, Campus Erasme CP 590/5, 808 route de Lennik, 1070 Bruxelles.

Dr P. Hooft, School voor Maatschappelijke Gezondheidszorg, Afdeling Gezondheidsecologie, Katholieke Universiteit Leuven, Kapucijnenvoer 35 niv 03, 3000 Leuven.

Luxembourg

Dr D. Hansen-Koenig, Directeur Général de la Santé, 57 boulevard de la Pétrusse, 2320 Luxembourg.

Federal Republic of Germany

Dr K. Kern, Ministerium für Arbeit, Soziales, Familie und Gesundheit, Bauhofstrasse 9, 55116 Mainz.

Dr B. Häussler, Institut für Gesundheits und Sozialforschung (IGES), Otto-Suhr-Allee 18, D-10585 Berlin.

Denmark

Dr K. Juel, Danish Institute for Clinical Epidemiology, 25 Svanemøllevej, 2100 Copenhagen.

France

Madame M. H. Bouvier-Colle, INSERM U-149, 16 av. P. Vaillant-Couturier, 94807 Villejuif Cedex, Paris.

Madame le Docteur F. Hatton, Service d'Information sur les Causes Médicales de Décès, 44 Chemin de Ronde - BP 34, 78110 Le Vésinet, Paris.

Mr E. Jougla, Service d'Information sur les Causes Médicales de Décès, 44 Chemin de Ronde-BP 34, 78110 Le Vésinet, Paris.

Greece

Professor G. Papaevangelou, Professor of Epidemiology and Medical Statistics, Athens School of Hygiene, 196 Alexandras Avenue, PO Box 14085, 11521 Athens.

Dr C. Tsimbos, Department of Statistics and Actuarial Studies, University of Piraeus, 40 Karaoli and Dimitriou Street, 18532 Piraeus.

Italy

Professor P. L. Morosini, Laboratorio di Epidemiologia e Biostatistica, Istituto Superiore di Sanita, Viale Regina Elena 299, 00161 Roma.

Dr P. Lauriola, Servizio Igiene Pubblica USL n16, Via Canaletto 15, 41100 Modena.

Dr E. Magliola, Dipartimento di Demografia, Via Nomentama 41, 00161 Roma.

Dr G. Feola, ISTAT, Reparto Statistiche Sanitarie, Viale Liegi 13, 00198 Roma.

Ireland

Dr J Barry, Eastern Health Board, Baggot Street Community Hospital, 18 Upper Baggot St, Dublin 4.

The Netherlands

Dr J. P. Mackenbach, Instituut Maatschappelijke, Gezondheidszorg, Erasmus Universiteit, PO Box 1738, 3000 DR Rotterdam.

United Kingdom: England, Wales, and Northern Ireland

Project director and members of co-ordinating team from the Department of Public Health Medicine, United Medical and Dental Schools of Guy's and St Thomas's (UMDS), St Thomas's Hospital, London SE1 7EH.

Project Director: Professor W. W. Holland

Mr J. Charlton–Statistician (from November 1983–January 1986)
Mr A. Fitzgerald–Statistician (from October 1990–August 1995)
Ms E. Paul–Statistician (from March 1986–June 1990)
Mr S. Phillips–Research Assistant (from January 1990)
Mr R. Wood–Editorial Assistant (from February 1994)

United Kingdom–Scotland

Mrs V. Carstairs, Health Services Research Network National Co-ordinator, Edinburgh University, 12 Buccleuch Place, Edinburgh EH8 9AG.

Portugal

Professor L. Cayolla da Motta, Escola Nacional de Saúde Pública, Avenida Padre Cruz, 1699 Lisboa Codex.

Dr M. L. Sequeira, Departmente de Estudos e Planeamento da Saúde, Av Alvares Cabral 25-30, 1200 Lisboa.

Dr A. Dias, Division of Epidemiology and Biostatistics, Ministério da Saúde, Alameda D. Afonso Henriques, 45, 1056 Lisboa Codex.

Spain

Dr M. J. Medrano, Instituto de Salud 'Carlos III', Centro Nacional de Epidemiologia, Sinesio Delgado 6, 28029 Madrid.

Commission of The European Communities

Dr A. Baert, Commission of the European Community, DG XII/E4, Rue de la Loi 200, 1049 Brussels, Belgium.

Dr G. Fracchia, Secretary of COMAC-HSR, Commission of the European Community, DG XII/F/6 Office SDM 2/37, Rue de la Loi 200, 1049 Brussels, Belgium.

LIST OF DISEASES MAPPED

Cause of death	Age range	Abbreviation on tables	ICD 9th revision (all countries except Denmark)	ICD 8th revision (Denmark only)
Tuberculosis	5-64	TUB	010–018, 137	010–019
Malignant neoplasm of cervix uteri	15–64	CERV	180	180
Malignant neoplasm of cervix and body of uterus	15–54	UTER	179, 180, 182	180, 182
Hodgkin's disease	5–64	HODG	201	201
Chronic rheumatic heart disease	5–44	CRHD	393–398	393–398
All respiratory diseases	1–14	RESP	460–519	460–519
Asthma	5–44	ASTH	493	493
Appendicitis	5–64	APP	540–543	540–543
Abdominal hernia	5–64	HERN	550–553	550–553
Cholelithiasis and cholecystitis	5–64	CHOLY	574–575.1, 576.1	574–575
Hypertensive and cerebrovascular diseases	35–64	HYP/S	401–405, 430–438	400–404, 430–438
Maternal mortality	all	MAT	630–676	630–678
Perinatal mortality	<1 week + still births	PER	all	all
Cancer of the breast	25–64	BREAST	174	174
Ischaemic heart disease	35–64	ISHD	410–414, 429.2	410–414
Peptic ulcers	25–64	PEPTIC	531-534	531-534
All causes	5-64	ALL	all	all
All causes	all	ALL	all	all

Note: Portugal and Greece did not supply data for Asthma in the 1980–84 period.

Please note that in Spain, coding practices have changed between the 1980–84 and 1985–89 time periods for deaths involving cancers of the cervix and of the uterus. This leads to an increase in the number of deaths and mortality rates for cancer of the cervix and a parallel decrease in mortality for cancer of the uterus, between the two time periods. This should be borne in mind when examining the relevant data.

1. INTRODUCTION

In the absence of any intervention through health services, mortality would be determined purely by social, environmental and genetic factors. Health services, through preventive and remedial activities, and governments, through legislative policy, modify the influence of some of these factors, with the objective of reducing mortality and morbidity. For some diseases medical knowledge is sufficiently advanced to prevent almost all deaths in more resilient age groups. For such deaths to be prevented, however, timely action is necessary and the observation of an appreciable number of deaths suggests that such action may not have been taken. For example, even though effective means of early detection and effective treatment are available, in the period 1985–89 there were over 5000 deaths from cervical cancer in women aged 15–64 years and over 950 from tuberculosis amongst individuals aged 5–64 years in England and Wales, with wide variation between different parts of the country. The sequence of events leading up to avoidable disease, death, or disability of an individual can, however, be complex. For example, a case of diphtheria or poliomyelitis may be the consequence of failure by a government to introduce the necessary legislation to promote or fund immunization programmes; health service managers to implement such programmes; a doctor to immunize patients; parents to take their baby to a clinic because it is too far away or because of the family's religious views.

Diseases may be identified in which health education, immunization practices, continuity of care, surgical standards and many other particular aspects of the health care system are important in avoiding unnecessary deaths. Geographical comparison of these 'avoidable deaths' can pin-point areas with particular health care delivery problems. Comparison with areas where action has been effective in reducing such mortality may enable other areas to improve their performance.

It is difficult to assess the efficacy of health care services. Defining the outcome of health service intervention is a complex process and there are few relevant data available. An imaginative proposal to address this problem was put forward in the papers of the Preventable and Manageable Diseases Working Group (Rutstein *et al* 1976, 1980). They proposed an apparently practical and inexpensive method of devising outcome measures for health services by counting cases of 'unnecessary disease and disability, and unnecessary untimely deaths' as measures of the quality of medical care. Here medical care was defined in its broadest sense; that is, as prevention, cure, and care, including the application of all relevant medical knowledge, the services of all medical and allied personnel, the resources of governmental, voluntary and social agencies, and the co-operation of the individuals themselves. An excessive number of such unnecessary events was taken as a warning signal of possible shortcomings in the health care system which warranted further investigation. For certain diseases or disabilities even a single event could warrant attention.

This atlas, which examines a selection of unnecessary untimely deaths, is the third publication of the EC Concerted Action Project on Health Services and 'Avoidable Deaths'. It has been prepared by representatives from member countries of the EC (see List of Participants). The first edition of the atlas (OUP 1988) describes avoidable mortality in the EC for the years 1974–78. The second edition, Volumes I and II (OUP 1991,1993) describes mortality for the years 1980-84, and changes in mortality between 1974–78 and 1980–84. This third edition describes mortality for the years 1985–89 and changes in mortality between 1980–84 and 1985–89.

For most of the conditions, in the age-groups studied, mortality should be largely avoidable given appropriate and timely medical intervention, although some 'avoidable deaths' will occur even under optimal conditions. A high death rate in any of the conditions studied may serve as an indicator of some inadequacy or reason for investigation.

The aims of the EC Concerted Action Project were:

(1) to produce a set of maps illustrating 'avoidable' death rates from a number of selected conditions for specified age ranges;

(2) to make comparisons between and within the participating countries;

(3) to relate the resulting variation to differing levels or modes of delivery of health service inputs;

(4) to expand on the work already done in the previous editions of the atlas.

This atlas addresses aims (1), (2) and (4).

The England and Wales working group representatives formed the co-ordinating centre based at the United Medical and Dental Schools of Guy's and St Thomas's Hospitals, London. The centre received and analysed data from all participating countries.

The project was financed by the Commission of the European Communities, Directorate-General for Science, Research, and Development (XII).

This atlas contains the maps showing standardized mortality ratios (SMRs; see Definitions section) standardized to the average age-specific death rates of both the EC as a whole and the individual country and the percentage change in mortality from the early to late eighties. The role of this atlas is to make relevant data available to enable appropriate questions to be posed and to increase awareness of areas with potential problems. High SMRs should lead to further research at a local level to reveal the underlying cause of the observed excess.

1. INTRODUCTION

En l'absence de toute intervention des services de santé, la mortalité serait déterminée par des facteurs sociaux, des facteurs liés à l'environnement et des facteurs génétiques. Les services de santé, par le biais d'actions préventives et curatives, et les gouvernements, par leurs réglementations, modifient l'influence de certains de ces facteurs dans le but de réduire la mortalité et la morbidité. Pour les groupes d'âge les plus réceptifs, les connaissances médicales sur certaines maladies sont actuellement suffisamment avancées pour que la plupart des décès dus à ces pathologies puissent être prévenus. Néanmoins, pour que ces décès soient évités, une action appropriée doit être menée à temps; l'observation d'une certaine fréquence de décès peut révéler qu'une telle action n'a pas été menée. Par exemple, durant la période 1985–89, il est survenu en Angleterre-Galles, plus de 5000 décès dus au cancer du col de l'utérus parmi les femmes âgées de 15 à 64 ans et plus de 950 décès dus à la tuberculose parmi les sujets âgés de 5 à 64 ans (avec de larges variations régionales), alors même que les moyens d'un dépistage précoce et d'un traitement efficace étaient disponibles. La séquence des événements conduisant à une maladie, à un décès ou à une incapacité évitable peut être complexe. Par exemple, un cas de diphtérie ou de poliomyélite peut être la conséquence de différents types de carences: carence du gouvernement dans l'introduction de la législation nécessaire à la promotion ou à l'instauration des programmes de vaccination; carence des responsables des services de santé dans la mise en oeuvre de ces programmes; carence des médecins n'ayant pas vacciné leurs patients; carence des parents n'ayant pas conduit leur enfant à la clinique parce qu'elle était éloignée ou par conviction religieuse.

Il est ainsi possible d'identifier un certain nombre d'affections pour lesquelles l'éducation sanitaire, les pratiques vaccinales, la continuité des soins, la qualité de la chirurgie ainsi que d'autres aspects du système de soins ont une grande importance pour éviter les décès. La comparaison géographique de la fréquence de ces décès 'évitables' peut permettre de mettre en évidence des zones à problèmes. La comparaison avec d'autres régions, où la mortalité a pu être effectivement réduite, peut encourager ces zones à améliorer leur performance.

L'efficacité des services de santé est difficile à mesurer. Les résultats des interventions ne sont pas simples à définir et peu de données sont disponibles pour les analyser. Une solution ingénieuse a été proposée par le 'Preventable and Manageable Diseases Working Group' (Rutstein *et al.* 1976, 1980). Ce groupe a proposé une méthode pratique et peu coûteuse d'évaluation des services de santé qui consiste à dénombrer les cas de maladies, d'incapacité et de décès évitables et prématurés en tant qu'indicateur de la qualité des soins médicaux. Les soins médicaux sont ici définis dans un sens très large: prévention, cure et soins, incluant l'application de toute connaissance médicale appropriée, les services du personnel médical et auxiliaire, les ressources administratives, les actions sociales et la coopération des individus eux-mêmes. L'observation d'un nombre excessif de ces événements morbides doit permettre de donner l'alerte sur d'éventuelles imperfections du système de santé et entraîner des investigations supplémentaires. Pour certaines maladies ou incapacités, un seul événement peut même servir d'alerte.

La présente édition de cet atlas, qui repose sur une sélection de décès évitables et prématurés, est la troisième publication de l'Action Concertée de la Communauté Européenne sur les Services de Santé et les Morts Evitables. Elle a été préparée par des représentants des pays membres de la CEE (voir la liste des participants). La première édition de l'atlas (OUP 1988) décrivait la mortalité 'évitable' au sein de la Communauté Européenne durant les années 1974–78. La seconde édition, Volume I et II (OUP 1991, 1993) décrivait la mortalité pour les années 1980–84 et les évolutions observées entre 1974–78 et 1980–84. Cette troisième édition décrit la mortalité durant la période 1985–89 et les évolutions entre 1980–84 et 1985–89. Les variations des taux de décès par pays entre 1970–74 et 1985–89 y sont également présentées.

Pour la plupart des maladies retenues et pour les groupes d'âge considérés, une grande part des décès devrait pouvoir être évitée, compte-tenu d'interventions médicales appropriées en temps utile (certains décès peuvent cependant survenir même dans des conditions jugées optimales). Une fréquence élevée de décès pour ces pathologies peut ainsi servir de révélateurs de certaines inadaptations et justifier le déclenchement d'investigations.

Les objectifs de l'Action Concertée Européenne étaient:

(1) de produire un ensemble de cartes indiquant la fréquence des décès 'évitables' pour des états pathologiques sélectionnés et à des âges spécifiques,

(2) de réaliser des comparaisons entre pays et à l'intérieur de chaque pays,

(3) de mettre en relation les écarts observés et les différents niveaux et modes de délivrance des services de soins,

(4) de prolonger les analyses effectuées dans les précédentes éditions de l'atlas.

La présente édition répond aux objectifs (1), (2) et (4).

Les représentants anglais et gallois ont été chargés de la coordination de l'étude. Le centre coordinateur a été situé à l'Ecole de Médecine du Guy's et St Thomas's Hôpital à Londres. Ce centre a reçu et analysé les données statistiques fournies par tous les pays participant au projet.

Le projet a été financé par la Commission des Communautés Européennes, Direction Générale des Sciences, de la Recherche et du Développement (XII).

Cette troisième édition contient les cartes des indices de mortalité relative (SMR voir la section 'Définitions') standardisés selon les taux spécifiques par âge de la CEE entière et selon ceux de chaque pays. Sont également présentées, les variations de mortalité observées entre le début et la fin des années 80. Le but de cet atlas est de rendre disponibles des données permettant de soulever des questions relatives au fonctionnement du système de santé et d'attirer l'attention sur d'éventuelles zones géographiques à problème. Des SMR élevés doivent en effet conduire à des investigations supplémentaires au niveau local afin de mettre à jour les principaux facteurs responsables de l'excès des décès.

1. EINLEITUNG

Ohne eine effektive gesundheitliche Versorgung wäre die Sterblichkeit einer Bevölkerung ausschließlich durch soziale, umweltbezogene, und genetische Faktoren bestimmt. Das Gesundheitswesen soll durch vorbeugende und kurative Maßnahmen die Wirkung dieser Faktoren so beeinflussen, daß Mortalität und Morbidität in der Bevölkerung gesenkt werden. Regierungen und Behörden können die dazu erforderlichen gesetzlichen Rahmenbedingungen schaffen. Bei einigen Krankheiten ist das medizinische Wissen weit genug entwickelt, um nahezu alle Sterbefälle in den jungen und widerstandsfähigen Altersgruppen zu verhindern. Um solche Todesfälle zu verhindern, ist rechtzeitiges Handeln notwendig, und die Beobachtung einer nennenswerten Zahl von Sterbefällen läßt vermuten, daß ein solches Eingreifen möglicherweise versäumt worden ist. Um dies mit einem Beispiel zu verdeutlichen: Obwohl es wirksame Methoden der Früherkennung und der Behandlung gibt, wurden zwischen 1985–89 in England und Wales über 5000 Todesfälle an Cervix-Karzinom bei Frauen im Alter von 15–64 Jahren und über 950 Todesfälle an Tuberkulose bei Menschen im Alter von 5–64 Jahren registriert. Dabei wurden große Abweichungen zwischen verschiedenen Regionen einzelner Länder festgestellt. Die Folge von Ereignissen, die im Einzelfall zu einer vermeidbaren Erkrankung, zum Tode, oder zu einer Behinderung geführt hat, kann oft komplex sein. Zum Beispiel kann ein Fall von Diphtherie oder Poliomyelitis die Folge des staatlichen Versäumnisses sein, nicht die notwendigen Gesetze zur Einführung und Finanzierung von Impfprogrammen erlassen zu haben; der Nachlässigkeit der Gesundheitsverwaltungen bei der Durchführung solcher Programme; des Versäumnisses eines Arztes, den Patienten zu impfen; oder des Versäumnisses der Eltern, das Baby aufgrund großer Entfernungen oder aus religiösen Überzeugungen nicht zum Arzt zu bringen.

Es gibt Krankheiten, bei denen die Gesundheitserziehung; Verfahrensweisen beim Impfen, die Kontinuität der Betreuung, das Niveau der chirurgischen Versorgung, und zahlreiche weitere Aspekte des Gesundheitssystems für die Vermeidung bestimmmter Todesfälle eine wichtige Rolle spielen. Geographische Vergleiche dieser 'vermeidbaren Sterbefälle' können Regionen mit besonderen Versorgungsproblemen ausweisen. Ein Vergleich mit Regionen, die solche Sterbefälle erfolgreich zurückgedrängt haben, kann anderen Regionen eine Hilfe bei der Verbesserung ihrer Leistungsfähigkeit sein.

Die tatsächliche Wirksamkeit der gesundheitlichen Versorgung ist schwer einzuschätzen. Es ist ein komplexer Vorgang, den Ertrag der gesundheitlichen Versorgung zu bestimmen, und meist stehen nur wenige relevante Daten zur Verfügung. Die Beiträge der 'Arbeitsgruppe zu vermeidbaren und behandelbaren Krankheiten' (Rutstein *et al.* 1976, 1980) waren ein konstruktiver Vorschlag zur Lösung dieses Problems. Die Autoren haben eine offenbar praktische und kostengünstige Methode für die Beurteilung medizinischer Versorgungsleistungen vorgeschlagen, indem sie Fälle 'vermeidbarer Krankheit und Behinderung sowie vermeidbarer und vorzeitiger Sterbefälle' als Kriterium für die Qualität der medizinischen Versorgung gewertet haben. 'Medizinische Versorgung' wurde dabei im weitesten Sinne definiert, also als Prävention, Behandlung, und Betreuung unter Nutzung des gesamten medizinischen Wissens, der Arbeit aller medizinischen Berufe, der staatlichen Ressourcen sowie der freiwilligen und sozialen Organisationen einschließlich der Mitwirkung der Patienten selbst. Eine übermäßige Häufung von 'vermeidbaren' Ereignissen wurde als warnender Hinweis auf mögliche Defizite im medizinischen Vesorgungssystem gewertet und sollte Ausgangspunkt für weitere Untersuchungen sein. Bei bestimmten Krankheiten und Behinderungen sollte sogar ein einziger Fall eine besondere Beachtung finden.

Dieser Atlas der eine Auswahl 'vermeidbarer' und vorzeitiger Sterbefälle untersucht, ist die dritte Veröffentlichung des gemeinsamen EG–Projekts über die gesundheitliche Versorgung und 'Vermeidbare Sterbefälle'. Er wurde von Vertretern der teilnehmenden Länder vorbereitet (siehe Teilnehmerliste). Die erste Ausgabe des Atlasses (OUP 1988) beschreibt die 'vermeidbare Sterblichkeit' in der EG für den Zeitraum 1974–78. Bände I und II der zweiten Ausgabe (OUP 1991, 1993) stellen die Sterblichkeit für den Zeitraum 1980–84 dar sowie Veränderungen in der Sterblichkeit zwischen 1974–78 und 1980–84. Der vorliegende dritte Band ergänzt die Darstellung der Sterblichkeit um den Zeitraum 1985–89 sowie die Veränderungen in der Sterblichkeit zwischen 1980–84 und 1985–89.

Bei den meisten der in den jeweiligen Altersgruppen untersuchten Krankheiten sollte die Sterblichkeit durch geeignete und rechtzeitige medizinische Intervention verhindert werden können, auch wenn eine gewisse Zahl an 'vermeidbaren Todesfällen' selbst unter optimalen Bedingungen auftreten wird. Eine hohe Todesrate bei einer der hier untersuchten Krankheiten könnte als Indikator unzureichender Behandlung und darüber hinaus als Anlaß zu weiterer Untersuchung dienen.

Die Ziele des gemeinsamen EG-Projektes lauteten wie folgt:

(1) Erstellung eines Atlasses zur Prävalenz 'vermeidbarer Sterbefälle' an ausgewählten Gruppen von Todesursachen in bestimmten Altersgruppen;

(2) Vergleiche innerhalb und zwischen den beteiligten Ländern;

(3) Herstellung von Bezügen zwischen der Variation der Mortalität und Unterschieden der Ausstattung und Organisation der medizinischen Versorgung;

(4) Fortführung und Erweiterung der in den früheren Ausgaben des Atlasses geleisteten Arbeit.

Diese Atlas behandelt die Ziele (1), (2), und (4).

Das Koordinationszentrum wurde von Mitgliedern der Arbeitsgruppe England und Wales an den United Medical and Dental Schools of Guy's and St Thomas's Hospitals, London geführt. Das Zentrum sammelte und analysierte die Daten aller beteiligten Länder. Das Projekt wurde durch die Kommission der Europäischen Gemeinschaft, Generaldirektorat für Wissenschaft, Forschung, und Entwicklung (XII) finanziert.

Dieser Atlas enthält Karten mit standardisierten Mortalitätsquotienten (SMRs—siehe das kapitel 3, 'Definitionen');

standardisiert wurde auf die durchschnittliche altersspezifische Mortalitätsrate sowohl der gesamten EG, des einzelnen Landes wie auch des prozentualen Wandels in der Sterblichkeit in den frühen bis späten achtziger Jahren. Die Aufgabe dieses Atlasses besteht darin, die relevanten Daten verfügbar zu machen, damit angemessene Fragen gestellt werden können und die Aufmerksamkeit verstärkt auf Regionen mit möglichen Problemen gelenkt wird.

Hohe SMRs sollten zu weitere Forschung auf lokaler Ebene anregen um die tatsächlichen Ursachen des beobachteten Übermaßes offenzulegen.

2. METHODS

Selection of indicators for health care outcome

Indicators based on mortality from 17 disease groups are presented in this volume. These are a combination of conditions covered in the second edition Volumes I and II (OUP 1991, 1993), which were selected to measure the outcome of primary prevention, secondary prevention, and curative aspects of health services on the residents of defined geographical areas. For all the conditions considered it was reasonably certain that effective treatment or primary or secondary prevention could be provided by health care services.

The indicators, which are termed 'avoidable death indicators', are intended to provide warning signals of potential shortcomings in health care delivery, although there may be other explanations. Two uses were envisaged for the indicators in this atlas:

(a) to examine whether there is geographic equity of outcome for specific aspects of health service activity;

(b) to provide warning signals to be investigated by local studies, which would aim to identify avoidable factors and other problems so that management of local health services could be improved.

The selection of causes of death to be included as indicators of health care outcome began with a modified list of the 14 disease groups used by Charlton *et al.* in 1983 in their study of geographic variations in mortality in England and Wales. This was drawn from the list of 'sentinel health events' compiled by a working party on preventable and manageable disease in the United States, referred to above (Rutstein *et al.* 1980).

At the first workshop of the working party a list of disease groups was reviewed by participants from all the then EC countries, since different member countries may rank the importance of diseases differently. After review, 17 disease groups were agreed as indicators of primary and secondary prevention and curative care. These were covered in the first two editions of Volume I of the atlas (OUP 1988 and 1991). Following subsequent meetings of the working party, a further eight conditions were identified as being of interest and these eight conditions were covered in the second edition Volume II (OUP 1993). The first edition covered the period 1974–78, the second edition the period 1980–84. This edition covers the period 1985–89 and considers all those conditions mapped in the two editions of Volume I (tuberculosis, cervical cancer, cancer of the cervix and uterus, Hodgkin's disease, chronic rheumatic heart disease, childhood respiratory disease, asthma, appendicitis, abdominal hernia, cholecystectomy, hypertension and stroke, maternal and perinatal mortality) and three conditions from Volume II (cancer of the breast, ischaemic heart disease, peptic ulcers).

For the final three diseases the role of the health services is less certain; while not all deaths from these causes would be avoidable, the health services nevertheless, can make a substantial contribution to minimizing the level of mortality. The general principles underlying the choice of each disease group were that each should have identifiable effective interventions and health care providers. The tables in Appendix A show, for each of the disease groups selected, the ICD codes, age groups and diseases included, the reasons which led the working party to consider these deaths 'avoidable' (that is, modifiable factors which may contribute to mortality) and the health service and other interventions which could reduce mortality. Strict age limits were set for each disease group to enhance the validity of mortality as an indicator of health service outcome. These disease groups were intended to cover a range of different health services. They do not include all conditions for which death is avoidable by medical intervention, nor would every death from some of these causes be avoidable, although it is expected that a proportion could be prevented. Maps and tables were produced to show local geographical variations in mortality from the sixteen conditions listed above.

Owing to the problems with certification and coding in certain countries, data from cancer of the cervix and the body of the uterus were combined (Kelson and Farebrother 1987). Within the age range 15–54 years almost all deaths thus classified are likely to be from cervical cancer. Maps are presented both for deaths from cervical cancer and for deaths from cancer of the cervix and body of the uterus.

The data

The indicators are based on mortality data for 1985–89, except for The Netherlands, and Spain (1985–88). The population data are for 1985–89, except for France (1987), Greece (1987), Ireland (1986), The Netherlands (1985–88), and Spain (1986).

The time-trend analysis also uses data from the early 1980s. These mortality data cover the period 1980–84, except for Greece (1980–82), Spain (1979–83), Italy (1979–83), and England and Wales (1980–84) for all conditions except cancer of the breast, ischaemic heart disease and peptic ulcer (1982–84). Population data for the earlier time period are for 1980–84 except for France (1982), Greece (1981), Ireland (1981), Spain (1981), Italy (1979–83), and England and Wales (1980–82). Because Greece and Portugal did not supply asthma data for the early eighties they were not included in the time-trend analysis of asthma mortality.

The data originate from the official agencies, and population data, for example, are based on censuses, using official estimates of changes between censuses if available. The sources are listed in Appendix B. The participants from each country are responsible for the accuracy of their own country's data, which were supplied to the co-ordinating centre classified by age, sex, and administrative area. The aim was to have administrative areas with approximately 500000 population, but since existing administrative units had to be employed, areas vary in size. There were 552 administrative areas in the EC in 1985–89 for the purposes of this study. In order to gain clarity in the maps, larger area authorities (regional rather than district) were used for England and Wales. This reduced the total number of mapped areas to 368.

The 9th revision of the International Classification of Diseases was introduced in 1979. All countries have used this coding throughout the 1980s apart from Denmark, which has used ICD8.

The possible effect of this on Denmark's results was investigated using OPCS (England and Wales) 'bridge coding' results, where a 25 per cent sample of deaths occurring in 1978 was coded according to both ICD8 and ICD9. The difference in the number of deaths assigned to particular diseases was less than five per cent for each of the 'avoidable' causes except for chronic rheumatic heart disease, asthma, appendicitis, and abdominal hernia. The differences in classifications resulted in a fall of 39 per cent in deaths from chronic rheumatic heart disease, and a 9 per cent fall in deaths from abdominal hernia over the age ranges studied (from ICD8 to ICD9). Deaths from asthma and appendicitis increased by 9 per cent and 7 per cent respectively.

Analysis and presentation

The geographical distributions of 'avoidable' mortality over the administrative areas of the EC in 1985–89, and the change from 1980–84 to 1985–89, are presented in maps (368 areas) and tables (552 areas). EC maps of SMRs in 1985–89 and change in mortality over the 1980s are presented together so as to aid interpretation.

In The Netherlands the boundary between Overijssel and Flevoland has been redefined. The mortality data for the period 1980–84 has been adjusted so as to allow for this.

Analysis and presentation of data for 1985–89

Since local age- and sex-specific death rates would be unreliable due to the small numbers of deaths involved, indirect age standardization (standardized mortality ratios—SMRs) was employed (see Armitage 1994).

The two sexes were combined, since we did not consider that the avoidability of death should depend on gender. For gender-specific conditions, the deaths are age-standardized to the population of that gender.

For each disease group and each of the 552 areas included in the study, SMRs were calculated in two different ways:

(a) using the age-specific death rates for the EC as a whole for that disease;

(b) using the age-specific death rates pertaining to the area's own country.

The first method was used to show between-country variation with all data standardized to a common standard (whole EC = 100). The second method was used to show within-country variation (whole country = 100).

Statistical tests were carried out on the resulting SMRs to examine:

(a) whether SMRs validly describe the data;

(b) whether the degree of heterogeneity between different areas is greater than could be expected by chance;

(c) for each area, whether the SMR is significantly different than 100 (the standard).

Tests (a) and (b) above are chi-squared tests as described by Gail (1978). Test (c) is as described by Armitage (1994)—significance was calculated by regarding the observed number of deaths as following a Poisson distribution with mean equal to the expected number of deaths based on standard age-specific rates. A two-sided test was chosen in order to highlight all those areas in which the death rate differed significantly from the national/EC standard. Test (a) examines whether the death ratios (local/EC and local/national) for the different age groups are similar, this being a necessary requirement for the SMR to validly describe the data. There was no evidence of SMRs being inappropriate for any cause of avoidable mortality.

The SMR is a relative, not an absolute, measure of mortality. An SMR of 200 may indicate two deaths when one was expected or 300 deaths when 150 were expected. It is essential to consider not just the SMR but also the actual number of deaths. Tables of SMRs include the observed number of deaths. Maps indicate those areas where few deaths are expected. The SMRs measure mortality relative to EC and national standards, neither of which should be seen as a 'gold standard'. As such, a low SMR does not necessarily indicate satisfactory performance

Maps for the period 1985–89

Two set of maps were produced to show up different aspects of mortality variations. Six shading intervals were used for all maps. Shading is based on SMR size and does not reflect statistical significance. The darker shades represent higher mortality. Care is needed when interpreting maps illustrating conditions for which there are few deaths expected in the age range studied. Observed results are variable and a small difference between the number of deaths which occur and the expected number based on standard age-specific rates may yield extreme SMRs.

The two methods of allocating areas to intervals are described below. Histograms showing the distribution of SMRs are shown on each map.

(a) *Whole EC, sextile intervals*

These maps are intended to show between-country variations. They show the rankings of areas when mortality is compared with a common EC standard. Mortality data for each area were age standardized using the age-specific death rates of the EC as a whole (SMR for whole EC = 100), and these SMRs were then placed in rank order. Equal numbers of areas were placed in each shading interval with darker shades indicating higher SMRs. Striped shading indicates those areas where particular care is needed when interpreting extreme SMRs due to the uncertainty in estimates. Areas in which the number of deaths expected based on EC rates was five or less are striped.

In order to highlight between-country variation, a map showing SMRs by country, rather than small area is also presented inset. As before the SMR uses the EC standard.

On each EC map a histogram of frequencies of the SMRs is included to illustrate the amount of variability in the SMRs across small areas of the EC for mortality from the cause of death mapped. The histograms are based on a grouping interval of 20. The same grouping interval is used for every histogram to provide a common scale on which variability of SMRs for different disease groups can be compared. The histogram intervals are different from the SMR ranges used in shading the maps.

(b) *Individual countries, sextile intervals*

These maps are intended to show within-country variations in mortality, and separate maps have been produced for each country. Here the mortality data for each area have been standardized to the age-specific death rates of the country to which they belong (SMR for whole country = 100), so the SMR for a small area indicates the extent to which that area differs from the country as a whole.

Between-country comparisons of mortality levels should not be made using these maps. It was important that for each disease a common yardstick should be employed to show variation within the different countries, so the 368 small area SMRs based on national standards were ranked and divided into sextiles to create the shading intervals. The shading based on standardization using national rates illustrates the extent to which mortality in a small area differs from the average mortality in its own country compared with the extent to which other small areas in the EC differ from the average mortality in their countries.

Individual country maps are not striped because stripes would not be clearly visible against shades of grey background. However, results for areas in which few deaths occurred should be interpreted with caution. Table 8.2 presents SMRs along with the actual number of deaths.

A histogram of the frequencies of the SMRs based on a grouping interval of 20 is presented on each map. They show in grey the distribution of small-area SMR's based on national standards for the 368 areas of the whole EC, and in black the distribution of the SMRs for the country in the map. The histogram intervals are different from the SMR ranges used in shading the maps.

Tables for the period 1985–89

Tables showing the number of deaths for each cause and the mortality indicators (standardized both to the EC and to the individual country) and whether they significantly exceed 100 (the SMR for the standard population), are given for each area of each country in Table 8.2. Summaries at a national level are given in Table 8.3. Whether an SMR for an area differs significantly from the standard depends not only on the size of the SMR but also on the population size of the area and the overall death rate for the particular disease (both of which contribute to the 'expected' number of deaths in an area). The same SMR value in two areas that differ greatly in population size may be significantly different from the standard in the area with the larger population, but not from that in the area with the smaller population. Table 8.1 contains the populations for each area.

Changes in 'avoidable mortality' between 1980–84 and 1985–89

To make comparisons between levels of 'avoidable mortality' in 1980–84 and 1985–89, the mortality and population must relate to the same geographic areas. For England and Wales the second edition quoted results were at an Area Health Authority (AHA) level whereas this edition uses District Health Authorities (DHA). In this edition both AHAs and DHAs have been aggregated to Regional Health Authority level.

In The Netherlands the boundary between Overijssel and Flevoland has been redefined. This edition uses the redefined boundaries and data for the period 1980–84 have been adjusted so as to allow for this.

Maps of changes between 1980–84 and 1985–89

The shading in these maps is based on the percentage change in age-standardized mortality rates (standardized to the EC 1985–89 rate). Areas were divided into two groups according to whether there was or was not an increase in age-standardized mortality. Those areas in which there was no change are included in the second group. Areas were ranked according to the annual percentage change in mortality from 1980–84 to 1985–89. Most maps use four shades of blue and two shades of red. A quarter of the areas in which there was no increase in mortality were placed in each blue shading interval. Half of the areas in which there was an increase were placed in each red shading interval.

There was an increase in the overall death rate from asthma and breast cancer. For all other conditions there was an overall decrease. The shading scheme used when mapping the percentage change in mortality from asthma and breast cancer reflects this. One-third of the areas which experienced no increase in mortality were placed in blue shade. One-third of the areas where there was an increase were placed in each red shading interval.

Striped shading indicates those areas where particular care is needed when interpreting extreme percent change due to the increased uncertainty in the estimates of rate of change. Those areas where there were five or less deaths observed in both time-periods are striped. In order to highlight the between-country variation in percentage change, results are also displayed inset at a country level.

Tables of changes between 1980–84 and 1985–89

Changes in avoidable mortality at a national level are shown in Tables 9.1 and 9.3 (p. 276 and p. 288). The overall change in mortality is given in Table 9.1. This gives the number of deaths, crude death rate, age-standardized death rate for each disease in each country from 1980–84 to 1985–89, and the annual percentage change in death rate from 1980–84 to 1985–89. The age-standardized death rate is taken to be the SMR (standardized to the EC 1985–89 rate) multiplied by the EC crude death rate for 1985–89. In the EC as a whole there has been a decline in mortality from all conditions with the exception of asthma for which there has been a slight increase. National changes in age-specific mortality are given in Table 9.3. The number of deaths observed and the age-standardized death rate are given for both periods together with the change in death rates between the two time periods. Data on population change in the different age-groups is shown in Table 9.2.

2. MÉTHODES

Selection des indicateurs d'evaluation des soins

Les indicateurs présentés dans cet atlas reposent sur la mortalité due à dix-sept groupes de causes. Il s'agit d'un regroupement de pathologies prises en compte dans la deuxième édition de l'atlas, Volume I et II (OUP 1991, 1993). Ces indicateurs ont été choisis dans le but de mesurer le résultat des interventions des services de santé en matière de prévention primaire et secondaire et de soins, au sein des zones géographiques considérées. Pour l'ensemble de ces pathologies, il est pratiquement certain, que des traitements effectifs ou que des actions de prévention primaire et secondaire peuvent être assurés par les services de soins.

Ces 'indicateurs de morts évitables. doivent permettre de donner l'alerte en cas d'insuffisances dans la délivrance des soins, même si d'autres explications sont possibles. Deux utilisations distinctes de ces indicateurs ont été envisagées dans l'atlas:

(1) établir s'il existe une égalité géographique dans l'activité des services locaux de santé,

(2) fournir des signaux d'alarme qui peuvent permettre de déclencher des investigations locales ayant l'objectif d'identifier les facteurs évitables afin d'améliorer le fonctionnement des services de santé.

La sélection des causes de décès a pour origine la liste des quatorze groupements de maladies utilisés par Charlton et al. en 1983 pour l'étude des variations géographiques de la mortalité en Angleterre et au Pays de Galles. Celle liste était elle-même issue de la liste des 'événements sentinelles', proposée par un groupe de travail sur les maladies à prévenir et à traiter aux Etats-Unis (Rutstein *et al.* 1980).

Lors de la première réunion du groupe de travail, une liste de causes a été discutée par tous les participants de la Communauté, les membres des différents pays pouvant évaluer diversement le caractère plus ou moins évitable des différentes affections. Après cet examen, dix-sept groupes de maladies ont été retenus en tant qu'indicateurs de la prévention primaire, de la prévention secondaire et des soins curatifs. Ces pathologies ont fait l'objet des deux premières éditions du Volume I de l'atlas (OUP 1988 et 1991). Huit nouvelles affections ont été ajoutées lors de réunions ultérieures du groupe de travail. Ces huit maladies ont été prises en compte dans le Volume II (OUP 1993). La première édition a couvert la période 1974–78 et la seconde édition la période 1980–84. La présente édition concerne la période 1985–89 et se base sur l'ensemble des affections sélectionnées dans les deux éditions du Volume I (tuberculose, cancer du col de l'utérus, cancer du col et du corps de l'utérus, maladie d'Hodgkin, cardiopathies rhumatismales chroniques, maladies respiratoires des enfants, asthme, appendicite, hernie abdominale, cholélithiase et cholécystite, maladies hypertensives et maladies vasculaires cérébrales, mortalité maternelle et périnatale) et sur trois maladies incluses dans le Volume II (cancer du sein, cardiopathies ischémiques, ulcères peptiques).

En ce qui concerne ces trois dernières maladies, le rôle que peut jouer les services de santé est plus discutable. Tous les décès relevant de ces causes ne peuvent être considérés comme évitables mais les services de santé peuvent néanmoins contribuer dans une mesure non négligeable a la réduction du niveau de mortalité. La sélection des maladies a reposé sur deux principes généraux: des interventions connues et efficaces existaient et des soins appropriés pouvaient être dispensés. Les tableaux de l'annexe A présentent, pour chacun des groupes d'affections sélectionnées, les codes de la Classification Internationale des Maladies correspondant, les groupes d'âge considérés et les raisons qui ont conduit le groupe d'étude à considérer ces décès comme 'évitables': facteurs influençant la mortalité sur lesquels on peut agir, soins et autres types d'interventions qui peuvent réduire la mortalité. Pour chaque groupe d'affections, des limites d'âge ont été définies afin d'affiner les indicateurs de mortalité en tant qu'indice de la qualité des services de soins. Les groupes d'affections sélectionnées devaient couvrir l'ensemble des différents services de santé. Ils n'englobent cependant pas toutes les affections où des interventions médicales peuvent éviter les décès. De même, si chaque décès dû à ces causes ne peut-être considéré comme totalement évitable, on peut cependant penser qu'une proportion importante de ces décès peut être actuellement prévenue. Des cartes et des tableaux présentent les variations géographiques de la mortalité pour les seize affections mentionnées ci-dessus.

Compte-tenu de problèmes de certification et de codification spécifiques à certains pays, les données relatives aux cancers du corps et du col de l'utérus ont été regroupées (Kelson and Farebrother 1987). Dans la classe d'âge 15–54 ans, la plupart des décès sont des cancers du col. C'est pourquoi les cartes sont présentées simultanément pour les cancers du col et pour les cancers du col et du corps regroupés.

Les donnees

Les indicateurs présentés sont basés sur les données de mortalité de la période 1985–89, sauf pour la Hollande et l'Espagne (1985–88). Les données de population sont relatives à la période 1985–89 sauf pour le France (1987), la Grèce (1987), l'Irlande (1986), la Hollande (1985–88), et l'Espagne (1986).

Les analyses d'évolution dans le temps prennent également en compte des données du début des années 80. Pour la mortalité, il s'agit de la période 1980–84, excepté pour le Grèce (1980–82), l'Espagne (1979–83), l'Italie (1979–83) et l'Angleterre et Galles (1980–82) pour l'ensemble des pathologies sauf le cancer du sein, les cardiopathies ischémiques et les ulcères peptiques (1982–84). Les données de population du début des années 80 concernent la période 1980–84 à l'exception de la France (1982), la Grèce (1981), l'Irlande (1981), l'Espagne (1981), l'Italie (1979–83) et l'Angleterre et Galles (1980–82). La Grèce et le Portugal n'ont pas pu fournir les données de l'asthme pour le début des années 80. Ces deux pays ne sont donc pas pris en compte dans l'analyse des évolutions dans le temps de la mortalité par asthme.

Pour tous les pays, les données de mortalité proviennent des statistiques officielles et les données de population sont basées sur les recensements en utilisant éventuellement des estimations intercensitaires. Les sources de données sont répertoriées dans l'annexe B. Les participants de chaque pays sont responsables de la validité des données de leur propre pays. Ces données ont été fournies au centre coordinateur, regroupées par sexe, âge, et région administrative (de résidence pour la France). L'objectif était de constituer des régions comprenant environ 500000 habitants. Mais, comme il fallait se baser sur des circonscriptions administratives existantes, la taille des différentes régions varie sensiblement. Pour l'ensemble de la Communauté Européenne, 552 régions administratives ont été distinguées durant la période d'étude 1985–89. En Angleterre-Galles, pour améliorer la lisibilité des cartes, des zones sanitaires plus vastes (région plutôt que district) ont été utilisées. Le nombre total de régions cartographiées a été ainsi ramené à 368.

La 9ème révision de la Classification Internationale des Maladies (CIM) a été introduite en 1979. Tous les pays l'ont utilisée durant les années 80, à l'exception du Danemark qui a conservé la 8ème révision.

L'effet éventuel de l'utilisation de la CIM8 sur les résultats du Danemark, a été évaluée en se basant sur la table de correspondance établie par l 'Office of Population and Censuses and Surveys' (OPCS). Un échantillon de 25 pour cent des décès survenus en Angleterre-Galles en 1978, a été codé simultanément selon la 8ème et la 9ème révision. La différence dans les décès assignés à telle ou telle rubrique s'est avérée nettement inférieure à 10 pour cent pour la plupart des causes 'évitables', à l'exception des cardiopathies rhumatismales chroniques, de l'asthme, de l'appendicite et des hernies abdominales. Le changement de classification (CIM8-CIM9) s'est traduit, dans les groupes d'âge étudiés, par une diminution de 39 pour cent du nombre des décès par cardiopathies rhumatismales chroniques et de 9 pour cent des décès par hernies abdominales. Les décès par asthme et appendicite ont augmenté de respectivement 9 et 7%.

Analyse et presentation

Des cartes (368 régions) et des tableaux (552 régions) indiquent la distribution géographique des causes de mortalité 'évitable' selon les zones administratives de la Communauté Européenne pour les périodes 1980–84 et 1985–89 ainsi que les évolutions observées entre ces deux périodes. Les cartes relatives à la période 1985–89 et les évolutions sont présentées simultanément afin de faciliter les interprétations.

Pour la Hollande, la frontière entre Overijssel et Flevoland ayant été redéfinie, les données de mortalité de la période 1980–84 ont été ajustées en conséquence.

Analyse et presentation des donnees pour la periode 1985–89

En raison du faible effectif de décès par classe, les taux spécifiques de mortalité par sexe et âge, auraient été peu fiables au niveau local. Une standardisation indirecte par âge a donc été utilisée (indice de mortalité relative—SMR, voir Armitage 1994).

Le caractère évitable des décès ne devant pas dépendre du sexe des sujets, les analyses ont été effectuées à sexes regroupés. Pour les maladies spécifiques d'un sexe, les taux de décès ont été ajustés par âge en fonction de la population du sexe concerné.

Pour chacun des groupes de pathologies et pour chacune des 552 régions, les SMR ont été calculés de deux manières différentes:

(1) en utilisant les taux spécifiques par âge de la Communauté Européenne considérée comme un tout,

(2) en utilisant pour les analyses nationales, les taux spécifiques par âge du pays considéré.

La première méthode a été utilisée pour analyser les variations entre pays par rapport à une référence commune (ensemble de la CEE = 100). La deuxième méthode a été utilisée pour indiquer les variations régionales internes à chaque pays (ensemble du pays = 100).

Des tests statistiques ont été réalisés sur les indices de mortalité relative, pour vérifier:

(1) si l'utilisation du SMR était justifiée;

(2) si le degré d'hétérogénéité entre différentes régions était plus grand que celui dû au hasard;

(3) si le SMR était significativement différent de 100 (la référence) dans chaque région.

Les tests (1) et (2) sont des tests du chi-deux décrits par Gail (1978) et le test (3) a été proposé par Armitage (1994). Le degré de signification a été obtenue en considérant que, sous l'hypothèse d'absence de différence, le nombre de décès observé suivait une distribution de Poisson, dont la moyenne était égale au nombre des décès attendus sur la base des taux spécifiques par âge de référence. Des tests bilatéraux ont été utilisés (détermination des zones où les taux de mortalité différaient significativement des moyennes nationales et européenne). Le test (1) a permis de vérifier si les SMR ne différaient pas selon les groupes d'âge, condition nécessaire pour que l'utilisation du SMR soit valide (cette condition s'est vérifiée pour toutes les causes de décès évitables considérées).

Il faut rappeler que le SMR est une mesure relative de la mortalité (non absolue). Un SMR de 200 peut aussi bien indiquer 2 décès quand 1 était attendu que 300 décès quand 150 étaient attendus. C'est pourquoi, il est essentiel de considérer non seulement les SMR mais également l'effectif réel de décès. Les tableaux où figurent les SMR présentent également ces effectifs de décès. Des cartes indiquent les zones où peu de décès sont attendus. Les SMR mesurent les écarts relatifs de mortalité par rapport à la moyenne européenne ou par rapport à la moyenne du pays considéré. Ces moyennes ne doivent pas être considérées comme des normes (un SMR peu élevé n'indique pas forcément une situation favorable).

Cartes pour la periode 1985–89

Deux ensembles de cartes ont été réalisés afin d'illustrer différents aspects des variations de la mortalité. Six classes ont été utilisées pour toutes les cartes. Ces classes sont basées sur la valeur des SMR et non sur le degré de signification statistique des tests. Les régions à forte mortalité sont représentées par des trames foncées. Il faut interpréter avec prudence les cartes concernant des pathologies où les décès sont peu nombreux aux âges considérés. Les résultats observés peuvent en effet être instables et une différence minime entre le nombre de décès observés et le nombre de décès attendus peut conduire à des SMR très élevés ou, au contraire, très faibles.

Les méthodes utilisées pour la détermination des classes sont décrites ci-dessous. Des histogrammes indiquant la distribution des SMR sont présentés sur chaque carte.

(1) Communauté Européenne

Ces cartes ont pour objectif de mettre en évidence les variations interpays. Elles permettent de classer les différentes zones en fonction de leur niveau de mortalité par rapport à la moyenne européenne. Les données de mortalité de chaque zone ont été standardisées par âge selon les taux de décès spécifiques de l'ensemble de la Communauté Européenne (SMR de la Communauté Européenne = 100) et les SMR de chaque zone ont été ensuite ordonnés. Chacune des six trames correspond à un même nombre de zones, les trames les plus foncées indiquant les SMR les plus élevés. Des trames rayées permettent d'indiquer les zones pour lesquelles les résultats doivent être interprétés avec prudence du fait du faible effectif de décès concernés. Les zones dont l'effectif de décès attendus (sur la base des taux de décès européens) était égal ou inférieur à 5 ont été ainsi représentées avec des rayures.

Pour mettre en évidence les variations globales entre-pays, une carte indiquant les SMR par pays, et non plus par zones, a été également incluse (SMR se référant à la moyenne européenne).

Sur chaque carte de la Communauté Européenne, un histogramme de fréquences des SMR est présenté pour indiquer l'importance des variations entre zones des SMR de la cause cartographiée. Ces histogrammes comportent 20 classes. Le même mode de regroupement a été utilisé pour chaque histogramme, afin de disposer d'une échelle commune permettant de comparer la variabilité des SMR selon les différentes affections. Les intervalles définis pour ces histogrammes sont différents des classes de SMR utilisées pour la cartographie.

(2) Par pays

Ces cartes ont pour objectif la mise en évidence des variations entres zones d'un même pays. Des cartes distinctes ont été ainsi réalisées pour chaque pays. Les données de mortalité de chaque pays ont été standardisées en prenant pour référence les taux spécifiques par âge du pays concerné (SMR de l'ensemble du pays = 100). Le SMR de chaque zone indique l'écart de mortalité avec la moyenne nationale. Ces cartes ne doivent pas être utilisées pour comparer le niveau de la mortalité entre pays. Il était important d'utiliser, pour chaque affection, une mesure commune permettant de mettre en évidence les variations internes aux différents pays. Aussi, l'ensemble des SMR (avec référence nationale) relatifs aux 368 régions, ont été classés et subdivisés en sextiles afin de déterminer les intervalles de classes cartographiées. Les trames définies ainsi illustrent l'amplitude avec laquelle la mortalité des régions diffère de la mortalité moyenne nationale en comparaison de I'amplitude avec laquelle les autres régions de la Communauté Européenne diffèrent de la mortalité moyenne de leur propre pays.

Les cartes relatives aux différents pays ne comportent pas de zones rayées (des rayures ne seraient pas ressorties sur un fond gris). Cependant, les résultats concernant des régions pour lesquelles peu de décès sont observés doivent être interprétés avec prudence. Le Tableau 8.2 présente, avec les SMR, les effectifs de décès concernés.

Un histogramme de la fréquence des SMR, construit selon des intervalles d'une amplitude égale à 20, est présenté avec chaque carte. En gris, figure la distribution des SMR des 368 régions de la Communauté Européenne basés sur les taux nationaux, et, en noir, figure la distribution des SMR du pays considéré. Les intervalles définis pour les histogrammes sont différents des classes de SMR utilisées pour la cartographie.

Tableaux pour la periode 1985–89

Le Tableau 8.2 indique, pour chaque région de chaque pays, les effectifs de décès par cause, les indicateurs de mortalité (standardisation européenne et standardisation nationale) ainsi que le résultat des tests (SMR significativement supérieur à 100). Des synthèses des résultats sont présentées pour chaque pays dans le Tableau 8.3. Le degré de signification des tests relatifs aux SMR dépend non seulement du niveau du SMR mais également de la taille de la population de la région concernée et du taux de mortalité pour la cause considérée (chacun des deux contribue au nombre 'attendu' de décès dans la région). Un SMR de même valeur, observé dans deux régions de taille différente, peut ainsi être significatif pour la région de taille élevée et non significatif pour la région de taille faible. Le Tableau 8.1 présente les effectifs de population de chaque zone.

Variation de la 'mortalité évitable' entre les periodes 1980–84 et 1985–89

Pour pouvoir comparer le niveau de la mortalité évitable en 1980–84 et en 1985–89, les données de mortalité et les données de population doivent se rapporter aux mêmes zones géographiques. Pour l'Angleterre et Galles, les analyses figurant dans la deuxième édition concernaient les AHA (Area Health Authority) alors que l'édition présente prend en compte les DHA (District Health Authorities). AHA et DHA ont donc été regroupés à un niveau 'Regional Health Autorities'.

Pour la Hollande, la frontière entre Overijssel et Flevoland ayant été redéfinie, cette édition se base sur les nouvelles frontières et les données de la période 1980–84 ont été ajustées en conséquence.

Cartes indiquant les variations entre 1980–84 et 1985–89

Les trames de ces cartes sont basées sur le pourcentage de variation des taux de mortalité standardisés par âge (standardisation selon les taux européens de la période 1985–89). Les zones ont été d'abord divisées en deux groupes selon que les taux standardisés avaient augmenté ou diminué. Les zones pour lesquelles aucun changement n'a été constaté ont été incluses dans le deuxième groupe. Les zones ont été ensuite classées en fonction du pourcentage de variation de la mortalité entre 1980–84 et 1985–89. La plupart des cartes utilisent quatre trames de bleu et deux trames de rouge. Les zones pour lesquelles on a constaté une diminution, on été réparties en quatre groupes égaux (selon leur classement) correspondant à chacune des quatre trames de bleu. Les zones pour lesquelles on a constaté une augmentation, on été réparties en deux groupes égaux (selon leur classement) correspondant à chacune des deux trames de rouge.

Les seules causes pour lesquelles on a constaté une augmentation d'ensemble de la mortalité sont l'asthme et le cancer du sein. Pour toutes les autre pathologies, il y a eu une diminution globale de la mortalité. Le système de trames particulier utilisé pour représenter l'asthme et le cancer du sein reflète cette situation. Pour ces pathologies, un tiers des zones où la mortalité n'a pas augmenté a été représenté par chaque trame bleue. Un tiers des zones où la mortalité a augmenté a été représenté par chaque trame rouge.

Des trames rayées permettent d'indiquer les zones pour lesquelles les résultats doivent être interprétés avec prudence du fait d'une faible précision dans les estimations de variation de mortalité. Les zones où l'effectif de décès attendus était égal ou inférieur à 5, pour les deux périodes, ont été ainsi représentées avec des rayures. Pour comparer globalement les variations selon les différents pays, des résultats sont aussi présentés au niveau agrégé de chaque pays.

Graphiques

Des graphiques indiquent les taux de mortalité par pays pour les trois périodes 1974–78, 1980–84 et 1985–89. Ces résultats utilisent certaines données provenant des premières éditions de l'atlas. Les taux de décès par pays ont été standardisés par âge sur la base des taux de mortalité de l'Europe Communautaire en 1985–89. Les résultats sont présentés selon une échelle logarithmique afin de mettre en évidence le pourcentage de variation des taux de décès dans le temps. Des courbes illustrent les évolutions de la mortalité évitable.

Tableaux indiquant les variations entre 1980–84 et 1985–89

Les variations de la mortalité évitable par pays sont présentés en Tableux 9.1 et 9.3. Les variations d'ensemble de la mortalité sont présentés dans le Tableau 9.1. Ce tableau indique l'effectif des décès, les taux brut de décès, les taux de décès standardisés par âge pour chaque maladie et pour chaque pays en 1980–84 et 1985–89, ainsi que le pourcentage annuel de variation des taux de décès entre 1980–84 et 1985–89. Les taux de décès standardisés par âge ont été calculés en multipliant les SMR (standardisés sur la base européenne 1985–89) par les taux bruts européens de 1985–89. Les variations par pays des taux spécifiques par âge sont présentées dans le Tableau 9.3. Les effectifs de décès et les taux de décès standardisés par âge y sont indiqués pour l'ensemble des deux périodes ainsi que les variations des taux de décès entre les deux périodes. Les variations inter-période de l'effectif des populations selon les différents groupes d'âge sont indiquées dans le Tableau 9.2.

2. METHODEN

Auswahl von Indikatoren zur Leistungsbewertung der gesundheitlichen Versorgung

Im vorliegenden Band werden Indikatoren vorgestellt, die sich auf die Sterblichkeit bei insgesamt siebzehn Krankheitsgruppen beziehen. Sie stellen eine Kombination der in Band I und II der zweiten Ausgabe behandelten Todesursachen dar (OUP 1991, 1993). Diese Indikatoren wurden ausgewählt, um die Leistungen der Primär- und Sekundärprävention sowie der kurativen Sektoren der gesundheitlichen Versorgung in ihrem Ergebnis bei den Einwohnern definierter geographischer Gebiete zu messen. Bei all den hier betrachteten Krankheiten ist unstrittig, daß entweder eine wirksame medizinische Behandlung oder eine Primär-bzw. Sekundärprävention im System der gesundheitlichen Versorgung zur Verfügung steht. Diese Indikatoren, die wir 'Vermeidbarer- Tod-Indikatoren' genannt haben, sollen Warnsignale für mögliche Defizite der gesundheitlichen Versorgung setzen, obwohl stets auch andere Erklärungen in Frage kommen. In dem vorliegenden Atlas ist vorgesehen, daß die Indikatoren in zweierlei Hinsicht genutzt werden:

(1) zu prüfen, ob bestimmte Bereiche der gesundheitlichen Versorgung in den geographischen Regionen zu ausgeglichenen Resultaten führen;

(2) Warnsignale zu setzen, denen dann lokale Studien mit dem Ziel nachgehen sollten, 'vermeidbare" Faktoren und andere Probleme zu erkennen, so daß die örtliche gesundheitliche Versorgung verbessert werden kann.

Die Auswahl von Todesursachen, die als Indikatoren für die Bewertung der Leistungen der gesundheitlichen Versorgung benutzt werden sollten, begann mit einer überarbeiteten Liste der 14 Krankheitsgruppen, die Charlton *et al.* (1983) ihrer Studie über regionale Mortalitätsunterschiede in England und Wales zugrundegelegt hatten. Diese wiederum entstammt einer Liste von 'gesundheitlichen Ereignissen mit Signalfunktion', die von der oben erwähnten Arbeitsgruppe zu vermeidbaren und behandelbaren Krankheiten in den Vereinigten Staaten erstellt worden war (Rutstein *et al.* 1980).

Beim ersten Workshop der Arbeitsgruppe wurde eine Liste von Krankheitsgruppen mit Vertreten aller, der damals zehn teilnehmenden Länder diskutiert, um die möglicherweise unterschiedliche Beurteilung hinsichtlich der Bedeutung der Krankheiten zu berücksichtigen. Als Ergebnis der Diskussion wurden 17 Krankheitsgruppen als Indikatoren für primäre und sekundäre Prävention sowie für kurative Behandlung ausgewählt. Sie waren Gegenstand der ersten beiden Ausgaben von Band I des Atlasses (OUP 1988 und 1991). Bei den anschließenden Treffen der Arbeitsgruppe wurden acht weitere Krankheitsgruppen als relevant ausgewählt. Diese acht Krankheitsgruppen wurden in Band II der zweiten Ausgabe behandelt (OUP 1993). Während die erste Ausgabe den Zeitraum 1974–78, die zweite Ausgabe den von 1980–84 behandelte, widmet sich die vorliegende Ausgabe den Jahren zwischen 1985–1989 unter Berücksichtigung der in den beiden Ausgaben des Bandes I graphisch dargestellten Krankheiten (Tuberkulose, Cervix-Karzinom, Cervix- und Korpus-Krebs des Uterus, Hodgkinsche Krankheit, chronisch rheumatische Herzkrankheit, Asthma, Appendizitis, Abdominalhernie, Cholecystectomie, Hypertonie und Schlaganfall, Maternal- und Perinatalsterblichkeit) und drei Krankheiten aus Band II (Brustkrebs, ischämische Herzkrankheit, Magenschwüre).

Hinzuzufügen wäre, daß es bei den letzteren drei Krankheitsgruppen minder gewiß ist, wie ausschlaggebend die Rolle der Gesundheitsverwaltungen tatsächlich ist. Obgleich nicht alle Sterbefälle bei den erwähnten Krankheitsgruppen vermeidbar sind, können die Gesundheitsdienste dennoch beträchtliche Beiträge zur Verringerung der Sterblichkeit machen. Grundprinzip bei der Wahl der Krankheitsgruppen war, daß für jede Gruppe sowohl wirkungsvolle Interventionsverfahren als auch Träger der Versorgung vorhanden sein mußten. Die Tabellen im Anhang A zeigen für jede der ausgewählten Krankheitsgruppen die ICD- Codes, die Altersgruppen und die subsumierten Krankheiten; darüberhinaus werden die Gründe genannt, die die Arbeitsgruppe veranlaßten, diese Sterbefälle als 'vermeidbar' einzustufen (d. h. als veränderbare Faktoren, die unter gegebenen Bedingungen zur Gesamtmortalität beitragen) und es wird aufgeführt, welche Art gesundheitslicher Versorgung oder andere Intervention die Sterblichkeit verringern könnte. Bei jeder Krankheitsgruppe wurden strenge Altersgrenzen festgelegt, um die Validität des Mortalitätsmaßes als Indikator für die Leistungsfähigkeit der gesundheitlichen Versorgung zu erhöhen. Mit diesen Krankheitsgruppen sollte ein breiteres Band unterschiedlicher Versorgungsleistungen und - dienste abgedeckt werden. Sie umfassen jedoch weder alle Krankheiten, bei denen der Tod durch medizinische Intervention 'vermeidbar' ist, noch ist jeder einzelne Todesfall an den ausgewählten Todesursachen zu vermeiden. Es wird jedoch angenommen, daß ein gewisser Anteil dieser Sterbefälle verhindert werden könnte. Um die regionalen geographischen Mortalitätsunterschiede bei den acht genannten Todesursachen zu demonstrieren, wurden die Karten und Tabellen erstellt.

Wegen Kodierungsproblemen in einigen Ländern wurden die Daten für Cervix- und Korpus-Krebs des Uterus zusammengefaßt (Kelson und Farebrother 1987). Innerhalb der Altersgruppe von 15–54 Jahren sind damit fast alle der so klassifizierten Todesfälle auf Cervix-Karzinom zurückzuführen. Es werden Karten gezeigt, die sowohl die Sterbefälle an Cervix-Karzinom als auch die an Cervix- und Korpus-Krebs des Uterus wiedergeben.

Die Daten

Die Indikatoren basieren auf Mortalitätsdaten für 1985–89 mit Ausnahme der Niederlande und Spaniens (1985–88). Die Bevölkerungsdaten beziehen sich auf auf 1985–1989. Ausnahmen bilden: Frankreich (1987), und Griechenland (1987), Irland (1986), die Niederlande (1985–88), und Spanien (1986).

Die Zeittrend-Analyse verwendet außerdem Daten aus den frühen achtziger Jahren. Diese Mortalitätsdaten behandeln den Zeitraum 1980–1984 für alle Krankheiten außer Brustkrebs, ischämischer Herzkrankheit und Magengeschwüren (1982–84). Ausnahmen bilden:

Griechenland (1980–82), Spanien (1979–83), Italien (1979–83), und England und Wales (1980–84). Die Bevölkerungsdaten des füheren Zeitraumes beziehen sich auf 1980–84 mit Ausnahme Frankreichs (1982), Griechenlands (1981), Irlands (1981), Spaniens (1981), Italiens (1979–83), England und Wales (1980–82). Da Griechenland und Portugal keine Daten über Asthma für die frühen achtziger Jahre zur Verfügung stellten, konnten sie nicht in die Zeittrend-Analyse zur Asthmasterblichkeit aufgenommen werden.

Die Daten stammen aus amtlichen Statistiken; die Bevölkerungsdaten z.B. beruhen auf Volkszählungen, wobei amtliche Fortschreibungen für Zeiträume zwischen Volkszählungen—soweit vorhanden—zugrundedelegt werden. Die Datenquellen sind in Anhang B aufgeführt. Die Teilnehmer der einzelnen Länder sind für die Stimmigkeit der Daten ihres Landes verantwortlich, die dem Koordinationszentrum gegliedert nach Alter, Geschlecht, und Verwaltungsgebieten übermittelt wurden.

Angestrebt wurden Verwaltungsgebiete von ungefähr 500 000 Einwohnern. Da jedoch existierende administrative Einheiten benutzt werden mußten, variieren die Regionen in ihrer Größe. Im Zeitraum 1985–89 gab es in der EG 552 Verwaltungsbebiete, die für diese Studie in Frage kommen. Um die Übersichtlichkeit der Karten zu verbessern, wurden für England und Wales größere Regionaleinheiten benutzt ('regions' statt 'districts'). Dadurch verringerte sich die Zahl der in die Karten aufgenommen Regionen auf 368.

Die 9. Revision der Internationalen Klassifikation der Krankheiten (ICD9) wurde in 1979 eingeführt. Alle Länder haben diese Kodierung während der achtziger Jahren benutzt, mit Ausnahme von Dänemark, das die ICD8 zugrundegelegt hat. Ein möglicher Einfluß dieses Unterschiedes auf die Ergebnisse in Dänemark wurde unter Verwendung der erhaltenen Resultate bei Anwendung des Umsteigeschlüssels des OPCS (England und Wales) untersucht. Dort war eine Stichprobe von 25 prozent aller Todesfälle des Jahres 1978 sowohl nach ICD8 als auch nach ICD9 kodiert worden. Die Unterschiede in der Zahl der Todesfälle, die bestimmten Krankheiten zugeordnet wurden, betrugen für jede der 'vermeidbaren' Todesursachen weniger als 5 prozent mit Ausnahme der chronisch rheumatischen Herzkrankheiten, Asthma, Appendizitis, und Abdominalhernie. Dort führten die Klassifikationsunterschiede in den betrachteten Altersgruppen zu einer Verminderung der Zahl der Todesfälle um 39 prozent bei chronisch rheumatischer Herzkrankheit und 9 prozent bei Abdominalhernie (von ICD8 bis ICD9). Todesfälle aufgrund von Asthma und Appendizitis stiegen um 9 prozent beziehungsweise 7 prozent an.

Analyse und Präsentation

Die geographische Verteilung der 'vermeidbaren' Mortalität über die Verwaltungsgebiete der EG im Zeitraum 1985–89 sowie deren Veränderung zwischen 1980–84 und 1985–89 werden in Karten (368 Regionen) und Tabellen (552 Regionen) dargestellt. EG-Karten der SMRs von 1985–89 und der Mortalitätswandel während der achtziger Jahre werden zusammen dargestellt um die Interpretation zu erleichtern.

In den Niederlanden ist die Grenze zwischen Overijssel und Flevoland neu festgelegt worden. Die Mortalitätsdaten für 1980–84 sind entsprechend angepaßt worden.

Analyse und Präsentation der Daten für 1985–89

Da alters- und geschlechtsspezifische Mortalitätsraten für kleinräumliche Einheiten wegen der geringen Zahl von Todesfällen zu ungenau wären, wurde die indirekte Altersstandardisierung (standardisierte Mortalitätsquotienten—SMRs) angewandt (siehe Armitage 1993). Die Daten für beide Geschlechter wurden zusammengefaßt, da nicht davon auszugehen ist, daß die Vermeidbarkeit von Todesfällen geschlechtsabhängig ist. Bei geschlechtsspezifischen Erkrankungen bezieht sich die Altersstandardisierung auf den Bevölkerungsteil des betreffenden Geschlechts.

Für jede Kranheitsgruppe und jede der 552 in die Studie einbezogenen Regionen wurden die SMRs auf zwei verschiedene Arten berechnet:

(a) unter Zugrundelegung der altersspezifischen Mortalitätsraten für die EG insgesamt;

(b) unter Zugrundelegung der altersspezifischen Mortalitätsraten des Landes, dem die Region angehört.

Die erste Methode wurde angewandt, um Unterschiede zwischen den Ländern durch Standardisierung aller Daten auf eine gemeinsame Bezugsgröße (EG insgesamt = 100) zu zeigen. Die zweite Methode wurde gewählt, um Differenzen innerhalb eines Landes (gesamtes Land = 100) darzustellen.

Die ermittelten SMRs wurden statistischen Tests unterzogen, um zu prüfen:

(a) ob die SMRs die Daten zutreffend wiedergeben;

(b) ob das Ausmaß an Unterschiedlichkeit zwischen den Regionen das bereits zufällig zu erwartende übersteigt;

(c) ob in einer Region der Mortalitätsquotient (SMR) signifikant abweichend von 100 (Standardwert) ist.

Die Tests (a) und (b) sind Chi-Quadrat-Verfahren, wie sie von Gail (1978) beschrieben wurden. Test (c) wurde von Armitage (1993) dargestellt. Bei der Signifikanzbestimmung wurde unterstellt, daß die Zahl der beobachteten Todesfälle einer Poisson-Verteilung folgt, mit einem Mittelwert gleich der erwarteten Zahl von Sterbefällen aufgrund der altersspezifischen Raten der Referenzbevölkerung. Es wurde zweiseitig getestet, um alle Regionen herauszustellen, in denen die Mortalitätsrate signifikant vom nationalen bzw. EG-Standard abweicht. In früheren Ausgaben und Bänden des Atlasses wurden einseitige Tests durchgeführt. Der Test (a) prüft, ob die Mortalitätsquotienten (regional/EG und regional/national) für die verschiedenen Altersgruppen gleichartig sind. Dies ist eine Vorraussetzung für die valide Beschreibung der Daten durch den SMR. Bei keiner 'vermeidbaren' Todesursache wurde festgestellt, daß die SMRs ungeeignet wären.

Die SMR ist ein relatives und kein absolutes Maß der Mortalität. Eine SMR von 200 kann zwei Todesfälle indizieren, wo nur einer erwartet war, oder aber auch 300 bei nur 150 erwarteten Fällen. Es ist daher wichtig, nicht nur die SMR an sich sondern auch die tatsächliche Zahl der Todesfälle zu berücksichtigen. Die Tabellen der SMRs enthalten die registrierten Todesfälle. Karten deuten die Regionen an, in denen nur wenige Todesfälle erwartet werden. Die SMRs messen die Mortalität relativ zu den EG und nationalen Standards. Keiner dieser Standards sollte jedoch als das 'goldene Maß' angesehen werden. Eine niedrige SMR deutet deshalb nicht zwangsläufig auf eine zufriedenstellende Leistung hin.

Karten für den Zeitraum 1985–89

Um verschiedene Aspekte von Mortalitätsunterschieden aufzuzeigen, wurden auf diese Weise zwei Typen von Karten erzeugt. Sechs Schattierungen liegen allen Karten zugrunde. Die Schattierungen repräsentieren die Größe der SMR-Werte und sagen nichts über die statistische Signifikanz aus. Dunklere Schattierungen deuten eine höhere Mortalität an. Vorsicht ist geboten bei der Interpretation von Karten, die Krankheitsgruppen mit geringen Todesfallzahlen im betrachteten Altersbereich darstellen. Der Grund hierfür liegt darin, daß schon ein geringer Unterschied zwischen der Zahl der beobachteten Todesfälle und der aufgrund der altersspezifischen Mortalitätsraten der Referenzbevölkerung erwarteten Zahl, extreme SMRs zur Folge haben kann. Die beiden Methoden der Zuordnung von Regionen zu Abstufungsintervallen werden im folgenden beschrieben. Auf jeder Karte finden sich außerdem Histogramme, die die Verteilung der SMRs wiedergeben.

EG insgesamt, Sextil-Intervalle

Diese Karten sollen Unterschiede zwischen den einzelnen Ländern aufzeigen. Sie zeigen die Rangordnung der Regionen beim Vergleich der Mortalität mit einem gemeinsamen EG-Standard. Die Mortalitätsdaten jeder Region wurden unter Zugrundelegung der alterspezifischen Raten der EG insgesamt (SMR der EG = 100) altersstandardisiert, und diese SMRs wurden sodann der Größe nach geordnet. Jedem Abstufungsintervall wurde eine gleiche Zahl von Regionen zugeordnet, wobei eine dunklere Schattierung höhere SMRs andeutet. Eine gestreifte Schattierung weist auf Regionen hin, bei denen extreme SMRs mit besonderer Vorsicht aufgrund von Ungewißheit bei den Schätzungen interpretiert werden sollten. Regionen, in denen die erwartete Zahl an Todesfällen basierend auf EG-Raten 5 prozent und weniger betrugen, sind ebenfalls gestreift.

Um die Schwankungen zwischen den einzelnen Ländern hervorzuheben,befindet sich nebenan eine Karte, die SMRs länderweise statt nach kleineren Regionen darstellt.

Auf jeder Karte der EG ist ein Histogramm der Häufigkeiten der SMRs abgebildet, um für die jeweils betrachtete Todesursache das Ausmaß der Variabilität der SMRs für die kleinräumlichen Regionen der EG zu illustrieren. Die Histogramme basieren auf einer Gruppierung von 20 Prozentpunkten pro Intervall. Das gleiche Gruppierungsintervall liegt jedem Histogramm zugrunde, um die Variabilität der SMRs in den verschiedenen Krankheitsgruppen auf einem einheitlichen Maßstab vergleichen zu können. Die Histogramm-Intervalle unterscheiden sich von den SMR-Spannbreiten, die für die Schattierungen der Karten benutzt wurden.

Einzelne Länder, Sextil-/Quartil-Intervalle

Mit diesen Karten sollen die Mortalitätsunterschiede innerhalb eines Landes aufgezeigt werden; für jedes Land wurden eigene Karten angefertigt. Für jede Region wurden die Mortalitätsdaten auf die altersspezifischen Mortalitätsraten des zugehörigen Landes standadisiert (SMR des Landes = 100), somit drückt der SMR für eine Region das Ausmaß ihrer Abweichung vom Land als Ganzes aus. Vergleiche zwischen den Ländern sollten nicht mit diesen Karten angestellt werden. Um Variationsbreiten in den verschiedenen Ländern zu zeigen, war es wichtig bei jeder Krankheit einen gemeinsamen Maßstab anzulegen. Daher wurden die auf nationalen Standards beruhenden SMRs für die 368 kleinräumlichen Regionen in eine Rangfolge gebracht und Sextilen zugeornet, um daraus die Schattierungen abzuleiten. Die auf den Standardisierungen mittels nationaler Raten beruhende zeigt in welcher Größenordnung die Mortalität einer Region vom eigenen Landesdurchschnitt abweicht, gleichzeitig ersieht man das Spektrum der Abweichungen andere europäischer Regionen von ihren jeweiligen Landesdurchschnitten.

Individuelle Länderkarten sind nicht gestreift, da Streifen vor einem grauen Hintergrund nicht besonders gut erkennbar wären. Es sollten jedoch die Ergebnisse für Regionen, in denen nur wenige Todesfälle auftreten, mit Vorsicht interpretiert werden. Tabelle 8.2 stellt SMRs zusammen mit der tatsächlichen Zahl an Todesfällen dar.

Jede Karte enthält ein Histogramm der SMR-Häufigkeiten, basierend auf einem Gruppierungsintervall von 20. Sie zeigen in grau die Verteilung der SMRn kleiner Gebiete, auf einem für die 368 Gebiete der EG insgesamt beruhenden National-Standard, und in schwarz die Verteilung der SMRn für das jeweilige Land. Die Histogramm-Intervalle Unterscheiden sich von den SMR-Spannbreiten, die für die Schattierung der Karten benutzt wurde.

Tabellen für den Zeitraum 1985–89

Tabellen mit der Zahl der Todesfälle für jede Ursache und den Mortalitätsindikatoren (standardisiert sowohl auf die EG als auch auf das einzelne Land) und der Angabe, ob sie den Wert 100 (der SMR-Wert der Referenzbevölkerung) signifikant übersteigen, finden sich für jede Region jeden Landes in Tabelle 8.2. Zusammenfassungen auf nationaler Ebene werden in Tabelle 8.3 dargestellt. Ob der SMR einer Region signifikant von der Referenzbevölkerung abweicht, hängt nicht nur von der Größe des SMR ab, sondern auch von der regionalen Bevölkerungsgröße und der Gesamtmortalitätsrate der jeweiligen Krankheit (beide letzteren Faktoren nehmen Einfluß auf die Zahl 'erwarteter' Sterbefälle in einer Region). Ein identischer SMR-Wert in zwei Regionen mit stark unterschiedlicher Bevölkerungszahl kann für das Gebiet mit der größeren Bevölkerung eine signifikante Abweichung vom Standard bedeuten, jedoch nicht für jenes mit einer kleineren Bevölkerung. Tabelle 8.2 enthält die Bevölkerungen jeder einzelnen Region.

Veränderungen bei der 'vermeidbaren Sterblichkeit' zwischen 1980–84 und 1985–89

Um Vergleiche zwischen dem Ausmaß der 'vermeidbaren Mortalität' für 1980–84 gegenüber dem für 1985–89 anstellen zu können, müssen sich die Mortalitäts- und Bevölkerungsdaten auf die gleichen Gebietseinheiten beziehen. Die in der zweiten Ausgabe für England und Wales dargestellten Resultate bezogen sich auf die Ebene der Area Health Authority (AHA) während sich die vorliegende Ausgabe auf die District Health authorities (DHA) bezieht. Die Daten beider Ebenen (AHAs und DHAs) wurden auf Basis der Regional Health Authority zusammengefaßt.

In den Niederlanden ist die Grenze zwischen Overijssel und Flevoland neu festgelegt worden. Die vorliegende Ausgabe trägt diesem Umstand Rechnung, und die Daten für 1980–84 sind entsprechend angepaßt worden.

Karten zu den Veränderungen zwischen 1980–84 und 1985–89

Die Schattierung in den Karten beruht auf dem prozentualen Wandel der altersstandardisierten Mortalitätsraten (standardisiert nach der EG-Rate von 1985–89). Die einzelnen Regionen wurden entsprechend eines aufgetretenen oder nicht aufgetretenen Anstiegs in der altersstandardisierten Mortalität in zwei Gruppen eingeteilt. Regionen, in denen es keine Veränderung gab, wurden der zweiten Gruppe zugeteilt. Regionen wurden entsprechend des jährlichen prozentualen Wandels in der Mortalität von 1980–84 bis 1985–89 in eine Rangfolge eingeteilt. Die meisten Karten verwenden vier Arten von blauer und zwei Arten von roter Schattierung. Ein Viertel der Regionen, in denen kein Anstieg der Mortalität stattfand, wurden jeweils in ein blau schattiertes Intervall eingeordnet. Die Hälfte der Regionen mit einem Anstieg wurden jeweils in den beiden rot schattierten Intervallen eingeordnet.

Es wurde ein Anstieg der Gesamttodesrate bei Asthma und Brustkrebs festgestellt. Bei allen anderen Krankheiten wurde insgesamt ein Rückgang verzeichnet. Die Schattierungsweise der graphischen Darstellung des prozentualen Wandels in der Mortalität spiegelt dies wider. Ein Drittel der Regionen, die keinen Anstieg der Mortalität erfuhren, wurden in einen blau schattierten Bereich eingeordnet.

Eine gestreifte Schattierung weist auf Regionen hin, bei denen die Interpretation extremer prozentualer Schwankungen aufgrund der gestiegenen Unsicherheit bei den Schätzungen der Veränderungsrate besonderer Vorsicht bedarf. Regionen, in denen während den beiden betrachteten Zeiträumen fünf oder weniger Todesfälle auftraten, sind gestreift. Um die Unterschiede des prozentualen Wandels zwischen den einzelnen Ländern hervorzuheben, werden die Ergebnisse außerdem in einer Nebenkarte auf Länderebene dargestellt.

Tabellen zu den Veränderungen zwischen 1980–84 und 1985–89

Veränderungen bei der 'vermeidbaren' Mortalität auf nationaler Ebene werden in Tabelle 9.1 (S.000) und in Tabelle 9.3 (S.000) wiedergegeben. Die gesamte Veränderung der Mortalität wird in Tabelle 9.1 gezeigt. Hier wird die Anzahl der Todesfälle, die reine und altersstandardisierte Todesrate für jede Krankheit in jedem Land von 1980–84 bis 1985–89, sowie der jährliche prozentuale Wandel in der Todesrate von 1980–84 bis 1985–89 aufgeführt. Bei der altersstandardisierten Todesrate wird unterstellt, daß sie durch Multiplikation der SMR (standardisiert auf die EG-Rate von 1985–89) mit der reinen EG-Todesrate von 1985–89 ermittlet wird. In der gesamten EG gab es einen Rückgang der Mortalität bei jeder untersuchten Todesursache mit Ausnahme von Asthma, für das die Mortalität leicht anstieg. Nationale Veränderung bei der altersspezifischen Mortalität werden in Tabelle 9.1 gezeigt. Die Zahl der beobachteten Todesfälle und die altersstandardisierte Todesrate für beide Zeiträume werden zusammen mit dem Wandel in der Todesrate zwischen den beiden Zeiträumen dargestellt. Änderungen der Bevölkerungsdaten für die verschiedenen Altersgruppen werden in Tabelle 9.2 gezeigt.

3. DEFINITIONS

Age-specific death rate: the number of deaths in a specific age group per 100000 population in that age group.

Age-standardized death rate: the SMR for an area multiplied by the crude death rate of the reference population (whole of EC or individual country).

Areas: administrative areas for local health services in particular countries. These were chosen on the basis of availability of data. The populations of these areas were intended to be approximately 500000 but depend in practice on the organisation of health services or the availability of information on mortality in individual countries.

'Avoidable deaths': death from specific diseases (within selected age groups) for which mortality should be wholly or substantially avoidable when appropriate medical care is sought and provided in good time.

Expected deaths: expected deaths represents the number of deaths expected had the age-specific death rates for the reference population applied for the area studied.

Maternal death rate: the number of deaths associated with childbirth per 100000 live and still births.

Maternal 'SMR': the percentage ratio of the crude maternal death rate in the area studied to the crude maternal death rate in the reference population (whole EC or individual country).

ICD number: code assigned to cause(s) of death by the International Classification of Diseases/8th or 9th revision.

Annual percentage change in mortality: the percentage change in mortality from 1980–84 to 1985–89.

Perinatal death rate: the number of still births and deaths in the first week of life per 1000 live and still births.

Perinatal 'SMR': the percentage ratio of the crude perinatal death rate in the area studied to the crude perinatal death rate in the reference population (whole of EC or individual country).

Standardized mortality ratio (SMR): the percentage ratio of the number of deaths observed in the area studied to the number expected from the standard age-specific death rates.

3. DÉFINITIONS

Taux spécifiques de mortalité par âge: effectif de décès dans un groupe d'âge particulier pour 100000 habitants du groupe d'âge considéré.

Taux de mortalité standardisé par âge: SMR de la zone, multiplié par le taux brut de décès de la population de référence (Communauté Européenne tout entière ou pays individuel selon le cas).

Régions: zones administratives correspondant pour certains pays à des secteurs sanitaires. Ces zones ont été choisies en fonction de la disponibilité de données statistiques. Le nombre d'habitants de chaque zone devait être d'environ 500000 mais, en pratique, il varie fortement en fonction de l'organisation des services médicaux ou de la disponibilité des informations sur la mortalité propre à chaque pays.

Décès 'évitables': affections spécifiques pour lesquelles la mortalité peut être complètement ou en grande partie évitée à certains âges définis, à condition que des soins médicaux appropriés soient prodigués en temps utile.

Décès attendus: somme des produits des taux spécifiques par âge de la population de référence (Communauté tout entière ou pays individuel) par l'effectif de population correspondante de chaque zone étudiée.

Taux de mortalité maternelle: effectif de décès associés à une grossesse pour 100000 naissances totales.

SMR 'maternel': rapport (multiplié par 100) du taux de mortalité maternelle dans la zone étudiée sur le taux de mortalité maternelle dans la population de référence (Communauté tout entière ou pays individuel).

Code de la CIM: code attribué aux affections responsables des décès par la Classification Internationale des Maladies, 8ème ou 9ème révision.

Pourcentage annuel de variation de la mortalité: pourcentage de variation de la mortalité entre 1980–84 et 1985–89.

Taux de mortalité périnatale: effectif de mort-nés et de décès durant la première semaine de vie pour 1000 naissances totales.

SMR 'périnatal': rapport (multiplié par 100) du taux de mortalité périnatale dans la zone étudiée sur le taux de mortalité périnatale dans la population de référence (Communauté tout entière ou pays individuel).

Indice de mortalité relative (SMR): rapport (multiplié par 100) du nombre de décès observés dans la région étudiée au nombre de décès attendus sur la base des taux de décès par âge de la population de référence.

3. DEFINITIONEN

Alterspezifische Mortalitätsrate: die Zahl der Sterbefälle in einer spezifischen Altersgruppe, bezogen auf 100 000 der Bevölkerung dieser Altersgruppe.

Altersstandardisierte Mortalitätsrate: SMR für eine Gebietseinheit, multipliziert mit der rohen Mortalitätsrate der Referenzbevölkerung (EG insgesamt oder einzelnes Land.)

Regionen: Verwaltungseinheiten für die regionalen Gesundheitsdienste in einzelnen Ländern. Diese wurden nach dem Vorhandensein der Daten ausgewählt. Die Bevölkerung der Regionen sollte ungefähr 500 000 betragen; dies hängt jedoch von der Organisation der Gesundheitsdienste oder der Verfügbarkeit der Mortalitätsdaten in den einzelnen Ländern ab.

'Vermeidbare' Sterbefälle: Sterbefälle an spezifischen Krankheiten (innerhalb ausgewählter Altersgruppen) für die die Sterblichkeit ganz oder zum Grossteil vermeidbar sein sollte, wäre medizinische Behandlung in Anspruch genommen und rechtzeitig gewährt.

Erwartete Todesfälle: Die Zahl von Sterbefällen, die zu erwarten wäre, wenn die altersspezifischen Sterberaten der Referenzbevölkerung in der untersuchten Region gelten würden.

Müttersterblichkeit: die Zahl der im Zusammenhang mit Geburt verstorbenen Frauen, bezogen auf 100 000 Lebend- und Totgeburten.

Mütter 'SMR': Prozent-Quotient aus der rohen Mütter-Mortalitätsrate in der untersuchten Region, und der rohen Mütter-Mortalitätsrate der Referenzbevölkerung (EG insgesamt oder einzelnes Land.)

ICD-Kategorie: Todesursache/n zugeteilte/n Ziffer/n des Kodex der Internationalen Klassifikation der Krankheiten 8. oder 9. Revision.

Jährlicher prozentualer Wandel in der Sterblichkeit: der in Prozent gemessene Wandel in der Sterblichkeit in den Zeiträumen von 1980–84 bis 1985–89.

Perinatale Sterblichkeit: die Zahl von Totgeburten und Säuglingssterbefällen in der ersten Lebenswoche bezogen auf 1000 Lebend- und Totgeburten.

Perinatal 'SMR': Prozent-Quotient aus der rohen Perinatal-Mortalitätsrate der untersuchten Region, und der rohen Perinatal-Mortalitätsrate der Referenzbevölkerung (EG insgesamt oder einzelnes Land).

'Standardisierter Mortalitätsquotient' (SMR): Verhältniszahl in Prozenten, gebildet aus der Zahl der beobachteten Todesfälle in der untersuchten Region und der Zahl von Sterbefällen, wie sie nach den altersspezifischen Sterberaten des Standards zu erwarten wären.

4. INTERPRETATION OF THE MAPS/DATA AND SUGGESTIONS FOR FOLLOW-UP

Observed variation in mortality between countries and areas may be an artefact due to variations in data collection; that is, diagnosis, certification, and coding of deaths. The effect of inaccuracies in death certification and coding in Europe has been investigated for respiratory disease and cancer mortality. Doctors in each country were asked to complete death certificates for a series of case histories and certificates were then coded nationally and by a WHO reference centre. Kelson and Heller (1983), found that for acute respiratory disease there were marked differences in the recording of diagnosis between eight EC countries (for example, in the percentage of doctors certifying a particular case history as asthma varied from 54 per cent to 84 per cent). These differences were attributed to the way in which doctors complete death certificates and to coding. Mackenbach *et al.* (1987) concluded that for some conditions differences in certification and coding may be important in explaining difference in reported death rates. He stressed the need to consider certification and coding together, because in some cases national coding adapted to errors in certification. The further analysis of the data on chronic obstructive lung disease led Burney (1989) to conclude 'tentatively' that differences in coding, in particular when considering atypical and ambiguous cases, may explain more of the observed variation in death rates than was first thought. Apparent time trends may be due to changes in registration practice (Lindahl and Johansson 1994). The trend in reported death rates, from the early to late 1980s, should not have been directly affected by changes in ICD as all EC countries continued to use ICD9 with the sole exception of Denmark which continued to use ICD8. Although misclassification does not fully explain the observed levels of variation (Diehl and Gau 1982) it remains an important factor for many diseases and knowledge of its variation between areas should facilitate interpretation of results presented here.

Additionally the variation may be due to an uneven distribution of disease incidence or prevalence, or geographical variations in the provision and effectiveness of health services. Health services should react to need and target those areas where incidence is greatest and thus inner city areas where the incidence of TB is highest should provide more care than rural areas. For those diseases where not all deaths are avoidable by timely and appropriate intervention (for example, asthma, ischaemic heart disease) incidence or prevalence between areas should be taken into account when examining variation in mortality. For those diseases where deaths are substantially avoidable by adequate and timely health service intervention irrespective of the incidence or prevalence (for example, hypertension, breast cancer) variation in incidence or prevalence may explain but does not justify variation in mortality.

Case fatality may be influenced by the availability of services, the uptake of services and the effectiveness of services. The uptake of services may be influenced by their acceptability, ease of access to them, perception of need by patients, social factors, and family and social support. A confidential inquiry into death from stroke and hypertensive disease in patients under 75 years considered 123 deaths and identified avoidable factors which contributed to death (Payne *et al.* 1993).

Failure of health service to:

- detect hypertension
- follow-up and treat hypertension once diagnosed
- ensure that patients were recalled if they missed follow-up appointments
- diagnose and treat complications of hypertension.

Failure of the patient to:

- take drugs or agree to attend to follow-up
- stop smoking
- lose weight
- reduce alcohol consumption.

Inadequate follow-up and failure to stop smoking were the most common. For 56 of the 81 hypertensive patients it was agreed that minimum standards of care with regard to follow-up had not been met.

For all, conditions, the observed between-area variation in death rate and rate of fall is due in part to random variation. In particular for an area in which few deaths are expected due to a small population or a low death rate, the estimated SMR and percentage change in mortality will be highly unstable. For those conditions for which the death rate is low (such as maternal mortality), the between-area variation in mortality will largely reflect random variation as opposed to true heterogeneity in the underlying risk. Some authors have suggested the use of statistical techniques which smooth area statistics towards some average value (for example, national average) (Bernardinelli and Montomoli 1992). Smoothing has little effect on maps of conditions for which mortality is relatively common (for example, ischaemic heart disease), but has a major effect when mortality is rare (maternal mortality, for example). Although results presented here are not smoothed, the difficulties which small number of deaths present should not, however, be overlooked as maps are prone to over-interpretation when attention is drawn to extreme results in low population areas. EC maps present small-area results, without smoothing, but indicate those areas where few deaths are expected and the results are particularly uncertain. In addition, the more stable national results are also presented. Tabulated results always include the actual number.

A description of variation in potentially 'avoidable mortality' between areas is only the first step in a series of investigations (Charlton *et al.* 1984). Any explanation of this variation may require further investigation, and some examples of ways in which this might be done are outlined.

Trends in the indicators

Studies of the variation in mortality over time (see Appendix C) have revealed a fall in death rates for most of the conditions considered avoidable, but emphasise that the observed decline in avoidable mortality may be due to factors other than improved health care. Socio-economic factors are improving and for many of the conditions 'spontaneous' declines in incidence have been observed. In order to allow for possible confounding effects of these additional factors trends in mortality from avoidable conditions were compared to trends in mortality from other conditions. Mortality from amenable conditions declined faster than mortality from non-amenable conditions and these studies concluded that this indicated a partial association between the decline in avoidable mortality and the improvement in the quality of health care.

Macro-studies

An attempt may be made in these studies to explain variation in mortality between areas and countries using aggregate data (routinely available or specially collected) on disease incidence, prevalence, case fatality, treatment patterns, diagnosis, certification and coding patterns, socio-economic factors, health service provision and expenditure on health (Bauer and Charlton 1986; Charlton *et al.* 1984*a*, *b*; Charlton and Lakhani 1985). There are a number of problems in the reliability of aggregate data and comparability of data between areas and countries. There may also be interactions between the variables, which make the interpretation of such analyses difficult. For example, socio-economic factors may affect the uptake of services and their timely and appropriate use, and thus influence mortality. The availability of health services may directly influence mortality. However, socio-economic factors may also be associated with the availability of services, in that socially deprived areas may have a lower availability and quality of service.

Despite these problems with interpretation, such studies provide a useful and relatively inexpensive first line investigation of variation in mortality, particularly between areas at the two extremes of the distribution (that is, in comparing areas with high and low mortality).

Mackenbach *et al.* (1990) have reviewed 11 aggregate data studies on avoidable mortality and health services published since 1983. They concluded that:

- the low levels of mortality from amenable causes which presently prevail in industrialized countries do probably reflect, at least in part, the increased effectiveness of health services;
- geographical variation in mortality from amenable causes has not yet been shown to reflect differences of health services;
- if geographical variation in mortality does reflect such differences, the latter arise from circumstances other than the level of supply (for example, from more specific aspects of health care delivery), and are probably closely related to socio-economic circumstances.

More recent aggregate data studies which have considered the variation in 'avoidable mortality' rates have reached largely consistent results.

The lack of direct evidence for an association between preventable death rates and the supply of health care does not invalidate it as a measure of the efficiency and efficacy of health care delivery. Results have been based on crude measures of health care such as regional density of GPs, acute hospital beds, and consultants and reflect quantity not quality or access to existing services. The results may indicate, as suggested by many authors, that once a certain basic standard is achieved it is the accessibility of given services which determines, at least in part, the level of avoidable mortality, suggesting the need for improved targeting of services.

It is improbable that more aggregate data studies will contribute to a further understanding of the determinants of avoidable mortality. In-depth studies at the individual level are much more likely to produce new knowledge of factors limiting the effectiveness of health services.

Micro-studies

These studies may involve the investigation of individual deaths in an attempt to identify factors that either explain variation in mortality or identify 'avoidable factors' (such as aspects of service availability, uptake, appropriate use, efficiency and effectiveness that may have contributed to the mortality). There are several stages in such investigations. The first stage is an examination of death certificates and health records to check the diagnoses, certification, and coding of causes of death for each case. This will establish how many deaths may still be classified as 'avoidable', in keeping with the study definition. The next stage will be a detailed, confidential enquiry into each death, to identify potentially 'avoidable factors', for example, as previously described for hypertension. In order to help assess the importance of different 'avoidable factors', it will be necessary to study controls as well (that is, cases matched for age, sex, diagnosis, and area of residence, but who survived). A problem with these studies is that the evidence on 'avoidable factors' tends to be subjective and circumstantial. Before undertaking any confidential enquiry, criteria of what constitutes 'avoidable factors' should be established.

Standardized questionnaires, lists of potentially 'avoidable factors', and guide-lines for the classification of factors for each disease would have to be prepared. The confidential enquiry may be carried out by sending questionnaires to doctors and other health care professionals involved in the management of each case and also by extracting information from medical care records, if these are available. The questionnaires may then be examined by independent assessors, who would use the lists and guide-lines to determine the part each 'avoidable factor' plays in each case. Differences between cases and controls in 'avoidable factors', or common factors observed in a large number of cases and also for a number of diseases, may identify shortcomings in service provision and uptake that are amenable to intervention.

A major benefit of studies at the patient level is that they can assess a wide variety of outcome measures which encompass patient satisfaction and disability. Measures of excess mortality are irrelevant where services, such as those for the elderly, are focused mainly on relieving pain and improving the quality of life. The shift of emphasis from acute life-threatening conditions to chronic incurable illness necessitated a different approach to the measurement of need and outcome (Wilkin *et al.* 1992). For conditions such as diabetes, arthritis, or asthma, cure and survival are no longer adequate measures of health care performance. Appropriate measures must account for the severity of the condition. It is not enough to estimate the death rate from asthma or indeed its prevalence, it is essential to measure the severity of the condition. A major benefit of studies at a patient level is that they assess a wide variety of outcome measures which encompass patient satisfaction and disability. An on-going EC Biomed programme to investigate alternate measures of care for stroke patients was motivated by the observed variation in death rates but will describe patient outcome using measures of impairment, disability, and handicap, in addition to death.

Summary

The atlas presents results for a series of conditions for which mortality is considered largely avoidable given timely and appropriate medical intervention. The between-area variation in mortality from 1985–89, and the mortality change from 1980–84 to 1985–89 is presented so as highlight areas where further study is needed.

The atlas does not attempt to explain the levels of variation observed both within and between countries but rather hopes to motivate further research at a small area level which would examine in detail the variation in rates and identify possible causes, highlight failings in the health service, and suggest appropriate action to eliminate the observed excess.

Avoidable mortality is now accepted by the European Commission and by many member countries as an important indicator of performance. Motivated by previous work many other countries have analysed the regional variation in mortality from avoidable conditions and an atlas of 'avoidable mortality' in Eastern Europe is now being compiled. Ultimately however the success of this project will depend on the quality of the research which it motivates and the resulting improvements in individual health. In mind of this the EC Working Group on Health Services and 'Avoidable Deaths' supplied a series of brief accounts of recent research in this area (in their home countries) which is presented here.

4. INTERPRÉTATION DES CARTES ET DONNÉES: PROPOSITION POUR LA SUITE DES TRAVAUX

Les variations de mortalité observées entre pays ou entre régions peuvent être en partie artificielles et résulter de différences dans la collecte des données (diagnostic, certification et codage des décès). L'impact éventuel de pratiques de certification et de codification propres à certains pays a été étudié dans le cas des maladies respiratoires, du cancer et du diabète. Des médecins de différents pays ont certifié une série de cas cliniques identiques. L'ensemble des certificats a été ensuite codé dans chaque pays et par un centre OMS de référence. Kelson et Heller (1983) ont ainsi mis en évidence des différences importantes entre huit pays de la CEE dans la déclaration des maladies respiratoires aiguës: par exemple, le pourcentage de médecins attribuant le décès d'un même cas clinique à l'asthme variait de 54 à 84 per cent. Les divergences ont été attribuées à la fois à la certification médicale et au codage. Mackenbach *et al.* (1987) en ont conclu que, pour certaines pathologies, les différences de certification et de codification pouvaient être responsables d'une grande part des variations des taux de mortalité rapportés. Ils ont également insisté sur la nécessité d'analyser simultanément, dans ce type d'étude, les processus de certification et de codage car, dans certains cas, le codage peut compenser les erreurs de certification. Burney (1989) a réalisé une analyse complémentaire des résultats de l'étude sur les maladies respiratoires et a conclu que les différences de codification, en particulier pour des cas atypiques et ambigus, peuvent expliquer une grande part des variations de mortalité observées. Lindahl et Johanson (1994) ont montré que certaines évolutions de la mortalité dans le temps pouvaient être dues à des changements dans les pratiques d'enregistrement. Les tendances observées au cours des années 80 étudiées dans cet atlas, n'ont cependant pas pu être directement affectées par des changements de classification des maladies puisque l'ensemble des pays (excepté le Danemark qui a continué à utiliser la 8ème révision), ont utilisé durant cette période la même révision de la CIM (9ème révision). Si les erreurs de classements ne peuvent expliquer entièrement le niveau de variation de la mortalité (Diehl et Gau 1982), elles constituent cependant un facteur à prendre en compte pour de nombreuses maladies. L'analyse de ces variations de pratiques entre zones devrait faciliter l'interprétation des résultats présentés dans cet atlas.

Les différences mises en évidence peuvent également être dues à des variations de l'incidence et de la prévalence des maladies, de l'offre de soins et de l'efficacité des services de santé. Les services de santé devraient être adaptés aux besoins dans les zones où l'incidence est plus élevée. Par exemple, dans les zones urbaines, où l'incidence de la tuberculose est importante, les soins devraient être davantage développés que dans les zones rurales. Pour les maladies où tous les décès ne peuvent pas être considérés comme évitables (asthme, cardiopathie ischémique...), l'incidence et la prévalence devraient être prise en compte dans l'analyse des variations de la mortalité. Pour les maladies où une part importante des décès est évitable (hypertension, cancer du sein...), les variations d'incidence et de prévalence peuvent également expliquer une part des différences de mortalité.

Les décès peuvent également résulter de la disponibilité plus ou moins grande des services, de leur attractivité et de leur efficacité. Ces caractéristiques et leur acceptabilité par la population peuvent être liées, d'une part à leur accessibilité et à la perception par les patients du besoin qu'ils en ont, d'autre part à des facteurs sociaux et familiaux propres aux patients eux-mêmes. Une enquête confidentielle sur les décès par accidents vasculaires cérébraux et maladie hypertensive chez des patients âgés de moins de 75 ans (123 décès étudiés) a identifié les principaux facteurs évitables ayant contribué à la mort (Payne *et al.* 1993):

Défaillance des services de santé pour:

- dépister l'hypertension
- traiter et suivre l'hypertension une fois diagnostiquée
- s'assurer que les patients étaient reconvoqués s'ils manquaient leur rendez-vous de contrôle
- diagnostiquer et traiter les complications de l'hypertension.

Manquement du patient pour :

- prendre ses médicaments ou se présenter au suivi
- arrêter de fumer
- perdre du poids
- réduire sa consommation d'alcool.

Les facteurs principaux étaient l'inadaptation du suivi et l'échec de l'arrêt du tabagisme. Pour 56 des 81 patients hypertendus, il a été constaté que les soins de base, eu égard au suivi, n'avaient pas été prodigués.

Les écarts de mortalité observés entre zones (fréquence et évolution dans le temps), peuvent également résulter de variations aléatoires. En particulier, dans les zones où peu de décès sont attendus en raison de la faible taille de la population ou d'un taux de mortalité bas, les SMR et les pourcentages d'évolution peuvent être très instables. Pour les affections dont le taux de mortalité est faible (mortalité maternelle...), les différences de mortalité peuvent ainsi refléter des variations aléatoires plutôt qu'une véritable hétérogénéité du risque sous-jacent. Certains auteurs ont suggéré l'utilisation de techniques statistiques de lissage des données par zone vers une valeur moyenne, par exemple, moyenne nationale, (Bernadinelli et Montonoli 1992). Ce lissage aurait peu d'effets sur les cartes de pathologies dont la mortalité est élevée (cardiopathies ischémiques...) mais pourrait avoir de grandes conséquences quand la mortalité est rare (mortalité maternelle...). Bien que les résultats présentés dans cet atlas ne soient pas lissés, les biais liés à des petits effectifs de décès ne doivent pas être négligés, car les cartes sont propices à une sur-interprétation quand l'attention est attirée par des résultats extrêmes correspondant à des régions de population de petite taille.

Les cartes européennes présentent les résultats sans lissage, mais signalent les zones où les effectifs de décès sont faibles. De plus, les effectifs de décès sont toujours indiqués.

La description des variations entre régions de la mortalité 'évitable' constitue la première étape d'une série de recherches (Charlton *et al.* 1984). Les facteurs explicatifs de ces variations observées nécessitent des investigations supplémentaires du type de celles présentées ci-dessous.

Tendance des indicateurs

Les études des variations de la mortalité dans le temps (voir annexe C) révèlent une chute des taux de mortalité pour la plupart des affections considérées. Cependant, le déclin observé de la mortalité évitable peut être dû à d'autres facteurs que l'amélioration des soins. Les conditions socio-économiques progressent et, pour plusieurs des pathologies considérées, un déclin de l'incidence a été simultanément observé. Afin de contrôler les effets éventuels de facteurs de confusion, les tendances de la mortalité évitable ont été comparées aux tendances de la mortalité due à d'autres causes. Ces études ont montré que la mortalité due aux pathologies évitables a davantage décliné et en ont déduit que le déclin de la mortalité évitable est associé à une amélioration des soins.

Etudes macroscopiques

Ces études tentent d'expliquer les variations de la mortalité entre régions et pays, au moyen de données agrégées (disponibles en routine ou collectées spécialement): incidence, prévalence, létalité, modes de traitement, diagnostics, certification, codification, facteurs socio-économiques, disponibilité des services de santé, dépense de santé (Bauer et Charlton 1986; Charlton *et al.* 1984*a, b*; Charlton et Lakhani 1985). Il existe de nombreux problèmes relatifs à la fiabilité des données agrégées et à leur degré de comparabilité entre régions et pays. De plus, des interactions entre variables peuvent rendre difficile l'interprétation de ces analyses. Par exemple, les facteurs socio-économiques peuvent influer sur le mode de recours aux services de soins et donc sur le niveau de mortalité.

La disponibilité des services de santé peut influer directement sur la mortalité. Néanmoins, les facteurs socio-économiques sont également associés à la disponibilité des services, car dans les zones défavorisées socialement, il peut y avoir une moindre disponibilité et qualité des services.

En dépit de ces problèmes d'interprétation, les études macroscopiques constituent une première approche utile et peu coûteuse, des variations de la mortalité, en particulier pour les régions se trouvant aux deux extrémités de la distribution (comparaison des régions à haute et basse mortalité).

Mackenbach *et al.* (1990) ont fait la synthèse de onze études de données agrégées publiées depuis 1983 et analysant la relation entre mortalité évitable et services de santé. Ils ont conclu que:

- le faible niveau de la mortalité due à des causes 'évitables' dans les pays industrialisés, reflète en partie une amélioration de l'efficacité des services de santé. On ne peut cependant affirmer pour autant que les variations géographiques de la mortalité due à des causes 'évitables' reflètent des différences dans l'efficacité des services de santé;

- si les variations géographiques de la mortalité reflétaient de telles différences dans l'efficacité des services, cela serait dû à des facteurs autres que le niveau de l'offre, par exemple à des aspects plus spécifiques de la délivrance des soins vraisemblablement très liés au contexte socio-économique.

Des études plus récentes basées sur des données agrégées et orientées sur les variations des taux de mortalité évitable ont conduit à des résultats semblables.

Bien qu'il n'y ait pas une preuve directe de l'association entre taux de mortalité évitable et niveau de l'offre de soins, les taux ne doivent pas être invalidés en tant que mesure de l'efficacité de la délivrance des soins. Les indicateurs pris en compte ont été basés sur des mesures très globales du système de santé telles que les densités de généralistes et de spécialistes, le nombre de lits affectés au traitement des maladies aiguës.... Ils reflètent la quantité mais pas la qualité ou le niveau d'accès aux services existants. Or, comme l'ont suggéré plusieurs auteurs, lorsqu'un certain niveau de base d'offre de soins est atteint, c'est le niveau d'accès aux services concernés qui détermine surtout le niveau de la mortalité évitable.

Il est peu probable que des études supplémentaires se basant sur des données agrégées contribuent à une meilleure compréhension des déterminants de la mortalité. Des études approfondies au niveau individuel sont plus à même d'améliorer la connaissance des facteurs limitant l'efficacité des services de santé.

Etudes microscopiques

Ces études consistent en l'investigation des décès cas par cas afin d'identifier les facteurs 'évitables' qui expliquent les variations de la mortalité (disponibilité, rapidité, utilisation appropriée, efficacité des services...). La première étape de ce type de recherche consiste en l'examen des certificats de décès et des registres de morbidité pour vérifier les diagnostics, la certification et le codage des causes de décès pour chaque cas. Ceci doit permettre d'établir combien de décès peuvent toujours être classés comme véritablement 'évitable' eu égard à la définition de l'étude. L'étape suivante consiste en une enquête confidentielle précise sur chaque décès, afin d'identifier les facteurs évitables potentiels, par exemple, comme décrit antérieurement dans le cas des maladies hypertensives. De manière à déterminer le rôle spécifique de chacun des facteurs évitables, il est également important de constituer un groupe 'témoins' de survivants (appariés aux cas selon l'âge, le sexe, le diagnostic, la zone de résidence...).

La mise en évidence de facteurs évitables peut être cependant subjective et circonstancielle. Aussi, avant d'entreprendre toute enquête confidentielle, des critères relatifs au caractère 'évitable' de l'affection devraient être précisément établis.

Des questionnaires standardisés de listes de facteurs évitables potentiels et des guides pour le classement des facteurs pour chaque maladie doivent être préparés. L'enquête confidentielle peut être réalisée sur la base de questionnaires aux médecins et à d'autres professionnels de santé impliqués dans la gestion de chaque cas, et également en extrayant des informations des registres médicaux s'ils sont disponibles. Les questionnaires peuvent ensuite être analysés par des experts indépendants utilisant les listes et les guides pour déterminer la part jouée dans chaque décès par les facteurs évitables.

Les différences entre cas et témoins, en ce qui concerne ces facteurs évitables, peuvent alors permettre de mettre en évidence les insuffisances dans la disponibilité des soins et le type d'intervention nécessaire.

Un apport majeur des études microscopiques est la quantité d'informations précises qu'elles peuvent fournir (y compris concernant le degré de satisfaction du patient). Les mesures se basant sur la mortalité peuvent s'avérer inadaptées lorsque les services. Par exemple, ceux concernant des personnes âgées, sont principalement orientés vers les problèmes de douleur ou d'amélioration de la qualité de vie. L'analyse des états liés à des maladies chroniques incurables nécessite une approche différente pour mesurer les besoins et les résultats (Wilkin 1992). Pour des pathologies telles que le diabète, l'arthrite, l'asthme..., la guérison et la survie ne constituent pas des mesures adéquates de la performance des soins. Ces davantage le degré de sévérité des atteintes qui doit être pris en compte dans ce contexte.

Un programme européen (Biomed) est en cours visant à définir des mesures alternatives de soins pour les patients atteints d'accidents vasculaires. Il a été initié en raison des variations importantes des taux de mortalité observés, mais les résultats pour chaque patient seront analysés en utilisant également des données d'incapacité, de désavantages et de handicaps.

Résumé

Cet atlas présente la fréquence et l'évolution dans le temps d'une série de maladies pour lesquelles la mortalité peut être considérée comme évitable à condition qu'une intervention médicale appropriée soit dispensée en temps utile. Les variations de mortalité entre régions pour la période 1985–89 et les évolutions entre 1980–84 et 1985–89 sont présentées avec l'objectif de mettre en évidence les régions où des investigations complémentaires seraient nécessaires.

L'atlas ne cherche pas à expliquer les variations observées, ni à l'intérieur ni entre les pays, mais vise plutôt à encourager des études menées à un niveau plus fin analysant en détail la variation des taux afin d'identifier les causes. L'atlas vise également à mettre en évidence les défaillances des services de santé et à proposer des actions appropriées pour diminuer la surmortalité.

La mortalité évitable est désormais considérée par la Commission Européenne et par de nombreux pays membres, comme un indicateur de résultats important. Encouragés par les travaux antérieurs, de nombreux autres pays ont analysé les variations régionales de la mortalité due à des maladies évitables et un atlas de la mortalité évitable en Europe de l'Est est en cours de réalisation. Le succès de ces projets dépendra de la qualité des recherches qu'il aura suscitées et des améliorations obtenues sur la santé individuelle. Dans cet esprit, le groupe de travail de la Commission européenne sur les services de santé et les morts "évitables" présente ci-dessous une série de brefs rapports sur des recherches récentes qui ont été menées sur le sujet par les pays eux-mêmes.

4. INTERPRETATION DER KARTEN UND DATEN UND VORSCHLÄGE FÜR WEITERE UNTERSUCHUNGEN

Die festgestellten Mortalitätsunterschiede zwischen den Ländern und Regionen können ein Artefakt sein, das auf Unterschieden in der Praxis der Datensammlung beruht, d.h. der Diagnosestellung, der Bescheinigung und der Kodierung der Todesursachen. Die Auswirkung von Ungenauigkeiten in der Bescheinigung und Kodierung von Todesfällen in Europa ist bei Fällen von Atemwegserkrankungen und Krebssterblichkeit untersucht worden. Die Ärzte in den einzelnen Ländern wurden gebeten, Todesbescheinigungen einer Reihe von Fällen auszustellen, die dann national und zusätzlich von einem WHO-Beratungszentrum kodiert wurden. Kelson und Heller (1983) konnten für die akuten Atemwegserkrankungen ausgeprägte Unterschiede in der Diagnosendokumentation zwischen acht EG-Ländern zeigen (z.B. schwankte der prozentuale Anteil an Ärzten, die einen bestimmten Fall als Asthma bestätigten, zwischen 54 prozent und 84 prozent). Diese Unterschiede wurden der Art, wie Ärzte die Todesbescheinigungen ausfüllen und der Art und Weise der Kodierung zugeschrieben.

Mackenbach u. Mitarbeiter (1987) kamen zu dem Ergebnis, daß die Unterschiede in der Bescheinigung und Kodierung bestimmter Todesfälle Schwankungen in den registrierten Todesraten erklären könnten. Mackenbach betonte die Notwendigkeit, Bescheinigung und Kodierung zusammen zu berücksichtigen, da in manchen Fällen die nationale Kodierung Fehlern bei der Bescheinigung unterliegt. Die weitere Analyse der Daten über schwere chronische Lungenkrankheiten ließ Burney (1989) 'vorläufig' feststellen, daß Unterschiede in der Kodierung, insbesondere bei der Betrachtung atypischer, nicht eindeutig klassifizierbarer Fälle, die festgestellten Schwankungen in den Todesraten besser erklären könnten als zunächst angenommen. Offensichtliche, zeitliche Trends könnten auf den Wechsel in der Registrierungspraxis zurückzuführen sein (Lindahl und Johansson 1994). Der Trend bei den festgehaltenen Todesraten der frühen bis späten achtziger Jahre sollte nicht direkt von den Veränderungen der ICD betroffen worden sein, da alle EG-Länder weiterhin ICD9, mit Ausnahme Dänemarks, das ICD8 benutzte, anwendeten. Obwohl eine falsche Klassifikation die beobachteten Unterschiede nicht vollständig erklären kann (Diehl und Gau 1982), so bleibt dieser Umstand dennoch ein wichtiger Faktor für das Wissen um Krankheiten und ihrer Auftretensschwankungen in einzelnen Regionen. Dies sollte die Interpretation der hier dargestellten Ergebnisse erleichtern.

Zusätzlich können die Unterschiede auf ungleiche Verteilungen der Krankheitsinzidenz oder -prävalenz oder auf geographische Variationen des Grades und der Wirksamkeit der Versorgung durch das Gesundheitswesen zurückgehen. Das Gesundheitswesen sollte auf den Bedarf reagieren und gezielt diejenigen Regionen versorgen, wo die Krankheitsinzidenz am höchsten ist. Deshalb sollte in den innerstädtischen Bereichen, wo Fälle von TB am häufigsten sind, ein höherer Versorgungsgrad als in den ländlichen Regionen gegeben sein. Bei solchen Krankheiten, bei denen sich selbst durch zeitige und angemessene Intervention nicht all Sterbefälle vermeiden lassen (z.B. Asthma, ischämische Herzkrankheiten), sollten Inzidenz- und Prävalenzunterschiede zwischen den Regionen in Rechnung gestellt werden, wenn Mortalitätsunterschiede beurteilt werden sollen. Bei Krankheiten hingegen, bei denen Sterbefälle durch angemessene und rechtzeitige Versorgung und Behandlung ungeachtet der Inzidenz oder Prävalenz 'vermieden' werden können (z.B. Bluthochdruck, Brustkrebs), lassen sich Unterschiede in der Mortalität zwar durch Inzidenz und Prävalenz erklären, aber nicht rechtfertigen.

Die Letalität kann durch die Verfügbarkeit der Versorgungsangebote, ihre Inanspruchnahme sowie die Effizienz und Effektivität der gesundheitlichen Versorgungsleistungen beeinflußt werden. Die Inanspruchnahme von gesundheitlicher Versorgung kann durch den Grad ihrer Akzeptanz, leichte Zugänglichkeit, die Bedarfswahrnehmung der Patienten, soziale Faktoren sowie durch familiäre und soziale Unterstützung beeinflußt werden. Eine vertraulich angestellte Untersuchung von Todesfällen aufgrund von Schlaganfällen und hypertonischen Krankheiten bei Patienten unter 75 Jahren berücksichtigte 123 Todesfälle und identifizierte vermeidbare Faktoren, die zum Tod beitrugen (Payne u. Mitarbeiter 1993).

Versäumnis des Gesundheitswesens bei:

- dem Feststellen von Hypertonie
- der stetigen Nachuntersuchung und Behandlung bei diagnostizierter Hypertonie
- der Vergewisserung, daß Patienten erneut zu einem Nachfolgetermin eingeladen werden, falls sie den ersten versäumt haben
- der Diagnose und Behandlung auftretender Komplikationen bei Hypertonie.

Versäumnis des Patienten:

- bei der Einnahme von Medikamenten oder dem Einverständnis zu einer Nachfolgeuntersuchung zu erscheinen
- das Rauchen einzustellen
- Gewicht zu verlieren
- den Alkoholkonsums zu reduzieren.

Unzureichende Nachfolgeuntersuchungen und die Nichtaufgabe des Rauchens waren die häufigsten Versäumnisse. Bei 65 der 81 unter Hypertonie leidenden Patienten kam man zu dem Schluß, daß ein Minimumstandard der medizinischen Versorgung was die Nachfolgeuntersuchung angeht nicht erreicht worden ist.

Bei allen Krankheiten sind die beobachteten Unterschiede bei den Todes- und deren Abnahmeraten zwischen den einzelnen Regionen teilweise auf willkürliche Schwankungen zurückzuführen. Insbesondere sind die geschätzten SMR und die prozentuale Veränderung der Sterblichkeit in Regionen mit einer geringen Anzahl an Todesfällen aufgrund einer geringen Bevölkerungsdichte oder einer niedrigen Todesrate in hohem Maße instabil. Bei Krankheiten mit einer relativ niedrigen Todesrate (z.B. Müttersterblichkeit), spiegeln die Unterschiede in der Sterblichkeit zwischen den einzelnen

Regionen hauptsächlich willkürliche Schwankungen im Gegensatz zu der tatsächlichen Heterogenität der zugrundeliegenden Risiken wider. Einige Autoren haben den Gebrauch statistischer Techniken vorgeschlagen, die die Statistiken der betrachteten Regionen einem Durchschnittswert angleichen würden (z.B. nationaler Durchschnitt) (Bernardinelli und Montomoli 1992). Das Bereinigen von Statistiken hat nur eine geringe Auswirkung auf die Karten derjenigen Krankheiten, bei denen die Sterblichkeit relativ häufig vorkommt (z.B. ischämische Herzkrankheit). Große Auswirkungen lassen sich jedoch bei geringer Sterblichkeit feststellen (z.B. Müttersterblichkeit). Obwohl die hier dargestellten Ergebnisse nicht angeglichen sind, sollten jedoch die Schwierigkeiten, die eine geringe Zahl an Todesfällen stellt, nicht übersehen werden, da Karten leicht dem Fehler der Überinterpretation unterliegen, wenn sich die Aufmerksamkeit vor allem auf die extremen Ergebnisse in nur dünn besiedelten Regionen richtet. Die EG-Karten präsentieren die Ergebnisse kleiner Regionen ohne irgendwelche Datenbereinigung.

Gleichzeitig deuten sie aber auch die Regionen an, wo nur wenige Todesfälle erwartet werden und die Ergebnisse besonders ungewiß sind. Die tabellarisch dargestellten Ergebnisse beinhalten stets die wirklichen Zahlen.

Die Beschreibung der Unterschiede der potentiell 'vermeidbaren Mortalität' zwischen geographischen Regionen ist nur der erste Schritt in einer Reihe von Untersuchungen (Charlton *et al.* 1984*a*). Jede Erklärung für diese Unterschiede macht unter Umständen weitere Untersuchungen erforderlich, von denen einige beispielhaft im folgenden dargestellt werden:

Zeitliche Entwicklung der Indikatoren

Studien über die Schwankungen in der Sterblichkeit über die Jahre hinweg (s. Appendix C) haben einen Rückgang in den Todesraten für die meisten der als vermeidbar geltenden Krankheiten offenbart, unterstreichen jedoch den Umstand, daß dieser beobachtete Rückgang der vermeidbaren Sterblichkeit auf andere Faktoren als den des verbesserten Gesundheitswesens zurückzuführen sein könnten. Die sozioökonomischen Faktoren verbessern sich und bei vielen Krankheiten ist ein 'spontaner' Rückgang an Fällen festgestellt worden. Um einer das Bild möglicherweise verzerrenden Auswirkung dieser zusätzlichen Faktoren zuvorzukommen, wurden der Sterblichkeitstrend bei vermeidbaren Krankheiten mit dem anderer Krankheiten verglichen. Die Sterblichkeit aufgrund von behandelbaren Krankheiten fiel schneller als von nicht behandelbaren Leiden. Die Studien werteten dies als Andeutung eines partiellen Zusammenhangs zwischen dem Rückgang vermeidbarer Sterblichkeit und der qualitativen Verbesserung des Gesundheitswesens.

Makrostudien

Mit diesen Studien kann versucht werden, Mortalitätsunterschiede zwischen Regionen und Ländern auf der Basis von (routinemäßig gesammelten oder speziell erhobenen) aggregierten Daten zur Krankheitsinzidenz oder Prävalenz, Letalität, Behandlungsarten, Diagnosen, Dokumentations- und Kodierungspraktiken, sozioökonomischen Faktoren, sowie zu Versorgungsmustern und Ausgaben im Gesundheitswesen zu erklären (Bauer und Charlton 1986; Charlton *et al.* 1984 *a, b*; Charlton und Lakhani 1985). Hinsichtlich der Zuverlässigkeit aggregierter Daten und der Vergleichbarkeit dieser Angaben zwischen kleinräumlichen Gebieten und Ländern ergeben sich eine Reihe von Problemen. Darüberhinaus gibt es möglicherweise Wechselwirkungen zwischen den Variablen die eine Bewertung solcher Analysen erschweren. So können z.B. sozioökonomische Faktoren die Inanspruchnahme von Versorgungsleistungen sowie deren rechtzeitige und angemessene Anwendung beeinträchtigen und somit die Mortalität beeinflussen. Die Verfügbarkeit von gesundheitlicher Versorgung kann sich direkt auf die Mortalität auswirken; jedoch können sozioökonomische Faktoren auch in der Weise mit der Verfügbarkeit von Versorgungsleistungen verknüpft sein, daß in sozial benachteiligten Regionen das Angebot und die Qualität der Versorgung geringer sind.

Trotz dieser Schwierigkeiten der Interpretation stellen derartige Studien eine nützliche und relativ kostengünstige Methode für einen ersten Forschungszugang zu Mortalitätsunterschieden dar, der insbesondere für die Betrachtung von Regionen an den Extremen der Verteilung geeignet ist (d.h. Vergleiche zwischen Gebieten mit hoher gegenüber solchen mit niedriger Mortalität).

Mackenbach u. Mitarbeiter untersuchten 11 Studien mit Aggregatdaten über 'vermeidbare' Sterbefälle und Leistungen des Gesundheitswesens, die seit 1983 veröffentlicht worden sind. Sie kamen zu folgenden Schlüssen:

- die geringe Mortalität an behandelbaren Krankheiten, die gegenwärtig in den Industrieländern voherrscht, ist wahrscheinlich wenigstens teilweise auf die gewachsene Effektivität der gesundheitlichen Versorgung zurückzuführen.

- bislang konnte nicht gezeigt werden, daß regionale Unterschiede der Mortalität an behandelbaren Krankheiten auf Unterschiede in der gesundheitlichen Versorgung zurückzuführen sind.

- falls die regionale Variation doch Ausdruck solcher Unterschiede ist, so hat dies andere Gründe als das generelle Niveau der Versorgung; diese Unterschiede hängen beispielsweise mit spezifischeren Aspekten des gesundheitlichen Vesorgungsangebots zusammen und sind wahrscheinlich eng mit den sozioökonomischen Lebensbedingungen verknüpft.

Jüngst unternommene Gesamtdatenuntersuchungen zu den Schwankungen der vermeidbaren Sterblichkeit sind zu weitgehend übereinstimmenden Ergebnissen gekommen.

Das Fehlen direkter Beweise eines Zusammenhangs zwischen vermeidbaren Todesraten und der medizinischen Versorgung entwerten es nicht als Maß für die Effizienz medizinischer Versorgung. Die Ergebnisse basieren auf groben Maßstäben wie z.B. der regionalen Dichte an Allgemeinärzten, der genauen Anzahl an Krankenhausbetten und Chefärzten und spiegeln damit die Quantität und nicht die Qualität oder Zugänglichkeit der bestehenden Gesundheitsdienste wider. Wie einige Autoren unterstellt haben, könnten diese Ergebnisse darauf hinweisen, daß, sobald ein gewisser Basisstandard erreicht ist, die Zugänglichkeit zu bereits existierenden Gesundheitsdiensten zumindest in Teilen das Ausmaß der vermeidbaren Sterblichkeit bestimmt. Dies wiederum läßt auf die Notwendigkeit einer verbesserten Zielsetzung der Gesundheitsdienste schließen.

Es ist unwahrscheinlich, daß weitere Gesamtdatenuntersuchungen zu einem besseren Verständnis der Determinanten 'vermeidbarer Mortalität' beitragen Tiefergehende Studien auf der Basis von Individualdaten sind besser geeignet, neue Erkenntnisse über die Faktoren zu liefern, die die Wirksamkeit der gesundheitlichen Versorgung beschränken.

Mikrostudien

Diese Art von Studien sollte die Untersuchung einzelner Todesfälle umfassen, mit dem Ziel, entweder Faktoren zu identifizieren, die die Mortalitätsunterschiede erklären oder die selbst als 'vermeidbare Bedingungen' anzusehen sind (d.h. Aspekte der Verfügbarkeit, Inanspruchnahme, sinnvollen Nutzung, Effizienz, und Wirksamkeit der gesundheitlichen Versorgung, die alle für die Sterblichkeit eine Rolle spielen können). Es gibt mehrere Stufen bei solchen Untersuchungen: Die erste Stufe besteht im Sichten der Todesbescheinigungen und Krankenakten, um die Diagnosen, die Bescheinigungen, und die Kodierungen der Todesursachen für jeden Sterbefall zu überprüfen. Dabei klärt sich, wieviele Todesfälle nach Maßgabe der Definition der jeweiligen Studie schließlich noch als 'vermeidbar' bezeichnet werden können. Die nächste Stufe ist die detaillierte Einzelfallanalyse jedes einzelnen Todesfalls, die unter Wahrung der Vertraulichkeit durchgeführt wird, um mögliche 'vermeidbare Faktoren' zu finden, wie oben am Beispiel der Bluthochdruck-Fälle beschrieben. Um die Bedeutung einzelner 'vermeidbarer Faktoren' einschätzen zu können, wird es häufig notwendig sein, auch Kontrollfälle zu untersuchen (d.h. nach Alter, Geschlecht, Diagnose, und Wohnort parallelisierte Fälle, die aber überlebt haben). Die Problematik solcher Studien besteht darin, daß die Nachweisbarkeit 'vermeidbarer Faktoren' eher subjektiv und von den gegebenen Umständen abhängig ist. Bevor man mit einer Einzelfallanalyse beginnt, sollten Kriterien für 'vermeidbare Faktoren' festgelegt worden sein.

Standardisierte Fragebögen, Listen möglicher 'vermeidbarer Faktoren', und Richtlinien zur Klassifikation von Faktoren bei den einzelnen Krankheiten sind zu erstellen. Die vertrauliche Einzelfallanalyse kann durch Versendung von Fragebögen an die behandelnden Ärzte und andere im Gesundheitswesen arbeitende Personen durchgeführt werden, aber auch durch die Auswertung von Krankenakten, falls solche verfügbar sind. Die Fragebögen können sodann durch unabhängige Sachverständige ausgewertet werden, die anhand der vorbereiteten Listen und Richtlinien feststellen, welcher 'vermeidbare Faktor' in jedem Einzelfall eine Rolle gespielt hat. Unterschiede zwischen Todesfällen und Kontrollfällen bei den 'vermeidbaren Faktoren' oder aber Faktoren, die bei einer großen Zahl von Sterbefällen gleichzeitig und auch bei einer großen Zahl von Krankheiten beobachtet werden, können Defizite in Angebot und Inanspruchnahme von Leistungen der gesundheitlichen Versorgung markieren, die Interventionen zugänglich sind.

Ein großer Vorteil der Untersuchungen auf Patientenebene besteht in der Möglichkeit, eine weite Bandbreite an Ergebnismaßstäben beurteilen zu können, die sowohl die Zufriedenheit als auch die Behinderung von Patienten miteinbeziehen. Maßstäbe für eine besonders hohe Sterblichkeit sind bei Gesundheitsdiensten wie z.B. der Versorgung von alten Menschen, die sich hauptsächlich auf die Linderung von Schmerzen und der Verbesserung der Lebensqualität konzentrieren, irrelevant. Die Verlagerung des Schwerpunktes von akuten, lebensbedrohenden Krankheiten hin zu chronischen unheilbaren Leiden erforderte einen anderen Ansatz bei der Messung von Bedarf und Ergebnis (Wilkins u. Mitarbeiter 1994). Bei Krankheiten wie Diabetes, Arthritis oder Asthma sind die Heilung und das Überleben nicht länger angemessene Maßstäbe für die Leistungen des Gesundheitswesens. Geeignete Maßstäbe müssen der Schwere einer Krankheit Rechnung tragen. Es reicht nicht aus, die Todesrate oder gar die weite Verbreitung von Asthma zu schätzen. Wesentlich ist hier die Feststellung der Schwere eines Falles. Ein laufendes EG Biomed Programm zur Untersuchung sich abwechselnder Maßstäbe bei der Versorgung von Schlaganfallpatienten fand seine Motivation aufgrund der beobachteten Schwankungen der Todesraten. Es wird Ergebnisse auf der Ebene der Patienten beschreiben und dabei Maßstäbe an die gesundheitliche Beeinträchtigung und Behinderung legen.

Zusammenfassung

Dieser Atlas stellt die Ergebnisse für eine Reihe von Krankheiten dar, bei denen die Sterblichkeit bei rechtzeitigem und angemessenem medizinischen Eingreifen weitestgehend als vermeidbar angesegen wird. Die Unterschiede in der Sterblichkeit zwischen einzelnen Regionen in den Jahren von 1985–89, sowie deren Wandel in den Zeiträumen von 1980–84 und 1985–89 wird unter Hervorhebung derjenigen Regionen dargestellt, für die weitere Studien erforderlich sind.

Der Atlas versucht nicht, die Ebenen der beobachteten Unterschiede innerhalb und zwischen den Ländern zu erklären, sondern hofft vielmehr weitere Nachforschungen auf kleiner Gebietsebene anzuregen, die im Detail Ratenschwankungen untersuchen, mögliche Ursachen identifizieren, Versagen innerhalb des Gesundheitswesens hervorheben und angemessene Maßnahmen zur Beseitigung des beobachteten Übermaßes vorschlagen würden.

Die vermeidbare Sterblichkeit wird nun sowohl von der Europäischen Kommission als auch von vielen Mitgliedsländern als ein wichtiger Leistungsindikator anerkannt. Von früheren Arbeiten angeregt, haben viele andere Länder die regionalen Schwankungen der Sterblichkeit aufgrund von vermeidbaren Krankheiten untersucht und als Ergebnis wird nun ein Atlas der 'vermeidbaren Sterblichkeit' in Osteuropa zusammengestellt. Letzten Endes hängt der Erfolg dieses Projektes jedoch von der Qualität der angeregten Forschung und der hieraus folgenden Verbesserung der Gesundheit des einzelnen ab. Vor diesem Hintergrund stellte die EG-Arbeitsgruppe 'Gesundheitswesen und vermeidbare Sterblichkeit' eine Reihe kurzer Berichte über die jüngsten Forschungsarbeiten auf diesem Gebiet (in ihren Heimatländern) zur Verfügung, die hiermit dargestellt werden.

5. REFERENCES

Armitage, P. and Berry, G. (1994). *Statistical methods in medical research.* Blackwell Scientific, (3nd edn). Oxford.

Bauer, R.L. and Charlton, J.R.H. (1986). Area variation in mortality from diseases amenable to medical intervention: the contribution of differences in morbidity. *International Journal of Epidemiology*, **15**, 408–12.

Bernardinelli, L. and Montomoli, C. (1992). Empirical Bayes versus fully Bayesian analysis of geographical variation in disease risk. *Statistics in Medicine,* **11**, 983–1007.

Burney, P.G.J. (1989). Effet de la certification des décès sur les taux nationaux de mortalité déclarée par l'asthme. *Revue d'Épidémiologie et de Santé Publique*, **37**, 385–9.

Charlton, J.R.H. and Lakhani, A. (1985). Is the Jarman underprivileged area score valid? *British Medical Journal,* **290**, 1714–16.

Charlton, J.R.H., Bauer, R., and Lakhani, A. (1984*a*). Outcomes measures for district and regional health care planners. *Community Medicine,* **6**, 306–15.

Charlton, J.R.H., Prochazka, A., and Lakhani, A. (1984*b*). Death from appendicitis outside hospital? *Lancet*, **ii**, 399.

Diehl, A.K. and Gau, D.W. (1982). Death certification by British doctors: a demographic analysis. *Journal of Epidemiology and Community Health*, **36**, 146–9.

Gail, M. (1978). The analysis of heterogeneity for indirect standardized mortality ratios. *Journal of the Royal Statistical Society,* **A 141**(2), 224–34.

Holland, W.W. (ed.) (1988). *The European Community atlas of 'avoidable death',* (1st edn). Published by Oxford University Press for the European Community.

Holland, W.W. (ed.) (1991). *The European Community atlas of 'avoidable death',* Volume I (2nd edn). Published by Oxford University Press for the European Community.

Holland, W.W. (ed.) (1993). *The European Community atlas of 'avoidable death',* Volume II (2nd edn). Published by Oxford University Press for the European Community.

Kelson, M.C. and Farebrother, M. (1987). The effect of inaccuracies in death certification and coding practices in the European Economic Community (EEC) on international cancer mortality statistics. *International Journal of Epidemiology,* **16(3)**, 411–4.

Kelson, M.C. and Heller, R.F. (1983). The effect of death certification and coding practices on observed differences in respiratory disease mortality in eight EC Countries. *Revue d'Epidemiologie et de Sante Publique*, **31**, 423–32.

Lindahl, B.I. and Johansson, L.A. (1994). Multiple cause-of-death data as a tool for detecting artificial trends in the underlying cause statistics: a methodological study. *Scandinavian Journal of Social Medicine*, **22**, 45–58.

Mackenbach, J.P., Bouvier-Colle, M.H., and Jougla, E. (1990). 'Avoidable' mortality and health services: a review of aggregate data studies. *Journal of Epidemiology and Community Health*, **44**, 106–11.

Mackenbach, J.P., Van Duyne, W.M., and Kelson, M.C., (1987). Certification and coding of two underlying causes of death in The Netherlands and other countries of the European Community. *Journal of Epidemiology and Community Health,* **41(2)**, 156–60.

Payne, J.N., Milner, P.C., Saul, C., Bowns, I.R., Hannay, D.R., and Ramsay, L.E. (1993). Local confidential inquiry into avoidable factors in deaths from stroke and hypertensive disease. *British Medical Journal,* **307(6911)**, 1027–30.

Rutstein, D.D., Berenberg, W., Chalmers, T.C., Child, C.G. *et al.* (1976). Measuring the quality of medical care. *New England Journal of Medicine,* **294**, 582–8.

Rutstein, D.D., Berenberg, W., Chalmers, T.C., Fishman, A.P., *et al.* (1980). Measuring the quality of medical care: second revision of tables and indexes. *New England Journal of Medicine*, **302**, 1146.

Wilkin, D. (1993). Longitudinal studies of patients with chronic illness problems of linking process and outcome. *Scandinavian Journal of Primary Health Care–Supplement,* **2**, 54–7

6. STUDIES ON 'AVOIDABLE DEATH' WITHIN THE EUROPEAN COMMUNITY

STUDIES ON 'AVOIDABLE DEATH' IN BELGIUM

R. Lagasse and P. Hooft

The study of 'avoidable death' in Belgium has been developed within the general framework of the European project. Its first objective was to provide the co-ordinating centre with the available data for relevant causes of death. This has led to certain difficulties as the data for 1988 and 1989 has only recently been made available.

The more specific objectives of the study at a national level were:

(a) The publication of more detailed atlases for Belgium, at a district level, including the maps for those causes of death presented in the European atlases. This has been published for the period 1980–84 (Lagasse *et al.* 1992). Similar work is presently going on with the purpose of publishing a third edition for the period 1985–89.

(b) To study the reliability of the mortality data from a certification and coding point of view. This work has been made possible thanks to a collaboration with the Flemish Community Department in charge of the coding process (Aelvoet *et al.* 1991). A feasibility study has been performed for the EC (DG XII–Comac HSR) which should lead to a concerted action in Europe with the aim of assessing the comparability of the specific mortality statistics, and to progressively build up a European network which would bring together the administrative and academic actors operating in this field (Lagasse 1993).

(c) To examine the variation in premature mortality using the PYLL (Potential Years of Life Lost) methodology (Leveque *et al.* 1992).

(d) To investigate, in depth, the data on suicide in Belgium. The various aspects covered by these investigations concern the possible prevention of this cause of death, its epidemiological pattern, as well as the availability and reliability of the information (Moens 1988*a*, *b*; Moens *et al.* 1988, 1989; Moens and Vandevoorde 1989; Hooft *et al.* 1993).

The future work of the Belgian team will go on with the publication of the third edition of the Belgian atlas (1985–89). It will also develop the analysis of time trends over the three five-year periods covered by the successive editions. Finally, it will focus on specific problems like the one of premature mortality in adolescents and young adults: road traffic accidents, violent deaths, suicide, and AIDS, which show a greater impact in terms of PYLL as they mostly concern people of a very young age.

References

Aelvoet, W., Humblet, P.C., and Lagasse, R. (1991). Het in routine gebruikmaken van een geinformatiseerd controle programma als middel tot kwaliteitsbewaking van de statistieken van de burgerlijke stand in Vlaanderen. *Archives of Public Health,* **49**, 1–7.

Hooft, P., Vandevoorde, H., and Mulkers, U. (1993). On the influence of data source in aggregated data studies: a comparative study of suicide information based on death certificates and judicial files. *Journal of Epidemiology and Community Health*, **47**, 73–5.

Lagasse, R. (1993). Evaluation of death certificates' quality: report of the study. In *Health services research, (*ed. G.N. Fracchia, M. Theofilatou), p. 31–41. I.O.S. Press, Amsterdam.

Lagasse, R., Humblet, P.C., Hooft, P., Vandevoorde, H., and Wollast, E. (1992). Atlas of avoidable mortality in Belgium 1980–1984. *Archives of Public Health,* **50**, 1–97.

Leveque, A., Berghmans, L., Dramaix, M., and Lagasse, R. (1992). Premature mortality in Belgium (Walloon area): potential years of life lost as an indicator of importance and trends (1976–1986). *Archives of Public Health,* **50**, 141–57.

Moens, G. (1988*a*). Aspects of the epidemiology and prevention of suicide. Acta Biomedica Lovaniensis, Leuven University Press 28.

Moens, G. (1988*b*). Evaluatie van het effect van een gezondheidsvoorziening via een ecologische methode. *Tijdschr. Soc. Gezondheidszorg*, **65**, 764–5.

Moens, G., Haenen, W., and Vandevoorde, H. (1988). Suicide bij jongeren in Belgi °/oo: epidemiologische aspecten. *Tijdschr. Soc. Gezondheidszorg*, **66**, 239–44.

Moens, G., and Vandevoorde, H. (1989). Avoidability of psychotropic drugs and suicidal self-poisoning mortality in Belgium. *Acta Psychiatrica Scandinavica*, **79**, 444–9.

Moens, G., Loysch, M., Honggokoesoemo, S., and Vandevoorde, H. (1989). Recent trends in methods of suicide. *Acta Psychiatrica Seandinavica,* **79,** 207–15.

ETUDE SUR LES 'MORTS EVITABLES' EN BELGIQUE

R. Lagasse et P. Hooft

L'étude de la mortalité évitable en Belgique a été développée dans le cadre général du projet européen. Son premier objectif était de fournir des données disponibles sur les causes de décès concernées à un centre coordinateur. Ceci s'est heurté à quelques difficultés car les données de 1988 ont été disponibles seulement récemment et celles de 1989 ne furent pas obtenues à temps.

Les objectifs spécifiques de l'étude au niveau national étaient :

(a) La publication d'atlas plus détaillés pour la Belgique, incluant les cartes des causes de décès présentées dans les atlas européens, au niveau des districts. Ceci a été publié pour la période 1980–84 (Lagasse *et al.* 1992). Un travail similaire est actuellement poursuivi dans le but de publier une 3ème édition pour la période 1985–89.

(b) Etudier la validité des données de mortalité du point de vue de la certification et du codage. Ce travail a été possible grâce à la collaboration avec le Département communautaire flamand responsable du codage (Aelvoet *et al.* 1991). Une étude de faisabilité a été faite pour la communauté (DG XII–Comac HSR) qui aurait pu conduire à une action européenne concertée avec l'objectif d'établir la comparabilité des statistiques de mortalité et de construire progressivement un réseau européen qui aurait réuni les acteurs administratifs et scientifiques opérant dans ce domaine (Lagasse 1993).

(c) Examiner les fluctuations de la mortalité prématurée en utilisant la méthode des années potentielles de vie perdue (APVP) (Leveque *et al.* 1992).

(d) Etudier en profondeur les données sur le suicide en Belgique. Les aspects variés recouverts par ces investigations concernent la prévention éventuelle de cette cause, sa structure épidémiologique, aussi bien que la disponibilité et la validité de l'information (Moens, 1988*a*, *b*; Moens *et al.* 1988, 1989; Hooft *et al.* 1993).

Le travail ultérieur de l'équipe belge se prolongera par l'édition de la troisième édition de l'atlas belge (1985–89). L'équipe développera également l'analyse des évolutions chronologiques sur les trois périodes quinquennales couvertes par les éditions successives. Finalement il se centrera sur des problèmes spécifiques tels que la mortalité prématurée des adolescents et jeunes adultes : accident de la circulation routière, morts violentes, suicide et Sida qui ont un impact important en terme d'APVP puisque ces causes concernent principalement la population jeune.

Références

Aelvoet, W., Humblet, P.C., and Lagasse, R. (1991). Het in routine gebruikmaken van een geinformatiseerd controle programma als middel tot kwaliteitsbewaking van de statistieken van de burgerlijke stand in Vlaanderen. *Archives of Public Health*, **49**, 1–7.

Hooft, P., Vandevoorde, H., and Mulkers, U. (1993). On the influence of data source in aggregated data studies: a comparative study of suicide information based on death certificates and judicial files. *Journal of Epidemiology and Community Health*, **47**, 73–5.

Lagasse, R. (1993). Evaluation of death certificates' quality: report of the study. In *Health services research, (*ed. G.N. Fracchia, M. Theofilatou), p. 31–41. I.O.S. Press, Amsterdam.

Lagasse, R., Humblet, P.C., Hooft, P., Vandevoorde, H., and Wollast, E. (1992). Atlas of avoidable mortality in Belgium 1980–1984. *Archives of Public Health*, **50**, 1–97.

Leveque, A., Berghmans, L., Dramaix, M., and Lagasse, R. (1992). Premature mortality in Belgium (Walloon area): potential years of life lost as an indicator of importance and trends (1976–1986). *Archives of Public Health*, **50**, 141–57.

Moens, G. (1988*a*). Aspects of the epidemiology and prevention of suicide. Acta Biomedica Lovaniensis, Leuven University Press 28.

Moens, G. (1988*b*). Evaluatie van het effect van een gezondheidsvoorziening via een ecologische methode. *Tijdschr. Soc. Gezondheidszorg*, **65**, 764–5.

Moens, G., Haenen, W., and Vandevoorde, H. (1988). Suicide bij jongeren in Belgi °/oo: epidemiologische aspecten. *Tijdschr. Soc. Gezondheidszorg*, **66**, 239–44.

Moens, G., and Vandevoorde, H. (1989). Avoidability of psychotropic drugs and suicidal self-poisoning mortality in Belgium. *Acta Psychiatrica Scandinavica*, **79**, 444–9.

Moens, G., Loysch, M., Honggokoesoemo, S., and Vandevoorde, H. (1989). Recent trends in methods of suicide. *Acta Psychiatrica Seandinavica*, **79**, 207–15

STUDIEN ÜBER 'VERMEIDBARE' TODESFÄLLE IN BELGIEN

R. Lagasse und P. Hooft

Die Untersuchung 'vermeidbarer' Todesfälle in Belgien wurde im Rahmen des europäischen Projektes entwickelt. Oberstes Ziel war die Versorgung des koordinierenden Zentrums mit den verfügbaren Daten der in Frage kommenden Todesursachen. Dabei erwies sich die Beschaffung der Daten für 1988 und 1989 schwieriger als erwartet, da diese erst seit kurzem zur Verfügung stehen.

Die genauere Zielsetzung dieser Untersuchung auf nationaler Ebene lautete:

(a) Die Veröffentlichung eines detaillierteren Atlas für Belgien auf Bezirksebene, der die Karten derjenigen Todesursachen enthält, die auch im europäischen Atlas enthalten sind. Eine Veröffentlichung, die den Zeitraum von 1980–84 behandelt, ist bereits erschienen (Lagasse *et al.* 1992). Ähnliche Arbeiten sind in Vorbereitung mit dem Ziel, eine dritte Ausgabe für den Zeitraum von 1985–89 zu veröffentlichen.

(b) Die Untersuchung der Zuverlässigkeit der Mortalitätsdaten aus der Sicht der Zertifikatausstellung und Kodierung. Diese Arbeit wurde dank der Zusammenarbeit mit dem flämischen Gemeindeamt (Flemish Community Department), das für das Kodierungsverfahren verantwortlich ist, ermöglicht (Aelvoet *et al.* 1992). Es wurde eine Tauglichkeitsstudie für die EG vorgenommen (DG XII-Comac HSR), die wiederum zu einer europaweiten Aktion führen soll. Ziel ist es, eine Bewertung der Vergleichbarkeit bestimmter Sterblichkeitsstatistiken zu ermöglichen und Schritt für Schritt ein europäisches Netzwerk aufzubauen, das die administrativen wie akademischen Akteure auf diesem Gebiet zusammenbringen würde (Lagasse 1993).

(c) Die Untersuchung der Schwankungen bei der vorzeitigen Sterblichkeit unter Verwendung der PYLL (Potential Years of Life Lost)- Methodik.

(d) Die eingehende Untersuchung des Datenmaterials über Selbstmord in Belgien. Die verschiedenen Aspekte, die durch diese Untersuchung abgedeckt werden, betreffen die mögliche Verhinderung dieser Todesursache, ihres epidemologischen Musters sowie der Verfügbarkeit und Zuverlässigkeit von Informationen (Moens 1988*a, b*, Moens *et al.* 1988, 1989; Moens and Vandevoorde 1989; Hooft *et al.* 1993).

Die zukünftige Arbeit des belgischen Teams wird mit der Veröffentlichung der dritten Ausgabe des belgischen Atlas fortgesetzt (1985–89). Sie wird zudem eine Zeittrend-Analyse der drei Fünf-Jahres-Abschnitte, die in den nacheinander veröffentlichten Ausgaben enthalten sind, zusammenstellen. Im Mittelpunkt werden abschließend so spezifische Probleme wie die der vorzeitigen Sterblichkeit bei Heranwachsenden und jungen Erwachsenen stehen: Straßenverkehrsunfälle, gewaltsamer Tod, Selbstmord und Aids. Diese lassen einen stärkeren Einfluß was PYLL angeht erkennen, da sie zumeist sehr junge Menschen betreffen.

Quellenangabe

Aelvoet, W., Humblet, P.C., and Lagasse, R. (1991). Het in routine gebruikmaken van een geinformatiseerd controle programma als middel tot kwaliteitsbewaking van de statistieken van de burgerlijke stand in Vlaanderen. *Archives of Public Health,* **49**, 1–7.

Hooft, P., Vandevoorde, H., and Mulkers, U. (1993). On the influence of data source in aggregated data studies: a comparative study of suicide information based on death certificates and judicial files. *Journal of Epidemiology and Community Health*, **47**, 73–5.

Lagasse, R. (1993). Evaluation of death certificates' quality: report of the study. In *Health services research, (*ed. G.N. Fracchia, M. Theofilatou), p. 31–41. I.O.S. Press, Amsterdam.

Lagasse, R., Humblet, P.C., Hooft, P., Vandevoorde, H., and Wollast, E. (1992). Atlas of avoidable mortality in Belgium 1980–1984. *Archives of Public Health,* **50**, 1–97.

Leveque, A., Berghmans, L., Dramaix, M., and Lagasse, R. (1992). Premature mortality in Belgium (Walloon area): potential years of life lost as an indicator of importance and trends (1976–1986). *Archives of Public Health,* **50**, 141–57.

Moens, G. (1988*a*). Aspects of the epidemiology and prevention of suicide. Acta Biomedica Lovaniensis, Leuven University Press 28.

Moens, G. (1988*b*). Evaluatie van het effect van een gezondheidsvoorziening via een ecologische methode. *Tijdschr. Soc. Gezondheidszorg*, **65**, 764–5.

Moens, G., Haenen, W., and Vandevoorde, H. (1988). Suicide bij jongeren in Belgi o/oo: epidemiologische aspecten. *Tijdschr. Soc. Gezondheidszorg,* **66,** 239–44.

Moens, G., and Vandevoorde, H. (1989). Avoidability of psychotropic drugs and suicidal self-poisoning mortality in Belgium. *Acta Psychiatrica Scandinavica*, **79**, 444–9.

Moens, G., Loysch, M., Honggokoesoemo, S., and Vandevoorde, H. (1989). Recent trends in methods of suicide. *Acta Psychiatrica Seandinavica,* **79,** 207–15

STUDIES ON 'AVOIDABLE DEATH' IN THE FEDERAL REPUBLIC OF GERMANY

K. Kern

Since 1991 a series of reports and studies have been published in Germany as a result of the EC project on 'avoidable death':

1. The state of Rheinland-Pfalz (Rhineland-Palatinate) published a report on 'avoidable' deaths in the state's districts between 1980 and 1988 (Häussler and Reschke 1991). The report demonstrated a marked increase in mortality for 'avoidable' deaths caused by hypertension and stroke compared to west Germany, and an excess mortality for this condition in the south-eastern parts of the state. An update of the report is planned for the years 1989–1993.

2. The report was widely accepted as a useful element of state-based health reporting routines, and the underlying original EC methodology was adopted by all states (AGLMB 1991).

3. Discussion of the results led to a study of stroke care in Rheinland–Pfalz (Häussler and Mall 1994). It consisted of a comparison between estimated epidemiological figures on the one hand, and of capacities for acute and rehabilitative care on the other. The report described the lack of rehabilitative resources mainly in the ambulatory sector. Following this a longitudinal study is being carried out in four centres in Rheinland-Pfalz to describe patterns of care for stroke patients, the use of resources, and outcome. The study is part of the EC project 'Resource use, costs and outcome of different packages of care for stroke'. Results will be used to develop an advanced model of stroke care.

4. A recent study considered the differences in avoidable mortality between the old western and the new eastern states of Germany post-reunification (Häussler *et al.* 1995).

References

Ausschuß für Gesundheitsberichterstattung der Arbeitsgemeinschaft Leitender Medizinalbeamter (AGLMB) (1991). Indikatorensatz für den Gesundheitsrahmenbericht der Länder. Gebundenes Manusskript.

Häussler, B. and Reschke, P. (1991). *Vermeidbare Todesfälle in Rheinland-Pfalz 1980–88.* Herausgegeben vom Ministerium für Arbeit, Soziales, Familie und Gesundheit Rheinland-Pfalz.

Häussler, B. and Mall, W. (1994). Schlaganfallversorgung in Rheinland-Pfalz. Teil 1: Bestandsaufnahme und Versorgungsstruktur. In *Schriftenreihe 'Gesundheitswesen/Gesundheitsberichterstatfung' des Ministerium für Arbeit, Soziales, Familie und Gesundheit des Landes Rheinland-Pfalz, Mainz.*

Häussler, B., Hempel, E., and Reschke, P. (1995). Die Entwicklung von Lebenserwartung und Sterblichkeit in Ostdeutschland nach der Wende (1989–92). In *Das Gesundheitswesen,* **57**, 7, 365–72.

ETUDE SUR LES 'MORTS EVITABLES' EN ALLEMAGNE

K. Kern

Depuis 1991 une série de rapports et d'études publiées en Allemagne, résultent du projet européen sur 'les décès évitables'.

1. L'état de Rhénanie-Palatinat a publié un rapport sur les "morts évitables" des districts entre 1980 et 1988 (Häussler *et al.* 1991). Le rapport démontrait une augmentation marquée des décès causés par l'hypertension et les accidents vasculaires cérébraux (AVC) comparativement à l'Allemagne de l'ouest et une surmortalité pour ces conditions dans les parties sud-est de l'état. Une mise à jour de ce rapport est prévue pour les années 1990–93).

2. Le rapport fut largement accepté comme un élément utile des rapports de santé réguliers et de base au niveau des états, et la méthodologie originale sous-jacente européenne fut adoptée par tous les états (AGLNMB 1991).

3. Une discussion des résultats conduisit à une étude des soins des AVC en Rhénanie-Palatinat (Häussler *et al.* 1994). Elle consistait en une comparaison entre les résultats épidémiologiques attendus d'un côté et les capacités de traitement aigu et de réadaptation d'autre part. Le rapport décrivait l'absence de ressources pour la réadaptation, principalement en secteur ambulatoire. Consécutivement, une étude longitudinale a été entreprise dans 4 centres de Rhénanie-Palatinat pour décrire les types de soin vis-à-vis des patients victimes d'AVC, l'utilisation des ressources, et les résultats. L'étude constitue une partie du projet européen 'Ressources, coûts et résultats des différents types de soin des AVC'. Les résultats seront utilisés pour développer un nouveau modèle de soins de ces maladies.

4. Une étude récente a considéré les différences de mortalité évitable entre les états de l'ouest et les états orientaux de l'Allemagne réunifiée (Häussler *et al.* 1995).

Références

Ausschuß für Gesundheitsberichterstattung der Arbeitsgemeinschaft Leitender Medizinalbeamter (AGLMB) (1991). Indikatorensatz für den Gesundheitsrahmenbericht der Länder. Gebundenes Manusskript.

Häussler, B. and Reschke, P. (1991). *Vermeidbare Todesfälle in Rheinland-Pfalz 1980–88.* Herausgegeben vom Ministerium für Arbeit, Soziales, Familie und Gesundheit Rheinland-Pfalz.

Häussler, B. and Mall, W. (1994). Schlaganfallversorgung in

Rheinland-Pfalz. Teil 1: Bestandsaufnahme und Versorgungsstruktur. In *Schriftenreihe 'Gesundheitswesen/Gesundheitsberichterstatfung' des Ministerium für Arbeit, Soziales, Familie und Gesundheit des Landes Rheinland-Pfalz, Mainz.*

Häussler, B., Hempel, E., and Reschke, P. (1995). Die Entwicklung von Lebenserwartung und Sterblichkeit in Ostdeutschland nach der Wende (1989–92). In *Das Gesundheitswesen,* 57, 7, 365–72.

STUDIEN ÜBER 'VERMEIDBARE' TODESFÄLLE IN DER BUNDESREPUBLIK DEUTSCHLAND

K. Kern

Seit 1991 ist eine Reihe von Berichten und Studien in Deutschland veröffentlicht worden als Ergebnis des EG-Projektes 'Vermeidbare Todesfälle':

1. Das Bundesland Rheinland-Pfalz veröffentlichte einen Bericht über 'vermeidbare' todesfälle in den landeseigenen Bezirken zwischen 1980 und 1988 (Häussler und Reschke 1991). Dieser Bericht wies einen deutlichen Anstieg der Sterblichkleit bei vermeidbaren Todesfällen aufgrund von Bluthochdruck und Schlaganfällen nach im Gesamtvergleich zu Westdeutschland. Es wurde sogar eine außerordentlich hohe Sterblichkeit im südöstlichen Teil des Bundeslandes festgestellt. Eine Aktualisierung dieses Berichtes für den Zeitraum 1989–93 ist beabsichtigt.

2. Der Bericht wurde durchweg als ein nützliches Element der in einem Bundesland angewandten Verfahren der Gesundheitsberichterstattung anerkannt. Die diesem Bericht zugrundeliegende, ursprüngliche EG-Methodik wurde von allen Bundesländern übernommen (AGLMB 1991).

3. Die Diskussionen über diese Ergebnisse führten zu einer Studie der Versorgung nach einem Schlaganfall in Rheinland-Pfalz (Häussler und Mall 1994). Diese bestand aus einem Vergleich zwischen geschätzten epidemologischen Zahlen einerseits und der Leistungsfähigkeit akuter und wiederherstellender Versorgung andererseits. Dieser Bericht schilderte den Mangel an Mitteln zur Rehabilitation im ambulanten Sektor. In der Folge werden zur Zeit Langzeitstudien in vier Zentren von Rheinland-Pfalz durchgeführt, um die Strukturen medizinischer Versorgung von Schlaganfallpatienten, die Nutzung von Mitteln und Ergebnisse zu beschreiben. Diese Studie ist Teil des EG-Projektes 'Nutzung von Mitteln, Kosten und Ergebnis verschiedener Ansätze der Versorgung von Schlaganfallpatienten'. Die Ergebnisse dieser Studie sollen der Entwicklung eines fortschrittlichen Modells der Versorgung nach einem Schlaganfall dienen.

4. Eine kürzlich erschienene Studie berücksichtigte die Unterschiede in der vermeidbaren Sterblichkeit zwischen den alten westlichen und den neuen östlichen Bundesländern nach der deutschen Wiedervereinigung (Häussler *et al.* 1994).

Quellenangaben

Ausschuß für Gesundheitsberichterstattung der Arbeitsgemeinschaft Leitender Medizinalbeamter (AGLMB) (1991). Indikatorensatz für den Gesundheitsrahmenbericht der Länder. Gebundenes Manusskript.

Häussler, B. and Reschke, P. (1991). *Vermeidbare Todesfälle in Rheinland-Pfalz 1980–88.* Herausgegeben vom Ministerium für Arbeit, Soziales, Familie und Gesundheit Rheinland-Pfalz.

Häussler, B. and Mall, W. (1994). Schlaganfallversorgung in Rheinland-Pfalz. Teil 1: Bestandsaufnahme und Versorgungsstruktur. In *Schriftenreihe 'Gesundheitswesen/Gesundheitsberichterstatfung' des Ministerium für Arbeit, Soziales, Familie und Gesundheit des Landes Rheinland-Pfalz, Mainz.*

Häussler, B., Hempel, E., and Reschke, P. (1995). Die Entwicklung von Lebenserwartung und Sterblichkeit in Ostdeutschland nach der Wende (1989–92). In *Das Gesundheitswesen,* 57, 7, 365–72.

STUDIES ON 'AVOIDABLE DEATH' IN DENMARK

K. Juel

An analysis of 'avoidable' mortality in Denmark for the period 1970–83 was published in 1986 (Juel and Kamper-Jørgensen 1986). In this analysis regional and temporal variations were studied. Sixteen hospital districts and three time periods were used and 22 different disease groups were included. Both regional and temporal variations were found. It was concluded that in order to analyse the problem further, other determinants of mortality had to be considered, e.g. socio-economic conditions, life style and morbidity.

The concept of 'avoidable death' was later used in a study of mortality in Greenland for the period 1968–85 (Bjerregaard and Juel 1990). The purpose of this was to establish a base-line for health planning in Greenland. The list of 'avoidable deaths' to be studied was chosen by considering the situation of the local community as well as the mortality pattern. Several of the disease groups showed an increasing trend towards the end of the period. Regional patterns were particularly clear for infectious diseases, suicides and accidents.

Every year The National Bureau of Health publishes statistics on causes of death in Denmark. In recent years a section on 'avoidable deaths' has been included.

An update of the Danish study from 1986 with a longer time period has been planned.

References

Bjerregaard, P. and Juel, K. (1990). 'Avoidable deaths' in Greenland 1968–1985: variations by region and period. *Arctic Medical Research*, **49**, 119–127.

Juel, K. and Kamper-Jørgensen, F. (1986). 'avoidable deaths' in Denmark 1970–1983. Variations with hospital district and period. *Ugesker Laeger*, **148**, 1981–1985.

ETUDE SUR LES 'MORTS EVITABLES' AU DANEMARK

K. Juel

Une analyse de la mortalité "évitable" au Danemark, pour la période 1970–83 fut publiée en 1986 (Juel et Kamper-Jørgensen 1986). Dans cette analyse les variations régionales et temporelles furent étudiées. Seize hôpitaux de district en trois périodes et 22 groupes différents de causes ont été inclus. Des variations à la fois temporelles et régionales furent trouvées.

Il en a été conclu que pour analyser davantage le problème, d'autres déterminants de la mortalité devaient être pris en compte, c'est-à-dire: conditions socio-économiques, style de vie et morbidité.

Le concept de 'mort évitable' fut utilisé également pour une étude de la mortalité au Groenland durant la période 1968–85 (Bjerregaard et Juel 1990). Son objectif était d'établir un niveau de base pour la planification sanitaire du Groenland. La liste des morts évitables a retenir a été choisie en fonction des populations locales aussi bien qu'en fonction du schéma de la mortalité. Plusieurs des groupes de maladie montrèrent une augmentation vers la fin de la période. Des schémas régionaux étaient particulièrement évidents pour les maladies infectieuses, les suicides et les accidents.

Chaque année le Bureau national de la santé publie des statistiques de causes de décès au Danemark. Dans les années récentes, une section sur les morts évitables a été introduite.

Une mise à jour de l'étude danoise à partir de 1986 avec une période plus longue a été programmée.

Références

Bjerregaard, P. and Juel, K. (1990). 'Avoidable deaths' in Greenland 1968–1985: variations by region and period. *Arctic Medical Research*, **49**, 119–127.

Juel, K. and Kamper-Jørgensen, F. (1986). 'avoidable deaths' in Denmark 1970–1983. Variations with hospital district and period. *Ugesker Laeger*, **148**, 1981–1985.

STUDIEN ÜBER 'VERMEIDBARE' TODESFÄLLE IN DÄNEMARK

K. Juel

Eine Analyse der 'vermeidbaren' Sterblichkeit in Dänemark für den Zeitraum von 1970–83 ist 1986 veröffentlicht worden (Juel und Kamper-Jørgensen 1986). In dieser Analyse, die regionale und zeitliche Veränderungen untersuchte, wurden sechzehn Krankenhausbezirke und drei Zeiträume unter Berücksichtigung von 22 verschiedenen Krankheitsgruppen erfaßt. In der Tat wurden sowohl regionale als auch zeitliche Schwankungen festgestellt. Um dieses Problem besser analysieren zu können, mußten andere Determinanten wie z.B. sozio-ökonomische Verhältnisse, Lebensweise und Morbidität in Betracht gezogen werden.

Das Konzept der 'vermeidbaren Todesfälle' ging später in eine Studie über die Sterblichkeit in Grönland im Zeitraum von 1968–85 ein (Bjerregaard und Juel 1990). Der Zweck dieser Studie war die Ermittlung einer Grundlinie für die Gesundheitsplanung in Grönland. Die Liste der zu untersuchenden 'vermeidbaren Todesfälle' wurde unter Berücksichtigung der Situation örtlicher Gemeinden und des Sterblichkeitsmusters zusammengestellt. Einige der Krankheitsgruppen wiesen einen ansteigenden Trend gegen Ende des betrachteten Zeitraums auf. Im besonderen zeichneten sich regionale Muster bei Infektionskrankheiten, Selbstmorden und Unfällen ab.

Jedes Jahr veröffentlicht das nationale Gesundheitsministerium Statistiken zu den Todesursachen in Dänemark. In den vergangenen Jahren wurde ein Abschnitt über die 'vermeidbaren Todesfälle' hinzugefügt.

Eine Neuauflage der dänischen Studie von 1986 mit einem längeren Beobachtungszeitraum ist beabsichtigt.

Quellenangabe

Bjerregaard, P. and Juel, K. (1990). 'Avoidable deaths' in Greenland 1968–1985: variations by region and period. *Arctic Medical Research,* **49,** 119–127.

Juel, K. and Kamper-Jørgensen, F. (1986). 'avoidable deaths' in Denmark 1970–1983. Variations with hospital district and period. *Ugesker Laeger*, **148**, 1981–1985.

STUDIES ON 'AVOIDABLE DEATH' IN FRANCE

M.H. Bouvier-Colle and E. Jougla

Three main types of studies relevant to avoidable death were carried out in France:

- aggregate data analyses on the relationship between avoidable mortality and health services
- avoidable causes of death as general indicators of the population health status
- confidential enquiries into maternal deaths.

Aggregate data studies on the relationship between avoidable mortality and health services

We have attempted to relate the variations in the causes of avoidable mortality to health service input among the 95 French departments (Jougla *et al.* 1990; Mackenbach *et al.* 1991). This analysis controlled for social factors. At first, we performed independent two factors analysis of the departmental variations in health care variables (level of supply, consumption) and in social factors. These studies were undertaken with the aim of creating new discriminant and independent variables. Multiple stepwise regressions were then used to analyse the independent and joint associations of these new variables with mortality differences. The data highlight the considerable importance of social factors in explaining mortality differences and, in contrast, the marginal importance of health service characteristics. The aggregate indicators entered in these analyses are discussed. In particular, differences in effectiveness of health services might arise more easily from variables other than general level of supply, for example, from more specific aspects of use and access to health care delivery (Jougla *et al.* 1987).

Avoidable causes of death as general indicators of the population health status

In 1994 the Haut Comité de la Santé Publique produced an official report on the health of the French population. It is planned that the report will be widely distributed to the overall community (public health professionals, teachers, students, general population). One of the main objectives of this task was to produce operational indicators. In this context, avoidable death rates were recommended as indicators. In the first publication, 'Stratégie pour une politique de santé', the general concept of avoidable mortality was retained in order to assess the efficacy of prevention policy and health care services (Haut Comité de la Santé Publique 1992).

In the final report, the chapter 'Length of Life' is mainly based on the avoidable mortality indicators (Haut Comité de la Santé Publique 1995). This chapter has three specific objectives: to analyse the time trends in mortality over the last twenty years, to highlight the inequalities in health status, and to compare mortality among European countries. The history of the avoidable mortality concept is recalled (EC concerted action on health service research, atlases production). The health service indicators and the primary prevention indicators are distinguished in the report. The results show that the trends in primary prevention indicators are not good in France compared with other countries (lung cancer, violent deaths), and that inequalities by sex, residence, and social categories, do not decrease in France. In contrast, trends in health service indicators are similar in France and in several other countries. Finally, an important issue raised by this work was to establish a set of health indicators to guide public health policy in the future.

Confidential enquiries into maternal deaths

In the context of the European Avoidable Death Group, maternal mortality was selected as one of the health care services outcomes. The first two editions of the European atlas revealed an excessive number of maternal deaths in France. This was considered as a warning signal of possible shortcomings in the perinatal care system. As a result, confidential enquiries were carried out in order to tackle this problem. A survey was produced in selected volunteered regions (Bouvier-Colle *et al.* 1993; 1995*a*). All maternal deaths, according to the WHO definition, that occurred in these regions over a period of at least one year were studied. A specialist completed a full medical questionnaire for each death. Then a committee of medical experts determined the reasons for the death and whether it might have been avoided. Forty-six deaths were recorded, 39 of which were classified as maternal. Haemorrhages were the leading underlying cause, then embolisms and hypertensive diseases. Among the 39 deaths, 17 were determined by the committee to have been certainly 'avoidable deaths'; nine others were probably avoidable. The proportion of 'avoidable deaths' varied according to the cause of death. Of the 11 haemorrhage deaths, ten were considered avoidable as well as six hypertension deaths. None of the deaths from an amniotic embolism was considered avoidable.

The reasons why the deaths were preventable were grouped in three categories. More than half the deaths were related to inappropriate or substandard care; a third, to excessive delay; and four cases were linked to the patient's own negligence. For haemorrhages, an excessive delay in intervention was generally associated with insufficient transfusions. In the case of hypertensive and infectious diseases, inadequate care was more common than excessive delay.

This work illustrates the strength of confidential enquiries of this type in the assessment of health care quality, specifically when deaths are infrequent. Furthermore, to complete the knowledge on maternal mortality concerning the quality of care, we have recently studied the cases of pregnant women who need treatment in intensive care units (and risk factors) (Bouvier-Colle *et al.* 1995*b*).

This study has led to research at a European level. Indeed, important discrepancies in maternal death rates are recorded amongst the EC. We do not know if these differences are related to the notification and registration of deaths or to the deficiency of health care systems. A European concerted action aimed at analysing the role of these different factors is currently being undertaken in the context of the Biomed Programme (European Concerted Action 'M.O.M.S'. Contract No PL 931064).

References

Bouvier-Colle, M.H., Varnoux, N., and Breart, G. (1993). Facteurs évitables de la mortalité maternelle-Résultats de l'enquête INSERM.

In *Mises à jour en gynécologie et obstétrique,* (ed. M Tournaire) pp. 329–49. CNGOF-Vigot, Paris.

Bouvier-Colle, M.H., Varnoux, N., and Breart, G. (1995*a*). Maternal deaths and substandard care: the results of a confidential survey in France, submitted to *European Journal of Obstetrics, Gynecology, and Reproductive Bio*logy, **58**, 3–7.

Bouvier-Colle, M.H., Salanare, B., Ancel, P.Y., and Varnoux, N. (1995*b*). Obstetric patients treated in intensive care units and maternal mortality. Submitted to *European Journal of Obstetrics, Gynaecology, and Reproductive Biology*.

European Concerted Action 'M.O.M.S': Frequency and risk factors of maternal morbidity and mortality 'avoidable' deaths and evaluation of care. Contract No PL 931064.

Haut Comité de la Santé Publique. (1992). *Stratégie pour une politiqué de santé-Premières propositions.* Rapport au Ministre de la Santé et de l'Action Humanitaire, Paris, Octobre 1992, 68 pages.

Haut Comité de la Santé Publique. (1995). La santé en France. Rapport au Ministre de la Santé et de l'Action Humanitaire, Paris, 1995.

Jougla, E., Ducimetiere, P., Bouvier-Colle, M.H., and Hatton, F. (1987). Relation entre le niveau de développement du système de soins et le niveau de la mortalité 'évitable' selon les départements francais. *Revue d'Epidémiologie et de Santé Publique*, **35**, 365–77.

Jougla, E., Hatton, F., and Bouvier-Colle, M.H. (1990). Relation entre le niveau de l'état de santé et le niveau des densités médicales. *La Revue de Praticien-Médecine générale,* **86,** 71–4.

Mackenbach, J.P., Bouvier-Colle, M.H., and Jougla, E. (1991). 'Avoidable' mortality and health services: a review of aggregate data studies. *Journal of Epidemiology and Community Health,* **44**, 106–11.

ETUDE SUR LES 'MORTS EVITABLES' EN FRANCE

M.H. Bouvier-Colle et E. Jougla

Trois catégories d'études directement liées aux morts évitables ont été réalisées en France

- analyse de données agrégées sur la relation entre mortalité évitable et services de santé
- étude des causes de décès évitables en tant qu'indicateurs de l'état de santé des populations
- enquête confidentielle sur les morts maternelles.

Analyse de données agrégées sur la relation entre mortalité évitable et services de santé

Nous avons étudié la relation entre les variations des causes de mortalité 'évitable' et la fourniture des services de santé dans les 95 départements français (Jougla *et al.* 1990; Mackenbach *et al.* 1991). Cette analyse a pris en compte les caractères socio-démographiques. Nous avons d'abord réalisé deux analyses factorielles des populations sur les variations départementales des variables des systèmes de soins (niveau de l'offre et consommation) et sur les variations des facteurs socio-économiques. Ces études furent entreprises avec l'objectif de créer de nouvelles variables indépendantes et discriminantes. Ensuite des régressions multiples pas à pas furent mises en oeuvre pour analyser les relations d'indépendance ou d'association de ces nouvelles variables avec les différences de mortalité. Les données mirent en lumière l'importance considérable des facteurs socio-économiques dans l'explication des différences de mortalité et, en contraste, l'importance marginale des caractèristiques des services de santé.

Les indicateurs agrégés intégrés dans cette analyse sont discutés. En particulier des différences dans l'efficacité des services de santé peuvent provenir plus aisément d'autres facteurs que le niveau général de l'offre et par exemple, d'aspects plus spécifiques de l'utilisation et de l'accès à la délivrance des soins (Jougla et al. 1987).

Causes de décès évitables en tant qu'indicateurs généraux de la santé des populations

En 1994, le Haut Comité de la Santé publique a produit un rapport officiel sur la santé de la population française. Il a été prévu que le rapport soit largement distribué à l'ensemble du public: professionnels de santé publique, enseignants, étudiants, population générale. L'un des principaux objectifs de cette tâche était de produire des indicateurs opérationnels. Dans ce contexte, les taux de mortalité évitable furent recommandés comme indicateurs. Dans la première publication 'Stratégie pour une politique de santé', le concept général de mortalité évitable a été retenu pour établir l'efficacité de la politique de prévention et les services de santé (Haut Comité de la Santé Publique 1992).

Dans le rapport final, le chapitre 'Durée de vie' repose principalement sur les indicateurs de mortalité évitable (Haut Comité de Santé Publique 1995).

Ce rapport a trois objectifs spécifiques: analyser les tendances temporelles de la mortalité durant les 20 dernières années, éclairer les inégalités de l'état de santé et comparer la mortalité entre les pays européens. L'histoire du concept de mortalité évitable est rappelé (Action concertée de la Communauté Européenne de recherche sur les services de santé, et production d'atlas). Les indicateurs des services de santé sont distingués des indicateurs de prévention primaire. Les résultats montrent que les tendances des indicateurs de prévention primaire ne sont pas bons en France comparés à d'autres pays (cancer du poumon, morts violentes) et que les inégalités par sexe, résidence et catégories sociales, ne se réduisent pas. Au contraire, les tendances des indicateurs des services de santé sont similaires en France et dans plusieurs autres pays. Finalement, l'un des résultats importants de ce travail fut d'établir un ensemble d'indicateurs de santé pour guider la politique de santé publique dans le futur.

Enquêtes confidentielles sur les morts maternelles

Au sein du groupe européen des décès évitables, la mortalité maternelle avait été sélectionnée comme une mesure des services de soins. Les deux premières éditions de l'atlas européen ont révélé un nombre excessif de décès maternels en France. Ceci fut considéré comme un signal d'alarme d'éventuelles insuffisances du système de soins périnatals, aussi des enquêtes confidentielles ont été entreprises de manière à prendre ce problème à bras le corps. Une enquête a été menée dans des régions sélectionnées et volontaires (Bouvier-Colle et al. 1993; 1995*a*). Tous les décès maternels, selon la définition de l'Organisation Mondiale de la Santé (OMS), qui étaient survenus dans ces régions, sur une période d'un an au moins, furent étudiés. Un enquêteur spécialisé complétait un dossier médical pour chaque décès. Ensuite un Comité d'experts médicaux déterminait les causes du décès et jugeait s'il aurait pu être évité. Sur 46 décès étudiés, 39 furent classés maternels. Les hémorragies constituaient la plus fréquente des causes initiales de décès, ensuite les embolies et les maladies hypertensives de la grossesse. Parmi ces 39 décès, 17 furent jugés certainement évitables par le comité et 9 probablement. La proportion de morts évitables variait en fonction des pathologies; sur les 11 décès par hémorragie, 10 furent considérés évitables ainsi que 6 morts liées à l'hypertension. Aucun des décès par embolie n'a été jugé évitable.

Les raisons pour lesquelles les décès étaient jugés évitables ont été réunies en trois groupes. Plus de la moitié des décès étaient associés à des soins inappropriés ou limites; un tiers était dû au délai excessif des soins, et quatre cas étaient liés à la négligence de la patiente. Pour les hémorragies, un délai excessif d'intervention était généralement associé à l'insuffisance des transfusions. Dans les cas de l'hypertension et des maladies infectieuses, des soins inadéquats étaient plus fréquents que le délai excessif.

Ce travail illustre l'importance des enquêtes confidentielles de ce type dans l'établissement de la qualité des soins, en particulier quand les décès sont rares.

Cette étude est actuellement prolongée par une recherche au niveau européen. De grandes divergences des taux de mortalité maternelle sont enregistrées dans la Communauté Européenne. Nous ne savons pas encore si ces différences sont liées à la déclaration et à l'enregistrement des décès, ou à la déficience des systèmes de soin. Une action concertée européenne, dont nous sommes le chef de projet, est actuellement en cours pour analyser le rôle des différents facteurs, programme Biomed (action concertée européenne, contrat PL 931064).

Références

Bouvier-Colle, M.H., Varnoux, N., and Breart, G. (1993). Facteurs évitables de la mortalité maternelle-Résultats de l'enquête INSERM. In *Mises à jour en gynécologie et obstétrique,* (ed. M Tournaire) pp. 329–49. CNGOF-Vigot, Paris.

Bouvier-Colle, M.H., Varnoux, N., and Breart, G. (1995*a*). Maternal deaths and substandard care: the results of a confidential survey in France, submitted to *European Journal of Obstetrics, Gynecology, and Reproductive Biology*, **58**, 3–7.

Bouvier-Colle, M.H., Salanare, B., Ancel, P.Y., and Varnoux, N. (1995*b*). Obstetric patients treated in intensive care units and maternal mortality. Submitted to *European Journal of Obstetrics, Gynaecology, and Reproductive Biology.*

European Concerted Action 'M.O.M.S': Frequency and risk factors of maternal morbidity and mortality 'avoidable' deaths and evaluation of care. Contract No PL 931064.

Haut Comité de la Santé Publique. (1992). *Stratégie pour une politiqué de santé-Premières propositions.* Rapport au Ministre de la Santé et de l'Action Humanitaire, Paris, Octobre 1992, 68 pages.

Haut Comité de la Santé Publique. (1995). La santé en France. Rapport au Ministre de la Santé et de l'Action Humanitaire, Paris, 1995.

Jougla, E., Ducimetiere, P., Bouvier-Colle, M.H., and Hatton, F. (1987). Relation entre le niveau de développement du système de soins et le niveau de la mortalité 'évitable' selon les départements francais. *Revue d'Epidémiologie et de Santé Publique*, **35**, 365–77.

Jougla, E., Hatton, F., and Bouvier-Colle, M.H. (1990). Relation entre le niveau de l'état de santé et le niveau des densités médicales. *La Revue de Praticien-Médecine générale,* **86,** 71–4.

Mackenbach, J.P., Bouvier-Colle, M.H., and Jougla, E. (1991). 'Avoidable' mortality and health services: a review of aggregate data studies. *Journal of Epidemiology and Community Health,* **44**, 106–11.

STUDIE ÜBER 'VERMEIDBARE TODESFÄLLE' IN FRANKREICH

M.H. Bouvier-Colle, E. Jougla

In Frankreich wurden drei Hauptarten von Studien durchgeführt, die wichtig für die Untersuchung 'Vermeidbarer Todesfälle' sind:

- GesamtdatenanaÏysen über das Verhältnis zwischen vermeidbarer Sterblichkeit und den Gesundheitsdiensten
- vermeidbare Todesursachen als allgemeine Indikatoren für den Gesundheitszustand der Bevölkerung.
- vertraulich angestellte Nachforschungen zur Müttersterblichkeit.

Gesamtdatenstudien über das Verhältnis zwischen vermeidbarer Sterblichkeit und den Gesundheitsdiensten

Wir haben versucht, die Veränderungen in den Ursachen der vermeidbaren Sterblichkeit in Verbindung mit der Leistungsfähigkeit der Gesundheitsdienste innerhalb der 95 französischen Departments zu stellen (Jougla *et al.* 1990; Mackenbach *et al.* 1991). Diese Analyse war von sozialen Faktoren bestimmt. Zunächst wurden unabhängig voneinander zwei Faktoren untersucht: zum einen die für die Schwankungen der Variablen im Gesundheitsdienst

(Versorgungsniveau, Verbrauch) zuständigen, zum anderen die sozialen Faktoren. Diese Studien wurden mit dem Ziel unternommen, neue kritisch unterscheidende und unabhängige Variablen zu definieren. Mehrfache schrittweise vorgenommene Regressionen wurden angewendet, um die Ab- bzw. Unabhängigkieten dieser neuen Variablen von den Unterschieden in der Sterblichkeit analysieren zu können. Diese Daten unterstreichen die Bedeutung der sozialen Faktoren bei dem Versuch, Sterblichkeitsschwankungen zu erklären und zeigen im Gegensatz hierzu die geringe Bedeutung der Charakteristika des Gesundheitsdienstes. Die Gesamtheit der in diese Analysen eingegangenen Indikatoren wird besprochen. Insbesondere dürften sich Unterschiede in der Effektivität der Gesundheitsdienste weniger durch die Variablen des allgemeinen Versorgungsniveaus ergeben als vielmehr durch bestimmte Aspekte der Nutzung und der Zugänglichkeit von Einrichtungen der Gesundheitsversorgung (Jougla *et al.* 1987).

Vermeidbare Todesursachen als allgemeine Indikatoren des Gesundheitszustandes der Bevölkerung

1994 legte das Haut Comité de la Santé Publique einen offiziellen Bericht über den Gesundheitszustand der französischen Bevölkerung vor. Man beabsichtigt seine landesweite Verteilung an alle Gemeindemitglieder (Angestellte im Gesundheitswesen, Lehrer, Studenten, allgemeine Bevölkerung). Eines der Hauptziele dieses Vorhabens war die Aufstellung einsatzfähiger Indikatoren. In diesem Zusammenhang wurde empfohlen, die vermeidbare Sterblichkeitsrate als Indikator zu bewerten. In der ersten Veröffentlichung 'Stratégie pour une politique de santé' wurde das allgemeine Konzept der vermeidbaren Sterblichkeit bewußt zurückbehalten, um die Wirksamkeit von Vorbeugungsmaßnahmen und den Gesundheitsdiensten beurteilen zu können (Haut Comité de la Santé Publique 1992).

Das Kapitel 'Length of Life' des Abschlußberichtes beruht in der Hauptsache auf den Indikatoren vermeidbarer Sterblichkeit (Haut Comité de la Santé Publique, im Druck). Dieses Kapitel verfolgt drei bestimmte Ziele:

- eine Zeittrendanalyse der Sterblichkeit während der letzten zwanzig Jahre;
- die Hervorhebung der Ungleichheiten im Gesundheitszustand;
- einen Vergleich der Sterblichkeitsraten zwischen den europäischen Ländern.

Dies erinnert an die Geschichte des Konzepts der vermeidbaren Sterblichkeit (EG-weit abgestimmte Aktion zur Untersuchung der Gesundheitsdienste, Produktion von Atlanten). Der Bericht unterscheidet die Indikatoren des Gesundheitsdienstes von denen der primären Vorbeugung. Die Ergebnisse weisen einen schlechten Trend der Indikatoren primärer Vorbeugung (Lungenkrebs, gewaltsamer Tod) in Frankreich im Vergleich mit anderen Ländern nach. Außerdem ist keine Abnahme der Ungleichheiten bezüglich Geschlecht, Wohnsitz und sozialer Kategorien festzustellen. Im Gegensatz dazu zeichnen sich aber ähnliche Trends in Frankreich wie auch in mehreren anderen Ländern bei den Indikatoren des Gesundheitsdienstes ab. Die durch diese Arbeit aufgeworfenen wichtigen Fragen führten schließlich zur Festlegung einer Zahl von Gesundheitsindikatoren, die dem öffentlichen Gesundheitswesen in der Zukunft als Richtschnur dienen soll.

Vertraulich angestellte Nachforschungen zur Müttersterblichkeit

In Zusammenhang mit der European Avoidable Death Group wurde die Müttersterblichkeit als eines der im Bereich des Gesundheitsdienstes festgestellten Ergebnisse ausgewählt. Die ersten beiden Ausgaben des europäischen Atlas offenbarten eine außergewöhnlich hohe Müttersterblichkeitsrate in Frankreich. Man verstand dies als Warnsignal, das auf mögliche Unzulänglichkeiten im System der perinatalen Versorgung hinwies. Es folgten vertraulich angestellte Untersuchungen, um dieses Problem in Angriff zu nehmen. In ausgewählten, freiwillig dazu bereiten Regionen wurde eine Umfrage veranstaltet (Bouvier-Colle *et al.* 1993, 1995*a*). Den Definitionen der WHO entsprechend wurden alle Todesfälle von Müttern in diesen Regionen über einen Zeitraum von einem Jahr untersucht. Ein Facharzt füllte hierbei einen vollständigen medizinischen Fragebogen für jeden Todesfall aus. Ein Expertenausschuß bestimmte dann die Gründe für den Tod und beantwortete die Frage, ob dieser Tod hätte vermieden werden können. Von den 46 festgehaltenen Todesfällen handelte es sich bei 39 um in Zusammenhang mit einer Geburt verstorbenen Frauen. Blutungen lagen an erster Stelle bei den eigentlichen Todesursachen, gefolgt von Embolien und hypertonischen Krankheiten. Von den 39 Todesfällen wurden vom Ausschuß 17 als mit Sicherheit vermeidbar und neun als mit Wahrscheinlichkeit vermeidbar eingestuft. Der Anteil 'vermeidbarer Todesfälle' veränderte sich je nach Todesursache. 10 der 11 Todesfälle durch Blutungen wären vermeidbar gewesen, ebenso wie 6 Todesfälle in Zusammenhang mit Bluthochdruck. Hingegen wurde keiner der Tode durch amniotische Embolie als vermeidbar betrachtet.

Die Gründe, die eine Vermeidung dieser Todesfälle hätten bewirken können, wurden in drei Kategorien eingeteilt. Mehr als die Hälfte aller Todesfälle stand in Zusammenhang mit unangemessener oder unzulänglicher Versorgung. Ein Drittel aller Fällle war auf übermäßige Verzögerung zurückzuführen, während vier Fälle mit der Nachlässigkeit des Patienten selbst in Verbindung stehen. Bei Blutungen wurden übermäßige Verzögerungen bis zum Eingreifen im allgemeinen mit unzureichenden Transfusionen in Verbindung gebracht. Im Falle hypertonischer und infektiöser Krankheiten waren unzulängliche Versorgung weiter verbreitet als verspätetes Eingreifen.

Diese Arbeit veranschaulicht die Stärke vertraulich durchgeführter Befragungen dieser Art in der qualitativen Bewertung gesundheitlicher Versorgung ganz besonders dann, wenn Todesfälle vereinzelt auftreten. Um außerdem unser Wissen über Müttersterblichkeit in Zusammenhang mit der Qualität medizinischer Versorgung zu vervollständigen, haben wir jüngst die Fälle schwangerer Frauen untersucht, die auf Behandlung in Intensivstationen angewiesen sind (und Risiko-Faktoren) (Bouvier-Colle *et al.* 1995*b*).
Diese Studie hat zur Forschung auf europaweiter Ebene geführt. Tatsächlich wurden wichtige Unterschiede in der Müttersterblichkeitsrate innerhalb der EG festgehalten. Wir wissen nicht, ob diese Unterschiede auf Meldung und Registrierung der Todesfälle oder den Mangel an Gesundheitseinrichtungen zurückzuführen sind. Eine europaweit angelegte Aktion mit dem Ziel, die Rolle dieser verschiedenen Faktoren zu analysieren, wird zur Zeit in Zusammenhang mit dem Biomed Programme (European Concerted Action 'M.O.M.S' Contract No PL 931064) durchgeführt.

Quellenangabe

Bouvier-Colle, M.H., Varnoux, N., and Breart, G. (1993). Facteurs évitables de la mortalité maternelle-Résultats de l'enquête INSERM. In *Mises à jour en gynécologie et obstétrique*, (ed. M Tournaire) pp. 329–49. CNGOF-Vigot, Paris.

Bouvier-Colle, M.H., Varnoux, N., and Breart, G. (1995*a*). Maternal deaths and substandard care: the results of a confidential survey in France, submitted to *European Journal of Obstetrics, Gynecology, and Reproductive Biology*, **58**, 3–7.

Bouvier-Colle, M.H., Salanare, B., Ancel, P.Y., and Varnoux, N. (1995*b*). Obstetric patients treated in intensive care units and maternal mortality. Submitted to *European Journal of Obstetrics, Gynaecology, and Reproductive Biology*.

European Concerted Action 'M.O.M.S': Frequency and risk factors of maternal morbidity and mortality 'avoidable' deaths and evaluation of care. Contract No PL 931064.

Haut Comité de la Santé Publique. (1992). *Stratégie pour une politiqué de santé-Premières propositions.* Rapport au Ministre de la Santé et de l'Action Humanitaire, Paris, Octobre 1992, 68 pages.

Haut Comité de la Santé Publique. (1995). La santé en France. Rapport au Ministre de la Santé et de l'Action Humanitaire, Paris, 1995.

Jougla, E., Ducimetiere, P., Bouvier-Colle, M.H., and Hatton, F. (1987). Relation entre le niveau de développement du système de soins et le niveau de la mortalité 'évitable' selon les départements francais. *Revue d'Epidémiologie et de Santé Publique*, **35**, 365–77.

Jougla, E., Hatton, F., and Bouvier-Colle, M.H. (1990). Relation entre le niveau de l'état de santé et le niveau des densités médicales. *La Revue de Praticien-Médecine générale,* **86,** 71–4.

Mackenbach, J.P., Bouvier-Colle, M.H., and Jougla, E. (1991). 'Avoidable' mortality and health services: a review of aggregate data studies. *Journal of Epidemiology and Community Health,* **44**, 106–11.

STUDIES ON 'AVOIDABLE DEATH' IN GREECE

G. Papaevangelou and C. Tsimbos

Since the Second World War several socio-economic and cultural changes have occurred in this country which have had a significant impact on aspects of the socio-demographic milieu of the Greek population. The most important events observed during the post-war period are:

(a) the high and disproportionate urbanization process;

(b) the high emigration of the 1960s, the return migration of the 1970s and the immigration of Asian and Eastern European people since the late 1980s;

(c) the decline in period fertility and the mean family size;

(d) the gradual reduction of mortality due mainly to dramatic decrease in infant mortality and mortality from infectious diseases; and

(e) the increase in morbidity from chronic diseases such as cardiovascular diseases and neoplasms for both males and females.

Mortality

Between 1950 and 1990 the expectation of life at birth increased from 63.4 to 74.6 years for males and from 66.7 to 80.0 years for females. Although regional mortality differentials diminished over time, real inequalities, with respect to the socio-economic characteristics of the population and the distribution of the health services, still exist. Life table analysis has shown that the worst mortality conditions are observed in the region of Thrace, while the most favourable ones in the Island of Crete, the Aegian Islands, in Central Greece, and the Island of Eubea (Papadakis and Tsimbos 1993). Despite the long-term reductions in death rates, mortality from cardiovascular diseases and malignant neoplasms are following a rising trend so that nowadays these causes represent about three-quarters of the overall mortality. Mortality from circulatory diseases, respiratory diseases, and car accidents have shown clear seasonal variations. It should be noted that road accidents are the leading cause of death in the age group 15–44 years representing about 30 per cent of the mortality of these ages (Tsimbos and Papaevangelou 1994).

Health services

According to Greek constitution the state is responsible for the provision of health care to all citizens. The Ministry of Health, Welfare and Social Security has the responsibility of programming, co-ordinating and executing all health-related activities as well as activities regarding social welfare and social security. All health services in the public sector operate under a National Health System (ESY) which is an intermediate form of a system of social insurance and of a national health service. Greece is divided into 52 administrative departments and nine health regions. At least one regional university hospital is planned to serve each health region providing tertiary medical care; at least one hospital in each administrative department covers the needs for secondary health care. In rural and semi-urban areas primary health care is provided through health care centres. Young doctors are obliged to serve for at least one year in health stations in rural areas before starting any specialisation. More than 50 per cent of all specialized physicians practice in Greater Athens and another 25 per cent in large towns. Patients are free to move within the health system without geographical restrictions. The observed movement of patients to the health units of the big urban centres is related to the lack of technical facilities and specialized doctors in provincial hospitals. It should also be noted that the private sector also makes a significant contribution. A considerable number of private hospitals, diagnostic centres, and doctors of all kind of specialities are practising all over Greece. According to official data, in 1992 the total number of hospitals (excluding military ones) was 375 (public 140; non-Governmental 235), but from the total number of hospital beds (41575) over 70 per cent belong to the public sector. In 1992 there was a rate of 500 beds per 100000 population (Ministry of Health 1992).

Immunization programme

The Ministry of Health is responsible for the provision and quality of vaccines and their administration. All vaccines except those for typhoid and paratyphoid fever are imported from European and American companies, and their registration for human use is provided by the National Drug Organization. The effect of the systematic immunization of Greek children on the reduction of the morbidity and mortality from childhood's diseases is remarkable; however, there is not a national network for reporting all regular vaccinations in this country; in fact about half of the infant vaccines are administered by private paediatricians. According to epidemiological sampling surveys carried out in 1993, the national average immunization coverage at the age of two years of age, is estimated to be 95 per cent for poliomyelitis, 89 per cent for diphtheria and tetanus, 78 per cent for pertussis, 72 per cent for measles, 50 per cent for tuberculosis, and 18 per cent for hepatitis B. Up to now hepatitis B immunization has been recommended by the Ministry of Health to high risk groups only.

New trends and developments

AIDS was first reported in Greece in 1984. Greece was among the first nations to establish a national committee on AIDS. During the last ten years Greece has managed to have the lowest prevalence rates among western European countries. According to official statistics (in September 1994) a total of 999 AIDS cases have been reported. It is interesting to note that the prevalence of HIV in drug-users has remained very low compared to our European neighbours. However, the increase in the frequency of heterosexual transmission needs to be examined further using special monitoring. Finally, there have been problems with infectious and sexually transmitted diseases in relation to the health status and the poor living conditions of Asian and Eastern European migrants (Papaevangelou 1995).

References

Ministry of Health (1992). *Experts committee report on the health status of the Greek population*. Athens.

Papadakis, M. and Tsimbos, C. (1993). *Regional life tables for Greece, 1960–62, 1970–72, 1980–82*. BHTA Publishers, Athens.

Papaevangelou, G. (1995). AIDS: past, present and future. *Hellenic Archives of AIDS*, **3**, 15–19.

Tsimbos, C. and Papaevangelou, G. (1994). *Mortality of the Greek population by cause of death 1960–1990*. Greek Demographic Conference, Athens, 5–6 October 1992, pp. 157–69. Nea Synora, Livanis, Athens.

ETUDE SUR LES 'MORTS EVITABLES' EN GRÉCE

G. Papaevangelou et C. Tsimbos

Depuis la deuxième guerre mondiale, plusieurs changements socio-économiques et culturels sont intervenus dans ce pays qui eurent un impact significatif sur le milieu socio-démographique de la population grecque. Les événements les plus importants observés durant la période d'après guerre sont :

(a) le processus intense et déséquilibré de l'urbanisation ;

(b) une émigration élevée dans les années soixante, le retour de migration dans les années 1970 et l'immigration des populations d'Asie et d'Europe de l'est depuis la fin des années 1980 ;

(c) le déclin de la fécondité et de la taille moyenne des familles ;

(d) la réduction graduelle de la mortalité due principalement à la chute considérable de la mortalité infantile et de la mortalité dues aux maladies infectieuses;

(e) l'augmentation de la morbidité due aux maladies chroniques telles que maladies cardio-vasculaires et cancers pour les hommes et les femmes.

Mortalité

Entre 1950 et 1990, l'espérance de vie à la naissance a augmenté de 63,4 à 74,6 ans pour les hommes et de 66,7 à 80,0 pour les femmes. Bien que les différences de mortalité régionale aient diminué à travers le temps, de réelles inégalités, compte tenu des caractères socio-économiques de la population et de la distribution des services de santé, existent toujours. L'analyse des tables de mortalité a montré que les conditions de mortalité les pires sont observées en Thrace, tandis que les plus favorables se rencontrent dans les îles de Crète, et d'Egée, dans la Grèce centrale, et dans l'île d'Eubée (Papadakis et Tsimbos 1993). En dépit de la réduction des taux de mortalité sur le long terme, la mortalité cardio-vasculaire et par tumeurs malignes suit une tendance ascendante si bien qu'aujourd'hui ces causes représentent environ les trois-quarts de la mortalité totale. La mortalité par maladies circulatoires, ou infectieuses et par accidents de la route a montré de nettes variations saisonnières. Il faut noter que les accidents sont la cause principale de décès des groupes d'âge 15–44 ans, représentant environ 30 pour cent de la mortalité à ces âges (Tsimbos et Papaevangelou 1994).

Services de santé

Selon la constitution grecque, l'état est responsable de la prestation des soins à tous les citoyens. Le ministre de la santé, du bien être et de la sécurité sociale a la responsabilité de programmer, coordonner et exécuter toutes les activités liées à la santé, aussi bien que celles qui concernent le bien être social et la sécurité sociale. Tous les services de santé du secteur public opèrent dans le cadre d'un Système national de santé (ESY) qui est une forme intermédiaire entre un système d'assurance sociale et un service national de santé. La Grèce est divisée en 52 départements administratifs et 9 régions sanitaires. Il est prévu qu'au moins un hôpital régional procurant des soins de niveau III desserve chaque région sanitaire; au moins un hôpital de niveau secondaire couvre les besoins dans chaque département administratif. Dans les zones rurales et semi-urbaines, les soins primaires sont fournis à partir des centres de santé. Les jeunes médecins sont tenus d'exercer au moins un an en zone rurale, dans les centres de santé, avant de démarrer une spécialisation. Plus de 50 pour cent des médecins spécialistes exercent dans le grand Athènes et 25 pour cent supplémentaires dans les grandes villes. Les patients sont libres de se déplacer à l'intérieur du système de santé sans restriction géographique. Les mouvements des patients observés vers les services de santé des grands centres urbains sont liés à l'absence de facilités techniques et de médecins spécialisés dans les hôpitaux provinciaux. Il faut aussi noter que le secteur privé opère une contribution significative. Un nombre considérable d'hôpitaux privés, de centres de diagnostic et de médecins de toutes sortes de spécialités pratiquent tout à travers la Grèce. Selon les données officielles, en 1992, le nombre total d'hôpitaux (excluant les établissements militaires) était de 375 (public 140; non gouvernemental 235) mais sur le nombre total de lits d'hôpitaux (41 575) plus de 70 pour cent appartiennent au secteur public. En 1992, il y avait un taux de 500 lits pour 100 000 habitants (Ministère de la Santé 1992).

Programme de vaccination

Le ministère de la santé est responsable de la fourniture et de la qualité des vaccins et de leur administration. Tous les vaccins, exceptés ceux des fièvres typhoïde et paratyphoïde, sont importés d'Europe et des compagnies américaines, et leur enregistrement pour l'utilisation humaine est faite par l'Organisation nationale du médicament. L'effet de la vaccination systématique des enfants grecs sur la diminution de la morbidité et de la mortalité des maladies infantiles est remarquable; néanmoins il n'y a pas de réseau national de déclaration des vaccinations régulières dans ce pays. En fait à peu près la moitié des vaccins infantiles sont administrés par les pédiatres privés. Selon les enquêtes épidémiologiques sur échantillon, réalisées en 1993, le taux national moyen de couverture vaccinale à l'âge de 2 ans, est estimé à 95 pour cent pour la poliomyélite, 89 pour cent pour la diphtérie et le tétanos, 78 pour cent pour la coqueluche,72 pour cent pour la rougeole, 50 pour cent pour la tuberculose et 18 pour cent pour l'hépatite B. Jusqu'à maintenant la vaccination contre l'hépatite B a été recommandée par le ministère de la santé seulement aux groupes à risque élevé.

Développements et tendances à venir

Le Sida a été rapporté pour la première fois, en Grèce, en 1984. La Grèce fut parmi les premières nations à établir un comité national sur le Sida. Durant les dix dernières années la Grèce a agi de manière à avoir le taux de prévalence le plus bas parmi les pays européens de l'ouest. D'après les statistiques officielles (Septembre 1994) un total de 999 cas de Sida a été déclaré. Il est intéressant de noter que la prévalence du virus VIH parmi les toxicomanes est restée très basse comparativement à nos voisins européens. Néanmoins l'accroissement de la fréquence de la transmission hétérosexuelle suppose davantage d'études en utilisant un suivi particulier. Finalement, il y a des problèmes infectieux de santé et de maladies sexuellement transmissibles en relation avec l'état de santé et les conditions de pauvreté des migrants asiatiques et européens de l'est (Papaevangelou 1995).

Références

Ministry of Health (1992). *Experts committee report on the health status of the Greek population*. Athens.

Papadakis, M. and Tsimbos, C. (1993). *Regional life tables for Greece, 1960–62, 1970–72, 1980–82*. BHTA Publishers, Athens.

Papaevangelou, G. (1995). AIDS: past, present and future. *Hellenic Archives of AIDS*, **3**, 15–19.

Tsimbos, C. and Papaevangelou, G. (1994). *Mortality of the Greek population by cause of death 1960–1990*. Greek Demographic Conference, Athens, 5–6 October 1992, pp. 157–69. Nea Synora, Livanis, Athens.

STUDIEN ÜBER 'VERMEIDBARE TODESFÄLLE' IN GRIECHENLAND

G. Papaevangelou und C. Tsimbos

Seit dem Zweiten Weltkrieg sind in diesem Land mehrere sozioökonomische und kulturelle Veränderungen aufgetreten, die einen bedeutenden Einfluß auf Aspekte des sozio-demographischen Milieus der griechischen Bevölkerung ausgeübt haben. Die während der Nachkriegszeit wichtigsten Ereignissse waren:

(a) die hohe und unverhältnismäßige Urbanisierung;

(b) die hohe Auswanderungsrate in den sechziger Jahren, die Rückwanderung in den siebziger Jahren und die Einwanderung von Menschen aus Asien und Osteuropa seit den späten achtziger Jahren;

(c) der Rückgang periodischer Fruchtbarkeit und die mittlere Familiengröße;

(d) der allmähliche Rückgang der Sterblichkeit hauptsächlich aufgrund einer dramatischen Abnahme der Säuglingssterblichkeit und der Sterbluichkeit durch Infektionskrankheiten;

(e) die Zunahme chronischer Krankheiten wie Herzkranzgefäßerkrankungen und Neoplasmen bei Männern und Frauen.

Sterblichkeit

Zwischen 1950 und 1990 stieg die Lebenserwartung der in diesem Zeitraum geborenen Personen von durchschnittlich 63,4 auf 74,6 Jahren bei Männern und von 66,7 auf 80,0 Jahren bei Frauen an.

Obwohl regionale Unterschiede in der Sterblichkeit über die Jahre hinweg abgenommen haben, so bestehen jedoch weiterhin wirkliche Ungleichheiten, was die sozio-ökonomischen Charakteristika der Bevölkerung und die Verteilung von Gesundheitsdiensten angeht. Analysen von Lebenstabellen weisen die schlimmsten Sterblichkeitsverhältnisse in der Region Thrakien nach, während die Insel Kreta, die Ägäischen Inseln, Zentralgriechenland, und die Insel Eubea am besten abschneiden (Papadakis und Tsimbos 1993). Trotz der auf lange Sicht hin abnehmenden Sterberate befindet sich die Sterblichkeit aufgrund von Herzkranzgefäßerkrankungen und bösartigen Neoplasmen in einem Aufwärtstrend, so daß diese Ursachen heutzutage drei Viertel aller Todesursachen ausmachen. Todesfälle aufgrund von Kreislaufkrankheiten, Atemwegserkrankungen und Autounfällen haben deutlich saisonale Unterschiede aufgewiesen. Es sollte beachtet werden, daß Straßenunfälle die Haupttodesursache in der Altersgruppe von 15–40 Jahren ist und damit für 30 prozent aller Todesfälle in dieser Altersgruppe verantwortlicht ist (Tsimbos und Papaevangelou 1994).

Gesundheitsdienste

Laut der griechischen Verfassung ist der Staat für die medizinische Versorgung aller Bürger verantwortlich. Das Ministerium für Gesundheit, Wohlfahrt und Soziale Sicherheit trägt die Verantwortung für die Planung, Koordination und Ausführung aller Aktivitäten auf dem Gesundheitssektor ebenso wie im Bereich sozialer Wohlfahrt und Sicherheit. Alle Gesundheitsdienste im öffentlichen Sektor agieren unter dem Nationalen Gesundheitssystem (ESY), das als die Mischform eines Systems sozialer Versicherung und nationalem Gesundheitswesens zu beschreiben ist. Griechenland ist in 52 Verwaltungsbezirke und neun Gesundheitsregionen eingeteilt. Jede Gesundheitsregion ist zumindest von einem Universitätskrankenhaus mit tertiärer medizinischer Versorgung ausgestattet. Jeder Verwaltungsbezirk ist zumindest von einem Krankenhaus mit sekundärer medizinischer Versorgung bedient. In ländlichen und semiurbanen Gegenden wird die primäre gesundheitliche Versorgung von medizinischen Versorgungszentren übernommen. Junge Ärzte sind verpflichtet, für zumindest ein Jahr in den Gesunheitszentren ländlicher Regionen zu arbeiten, bevor sie sich spezialisieren. Mehr als 50 prozent aller Fachärzte praktizieren im Großraum Athen und nochmals 25 prozent in anderen großen Städten. Allen Patienten ist es freigestellt, sich innerhalb des Gesundheitswesens frei und von geographischen Einschränkungen unabhängig zu bewegen. Die beobachtete Abwanderung von Patienten in die Gesundheitseinrichtungen großer urbaner Zentren hängt mit dem Mangel an technischen Einrichtungen und Fachärzten in den Krankenhäusern der Provinz zusammen. Man sollte zudem den bedeutenden Beitrag des privaten Sektors beachten. Eine beträchtliche Zahl an privaten Krankenhäusern, Diagnosezentren und Ärzten jeglicher Fachrichtungen praktizieren in ganz Griechenland. Laut offizieller Daten betrug 1992 die Zahl der Krankenhäuser (mit Ausnahme der militärischen) 375 (öffentlich 140; nicht-staatlich: 235), jedoch gehörten aus der Gesamtanzahl aller Krankenhausbetten (41 575) 70 prozent zum öffentlichen Sektor. 1992 lautete das Verhältnis 500 Betten pro 100 000 Menschen in der Bevölkerung (Gesundheitsministerium 1992).

Immunisierungsprogramm

Das Gesundheitsministerium trägt die Verantwortung für die Bereitstellung und Qualität von Impfstoffen sowie deren Verabreichung. Alle Impfstoffe außer denen gegen Typhus und Paratyphus werden von europäischen und amerikanischen Firmen importiert. Ihre Registrierung für den Gebrauch am Menschen wird von der Nationalen Arzneimittel Organisation übernommen. Die Auswirkung systematischer Immunisierung griechischer Kinder auf den Rückgang der Morbidität und Sterblichkeit aufgrund von Kinderkrankheiten ist bemerkenswert. Es existiert allerdings kein nationales Netzwerk, das alle regelmäßigen Impfungen meldet. Tatsächlich wird ungefähr die Hälfte aller Kinderimpfungen von privaten Kinderärzten verabreicht. Den Ergebnissen einer 1983 ausgeführten epidemologischen Querschnittsuntersuchung zufolge wird der durchschnittliche Impfschutz bei Zweijährigen auf 95 prozent gegen Poliomyelitis, 89 prozent gegen Diphterie und Tetanus, 78 prozent gegen Keuchhusten, 72 prozent gegen Masern, 50 prozent gegen Tuberkulose und 18 prozent gegen Hepatitis B geschätzt. Bis jetzt wurde eine Impfung gegen Hepatitis B vom Gesundheitsministerium nur besonders gefährdeten Risikogruppen anempfohlen.

Neue Trends und Entwicklungen

AIDS wurde in Griechenland erstmals 1984 festgestellt. Griechenland gehörte zu den ersten Nationen, die einen nationalen AIDS-Ausschuß gründeten. Während der letzten zehn Jahre gelang es Griechenland, das niedrigste Ausbreitungsniveau unter den westlichen europäischen Ländern zu ereichen. Offiziellen Statistiken zufolge (im September 1994) wurde ein Gesamtzahl von 999 AIDS-Fällen registriert. Interessanterweise ist die Verbreitung von HIV bei Drogenkonsumenten sehr niedrig geblieben im Vergleich zu unseren europäischen Nachbarn. Jedoch verlangt die ansteigende Häufigkeit heterosexueller Übertragung einer eingehenden Untersuchung mit Hilfe spezieller Überwachung. Abschließend wurden Probleme mit infektiösen und sexuell übertragenen Krankheiten in Verbindung mit dem Gesundheitszustand unter den ärmlichen Lebensbedingungen asiatischer und osteuropäischer Einwanderer festgestellt (Papaevangelou 1995).

Quellenangaben

Ministry of Health (1992). *Experts committee report on the health status of the Greek population*. Athens.

Papadakis, M. and Tsimbos, C. (1993). *Regional life tables for Greece, 1960–62, 1970–72, 1980–82*. BHTA Publishers, Athens.

Papaevangelou, G. (1995). AIDS: past, present and future. *Hellenic Archives of AIDS*, **3**, 15–19.

Tsimbos, C. and Papaevangelou, G. (1994). *Mortality of the Greek population by cause of death 1960–1990*. Greek Demographic Conference, Athens, 5–6 October 1992, pp. 157–69. Nea Synora, Livanis, Athens.

STUDIES ON 'AVOIDABLE DEATH' IN ITALY

P. Lauriola

In 1990 a review on the methodology and the results of the first two European atlases of 'avoidable death' was published with focus on the Italian experience (Morosini *et al.* 1990). It emphasized the relative excess of deaths from cholecystitis and cholelithiasis all over Italy, as well as deaths from Hodgkin's disease in the north, and chronic rheumatic heart disease in the south.

In the same year two local studies appeared, a general one on some Italian regions (de Marco and Zanolin 1990), and one related to some particular groups of people (children, women, etc.) (Donzelli *et al.* 1990; Parazzini *et al.* 1990).

More recently, detailed analysis on surgical deaths (appendicitis, cholecystitis, abdominal hernia), extending from 1976 to 1989 (Lauriola *et al.*, in press), has shown a general decrease for all causes all over Italy, that continued in the period 1985–89. Generally speaking, the picture was better in the north and in the centre, but some regions in the north (that is, Piedmont and Liguria) had relatively unfavourable rates.

Some studies on the relations between asthma prevalence and asthma deaths are under way (Marinoni *et al.* 1993).

On-going works

Two confidential enquiries are being carried out; one on cholecystitis and cholelithiasis (Manenti *et al.* 1994), showing a good collaboration by clinicians and a poor reporting by local death registers, and the other which has just begun on traffic accident deaths, investigating both emergency practices and traffic conditions.

References

Donzelli, G.P., Profeti, C., Moroni, M., Piumelli, R., Rapisardi, G. and Scarano, E. (1990). Morti neonatali evitabili: verifica e revisione di qualità dell'assistenza perinatale. Atti 5° Convegno nazionale sugli studi di mortalità Firenze 24–25 Ottobre 1990.

Lauriola, P., Magliola, E., Cassindra, M., and Morosini, P. La mortalità evitabile in chirurgia. Analisi dettagliata ed aggiornamento della mortalità evitabile per cause 'chirurgiche' dell'atlante Europeo. Federazione Medica, in press.

Manenti, F., Trande, P., Luppi, G., Lauriola, P., Goldoni, C.A., Morosini, P., Collini, P., and Curcio Rubertini, B. (1994). VRQ of a 'confidential study' about undue deaths for cholecystitis-cholelithiasis in Emilia-Romagna (ITALY). Health care quality: The role of professionals and citizens and the influence of market forces. Venice, May 24–28, 1994.

De Marco, R. and Zanolin, E. (1990). Mortalità per cause riconducibili all'intervento medico nelle U.s.l. lombarde (1980–85). *Epidemiologia e Prevenzione,* **45**, 24–32.

Marinoni, A., de Marco, R., Basso, O., *et al.* (1993). Prevalence of respiratory symptoms and current asthma in a general population sample of northern Italy. *European Respiratory Journal,* **6**, 339s.

Morosini, P., Lauriola, P., Magliola, E., Feola, G., and Feola, E.M. (1990). Le morti evitabili nella valutazione della atività del servizio sanitario nazionale. *Epidemiologia e Prevenzione,* **45**, 48–58.

Parazzini, F., Grilli, R., Bruzzi, P., and Liberati, A. (1990). La mortalità prevenibile con la terapia in ambito oncologico: il caso del tumore della mammemlla, del'ovaio e del grosso intestino. Atti 5° Convegno nazionale sugli studi di mortalità, Firenze 24–25 Ottobre 1990.

ETUDE SUR LES 'MORTS EVITABLES' EN ITALIE

P Lauriola

En 1990, une revue de la méthodologie et des résultats des deux premiers Atlas européens sur 'les morts évitables' fut publié, l'accent étant mis sur l'expérience italienne (Morosini *et al.* 1990). Cette revue soulignait l'excès relatif des décès par cholélithiase et cholécystite à travers toute l'Italie, ainsi que les décès par maladie de Hodgkin dans le nord, et les cardiopathies rhumatismales chroniques dans le sud.

La même année, deux études locales ont été publiées, l'une générale, sur quelques régions italiennes (de Marco *et al.* 1990) et l'autre liée à certains groupes particuliers de population (femmes, enfants, etc.) (Donzelli *et al.* 1990 ; Parazzini *et al.* 1990).

Plus récemment une analyse détaillée des décès chirurgicaux (appendicite, cholécystite, hernie abdominale) s'étendant de 1976 à 1989 (Lauriola *et al.* in press) a montré un déclin général pour toutes les causes, dans toute l'Italie, qui se poursuit dans la période 1985–89. Généralement on peut dire que le tableau est meilleur dans le nord et au centre, mais quelques régions du nord (Piedmont et Ligurie) ont des taux relativement mauvais.

Quelques études sur la relation entre prévalence de l'asthme et décès par asthme sont en cours (Marinoni *et al.* 1993).

Travaux en cours

Deux enquêtes confidentielles ont été entreprises; l'une sur les cholécystites et cholélithiases (Manenti *et al.* 1994) montrant une bonne collaboration des cliniciens et une mauvaise déclaration des registres locaux de décès ; l'autre, qui démarre à peine, sur les accidents de la route, étudiant à la fois les pratiques d'urgence et les conditions de circulation.

Références

Donzelli, G.P., Profeti, C., Moroni, M., Piumelli, R., Rapisardi, G. and Scarano, E. (1990). Morti neonatali evitabili: verifica e revisione di qualità dell'assistenza perinatale. Atti 5° Convegno nazionale sugli studi di mortalità Firenze 24–25 Ottobre 1990.

Lauriola, P., Magliola, E., Cassindra, M., and Morosini, P. La mortalità evitabile in chirurgia. Analisi dettagliata ed aggiornamento della mortalità evitabile per cause 'chirurgiche' dell'atlante Europeo. Federazione Medica, in press.

Manenti, F., Trande, P., Luppi, G., Lauriola, P., Goldoni, C.A., Morosini, P., Collini, P., and Curcio Rubertini, B. (1994). VRQ of a 'confidential study' about undue deaths for cholecystitis-cholelithiasis in Emilia-Romagna (ITALY). Health care quality: The role of professionals and citizens and the influence of market forces. Venice, May 24–28, 1994.

De Marco, R. and Zanolin, E. (1990). Mortalità per cause riconducibili all'intervento medico nelle U.s.l. lombarde (1980–85). *Epidemiologia e Prevenzione,* **45**, 24–32.

Marinoni, A., de Marco, R., Basso, O., *et al.* (1993). Prevalence of respiratory symptoms and current asthma in a general population sample of northern Italy. *European Respiratory Journal,* **6**, 339s.

Morosini, P., Lauriola, P., Magliola, E., Feola, G., and Feola, E.M. (1990). Le morti evitabili nella valutazione della atività del servizio sanitario nazionale. *Epidemiologia e Prevenzione,* **45**, 48–58.

Parazzini, F., Grilli, R., Bruzzi, P., and Liberati, A. (1990). La mortalità prevenibile con la terapia in ambito oncologico: il caso del tumore della mammemlla, del'ovaio e del grosso intestino. Atti 5° Convegno nazionale sugli studi di mortalità, Firenze 24–25 Ottobre 1990.

STUDIEN ÜBER 'VERMEIDBARE TODESFÄLLE' IN ITALIEN

P. Lauriola

1990 wurde eine Übersicht über die Methodik und die Ergebnisse der ersten beiden europäischen Atlanten über 'Vermeidbare Todesälle' veröffentlicht, in dessen Mittelpunkt die Erfahrungen Italiens standen (Morosoni *et al.* 1990). Diese Veröffentlichung betonte die relativ hohe Anzahl von Todesfällen Gallenblase entzündung und Gallenblase steine in ganz Italien, ebenso wie die Sterbefälle aufgrund der Hodgkinschen Krankheit im Norden und chronisch rheumatischer Herzkrankheiten im Süden Italiens.

Im selben Jahr erschienen zwei lokale Studien: eine allgemeine Studie, die sich mit einigen Regionen Italiens beschäftigte (de Marco und Zanolin 1990) sowie eine zweite Studie, die sich mit bestimmten Personengruppen befaßte (Kinder, Frauen, etc.) (Donizelli *et al.* 1990; Parazzini *et al.* 1990).

In der letzten Zeit wiesen detailierte Analysen der Todesfälle bei chirurgischen Eingriffen (Appendizitis, Gallenblase entzündung, Abdomnialhernie) im Zeitraum von 1976–89 (Lauriola *et al.* im Druck) eine allgemeine Abnahme aller Todesursachen in ganz Italien nach, die sich auch in den Jahren von 1985–89 fortsetzte. Im allgemeinen zeichnet sich im Norden und im Zentrum Italiens ein besseres Bild ab, wobei jedoch in einzelnen Regionen im Norden (z.B. Piedmont und Liguria) verhältnismäßig ungünstige Raten festzustellen sind.

Einzelne Studien zum Verhältnis zwischen der Ausbreitung und den Todesfällen durch Asthma sind im Gange (Marinoni *et al.* 1993).

Weiterführende Arbeiten

Zur Zeit werden zwei vertraulich angestellte Umfragen vorgenommen (Manenti *et al.* 1994). Eine dieser Umfragen weist auf eine gute Zusammenarbeit mit den Kliniken, jedoch auf enttäuschende Resultate bei der lokalen Todesfallregistrierung hin. Die zweite, eben erst begonnene Umfrage über Unfalltode untersucht sowohl die Praktiken der Notfalldienste als auch die Verkerhrsbedingungen.

Quellenangabe

Donzelli, G.P., Profeti, C., Moroni, M., Piumelli, R., Rapisardi, G. and Scarano, E. (1990). Morti neonatali evitabili: verifica e revisione di qualità dell'assistenza perinatale. Atti 5° Convegno nazionale sugli studi di mortalità Firenze 24–25 Ottobre 1990.

Lauriola, P., Magliola, E., Cassindra, M., and Morosini, P. La mortalità evitabile in chirurgia. Analisi dettagliata ed aggiornamento della mortalità evitabile per cause 'chirurgiche' dell'atlante Europeo. Federazione Medica, in press.

Manenti, F., Trande, P., Luppi, G., Lauriola, P., Goldoni, C.A., Morosini, P., Collini, P., and Curcio Rubertini, B. (1994). VRQ of a 'confidential study' about undue deaths for cholecystitis-cholelithiasis in Emilia-Romagna (ITALY). Health care quality: The role of professionals and citizens and the influence of market forces. Venice, May 24–28, 1994.

De Marco, R. and Zanolin, E. (1990). Mortalità per cause riconducibili all'intervento medico nelle U.s.l. lombarde (1980–85). *Epidemiologia e Prevenzione,* **45**, 24–32.

Marinoni, A., de Marco, R., Basso, O., *et al.* (1993). Prevalence of respiratory symptoms and current asthma in a general population sample of northern Italy. *European Respiratory Journal,* **6**, 339s.

Morosini, P., Lauriola, P., Magliola, E., Feola, G., and Feola, E.M. (1990). Le morti evitabili nella valutazione della atività del servizio sanitario nazionale. *Epidemiologia e Prevenzione,* **45**, 48–58.

Parazzini, F., Grilli, R., Bruzzi, P., and Liberati, A. (1990). La mortalità prevenibile con la terapia in ambito oncologico: il caso del tumore della mammemlla, del'ovaio e del grosso intestino. Atti 5° Convegno nazionale sugli studi di mortalità, Firenze 24–25 Ottobre 1990.

STUDIES ON 'AVOIDABLE DEATH' IN IRELAND

J. Barry

In April 1994 the Department of Health published a document called 'Shaping a healthier future', a strategy for effective health care in the 1990s. The document is a watershed document in the Irish Health Services in that it takes a long-term view and explicitly sets targets in reorienting and reshaping the Irish Health Service so as to improve the health of the population. Three principles underpin the strategy: equity, quality of services, and accountability. Within these principles there is scope for the findings in the *European Community atlas of 'avoidable death'* to inform the development of the health services in Ireland. A greater role is envisaged for epidemiology and public health medicine and the application of health information to the health services.

Death rates from cardiovascular disease and various cancers are highlighted in the report, and while the focus in the report is on avoiding premature mortality, initiatives that should lead to a reduction in avoidable mortality will obviously also be welcomed. The document is an aspirational document and the extent at which this aspiration becomes reality will depend on a number of factors, in particular the setting up of departments of public health in the Health Boards and the necessary organizational and legislative changes that have to take place within the Irish Health Service to improve decision making and linkage between primary and secondary care.

There has been one publication as a result of the series of European atlases (Barry 1992). The poor performance of the Irish Health Service in terms of tuberculosis control is highlighted in this publication. Currently a national tuberculosis committee is sitting and recommendations are expected shortly, which should improve services aimed at reducing the burden of tuberculosis on the Irish population. There is presently no centralized communicable disease reporting system within Ireland and public health practices within different health authorities vary in terms of tuberculosis control.

These are exciting times for the Irish health service and from now on much attention will focus on the extent to which the framework for implementing the principles in 'Shaping a healthier future' will be put in place and the extent to which this will result in improved health of the population.

Reference

Barry, J. (1992). 'Avoidable Mortality' as an index of health care outcome: results from the European Community Atlas of 'Avoidable Death'. *Irish Journal of Medical Science*, August, **161,** No. 8, 490–2.

ETUDE SUR LES 'MORTS EVITABLES' EN IRLANDE

J. Barry

En avril 1994 le département de la Santé a publié un document appelé 'Façonner un avenir en meilleure santé' 'Shaping a healthier future', une stratégie pour des soins efficaces dans les années 90. Le document est une ligne de partage dans les services de santé irlandais, en ce qu'il prend une visée à long terme et établit explicitement les buts de réorientation et de refaçonnage du service sanitaire irlandais de manière à améliorer la santé de la population. Trois principes étayent la stratégie: équité, qualité des services et responsabilité. Dans ces trois principes il y a place pour les apports de l'Atlas européen des morts évitables d'informer le développement des services de santé en Irlande. Un rôle plus important de l'épidémiologie et de la médecine de santé publique est envisagé, ainsi que l'application de l'information sanitaire aux services de santé.

Les taux de mortalité par maladie cardio-vasculaire et par différents cancers sont présentés dans le rapport, et tandis que l'accent est mis sur la mortalité prématurée, les initiatives, qui devraient conduire à une réduction de la mortalité évitable, seront aussi bienvenues. Le document est ambitieux et l'extension selon laquelle les aspirations deviennent réalité dépendra de nombreux facteurs, et en particulier de l'édification de départements de santé publique au sein du ministère de la santé, et de nécessaires changements législatifs et d'organisation qui auront à prendre place au sein du Service irlandais de santé pour améliorer la prise de décision et le lien entre soins primaire et secondaire.

Une publication a résulté des séries de l'Atlas européen (Barry 1992). La faible performance du service de santé Irlandais en terme de lutte contre la tuberculose est soulignée dans cette publication. Un comité national de la tuberculose siège couramment et l'on attend des recommandations rapidement, qui devraient améliorer les services destinés à réduire la charge de la tuberculose sur la population irlandaise. Il n'y a pas actuellement de système centralisé de déclaration des maladies contagieuses en Irlande, et les pratiques de contrôle de la tuberculose varient d'une région sanitaire à une autre.

Ce sont des temps importants pour le service irlandais de santé, et désormais davantage d'attention sera portée à l'extension et à la mise en place du programme 'Shaping a healthier future' et sur la manière dont en résultera une meilleure santé de la population.

Références

Barry, J. (1992). 'Avoidable Mortality' as an index of health care outcome: results from the European Community Atlas of 'Avoidable Death'. *Irish Journal of Medical Science*, August, **161,** No. 8, 490–2.

STUDIEN ÜBER 'VERMEIDBARE TODESFÄLLE' IN IRLAND

J. Barry

Im April 1994 veröffentlichte das Department of Health ein Dokument mit dem Namen 'Shaping a healthier future'. Es handelt sich um eine Strategie wirksamer medizinischer Versorgung in den neunziger Jahren. Dieses Dokument stellt insofern einen Wendepunkt für das irische Gesundheitswesen dar, als es sich auf einen langen Zeitraum bezieht und ausdrücklich Ziele in der Neuorientierung und Umformung des irischen Gesundheitswesens setzt, um dadurch das Gesundheitsniveau der Bevölkerung zu verbessern. Diese Strategie beruht auf drei Prinzipien: Gerechtigkeit, Qualität der angebotenen Dienste und Verantwortlichkeit. Zukünftig werden die Epidemologie und die allgemeine Gesundheitsmedizin sowie die Umsetzung von Informationen zur Gesundheit im Gesundheitswesen eine bedeutendere Rolle spielen.

Die Sterberaten bei Herzkranzgefäßerkrankungen und verschiedenen Krebsarten werden im Bericht hervorgehoben. Während sich sein Augenmerk auf die Vermeidung vorzeitiger Todesfälle richtet, sind Initiativen, die zu deren Reduzierung führen sollten, selbstverständlich willkommen. Mit diesem Dokument werden Zielvorgaben gesetzt. Das Ausmaß, in dem diese Ziele erreicht werden, hängt von einer Anzahl von Faktoren ab, im besonderen jedoch von der Einführung von departments of public health im Rahmen der Health Boards. Außerdem sind organisatorische und legislative Veränderungen innerhalb des irischen Gesundheitswesens notwendig, um die Entscheidungsfähigkeit sowie die Verbindung zwischen primärer und sekundärer medizinischer Versorgung zu verbessern.

Eine alsAntwort auf die Reihe der europäischen Atlanten erschienene Veröffentlichung (Barry, 1992) hebt das schlechte Abschneiden des irirschen Gesundheitswesen in der Bekämpfung von Tuberkulose hervor. Zur Zeit tagt ein nationaler Tuberkulose-Ausschuß, dessen Empfehlungen in Kürze erwartet werden und die Gesundheistdienste verbessern soll, die sich mit der Entlastung der Bevölkerung Irlands von der Bürde der Tuberkulose befassen. Leider existiert in Irland noch kein zentralisiertes Kommunikationssystem der Krankheitserfassung. Die Praktiken der Tuberkulosebekämpfung unterscheiden sich innerhalb verschiedener Einrichtungen.

Für das irische Gesundheitswesen sind dies aufregende Zeiten. Von nun an wird sich das Interesse auf die Umsetzung der in dem Dokument 'Shaping a healthier future' genannten Prinzipien, sowie auf das Ausmaß, in dem sich der Gesundheitszustand der Bevölkerung verbessert, richten.

Quellenangabe

Barry, J. (1992). 'Avoidable Mortality' as an index of health care outcome: results from the European Community Atlas of 'Avoidable Death'. *Irish Journal of Medical Science*, August, **161,** No. 8, 490–2.

STUDIES ON 'AVOIDABLE DEATH' IN ENGLAND AND WALES

W.W. Holland

The following selection of studies illustrates some of the work on 'avoidable death' being undertaken by the Department of Public Health Medicine of United Medical and Dental Schools of Guy's and St Thomas's.

Our studies on stroke in three local districts began with a description of the incidence and case fatality of stroke in the three districts (Wolfe *et al.* 1993*a*, *b*). The observed variation in stroke mortality did not result from differences in case fatality but rather from differences in incidence. The district with the highest standardized mortality ratio also had the highest incidence of stroke and the highest frequency of individuals of Afro-Caribbean origin, a group which may be particularly at risk of hypertension and consequently stroke. It was concluded that preventive services and methods for identifying risk factors for stroke require improvement as do services providing treatment for individuals with stroke. Following this we are now undertaking randomized controlled trials to determine the most cost-effective means of managing patients, both before and after discharge from hospital with stroke. This is linked to practical studies to determine the deficiencies in care and to a European BIOMED programme in which we are co-ordinating a series of studies to determine the relationship between resource use, cost, and outcome of stroke care in different European countries.

The results of our original stroke study together with the government's concern about the health of ethnic minorities, led us to review the health problems of ethnic minorities. This has developed into a larger study of risk factors for stroke in the Afro-Caribbean ethnic minority group. The haemoglobinopathies are a particular problem of Afro-Caribbeans and we hope to extend this work with a study of the painful crises of sickle cell disease.

The provision of appropriate and effective preventive measures and clinical care often depends on an understanding of patients' beliefs about their medical conditions and treatments. This area has formed an important focus of social science research. Study of hypertensive patients provided new data on the beliefs and medication practices of the Afro-Caribbean community, thus assisting general practitioners in communicating better with this group of patients (Morgan and Watkins 1988). Similar research on parental meanings and management of childhood asthma is now under way and is concerned particularly with the reasons for low levels of compliance with treatment.

A recent study of asthma admission rates considered 20 areas in England and Wales, chosen so as to ensure a wide variation in mortality (Burney *et al.* 1991). The study considered asthma admission rates in men aged 20–44 years old. The authors concluded that asthma admission rates were not dictated solely by health service characteristics but also reflected need. A local study to evaluate community-based intervention to improve the management of asthma is now under way.

The department is currently co-ordinating an international survey, funded by the EC, to study the variation in asthma and asthma-like symptoms throughout Europe and other parts of the world (Burney *et al.* 1994).

Together with the Faculty of Public Health Medicine we have acted as the focus for producing a series of possible indicators for avoidable death and morbidity in order to try and identify the outcome of health services (McColl and Gulliford 1993). The first volume has recently been published and a second volume is currently being produced. These indicators may provide purchasing and providing authorities with more information on their achievements in improving the health of the nation.

Interpretation of indicators of health care outcome requires additional information concerning influences on the incidence and course of disease in populations. Cancer registry data were utilized as a sampling frame for a series of studies on the outcome of common cancers such as cancer of the bladder and oesophagus (Gulliford *et al.* 1991*a*, 1993*a*). These studies provided insights into the epidemiology of processes of health care and their associations with mortality but the results also underlined the difficulty of using observational data to evaluate the effectiveness of health care (Gulliford 1992) particularly when data collected within the health system may be unreliable or incomplete (Gulliford *et al.* 1991*b*, Gulliford *et al.* 1993*b*). The challenge now is to identify the critical information required to evaluate services and to put in place systems which can reliably capture these data over long periods of time, in diverse localities.

References

Burney, P.G.J., Luczynska, C., Chinn, S., and Jarvis, D. (1994). The European Community Respiratory Health Survey. *European Respiratory Journal,* **7**, 954–60.

Burney, P.G.J., Papacosta, A.O., Withey, C.H., Colley, J.R.T. *et al.* (1991). Hospital admission rates and the prevalence of asthma symptoms in 20 local authority districts. *Thorax*, **46**, 574–9.

Gulliford, M.C., Petruckevitch, A., and Burney, P.G.J. (1991*a*). Survival with bladder cancer, evaluation of delay in treatment, type of surgeon and modality of treatment. *British Medical Journal,* **302**, 437–40.

Gulliford, M.C., Petruckevitch, A., and Burney, P.G.J. (1991*b*). Hospital case notes and medical audit: evaluation of non-response. *British Medical Journal,* **302**, 1128–9.

Gulliford, M.C. (1992). Evaluating prognostic factors: implications for measurement of health care outcome. *Journal of Epidemiology and Community Health*, **46**, 323–6.

Gulliford, M.C., Barton, J.R., and Bourne, H. (1993*a*). Selection for oesophagectomy and post-operative outcome in a defined population. *Quality in Health Care*, **2**, 17–20.

Gulliford, M.C., Bell, J., Bourne, H., and Petruckevitch, A. (1993*b*). The reliability of cancer registry data. *British Journal of Cancer*, **67**, 819–21.

McColl, A.J. and Gulliford, M.C. (1993). *Population health outcome indicators for the NHS.* London: Faculty of Public Health Medicine and Department of Public Health Medicine, United Medical and Dental Schools of Guy's and St Thomas' Hospitals.

Morgan, M. and Watkins, C. (1988). Managing hypertension: beliefs and responses to medication among cultural groups. *Sociology Health and Illness*, **10**, 561–78.

Wolfe, C.D.A, Taub, N.A., Woodrow, J. *et al.* (1993*a*). Does the incidence, severity, or case fatality of stroke vary in southern England? *Journal of Epidemiology and Community Health*, **47**, 139–43.

Wolfe, C.D.A., Taub, N.A., Woodrow, J., *et al.* (1993*b*). Patterns of acute stroke in three districts of southern England. *Journal of Epidemiology and Community Health*, **47**, 144–8.

ETUDE SUR LES 'MORTS EVITABLES' EN ANGLETERRE ET GALLES

W.W. Holland

La sélection des études qui suit illustre quelques uns des travaux entrepris par le Département de Santé publique de l'Ecole dentaire et de médecine de Guy's et Thomas's Hôpital.

Nos études des accidents vasculaires cérébraux (AVC) commencèrent par une description de l'incidence et des cas mortels dans trois districts (Wolfe *et al.* 1993*a*, *b*). La variation observée de la mortalité par accident vasculaire cérébral ne résultait pas de différences de létalité mais bien plutôt de différences dans l'incidence. Le district ayant le rapport de mortalité standardisé le plus élevé avait aussi l'incidence la plus forte d'attaques et la plus forte fréquence de personnes d'origine afro-caraïbe, un groupe qui pourrait être particulièrement à risque d'hypertension et par conséquent d'attaque. Il en a été conclu que les services de prévention et les méthodes de dépistage des facteurs de risque devaient être améliorés ainsi que les services de soins à ces personnes. Nous menons actuellement des essais contrôlés randomisés afin de déterminer les moyens les plus efficaces de gérer les patients, à la fois avant et après la sortie de l'hôpital. Ceci est associé d'une part à des études pratiques pour déterminer les insuffisances des soins et d'autre part à un programme européen Biomed, dans lequel nous coordonnons une série d'études cherchant à déterminer la relation entre l'utilisation des ressources, le coût, et le résultat des soins des attaques, dans les différents pays européens.

Les résultats de notre étude originale, ainsi que les considérations gouvernementales sur les minorités ethniques, nous ont conduit à examiner les problèmes de santé de ces minorités. Ceci s'est développé dans une vaste étude des facteurs de risque d'attaques dans le groupe de la minorité ethnique afro-caraïbe. Les hémoglobinopathies sont un problème spécifique des afro-caraïbes et nous espérons étendre ce travail à l'étude des crises douloureuses de la maladie drépanocytose.

Une prévention appropriée et des soins cliniques efficaces dépendent souvent de la compréhension et des croyances des patients à propos de leur maladie et de son traitement médical. Ce domaine a constitué un objet important de recherche en science sociale. L'étude des patients hypertendus a fourni des informations nouvelles sur les croyances et les pratiques médicamenteuses des populations afro-caraïbes aidant ainsi les médecins généralistes à améliorer la communication avec ces groupes de patients (Morgan *et al.* 1988). Une recherche similaire sur les représentations parentales, et la gestion de l'asthme infantile, est maintenant entreprise et s'intéresse tout particulièrement aux raisons du faible niveau d'adhésion au traitement.

Une récente étude des taux d'admission pour asthme, a considéré 20 zones d'Angleterre et Galles, choisies de manière à représenter une large variation de la mortalité (Burney *et al.* 1991). L'étude a considéré les taux d'admission pour asthme des hommes âgés entre 20 et 44 ans. Les auteurs conclurent que les taux d'admission n'étaient pas seulement dictés par les caractères des services de santé, mais reflétaient également la demande. Une étude locale d'évaluation d'une intervention de santé publique pour améliorer le traitement de l'asthme est maintenant mise en route.

Le département coordonne actuellement une étude internationale, financée par la Communauté Européenne, pour étudier la variation de l'asthme et de la symptomatologie asthmatiforme, à travers l'Europe et d'autres parties du monde (Burney *et al.* 1994).

Ensemble, avec la Faculté de médecine de Santé publique, nous avons agi comme le centre de production d'une série d'indicateurs possibles pour les morts évitables et la morbidité de manière à essayer d'identifier la production des services de santé (McColl *et al.* 1993). Le premier volume a été récemment publié et un second est en cours de production.

Ces indicateurs peuvent fournir aux autorités davantage d'informations sur la réalisation de leur politique d'amélioration de la santé de la nation.

L'interprétation des indicateurs de santé requiert des informations supplémentaires concernant les influences sur l'incidence et le déroulement de la maladie dans les populations. Les données de registre du cancer furent utilisées à titre d'échantillon pour une série d'études sur l'issue de cancers courants tels que les cancers de la vessie et de l'oesophage (Gulliford *et al.* 1991*a*, 1993*a*). Actuellement le défi est d'identifier les informations critiques requises pour évaluer les services et mettre en place des systèmes qui pourraient capter sûrement de telles données sur longues périodes et dans différents sites.

Références

Burney, P.G.J., Luczynska, C., Chinn, S., and Jarvis, D. (1994). The European Community Respiratory Health Survey. *European Respiratory Journal*, **7**, 954–60.

Burney, P.G.J., Papacosta, A.O., Withey, C.H., Colley, J.R.T. *et al.* (1991). Hospital admission rates and the prevalence of asthma symptoms in 20 local authority districts. *Thorax*, **46**, 574–9.

Gulliford, M.C., Petruckevitch, A., and Burney, P.G.J. (1991*a*). Survival with bladder cancer, evaluation of delay in treatment, type of surgeon and modality of treatment. *British Medical Journal*, **302**, 437–40.

Gulliford, M.C., Petruckevitch, A., and Burney, P.G.J. (1991*b*). Hospital case notes and medical audit: evaluation of non-response. *British Medical Journal*, **302**, 1128–9.

Gulliford, M.C. (1992). Evaluating prognostic factors: implications for measurement of health care outcome. *Journal of Epidemiology and Community Health*, **46**, 323–6.

Gulliford, M.C., Barton, J.R., and Bourne, H. (1993*a*). Selection for oesophagectomy and post-operative outcome in a defined population. *Quality in Health Care*, **2**, 17–20.

Gulliford, M.C., Bell, J., Bourne, H., and Petruckevitch, A. (1993*b*). The reliability of cancer registry data. *British Journal of Cancer*, **67**, 819–21.

McColl, A.J. and Gulliford, M.C. (1993). *Population health outcome indicators for the NHS*. London: Faculty of Public Health Medicine and Department of Public Health Medicine, United Medical and Dental Schools of Guy's and St Thomas' Hospitals.

Morgan, M. and Watkins, C. (1988). Managing hypertension: beliefs and responses to medication among cultural groups. *Sociology Health and Illness*, **10**, 561–78.

Wolfe, C.D.A, Taub, N.A., Woodrow, J. *et al.* (1993*a*). Does the incidence, severity, or case fatality of stroke vary in southern England? *Journal of Epidemiology and Community Health*, **47**, 139–43.

Wolfe, C.D.A., Taub, N.A., Woodrow, J., *et al.* (1993*b*). Patterns of acute stroke in three districts of southern England. *Journal of Epidemiology and Community Health*, **47**, 144–8.

STUDIEN ÜBER 'VERMEIDBARE TODESFÄLLE' IN ENGLAND UND WALES

W.W. Holland

Die folgende Auswahl an Studien veranschaulicht einen Teil der Arbeiten über 'vermeidbare Todesfälle", die das Department of Public Health Medicine of United Medical and Dental Schools of Guy's and St Thomas's ausführt.

Unsere Studien zum Schlaganfall in drei örtlichen Bezirken begannen mit einer Beschreibung des Auftretens und des, in einigen Fällen, tödlichen Verlaufs (Wolfe *et al.* 1993*a*, *b*). Die beobachteten Unterschiede bei der Sterblichkeit ergaben sich nicht aufgrund von Unterschieden in der Anzahl der Todesfälle selbst, sondern durch Unterschiede in ihrem Auftreten. Der Bezirk mit der höchsten standardisierten Sterblichkeitsrate wies gleichzeitig das größte Vorkommen von Schlaganfällen und zudem die größte Zahl von Betroffenen afrikanisch-karibischen Ursprungs auf. Diese Gruppe mag besonders unter dem Risiko von Bluthochdruck und infolgedessen eines Schlaganfalls stehen. Man kam zu dem Schluß, daß sowohl vorbeugende Maßnahmen, Methoden zur Erkennung von Risikofaktoren als auch Einrichtungen zur Behandlung von Schlaganfallpatienten der Verbesserung bedürfen. Dementsprechend führen wir zur Zeit zufallsgeleitete Versuche durch, um das am kostenwirksamste Mittel bei der Behandlung von Schlaganfallpatienten vor und nach der Entlassung aus dem Krankenhaus zu bestimmen. Diese Versuche sind wiederum mit praktischen Studien zur Ermittlung von Mängeln bei der medizinischen Versorgung sowie dem europäischen BIOMED-Programm verbunden. Im Rahmen des BIOMED-Programms koordinieren wir eine Reihe von Studien, die das Verhältnis zwischen Resourcennutzung, Kosten und Ergebnissen der Betreuung nach einem Schlaganfall in verschiedenen Ländern Europas untersuchen.

Die Ergebnisse unserer ursprünglichen Schlaganfallstudie sowie die Sorge der Regierung um das gesundheitliche Wohl ethnischer Minderheiten veranlaßte uns zu einer Untersuchung der Gesundheitsprobleme in der letzteren Gruppe. Dies entwickelte sich zu einer umfangreicheren Studie der Risikofaktoren für einen Schlaganfall innerhalb der afro-karibischen, ethnischen Minderheitengruppe. Die Haemoglobinopathies ist ein besonderes Problem dieser Gruppe und wir hoffen, diese Arbeit um die Studie der Sichelzellenkrankheit zu erweitern.

Die Bereitstellung angemessener und wirksamer Maßnahmen der Vorbeugung und klinischen Betreuung hängt nicht selten vom Vetrauen der Patienten in die medizinischen Voraussetzungen und Behandlungsweisen ab. Dieses Gebiet ist zu einem wichtigen Gegenstand der sozialwissenschaftlichen Forschung geworden. Die Beobachtung unter Bluthochdruck leidender Patienten lieferte neue Informationen über Vorstellungen und Behandlungsmethoden innerhalb der afro-karibischen Gemeinde. Dadurch konnte den Allgemeinärzten geholfen werden, besser mit dieser Patientengruppe ins Gespräch zu kommen (Morgan und Watkins 1988). Ähnliche Untersuchungen über die Einstellung der Eltern und der Handhabung von Asthma bei Kindern finden zur Zeit statt und beschäftigen sich hauptsächlich mit den Gründen geringer Zustimmung zur Behandlung.

Eine jüngst unternommene Studie der Aufnahmeraten von Asthmapatienten in Krankenhäusern erstreckte sich über 20 Regionen von England und Wales um dadurch eine große Bandbreite an Todesfällen zu erfassen (Burney *et al.* 1991). Es wurden die Fälle von Männern zwischen 20 und 44 Jahren untersucht. Die Autoren stellten fest, daß Aufnahmeraten von Asthmapatienten nicht einzig und allein von den Eigentümlichkeiten der Gesundheitsdienste bestimmt waren, sondern auch den Bedarf wiederspiegelten. Es findet eine örtliche Studie zur Evaluierung des Eingreifens auf Gemeindebasis statt, um die Behandlung von Asthma zu verbessern.

Das Department koordiniert zur Zeit eine internationale, von der EG finanzierte Untersuchung der Unterschiede bei Asthma und asthmaähnlichen Symptomen in ganz Europa sowie anderen Teilen der Erde (Burney *et al.* 1994).

In Zusammenarbeit mit der Faculty of Public Health Medicine haben wir als Sammelpunkt gewirkt, eine Reihe von möglichen Indikatoren für vermeidbare Todesfälle und Morbidität zu ermitteln, um somit den Einfluß der Gesundheitsdienste zu erkennen (McColl und Gulliford 1993). Der erste Band ist kürzlich erschienen und ein zweiter Band ist in Bearbeitung. Diese Indikatoren könnten die Behörden mit mehr Informationen über deren Leistungen bezüglich der Verbeserung der Gesundheit in der Bevölkerung versorgen.

Die Interpretation von Indikatoren zu Ergebnissen gesundheitlicher Versorgung bedarf zusätzlicher Informationen, die sich mit den Einflüssen auf das Auftreten und den Verlauf von Krankheiten in der Bevölkerung auseinandersetzen. Die amtlich festgehaltenen Daten über Krebserkrankungen dienten als Musterrahmen für eine Reihe von Studien über weit verbreitete Krebsarten wie Blasenkrebs oder Speiseröhrenkrebs (Gulliford *et al.* 1991*a*, 1993*a*). Diese Studien gewährten Einblick in die Vorgänge innerhalb des Gesundheitswesens und deren Zussamenhang mit der Sterblichkeit. Die hieraus gewonnenen Ergebnisse unterstrichen jedoch gleichzeitig die Schwierigkeiten, die sich aus der Benutzung von Beobachtungsdaten zur Bewertung der Effektivität des

Gesundheitswesens ergeben (Gulliford 1992), insbesondere dann, wenn die innerhalb dieses Systems gesammelten Daten unzuverlässig oder unvollständig sein können (Gulliford *et al.* 1991*b*, Gulliford *et al.* 1993*b*). Die Herausforderung besteht nun in der Bestimmung der entscheidenden Informationen, die benötigt werden, um die Gesundheistdienste zu bewerten und Systeme der zuverlässigen Datenerfassung über längere Zeiträume hinweg an verschiedenen Orten zu installieren.

Quellenangabe

Burney, P.G.J., Luczynska, C., Chinn, S., and Jarvis, D. (1994). The European Community Respiratory Health Survey. *European Respiratory Journal,* **7**, 954–60.

Burney, P.G.J., Papacosta, A.O., Withey, C.H., Colley, J.R.T. *et al.* (1991). Hospital admission rates and the prevalence of asthma symptoms in 20 local authority districts. *Thorax*, **46**, 574–9.

Gulliford, M.C., Petruckevitch, A., and Burney, P.G.J. (1991*a*). Survival with bladder cancer, evaluation of delay in treatment, type of surgeon and modality of treatment. *British Medical Journal,* **302**, 437–40.

Gulliford, M.C., Petruckevitch, A., and Burney, P.G.J. (1991*b*). Hospital case notes and medical audit: evaluation of non-response. *British Medical Journal,* **302**, 1128–9.

Gulliford, M.C. (1992). Evaluating prognostic factors: implications for measurement of health care outcome. *Journal of Epidemiology and Community Health*, **46**, 323–6.

Gulliford, M.C., Barton, J.R., and Bourne, H. (1993*a*). Selection for oesophagectomy and post-operative outcome in a defined population. *Quality in Health Care*, **2**, 17–20.

Gulliford, M.C., Bell, J., Bourne, H., and Petruckevitch, A. (1993*b*). The reliability of cancer registry data. *British Journal of Cancer*, **67**, 819–21.

McColl, A.J. and Gulliford, M.C. (1993). *Population health outcome indicators for the NHS*. London: Faculty of Public Health Medicine and Department of Public Health Medicine, United Medical and Dental Schools of Guy's and St Thomas' Hospitals.

Morgan, M. and Watkins, C. (1988). Managing hypertension: beliefs and responses to medication among cultural groups. *Sociology Health and Illness*, **10**, 561–78.

Wolfe, C.D.A, Taub, N.A., Woodrow, J. *et al.* (1993*a*). Does the incidence, severity, or case fatality of stroke vary in southern England? *Journal of Epidemiology and Community Health*, **47**, 139–43.

Wolfe, C.D.A., Taub, N.A., Woodrow, J., *et al.* (1993*b*). Patterns of acute stroke in three districts of southern England. *Journal of Epidemiology and Community Health*, **47**, 144–8.

STUDIES ON 'AVOIDABLE DEATH' IN SCOTLAND

V. Carstairs

Scotland occupies a position at the adverse end of the spectrum of mortality—for all causes and many specific causes of death. It is inevitable that much of the research effort will focus on those causes, (for example, cancer of the lung, heart diseases), which account for large numbers of deaths. In general, such research is directed towards reduction in the levels of mortality from these major causes, rather than addressing any variation in rates: avoidable factors are mainly identified as life-style factors rather than quality of care. Heart conditions attract much of the research effort with population-based studies such as the Scottish Heart Health Study (Tunstall-Pedoe *et al.* 1989) and participation in the WHO MONICA project (WHO MONICA Project 1988) providing significant examples. Both primary and secondary prevention programmes are now in place in some areas of Scotland with particularly high mortality, and participation in the WHO Health Cities project provides an example of international collaboration (Glasgow Healthy City Project 1995). Further research will evaluate the outcomes of these programmes. In addition to population-based studies numerous enquiries are investigating the role of biochemical factors.

Scotland has participated in the EC Eurodiab Project; one phase, concerned with certification and coding practice for deaths where diabetes plays a contributory role, found that 36 per cent of the variation in mortality attributed to diabetes in the countries which took part could be explained by differences in certification or coding practice (EURODIAB Study Group 1993).

Research into avoidable causes, as defined in this project (that is, those conditions in which the delivery of medical care can be seen as a critical factor), for the most part recognizes that the condition presents a significant health problem rather than being concerned with regional variations within Scotland. In this context confidential enquiries into avoidable factors have been carried out into both maternal and perinatal deaths over a number of years (Scottish Office 1995), with maternal deaths now being reported on a UK basis in view of the low number of such events (Departments of Health of the United Kingdom 1995). Factors influencing the incidence of Sudden Infant Death Syndrome have also been the subject of investigation (Arneil *et al.* 1985). Despite a decrease of two-thirds in the rate since that time a current case–control study reports similar findings, smoking in pregnancy being identified as the main risk factor (OR 6.9 mother, 9.0 both parents). The increased risk of prone and side-sleep positions is also still evident (Gibson 1995).

More specific studies are in progress into other factors influencing early death; for example, to improve the identification of pregnancies at risk of a fetal chromosome abnormality by the assay of pregnancy specific markers in maternal serum. A further study is examining the antecedent obstetric factors influencing respiratory function in preterm infants, while another is concerned with the prediction and prevention of asthma in high-risk neonates. The prevalence of asthma in the population in general is also the subject of a number of enquiries.

Yet another confidential enquiry has been initiated into all deaths occurring in surgical units (Scottish Mortality Study 1994). In 1994 this was extended to the whole of Scotland; in that year the specialties of general surgery, vascular surgery, urology and neurosurgery were covered, and will be reported in 1995, other specialties are progressively being added into this continuing programme.

Screening programmes for the early detection of cancer of the breast and cancer of the cervix have been in operation for a number of years and monitoring of the incidence of and mortality from these diseases, and evaluation of the programmes is in progress.

Research into variations within Scotland focuses on antecedent factors rather than the quality of heath care; one enquiry will examine the influence of climate on morbidity and mortality while another is reporting on the association with socio-economic conditions in small areas (McLoone and Boddy 1994).

References

Arneil, G.C., Brooke, H., Gibson, A.A.M., *et al.* (1985). National post-perinatal infant mortality and cot death study, Scotland 1981–82. *Lancet*, **1**, 740–3.

Departments of Health of the United Kingdom. (1995). Reports on confidential enquiries into maternal deaths in the UK 1988–1990, 2nd UK report. HMSO, London.

EURODIAB Study Group. (1993). European study of the certification of causes of death in six case histories in diabetes patients. *International Journal of Epidemiology*, **22**, 116–26.

Gibson, A.A.M. (1995). Interim results. Personal communication.

Glasgow Healthy City Project. (1995). The health of the city: a shared concern. 1992. *Glasgow City Health Plan.*

McLoone, P. and Boddy, F.A. (1994). Deprivation and mortality in Scotland, 1981 and 1991. *British Medical Journal*, **309**, 1465–70.

Scottish Mortality Study (1994). Annual report 1994.

Scottish Office (1995). Report on maternal and perinatal deaths in Scotland. 1980–1990. HMSO, Edinburgh.

Tunstall-Pedoe, H., Smith, W.C.S., Crombie, K., and Tavendale, R. (1989). Coronary risk factors and life-style variations across Scotland: results from the Scottish heart health study. *Scottish Medical Journal*, **34**, 550–5, 556–60.

WHO MONICA Project. (1988). Geographical variations in major risk factors of coronary heart disease in men and women aged 35–64 years. *WHO Statistics Quarterly*, 1988, **43** (3, 4), 115–54.

ETUDE SUR LES 'MORTS EVITABLES' EN ECOSSE

V. Carstairs

L'Ecosse occupe une position défavorable à l'extrémité du spectre de la mortalité—pour toutes causes et plusieurs causes spécifiques de décès. Il est inévitable que beaucoup des efforts de recherche soient centrés sur ces causes, c'est-à-dire le cancer du poumon et les maladies cardiaques, qui rendent compte d'une grand nombre des décès. En général cette recherche est dirigée vers la réduction des niveaux de la mortalité due à ces causes majeures, plutôt que visant une quelconque variation des taux: les facteurs évitables sont principalement identifiés comme des facteurs de mode de vie plutôt que de qualité des soins. Les maladies cardiaques concentrent beaucoup de l'effort de recherche mené avec des études en population, telle que l'Etude écossaise de santé du coeur (Tunstall-Pedoe *et al.* 1989) et la participation au projet Monica de l'OMS (WHO Monica Project 1988) qui fournissent des exemples significatifs. Les programmes, à la fois de prévention primaire et de prévention secondaire, sont maintenant en place dans quelques une des régions écossaises à taux particulièrement élevés de mortalité, et la participation au projet de l'OMS sur la santé des villes procure un exemple de collaboration internationale (Glasgow Healthy City Project 1995). Des recherches supplémentaires évalueront l'effet de ces programmes. Outre les études en population, de nombreuses enquêtes mènent des investigations sur le rôle des facteurs biochimiques.

L'Ecosse a participé au Projet européen Eurodiab l'une des phases relative à la certification et la pratique du codage pour les décès où le diabète joue un rôle contributif, a trouvé que 36 pour cent des variations de la mortalité attribuée au diabète dans les pays participants, pouvaient être expliqués par des différences de certification ou le codage (Groupe d'Étude Eurodiab 1993).

La recherche sur les morts évitables, telle que définie dans le projet (c'est-à-dire les états dans lesquels la délivrance des soins médicaux peut être vue comme un facteur critique), considère, pour une grande part, l'état pathologique étudié en tant que problème de santé significatif plutôt que d'être lié à des variations régionales. Dans ce contexte, des enquêtes confidentielles sur les facteurs évitables ont été entreprises à la fois pour les décès maternels et périnatals sur plusieurs années (Office Écossais 1995), les décès maternels étant maintenant rapportés au niveau du Royaume-Uni à cause du faible nombre de ces événements (Department of Health of the United Kingdom 1995). Les facteurs influençant l'incidence du syndrome de mort subite du nourrisson ont également été l'objet d'investigations (Arneil *et al.* 1985). En dépit d'une décroissance des deux-tiers depuis cette époque, une étude cas–témoins en cours trouve de façon similaire que la tabagisme durant la grossesse est identifié comme le principal facteur (OR mère 6,9, les deux parents 9,0). Le risque accru dû à la position ventrale et latérale de sommeil reste toujours évident (Gibson 1995).

Des études plus spécifiques progressent sur d'autres facteurs intervenant dans les morts prématurées, c'est-à-dire pour améliorer l'identification des grossesses à risque d'anomalies chromosomiques foetales, par l'essai de marqueurs spécifiques dans le sérum maternel. Une autre étude examine les facteurs obstétriques influençant la fonction respiratoire des enfants prématurés, tandis qu'une autre est relative à la prévision et la prévention de l'asthme parmi les nouveau-nés à haut risque. La prévalence de l'asthme, dans la population en général, est aussi le sujet de nombreuses enquêtes.

Une autre enquête confidentielle a débuté sur tous les décès intervenant dans les unités chirurgicales. En 1994, celle ci fut étendue à la totalité de l'Ecosse. Cette année-là les spécialités de chirurgie générale, chirurgie vasculaire, urologie, et neurochirurgie ont été couvertes; elles feront l'objet de rapport en 1995; d'autres spécialités seront progressivement ajoutées dans ce programme en développement.

Les programmes de dépistage précoce du cancer de sein et du cancer du col ont été opérationnels depuis un bon nombre d'années, la surveillance de l'incidence et de la mortalité de ces pathologies et l'évaluation des programmes progressent.

La recherche des variations internes à l'Ecosse a été centrée sur les facteurs antécédents plutôt que sur la qualité de soins; une enquête examinera l'influence du climat sur la morbidité et la mortalité tandis qu'une autre porte sur leur association avec les conditions socio-économiques, dans les petites zones (McLoone *et al,* 1994).

Références

Arneil, G.C., Brooke, H., Gibson, A.A.M., *et al.* (1985). National post-perinatal infant mortality and cot death study, Scotland 1981–82. *Lancet*, **1**, 740–3.

Departments of Health of the United Kingdom. (1995). Reports on confidential enquiries into maternal deaths in the UK 1988–1990, 2nd U.K. report. HMSO, London.

EURODIAB Study Group (1993). European study of the certification of causes of death in six case histories in diabetes patients. *International Journal of Epidemiology*, **22**, 116–26.

Gibson, A.A.M. (1995). Interim results. Personal communication.

Glasgow Healthy City Project. (1995). The health of the city: a shared concern. 1992. *Glasgow City Health Plan.*

McLoone, P. and Boddy, F.A. (1994). Deprivation and mortality in Scotland, 1981 and 1991. *British Medical Journal*, **309**, 1465–70.

Scottish Mortality Study (1994). Annual report 1994.

Scottish Office (1995). Report on maternal and perinatal deaths in Scotland. 1980–1990. HMSO, Edinburgh.

Tunstall-Pedoe, H., Smith, W.C.S., Crombie, K., and Tavendale, R. (1989). Coronary risk factors and life-style variations across Scotland: results from the Scottish heart health study. *Scottish Medical Journal*, **34**, 550–5, 556–60.

WHO MONICA Project. (1988). Geographical variations in major risk factors of coronary heart disease in men and women aged 35–64 years. *WHO Statistics Quarterly*, 1988, **43** (3, 4), 115–54.

STUDIEN ÜBER 'VERMEIDBARE TODESFÄLLE' IN SCHOTTLAND

V. Carstairs

Schottland belegt eine der ungünstigsten Positionen im Spektrum der Sterblichkeit bezogen auf allgemeine und besondere Todesursachen. Es ist daher unvermeidlich, daß sich viele Forschungsarbeiten auf diese Ursachen wie z.B. Lungenkrebs und Herzerkrankungen konzentrieren, die für eine große Zahl von Todesfällen verantwortlich sind. Im allgemeinen richtet sich das Interesse dieser Art von Forschung auf die Verminderung der Todesfälle aufgrund oben genannter Hauptursachen, weniger jedoch auf die Schwankungen der Todesraten. Als vermeidbare Faktoren werden in der Hauptsache Merkmale der Lebensweise definiert und weniger die Qualität gesundheitlicher Versorgung. Herzleiden erfahren ein hohes Interesse in der Forschung mit bevölkerungsbezogenen Studien wie der Scottish Heart Health Study (Tunstall-Pedoe *et al.* 1989) und der Teilnahme am WHO MONICA Projekt (WHO MONICA Project 1988). In einigen Regionen Schottlands mit besonders hohen Sterblichkeitsziffern laufen nun Programme zur primären und sekundären Vorbeugung. Die Teilnahme am WHO Healthy Cities Project liefert ein Beispiel internationaler Zusammenarbeit (Glasgow Healthy City Project 1995). Weitere Untersuchungen werden die Ergebnisse dieser Programme beurteilen. In Ergänzung zu den bevölkerungsbezogenen Studien überprüfen zahlreiche Untersuchungen die Rolle biochemischer Faktoren.

Schottland hat am EG Eurodiab Projekt teilgenommen. Eine bestimmte Phase des Projektes, die sich mit der Ausstellung von Todesscheinen und der Praxis der Kodierung von Todesfällen befaßte, kam zu dem Ergebnis, daß inden teilnehmenden Ländern Fällen, wo Diabetes zum Tod beigetragen hat, 36 prozent der Schwankungen in der Sterblichkeit durch die Unterschiede bei der Zertifikatausstellung und Kodierungspraxis zu erklären waren (EURODIAB Study Group 1993).

Die im Rahmen dieses Projektes definierte Erforschung vermeidbarer Todesursachen wie z.B. den Umständen, in denen die Ausübung medizinischer Versorgung als wichtiger Faktor gesehen werden kann, anerkennt zum größten Teil, daß das Leiden selbst eine bedeutendes gesundheitliches Problem darstellt und eine Untersuchung regionaler Schwankungen innerhalb Schottlands eher in den Hintergrund tritt. In diesem Zusammenhang wurden vertraulich durchgeführte Nachforschungen zu Todesfällen von Müttern über einen Zeitraum mehrerer Jahre hinweg angestellt (Scottish Office 1995). Diese Todesfälle werden angesichts ihres seltenen Auftretens nun für das Vereinigte Königreich insgesamt festgehalten (Departments of Health of the United Kingdom 1995). Faktoren, die das Auftreten des plötzlichen Kindstodes (Sudden Infant Death Sybdrome) beeinflussen, waren ebenfalls Gegenstand der Forschung (Arneil *et al.* 1985). Trotz einer Verminderung der Todesraten um zwei Drittel seit diesem Zeitpunkt berichtet eine verbreitete Fallstudie von ähnlichen Ergebnissen, wonach Rauchen während der Schwangerschaft als Hauptrisikofaktor ausgemacht wurde (OR 6.9 Mutter, 9.0 beide Eltern). Das gesteigerte Risiko durch Bauch- und Seitenschlaflagen ist immer noch deutlich erkennbar (Gibson 1995).

Es finden zur Zeit genauere Studien zu weiteren Faktoren, die einen frühen Tod bewirken, statt. So soll beispielsweise die Erkennung von Schwangerschaften mit dem Risiko einer fötalen Chromosomen-Abnormalität durch eine Probe schwangerschaftsspezifischer Merkmale im Fruchtwasser verbessert werden. Eine weitere Studie untersucht die vorausgehenden Geburtshilfefaktoren, die die Atemwegsfunktionen bei Frühgeborenen beeinflussen. Wieder eine andere Studie beschäftigt sich mit der Vorhersage und Vermeidung von Asthma bei davon besonders gefährdeten Neugeborenen. Das Vorherrschen von Asthma in der Bevölkerung im allgemeinen ist ebenfalls Gegenstand einer Anzahl von Untersuchungen.

Eine weitere vertrauliche Untersuchung ist in die Wege geleitet worden, die sich mit allen Todesfällen in chirurgischen Abteilungen befaßt (Scottish Mortality Study 1994). 1994 wurde diese Untersuchung auf ganz Schottland ausgeweitet. In jenem Jahr wurden die Merkmale der allgemeinen und Gefäßchirurgie, der Urologie und Neurochirurgie abgedeckt und werden 1995 veröffentlicht. Andere Merkmale werden dem fortlaufenden Programm stetig hinzugefügt.

Untersuchungsprogramme zur Früherkennung von Brustkrebs und Cervix-Karzinom sind seit Jahren im Einsatz. Die Überwachung der Vorfälle von und der Todesfälle durch diese Krankheiten sowie eine Bewertung dieser Programme sind im Gange.

Die Untersuchung der Unterschiede innerhalb Schottlands konzentriert sich auf die vorausgehenden Faktoren und weniger auf die Qualität medizinischer Versorgung. Eine der Studien wird den Einfluß von Klima auf Erkrankungsziffern und Sterblichkeit prüfen, während eine andere über die Verbindung mit sozio-ökonomischen Bedingungen in kleineren Gebieten berichten wird (McLoone und Boddy 1994).

Quellenangabe

Arneil, G.C., Brooke, H., Gibson, A.A.M., *et al.* (1985). National post-perinatal infant mortality and cot death study, Scotland 1981–82. *Lancet*, **1**, 740–3.

Departments of Health of the United Kingdom. (1995). Reports on confidential enquiries into maternal deaths in the UK 1988–1990, 2nd U.K. report. HMSO, London.

EURODIAB Study Group (1993). European study of the certification of causes of death in six case histories in diabetes patients. *International Journal of Epidemiology*, **22**, 116–26.

Gibson, A.A.M. (1995). Interim results. Personal communication.

Glasgow Healthy City Project. (1995). The health of the city: a shared concern. 1992. *Glasgow City Health Plan.*

McLoone, P. and Boddy, F.A. (1994). Deprivation and mortality in Scotland, 1981 and 1991. *British Medical Journal*, **309**, 1465–70.

Scottish Mortality Study (1994). Annual report 1994.

Scottish Office (1995). Report on maternal and perinatal deaths in Scotland. 1980–1990. HMSO, Edinburgh.

Tunstall-Pedoe, H., Smith, W.C.S., Crombie, K., and Tavendale, R. (1989). Coronary risk factors and life-style variations across Scotland: results from the Scottish heart health study. *Scottish Medical Journal*, **34**, 550–5, 556–60.

WHO MONICA Project. (1988). Geographical variations in major risk factors of coronary heart disease in men and women aged 35–64 years. *WHO Statistics Quarterly*, 1988, **43** (3, 4), 115–54.

STUDIES ON 'AVOIDABLE DEATH' IN PORTUGAL

J. A. A. Dias

In recent years there has been a marked decrease in maternal mortality in Portugal. In fact, maternal death rates fell from 10.1 to 6.1/100000 live births (lb) from 1989 to 1993. Infant death rates have also declined from 12.1 to 8.6/1000 lb and perinatal mortality showed a similar trend, falling from 14.5 to 9.2/1000 lb in the same period (Araújo 1995; Serviço de Informação de Saúde 1994).

Policy developments from 1974 onwards have achieved a broad coverage through the health centres at the community level. The expenditure on perinatal surveillance and the increase in hospital delivery (Alves *et al.* 1994), as well as the creation of the National Commission for Maternal Health in 1988, have played a central role in reducing these avoidable causes of death (Departamento de Estudos e Planeamento da Saúde 1995).

During the five-year period of 1989–93 the standardized mortality rates of diabetes mellitus, lung, breast, colon, and prostrate cancers showed a steady increase, while cerebrovascular diseases, traffic accidents, and stomach cancer showed a slight decrease in their pattern of evolution (Departamento de Estudos e Planeamento da Saúde 1995; Dias 1993; Dias and Falcäo 1994; Serviço de Informação de Saúde 1993; Leitão 1993*a*, *b*; Marques 1993).

References

Alves, V., Pinto, E., and Fernanda, M. (1994). Incidência, mortalidade, morbilidade e desenvolvimento de recém-nascidos com idade gestacional inferior ou igual a 33 semanas. *Nascer e Crescer,* **3,** 25–39.

Araújo, M.P. (1995). Mortes maternas em Portugal: 1979–1993. *DGS–Ministério da Saúde,* 1–27.

Departamento de Estudos e Planeamento da Saúde. (1995). A saúde em Portugal. *DEPS–Ministério da Saúde,* 1–48.

Dias, J.A.A. (1993). Tumores malignos das principais localizações em Portugal. *Revista Portuguesa de Saúde Pública,* **11**, 15–31.

Dias, J.A.A. and Falcão, I.M. (1994). Análise da variação percentual das taxas de mortalidade por acidente vascular cerebral e doença isquémica do miocárdio nos triénios 1980–82 e 1990–92 a nivel distrital. *Saúde em Números,* **9**, 5–7.

Leitão, A.E. (1993*a*). Evolução recente da mortalidade em Portugal no grupo etário de 15 a 44 anos. *Saúde em Números,* **8**, 25–30.

Leitão, A.E. (1993*b*). Acidentes evitáveis; dia mundial da saúde. *DGS–Ministério da Saúde,* Abril, 1–24.

Marques, F.V.S. (1993). Rastreio dos cancros da mama e do colo do útero: opinião e prática de médicos de Clínica Geral. *Revista Portuguesa de Saúde Pública,* **11**, 5–14.

Seviço de Informação de Saúde. (1993). Risco de morrer em Portugal. *DGS–Ministério da Saúde,* 1–180.

Seviço de Informação de Saúde. (1994). Mortalidade infantil, perinatal e materna 1989–94. *DGS–Ministério da Saúde,* 1993 e 1994.

ETUDE SUR LES 'MORTS EVITABLES' AU PORTUGAL

J.A.A.Dias

Dans les années récentes il y a eu une baisse marquée de la mortalité maternelle au Portugal. Le taux de mortalité maternelle est tombé de 10,1 à 6,1 pour 100000 naissances vivantes de 1989 à 1993. Les taux de mortalité infantile, aussi, ont décliné de 12,0 à 5,6 pour 1000 et la mortalité périnatale a montré une tendance similaire, tombant de 14,5 à 9,2 pour 1000 durant la même période (Araújo 1995; Service d'Information sur la Santé 1994).

La politique développée depuis 1974 et ensuite, a atteint une bonne couverture de la population à travers les centres de santé au niveau communautaire. La dépense en surveillance périnatale et l'augmentation des accouchements à l'hôpital (Alves et al., 1994) aussi bien que la création de la Commission nationale sur la santé maternelle en 1988, ont joué un rôle central dans la réduction de ces causes de morts évitables (Département des études et de la planification sanitaire 1995).

Durant la période quinquennale 1989–93, les taux standardisés de mortalité par diabète, cancers du poumon, du sein, du colon, et de la prostate ont montré un accroissement régulier, tandis que les maladies cérébro-vasculaires, les accidents de la route et le cancer de l'estomac montrèrent une évolution en léger déclin (Département des études et du plan de santé, 1995; Dias 1993; Dias et Falcão 1994; Service d'information sur la santé 1993; Leitão 1993*a*, *b*; Marques 1993).

Références

Alves, V., Pinto, E., and Fernanda, M. (1994). Incidência, mortalidade, morbilidade e desenvolvimento de recém-nascidos com idade gestacional inferior ou igual a 33 semanas. *Nascer e Crescer,* **3,** 25–39.

Araújo, M.P. (1995). Mortes maternas em Portugal: 1979–1993. *DGS–Ministério da Saúde,* 1–27.

Departamento de Estudos e Planeamento da Saúde. (1995). A saúde em Portugal. *DEPS–Ministério da Saúde,* 1–48.

Dias, J.A.A. (1993). Tumores malignos das principais localizações em Portugal. *Revista Portuguesa de Saúde Pública,* **11**, 15–31.

Dias, J.A.A. and Falcão, I.M. (1994). Análise da variação percentual das taxas de mortalidade por acidente vascular cerebral e doença isquémica do miocárdio nos triénios 1980–82 e 1990–92 a nivel distrital. *Saúde em Números,* **9**, 5–7.

Leitão, A.E. (1993*a*). Evolução recente da mortalidade em Portugal no grupo etário de 15 a 44 anos. *Saúde em Números,* **8**, 25–30.

Leitão, A.E. (1993b). Acidentes evitáveis; dia mundial da saúde. *DGS–Ministério da Saúde,* Abril, 1–24.

Marques, F.V.S. (1993). Rastreio dos cancros da mama e do colo do útero: opinião e prática de médicos de Clínica Geral. *Revista Portuguesa de Saúde Pública,* **11**, 5–14.

Seviço de Informação de Saúde. (1993). Risco de morrer em Portugal. *DGS–Ministério da Saúde,* 1–180.

Seviço de Informação de Saúde. (1994). Mortalidade infantil, perinatal e materna 1989–94. *DGS–Ministério da Saúde,* 1993 e 1994.

STUDIEN ÜBER 'VERMEIDBARE TODESFÄLLE' IN PORTUGAL

J.A.A. Dias

In den vergangenen Jahren ist es zu einer merklichen Abnahme in der Müttersterblichkeit in Portugal gekommen. Tatsächlich fiel die Müttersterblichkeitsrate vom 10.1 auf 6.1/100000 Lebendgeburten (lb) zwischen 1989 und 1993. Ebenso ist die Sterblichkeitsrate bei Säuglingen von 12.1 auf 8.6/1000 lb abgesunken. Die perinatale Sterblichkeitsrate wies eine ähnliche Entwicklung auf und fiel von 14,5 auf 9,2 /1000 lb innerhalb desselben Zeitraums (Araújo 1995, Serviço de Informação de Saúde 1994).

Die Entwicklungen der Vorgehensweise haben seit 1974 einen weiten Verbreitungsgrad in den Gesundheitszentren auf Gemeindeebene erreicht. Die Ausgaben für perinatale Überwachung und die Zunahme an Geburten im Krankenhaus (Alves *et al.* 1994) sowie die Schaffung der Nationlen Kommisssion für Müttergesundheit 1988 haben eine zentrale Rolle bei der Reduzierung dieser vermeidbaren Todesursachen geführt (Departamento de Estudos e Planeamento da Saúde 1995).

Während des Zeitraums zwischen 1989–93 zeigte die standardisierte Sterblichkeitsrate für Diabetes Mellitus, Lungen-, Brust-, Dickdarm-, und Prostatakrebs einen stetigen Anstieg, während Gehirngefäßerkrankungen, Verkehrsunfälle und Magenkrebs eine leichte Abnahme in ihrem Evolutionsmuster aufwiesen (Departamento de Estudos e Planeamento da Saúde 1995; Dias 1993; Dias und Falcão 1994; Serviço de Informação de Saúde 1993; Leitão 1993*a*; Leitão 1993*b*; Marques 1993).

Quellenangabe

Alves, V., Pinto, E., and Fernanda, M. (1994). Incidência, mortalidade, morbilidade e desenvolvimento de recém-nascidos com idade gestacional inferior ou igual a 33 semanas. *Nascer e Crescer,* **3**, 25–39.

Araújo, M.P. (1995). Mortes maternas em Portugal: 1979–1993. *DGS–Ministério da Saúde,* 1–27.

Departamento de Estudos e Planeamento da Saúde. (1995). A saúde em Portugal. *DEPS–Ministério da Saúde,* 1–48.

Dias, J.A.A. (1993). Tumores malignos das principais localizações em Portugal. *Revista Portuguesa de Saúde Pública,* **11**, 15–31.

Dias, J.A.A. and Falcão, I.M. (1994). Análise da variação percentual das taxas de mortalidade por acidente vascular cerebral e doença isquémica do miocárdio nos triénios 1980–82 e 1990–92 a nivel distrital. *Saúde em Números,* **9**, 5–7.

Leitão, A.E. (1993*a*). Evolução recente da mortalidade em Portugal no grupo etário de 15 a 44 anos. *Saúde em Números,* **8**, 25–30.

Leitão, A.E. (1993*b*). Acidentes evitáveis; dia mundial da saúde. *DGS–Ministério da Saúde,* Abril, 1–24.

Marques, F.V.S. (1993). Rastreio dos cancros da mama e do colo do útero: opinião e prática de médicos de Clínica Geral. *Revista Portuguesa de Saúde Pública,* **11**, 5–14.

Seviço de Informação de Saúde. (1993). Risco de morrer em Portugal. *DGS–Ministério da Saúde,* 1–180.

Seviço de Informação de Saúde. (1994). Mortalidade infantil, perinatal e materna 1989–94. *DGS–Ministério da Saúde,* 1993 e 1994.

STUDIES ON 'AVOIDABLE DEATH' IN SPAIN

M.J. Medrano, M.V. Martínez de Aragón, and M.J. Barrado

In this report some of the most interesting characteristics of mortality in Spain will be presented and discussed. These findings are the results of several recent and on-going mortality studies with the common objective of serving as an epidemiological basis for public health intervention. Unfortunately, morbidity data available in our country are too scarce and incomplete to set priorities at a national level. The main studies on avoidable mortality carried out in Spain in the last few years are also commented upon.

General features of mortality in Spain

Spain enjoys one of the lowest general death rates and one of the highest life expectancies in Europe. The age, sex, and cause specific mortality pattern is as expected for developed countries, with most deaths occurring late in life and mostly due to cardiovascular diseases and cancer. However, new conditions have emerged causing a strong impact on mortality, especially amongst young adults through AIDS and motor vehicle injuries. Thus mortality in the age group 15–44 is very high when compared with rates in other EC countries, and in the last five years has increased in both sexes more than in any other country in Europe. Men exhibit higher death rates in all ages, the ratio of death rates in men and women being larger, probably due to social and cultural factors. Smoking related diseases, such as ischaemic heart disease (IHD), lung cancer and chronic respiratory disease, are the primary cause of death in Spain, but specific death rates for these conditions remain among the lowest in the EC. On the contrary, infectious diseases account only for 1 per cent of all deaths, but show high death rates in the European context.

Cardiovascular diseases are the most frequent cause of death in our country, representing 35 per cent in men and 48 per cent in women of the total number of deaths. Mortality from IHD was stable during the first half of the century, but rose sharply in the 1950–70 decades. Since 1975 mortality has fallen with a statistically significant decrease. This change in trends seems unrelated to time variations in prevalence of the main risk factors or competing causes of death, and age–period–cohort analyses show a decreasing period effect that could partially explain these trends. Moreover, spatial distribution of IHD mortality seems independent of age- and sex-related variables. Therefore, we believe that accessibility to qualified medical care is an effective intervention, mostly in provinces showing high rates such as the Canary Islands, Balearic Islands, and Andalucia.

Stroke mortality in Spain ranks on a medium level when compared with data from other European countries, and has been steadily falling since 1900 and more markedly since the mid-1970s, several years before anti-hypertensive drugs were widely available. A marked negative cohort effect has been identified. Again geographical areas located in the south and the Islands display rates in the highest quintile that are similar to those of European countries with the highest mortality (Barrado Lanzarote *et al.* in press). More in-depth studies are needed to explore potential roles of different factors in determining stroke mortality, including medical care.

Mortality from lung cancer in men is rising dramatically, whereas it is stable or even falling in northern European countries. Conversely, Spanish women have not increased their risk of dying from lung cancer. This trend may change in the future because of changing patterns in smoking habits; current data show that smoking prevalence is decreasing in men, mostly with the young, but sharply increasing in women. Accordingly, mortality in younger men tends to a plateau and younger cohorts show a lower risk of dying. As there are no outstanding improvements in lung cancer treatment, priorities set on prevention of smoking must be continued.

Spain has the lowest breast cancer death rates in Europe, but it is increasing in all age groups, whilst the rest of Europe, except Greece, shows a decrease with time. Given the improvement in survival derived from early detection and treatment, this increase in mortality reflects either a strong increase in incidence and/or severity, or poor access to secondary prevention. The period effect is stable, but risk by birth cohort has been increasing along the century. Current knowledge about risk factors for breast cancer is poor, so for the moment early detection programmes appear as the most effective strategy for prevention.

Spain presents high death rates for external causes in men, mostly due to motor vehicle accidents, which are the primary cause of death in young ages and the primary cause of potential years of life lost. Spain and Portugal are the only EC countries where this mortality increased in recent years, although the most recent data show a slight tendency towards stabilization. Alcohol seems an important factor implicated in mortality by motor vehicle accidents, and its consumption appears to have increased among the young population.

We conclude that efforts must be placed in tobacco and alcohol consumption prevention strategies, in promoting a healthy Mediterranean diet and in improvement of the accessibility to qualified medical care, especially for early diagnosis of breast cancer, cardiovascular risk factors, and ischaemic heart disease.

Research on avoidable mortality in Spain

It can be stated that the concept of avoidable mortality has reached a certain degree of popularity amongst Spanish epidemiologists and public health investigators. Several relevant studies have been published, and the 'avoidable death' indicators are now currently used by the health departments of some regions and at a national level. A few of these have made proposals for better use and understanding of this indicator as a public health tool, more than simply a method of medical care evaluation. There has also been some discussion about the real meaning of this indicator and its potential weakness to identify health care inequities. At least one case–control study has also been carried out to analyse the 'avoidability' of deaths by selected causes in young ages, its main results being that the main predictor of death was severity at admission to hospital, indicating that avoidable mortality is more an indicator of access to medical care than that of the performance of these services.

All this work has motivated the interest of the main source of finance for health research in Spain, which has given its support to this line of research.

In conclusion, avoidable mortality has been successfully incorporated into epidemiological work in Spain, and the EC Concerted Action Project on Health Services and 'Avoidable Deaths' has been a major stimulus for this interest.

References and further reading

Alfonso Sánchez, J., Sanchis Noguera, B., Prado del Baño, M.J., *et al.* (1993). Testing a new heath indicator: using aviodable causes of death and life expectancy for Spain between 1975–1986. *European Journal of Epidemiology*, **9**, 33–9.

Barrado Lanzarote, M.J., de Pedro Cuesta, J., and Almazán Isla, J. (1993). Stroke mortality in Spain, 1901–1986. *Neuroepidemiology*, **12**, 148–57.

Barrado Lanzarote, M.J., Medrano Albero, M.J., and de Pedro Cuesta, J. (1994*a*). Spatial distribution of stroke mortality in Spain. *Neuroepidemiology*, in press.

Barrado Lanzarote M.J., Medrano Albero M.J., and Almazán Isla J. (1994*b*) Mortalidad por cardiopatía isquémica. Serie temporal y distribución geográfica. *Revista Espanola de Cardiologia*, in press.

Barrado, M.J. and Medrano, M.J. Effect of age, birth cohort and period of death in mortality by stroke and ischaemic heart disease in Spain 1951–1991. Report in preparation.

Bernat Gil, L. and Rathwell, T. (1989). The effect of health services on mortality: amenable causes in Spain. *International Journal of Epidemiology*, **18**, 652–7.

Borrel i Thió, C., Plasència i Tardach, A., and Pañella i Noguera, H. (1991). Excés de mortalitat en una area urbana cèntrica: el cas de Ciutat Vella a Barcelona. *Gaceta Sanitaria*, **5**, 243–53.

Cerdeira, S., Abraira, L.,Alonso, J.M., *et al.* (1994). Mortalidad evitable en la Comunidad Autonoma Gallega. *Gaceta Sanitaria*, **8** (suppl), 50.

García Arcal, M.D., Pollán Santamaría, M., and López Abente, G. (1994). Mortalidad por cancer de mama en la Comunidad Europea (1970–1985). *Medicina Clinica (Barcelona)*, **102**, 125–8.

García Benavides, F.G., Orts, R., and Pérez, S. (1992). Adding years to life: effect of avoidable mortality on life expectancy at birth. *Journal of Epidemiology and Community Health*, **46**, 394–5.

García Benavides, F.G., Pérez, F., Cayuela, A., Nolasco, A., *et al.* (1990). Avoidable years of life lost ratio: an indicator to identify excess in mortality in health areas. *Gaceta Sanitaria*, **16**, 12–17.

Gispert, R. and Segura, A. (1990). La identificación de la mortalidad evitable y sus aplicaciones prácticas. *Gaceta Sanitaria*, **4**, 199–200.

Gispert, R., Moreno, C., and Rué, M. (1994). Es inevitable la mortalidad evitable? *Gaceta Sanitaria*, **8** (suppl), 51.

González Enriquez, J., Cerdá Mota, T., Regidor Poyatos, E., and Medrano Albero, M.J. (1989). Atlas de mortalidad evitable en España. *Ministerio de Sanidad y Consumo*. Madrid.

López Abente, G., Pollán Santamaría, M., Ruiz Tovar, M., *et al.* (1992). Cancer mortality in Spain 1952–1986. Effect of age, birth cohort and period of death. *Centro Nacional de Epidemiología*, Madrid.

Martínez de Aragón, M.V., Llácer Gil, A., Marín Rivero, M., and Martínez Navarro, F. (1993). Mortalidad en España 1989. Situacíon en el marco de la Unión Europea. *Ministerio de Sanidad y Consumo*. Madrid.

Pérez, J., Sanz, C., and Martínez, J.F. (1994). Análisis de la mortalidad por causas externas en España según el modelo de regresión de Preston. *Gaceta Sanitaria*, **44** (suppl), 208.

Regidor Poyatos, E. (1991). Acerca de la mortalidad evitable. *Gaceta Sanitaria*, **5**, 139–40.

ETUDE SUR LES 'MORTS EVITABLES' EN ESPAGNE

M.J. Medrano, M.V. Martínez de Aragón, et M.J. Barrado

Dans ce rapport, quelques unes des caractéristiques les plus intéressantes de la mortalité en Espagne seront présentées et discutées. Il s'agit des résultats de plusieurs études récentes, qui se poursuivent, sur la mortalité, dont l'objectif commun est de servir de base épidémiologique aux interventions de santé publique. Malheureusement, les données de morbidité disponibles dans notre pays sont trop rares et incomplètes pour établir des priorités à un niveau national. Les principales études sur les morts évitables traitées en Espagne dans les dernières années sont aussi commentées.

Caractères généraux de la mortalité en Espagne

L'Espagne a la chance d'avoir les taux les plus bas de mortalité générale et l'une des espérances de vie les plus élevées en Europe. L'âge, le sexe et la structure des causes de mortalité, sont ce que l'on attend dans les pays développés, avec la plupart des décès intervenant tard dans la vie, et principalement dus aux maladies cardio-vasculaires et aux cancers. Néanmoins de nouvelles conditions ont émergé, ayant un fort impact sur la mortalité spécialement parmi les jeunes adultes à travers le Sida et les traumatismes des accidents de la route. Ainsi la mortalité du groupe d'âge 15–44 est très élevée comparée aux taux des autres pays de la Communauté Européenne; elle a augmenté, au cours des cinq dernières années, pour les deux sexes davantage que dans les autres pays. Les hommes enregistrent des taux supérieurs de mortalité à tous les âges, l'indice de surmortalité masculine augmente, probablement en raison de facteurs culturels et sociaux. Les affections liées au tabagisme, telles que les cardiopathies ischémiques, le cancer du poumon, et les maladies respiratoires chroniques sont la première cause de mortalité en Espagne, mais les taux spécifiques de mortalité pour ces pathologies restent parmi les plus bas d'Europe. Au contraire, les maladies infectieuses qui comptent pour seulement 1 pour cent de tous les décès, ont des taux élevés pour un contexte européen.

Les maladies cardio-vasculaires sont la cause la plus fréquente de décès dans notre pays, représentant 35 pour cent du nombre total des décès des hommes et 48 pour cent des femmes. La mortalité par cardiopathies ischémiques était stable durant la première moitié du siècle, mais augmenta fortement dans les années 1950–70. Depuis 1975, la mortalité a diminué de manière statistiquement significative. Ce changement des tendances ne semble pas lié aux variations temporelles de la prévalence des principaux facteurs de risque, ou aux causes de décès concurrentes, et les analyses âge, période, et cohorte montrent un effet période, qui pourrait partiellement expliquer ces tendances. De plus la distribution spatiale des cardiopathies ischémiques semble indépendante des variables liées au sexe et à l'âge. Ainsi nous croyons que l'accessibilité à des soins médicaux qualifiés est une intervention efficace surtout dans les provinces montrant des taux élevés tels que les Iles Canaries, les Baléares, et l'Andalousie.

La mortalité due aux accidents vasculaires cérébraux (AVC), en Espagne, se range à un niveau moyen par comparaison aux données des autres pays européens ; elle a diminué régulièrement depuis 1900 et de manière plus marquée depuis le milieu des années 70, plusieurs années avant que les médicaments antihypertenseurs aient été largement disponibles. Un effet cohorte large et négatif a été identifié. De nouveau, des aires géographiques, situées dans le sud et les îles, montrent des taux dans les quintiles supérieurs qui sont similaires à ceux des pays européens aux taux les plus élevés. (Barrado Lanzarote *et al.*, in press). Des études plus approfondies sont nécessaires pour explorer le rôle potentiel des différents facteurs dans la survenue de la mortalité cérébro-vasculaire, y compris celui des soins.

La mortalité par cancer du poumon chez les hommes augmente dramatiquement, alors qu'elle est stable ou même diminue dans les pays européens du nord. Inversement, les femmes espagnoles n'ont pas augmenté leur risque de mourir par cancer du poumon. Cette tendance pourrait se modifier dans le futur en raison du changement des formes de tabagisme ; les données courantes montrent que la prévalence du tabagisme décroît chez les hommes surtout chez les jeunes, mais augmente de façon aiguë chez les femmes. De même la mortalité des jeunes hommes tend vers un plateau et les cohortes les plus jeunes montrent un risque plus faible de mourir. Comme il n'y a pas d'amélioration dans le traitement du cancer du poumon, la priorité doit être maintenue en faveur de la prévention.

L'Espagne a les taux de mortalité par cancer du sein les plus bas de l'Europe, mais ils sont en augmentation dans tous les groupes d'âge, tandis que les autres pays enregistrent une baisse, à l'exception de la Grèce. Etant donnée l'amélioration de la survie, grâce au dépistage précoce et au traitement, cette augmentation de la mortalité reflète soit un fort accroissement de l'incidence, ou de la sévérité, soit un accès insuffisant à la prévention secondaire. L'effet période est stable, mais le risque par cohorte de naissance a augmenté tout au long du siècle. Les connaissances courantes sur les facteurs de risque du cancer du sein étant limitées, le dépistage précoce apparaît comme la stratégie la plus efficace de prévention pour le moment.

L'Espagne présente des taux élevés de décès par cause extérieure de traumatismes, principalement dues aux accidents de véhicules, qui sont la première cause de décès des jeunes hommes et la première cause d'années potentielles de vie perdues. L'Espagne et le Portugal sont les deux seules nations de la Communauté Européenne où cette mortalité a augmenté dans les années récentes, bien que les plus récentes données indiquent une légère tendance à la stabilisation. L'alcool semble être un important facteur impliqué dans la mortalité par accidents de voiture et sa consommation paraît avoir augmenté parmi les jeunes.

Nous conclusons que les efforts doivent être portés sur la prévention de la consommation d'alcool et de tabac pour promouvoir la saine alimentation méditerranéenne, ainsi que l'amélioration de l'accès à des soins médicaux qualifiés, spécialement pour le diagnostic précoce du cancer du sein, les facteurs de risque cardio-vasculaires et les cardiopathies ischémiques.

Recherche sur la mortalité évitable en Espagne

On peut affirmer que le concept de mortalité évitable a atteint un certain degré de popularité parmi les épidémiologistes espagnols et les chercheurs en santé publique. Plusieurs études relatives à ce concept ont été publiées, et les indicateurs de mort évitable sont maintenant couramment utilisés par les départements de santé de certaines régions, et au niveau national. Des propositions ont été faites pour améliorer l'utilisation et la compréhension de cet indicateur en tant que règle de santé publique, et pas simplement comme méthode d'évaluation des soins médicaux. Il y a eu aussi quelques discussion à propos de la signification réelle de cet indicateur et sa faiblesse potentielle d'identification des inégalités de soins. Au moins un étude cas–témoins a été entreprise pour analyser 'l'évitabilité' des décès par certaines causes sélectionnées aux jeunes âges, ses principaux résultats étant que le principal prédicteur du décès était la sévérité de l'état à l'admission à l'hôpital, indiquant que la mortalité évitable est plus un indicateur d'accès aux soins qu'un indicateur de leur performance.

Tout ce travail a motivé l'intérêt de la principale source de financement pour la recherche en santé en Espagne, qui a donné son soutien à cette orientation de recherche.

En conclusion, la mortalité évitable a été incorporée avec succès dans les travaux épidémiologiques en Espagne, et le projet d'Action concertée européenne sur les services de santé et les morts évitables, a été un stimulant majeur pour l'intérêt qu'on lui a porté.

Références et à lire eventuellement

Alfonso Sánchez, J., Sanchis Noguera, B., Prado del Baño, M.J., *et al.* (1993). Testing a new heath indicator: using aviodable causes of death and life expectancy for Spain between 1975–1986. *European Journal of Epidemiology*, **9**, 33–9.

Barrado Lanzarote, M.J., de Pedro Cuesta, J., and Almazán Isla, J. (1993). Stroke mortality in Spain, 1901–1986. *Neuroepidemiology*, **12**, 148–57.

Barrado Lanzarote, M.J., Medrano Albero, M.J., and de Pedro Cuesta, J. (1994*a*). Spatial distribution of stroke mortality in Spain. *Neuroepidemiology*, in press.

Barrado Lanzarote M.J., Medrano Albero M.J., and Almazán Isla J. (1994*b*) Mortalidad por cardiopatía isquémica. Serie temporal y distribución geográfica. *Revista Espanola de Cardiologia*, in press.

Barrado, M.J. and Medrano, M.J. Effect of age, birth cohort and period of death in mortality by stroke and ischaemic heart disease in Spain 1951–1991. Report in preparation.

Bernat Gil, L. and Rathwell, T. (1989). The effect of health services on mortality: amenable causes in Spain. *International Journal of Epidemiology*, **18**, 652–7.

Borrel i Thió, C., Plasència i Tardach, A., and Pañella i Noguera, H. (1991). Excés de mortalitat en una area urbana cèntrica: el cas de Ciutat Vella a Barcelona. *Gaceta Sanitaria*, **5**, 243–53.

Cerdeira, S., Abraira, L.,Alonso, J.M., *et al.* (1994). Mortalidad evitable en la Comunidad Autonoma Gallega. *Gaceta Sanitaria*, **8** (suppl), 50.

García Arcal, M.D., Pollán Santamaría, M., and López Abente, G. (1994). Mortalidad por cancer de mama en la Comunidad Europea (1970–1985). *Medicina Clinica (Barcelona)*, **102**, 125–8.

García Benavides, F.G., Orts, R., and Pérez, S. (1992). Adding years to life: effect of avoidable mortality on life expectancy at birth. *Journal of Epidemiology and Community Health*, **46**, 394–5.

García Benavides, F.G., Pérez, F., Cayuela, A., Nolasco, A., *et al.* (1990). Avoidable years of life lost ratio: an indicator to identify excess in mortality in health areas. *Gaceta Sanitaria*, **16**, 12–17.

Gispert, R. and Segura, A. (1990). La identificación de la mortalidad evitable y sus aplicaciones prácticas. *Gaceta Sanitaria*, **4**, 199–200.

Gispert, R., Moreno, C., and Rué, M. (1994). Es inevitable la mortalidad evitable? *Gaceta Sanitaria*, **8** (suppl), 51.

González Enriquez, J., Cerdá Mota, T., Regidor Poyatos, E., and Medrano Albero, M.J. (1989). Atlas de mortalidad evitable en España. *Ministerio de Sanidad y Consumo*. Madrid.

López Abente, G., Pollán Santamaría, M., Ruiz Tovar, M., *et al.* (1992). Cancer mortality in Spain 1952–1986. Effect of age, birth cohort and period of death. *Centro Nacional de Epidemiología*, Madrid.

Martínez de Aragón, M.V., Llácer Gil, A., Marín Rivero, M., and Martínez Navarro, F. (1993). Mortalidad en España 1989. Situacíon en el marco de la Unión Europea. *Ministerio de Sanidad y Consumo*. Madrid.

Pérez, J., Sanz, C., and Martínez, J.F. (1994). Análisis de la mortalidad por causas externas en España según el modelo de regresión de Preston. *Gaceta Sanitaria*, **44** (suppl), 208.

Regidor Poyatos, E. (1991). Acerca de la mortalidad evitable. *Gaceta Sanitaria*, **5**, 139–40.

STUDIEN ÜBER 'VERMEIDBARE TODESFÄLLE' IN SPANIEN

M.J. Medrano, M.V. Martínez de Aragón, und M.J. Barrado

In diesem Bericht werden einige der interessantesten Merkmale der Sterblichkeit in Spanien dargelegt und diskutiert. Diese Ergebnisse stammen aus mehreren laufenden Studien mit dem allgemeinen Ziel, als epidemologische Basis für Maßnahmen des öffentlichen Gesundheitswesens zu dienen. Leider sind die verfügbaren Daten zu Morbidität in unserem Land zu knapp und unvollständig, um darauf aufbauend Prioritäten auf nationaler Ebene setzen zu können. Die Hauptstudien über vermeidbare Sterblichkeit, die in den letzten Jahren in Spanien unternommen wurden, werden ebenfalls kommentiert.

Allgemeine Merkmale der Sterblichkeit in Spanien

Spaniens Bevölkerung erfreut sich einer der niedrigsten allgemeinen Sterberaten und einer der höchsten Lebenserwartungen in Europa. Das alters-, geschlechts-, und ursachenspezifische Sterblichkeitsmuster entspricht den Erwartungen für entwickelte Länder, in denen der Todesfall spät im Leben eintritt und zumeist auf Herzgefäßerkrankungen und Krebs zurückzuführen ist. Jedoch hat das Auftreten neuer Leiden einen großen Einfluß auf die Sterblichkeit vor allem unter jungen Erwachsenenen durch AIDS, Auto- und Motorradunfälle geführt. Daher ist die Sterblichkeit in der Altersgruppe der 15–44 jährigen im Vergleich zu anderen EG-Ländern sehr hoch und hat in den letzten fünf Jahren bei beiden Geschlechtern mehr als in jedem anderen Land Europas zugenommen. Dabei weisen Männer eine höhere Sterberate in allen Altersgruppen auf. Das Verhältnis der Sterberate von Männern zu der von Frauen ist größer, wahrscheinlich augfgrund sozialer und kultureller Faktoren. Die mit Rauchen in Verbindung stehenden Krankheiten wie die ischämische Herzkrankheit (IHD), der Lungenkrebs und die chronischen Atemwegserkrankungen stellen die Haupttodesursachen in Spanien dar, jedoch gehören die entsprechenden Sterberaten zu den niedrigsten innerhalb der EG. Dagegen sind Infektionskrankheiten für nur prozent aller Todesfälle verantwortlich, verursachen jedoch im europäischen Gesamtzusammenhang sehr hohe Sterberaten.

Herzkranzgefäßerkrankungen sind die häufigsten Todesursachen in unserem Land und sind verantwortlich für 35 prozent der Todesfälle bei Männern und 48 prozent bei Frauen, bezogen auf die Gesamtsumme aller Todesfälle. Die Sterblichkeit bei IHD war während der ersten Hälfte diese Jahrhunderts unverändert, stieg jedoch in den Jahrzehnten von 1950–70 stark an. Seit 1975 ist die Sterblichkeit zurückgegangen, was sich in einer statistisch bedeutsamen Abnahme wiederspiegelte. Dieser Entwicklungswandel scheint unabhängig von den zeitlichen Unterschieden beim Vorherrschen der Hauptrisikofaktoren oder konkurrierenden Todesursachen zu sein. Alters–Zeitraum–Gruppen–Analysen weisen einen abnehmenden Einfluß des Zeitraums auf, was in Teilen diese Trends erklären könnte. Zudem scheint die räumliche Verteilung der IHD-Sterblichkeit von den alters- und geschlechtsbezogenen Variablen unabhängig zu sein. Wir glauben deshalb, daß der Zugang zu qualifizierter medizinischer Versorgung eine wirksame Vorbeugung darstellt, vor allem in Provinzen mit hohen Sterberaten wie den Kanarischen Inseln, den Balearen, und Andalusien.

Die Zahl der Todesfälle nach einem Schlaganfall in Spanien nimmt einen mittleren Wert im Vergleich zu den Daten anderer europäischer Länder ein. Sie ist seit 1900 ständig gefallen und hat Mitte der 70er Jahre einen weiteren bemerkenswerten Rückgang erfahren-mehrere Jahre bevor blutdrucksenkende Medikamente weitverbreitet erhältlich waren. Ein ausgeprägter negativer Gruppeneffekt ist erkannt worden. Wiederum weisen geographische Gebiete im Süden und auf den Inseln hohe Sterberaten im obersten Quintil auf, die denen der europäischen Länder mit der höchsten Sterblichkeit ähnlich sind (Barrado Lanzarote *et al.*, im druck) Weitere gründliche Studien sind notwendig um die mögliche Rolle verschiedener Faktoren bei der Bestimmung der Sterblichkeit nach einem Schlaganfall zu erforschen unter Berücksichtigung medizinischer Versorgung.

Die Sterblichkeit für Lungenkrebs bei Männern steigt dramatisch, während die der nördlichen europäischen Länder stabil bleiben oder sogar abnehmen. Umgekehrt haben Spanierinnen ihr Risiko, an Lungenkrebs zu sterben, nicht erhöht. Dieser Trend könnte sich in der Zukunft aufgrund von sich verändernden Mustern bei Rauchgewohnheiten ändern. Jetzige Daten bestätigen, daß die weite

Verbreitung des Rauchens bei Männern, vor allem bei den jüngeren, zurückgeht, bei den Frauen jedoch stark zunimmt. Dementsprechend scheint sich die Sterblichkeit bei jungen Männern auf einem gleichbleibenden Niveau zu bewegen und jüngere Gruppen weisen eine geringeres Risikos auf zu sterben.

Da es in den Behandlungsmethoden von Lungenkrebs keine außergewöhnlichen Verbesserungen gegeben hat, muß mit der auf die Vermeidung des Rauchens gesetzten Priorität fortgefahren werden.

Spanien hat die geringste Sterberate an Brustkrebs in Europa, die jedoch in allen Altersgruppen zunimmt, während diese im restlichen Europa, mit der Ausnahme Griechenlands, mit der Zeit eine Abnahme aufweist. Bedenkt man die verbesserten Überlebenschancen aufgrund frühzeitiger Entdeckung und Behandlung, spiegelt diese zunehmende Sterblichkeit entweder die starke Zunahme des Auftretens dieser Fälle und/oder deren Ausmaß, oder aber die geringe Zugänglichkeit sekundärer Vorbeugung wieder. Die Auswirkungen innerhalb eines Zeitraums sind stabil geblieben, aber das Risiko je Geburtsgruppe hat sich im Verlauf dieses Jahrhunderts erhöht. Das derzeitige Wissen über Risikofaktoren für Brustkrebs ist gering. Somit scheinen die Programme zur frühzeitigen Erkennung vorläufig die wirksamste Strategie der Vorbeugung zu sein.

Spanien verzeichnet hohe Sterbeziffern für externe Ursachen bei Männern hauptsächlich aufgrund von Verkehrsunfällen, die die Haupttodesursache in jungen Jahren und den potientiellen Verlust späterer Lebensjahre darstellt. Spanien und Portugal sind die einzigen EG Länder, in denen diese Sterblichkeit in den vergangenen Jahren zugenommen hat, obwohl die aktuellsten Daten eine leichte Tendenz hin zu Stabilisierung zeigen. Der Alkohol scheint ein wichtiger Faktor in Verbindung mit Todesfällen im Straßenverkehr zu sein, und sein Konsum in der jüngeren Bevölkerung scheint zugenommen zu haben.

Wir schließen hieraus die Notwendigkeit, sich um Strategien der Vermeidung des Tabak- und Alkoholkonsums, der Förderung einer gesunden, mediterranen Diät und der Verbesserung des Zugangs zu qualifizierter medizinischer Versorgung insbesondere im Hinblick auf die frühe Diagnose von Brustkrebs, den Risikofaktoren der Herzkranzgefäßerkrankungen und ischämischer Herzerkrankungen zu bemühen.

Nachforschungen zur vermeidbaren Sterblichkeit in Spanien

Man kann sagen, daß das Konzept der vermeidbaren Sterblichkeit einen gewissen Grad an Popularität unter spanischen Epidemologen und Untersuchungsbeamten des öffentlichen Gesundheitswesens gewonnen hat. Diesbezüglich sind mehrere Studien veröffentlicht worden. Die Indikatoren für 'vermeidbare Todesfälle' werden zur Zeit von den Gesundheitsämtern einzelner Regionen und auf nationaler Ebene angewendet. Es wurde von einigen Ämtern Vorschläge zum besseren Umgang und Verständnis dieser Indikatoren als Werkzeug des Gesundheitswesens gemacht, das diese zu mehr als nur einer Methode der Bewertung medizinischer Versorgung macht. Gleichzeitig setzte man sich mit der wirklichen Bedeutung dieser Indikatoren und ihrer potentiellen Schwächen bei der Erkennung von Ungerechtigkeiten in der medizinischen Versorgung auseinander. Es gab zumindest eine Fallstudie zur Untersuchung der 'Vermeidbarkeit' von Todesfällen aufgrund von ausgewählten Ursachen in jungen Jahren. Das wichtigste Ergebnis dieser Studie war die Feststellung, daß das Ausmaß und die Schwere einer Krankheit zum Zeitpunkt der Einlieferung eines Patienten in ein Krankenhaus der todesbestimmende Faktor sind. Dies läßt darauf schließen, daß vermeidbare Sterblichkeit eher ein Indikator für die Zugänglichkeit medizinischer Versorgungseinrichtungen als für deren Leistungsfähigkeit ist.

Die Gesamtheit dieser Arbeiten hat das Interesse der Hauptfinanzierungsquellen, aus denen die Gesundheitsforschung schöpft, zu weiterer Unterstützung dieser Forschungsarbeit angeregt.

Das Konzept der vermeidbaren Sterblichkeit ist in Spanien erfolgreich in die epidemologische Arbeit aufgenommen worden. Die EG-weit abgestimmte Aktion 'Project on Health Services and "Avoidable Deaths"' war ein wichtiger Anreiz.

Quellenangabe

Alfonso Sánchez, J., Sanchis Noguera, B., Prado del Baño, M.J., *et al.* (1993). Testing a new heath indicator: using aviodable causes of death and life expectancy for Spain between 1975–1986. *European Journal of Epidemiology*, **9**, 33–9.

Barrado Lanzarote, M.J., de Pedro Cuesta, J., and Almazán Isla, J. (1993). Stroke mortality in Spain, 1901–1986. *Neuroepidemiology*, **12**, 148–57.

Barrado Lanzarote, M.J., Medrano Albero, M.J., and de Pedro Cuesta, J. (1994*a*). Spatial distribution of stroke mortality in Spain. *Neuroepidemiology*, in press.

Barrado Lanzarote M.J., Medrano Albero M.J., and Almazán Isla J. (1994*b*) Mortalidad por cardiopatía isquémica. Serie temporal y distribución geográfica. *Revista Espanola de Cardiologia*, in press.

Barrado, M.J. and Medrano, M.J. Effect of age, birth cohort and period of death in mortality by stroke and ischaemic heart disease in Spain 1951–1991. Report in preparation.

Bernat Gil, L. and Rathwell, T. (1989). The effect of health services on mortality: amenable causes in Spain. *International Journal of Epidemiology*, **18**, 652–7.

Borrel i Thió, C., Plasència i Tardach, A., and Pañella i Noguera, H. (1991). Excés de mortalitat en una area urbana cèntrica: el cas de Ciutat Vella a Barcelona. *Gaceta Sanitaria*, **5**, 243–53.

Cerdeira, S., Abraira, L.,Alonso, J.M., *et al.* (1994). Mortalidad evitable en la Comunidad Autonoma Gallega. *Gaceta Sanitaria*, **8** (suppl), 50.

García Arcal, M.D., Pollán Santamaría, M., and López Abente, G. (1994). Mortalidad por cancer de mama en la Comunidad Europea (1970–1985). *Medicina Clinica (Barcelona)*, **102**, 125–8.

García Benavides, F.G., Orts, R., and Pérez, S. (1992). Adding years to life: effect of avoidable mortality on life expectancy at birth. *Journal of Epidemiology and Community Health*, **46**, 394–5.

García Benavides, F.G., Pérez, F., Cayuela, A., Nolasco, A., *et al.* (1990). Avoidable years of life lost ratio: an indicator to identify excess in mortality in health areas. *Gaceta Sanitaria*, **16**, 12–17.

Gispert, R. and Segura, A. (1990). La identificación de la mortalidad evitable y sus aplicaciones prácticas. *Gaceta Sanitaria*, **4**, 199–200.

Gispert, R., Moreno, C., and Rué, M. (1994). Es inevitable la mortalidad evitable? *Gaceta Sanitaria*, **8** (suppl), 51.

González Enriquez, J., Cerdá Mota, T., Regidor Poyatos, E., and Medrano Albero, M.J. (1989). Atlas de mortalidad evitable en España. *Ministerio de Sanidad y Consumo*. Madrid.

López Abente, G., Pollán Santamaría, M., Ruiz Tovar, M., *et al.* (1992). Cancer mortality in Spain 1952–1986. Effect of age, birth cohort and period of death. *Centro Nacional de Epidemiología*, Madrid.

Martínez de Aragón, M.V., Llácer Gil, A., Marín Rivero, M., and Martínez Navarro, F. (1993). Mortalidad en España 1989. Situacíon en el marco de la Unión Europea. *Ministerio de Sanidad y Consumo*. Madrid.

Pérez, J., Sanz, C., and Martínez, J.F. (1994). Análisis de la mortalidad por causas externas en España según el modelo de regresión de Preston. *Gaceta Sanitaria*, **44** (suppl), 208.

Regidor Poyatos, E. (1991). Acerca de la mortalidad evitable. *Gaceta Sanitaria*, **5**, 139–40.

7. MAPS AND HISTOGRAMS

Whole EC maps for the period 1985–89

1. These maps show SMRs (based on the EC standard) by disease and small area and are intended to show between-country variation.

2. Sextile intervals were used. The SMRs for each small area were ranked and one-sixth of the areas placed in each shading interval.

3. Striped shading indicates those areas where particular care is needed when interpreting extreme SMRs due to uncertainty in SMR estimates.

4. In order to highlight between-country variation, a map showing SMRs by country, rather than small area, is presented inset.

5. The histograms presented with the maps show the frequency distributions of the SMRs and are based on a grouping interval of 20. The same grouping interval is used for every histogram to provide a common scale on which variability of SMRs in different disease groups can be compared.

Whole EC maps of changes between 1980–84 and 1985–89

1. These maps show annual percentage change in age-standardized mortality rates (standardized to the EC 1985–89 rate) by disease and small area.

2. Areas were divided into two groups according to whether there was or was not an increase in age-standardized mortality. In each group, areas were ranked according to the annual percentage change in mortality from 1980–84 and 1985–89 and an equal number of areas placed in each shading interval within the group.

3. Striped shading indicates those areas where particular care is needed when interpreting extreme per cent change due to the increased uncertainty in the estimates of rates of change.

4. In order to highlight between-country variation, a map showing results by country rather than small area, is presented inset.

Individual country maps

1. These maps show SMRs (based on each country's own standard) by disease and small area and are intended to show within-country variation in an EC context.

2. Sextile intervals were used. The SMRs for each small area were ranked and one-sixth of the areas placed in each shading interval.

3. The histograms presented with the maps show the frequency distributions of the SMRs and are based on a grouping interval of 20. The same grouping interval is used for every histogram to provide a common scale on which variability of SMRs in different disease groups can be compared. The histograms show in grey the distribution of small area SMRs based on national standards for all the small areas of the EC, and in black the distributions of SMRs for the country in the map.

TUBERCULOSIS MORTALITY AGES 5–64: 1985–89

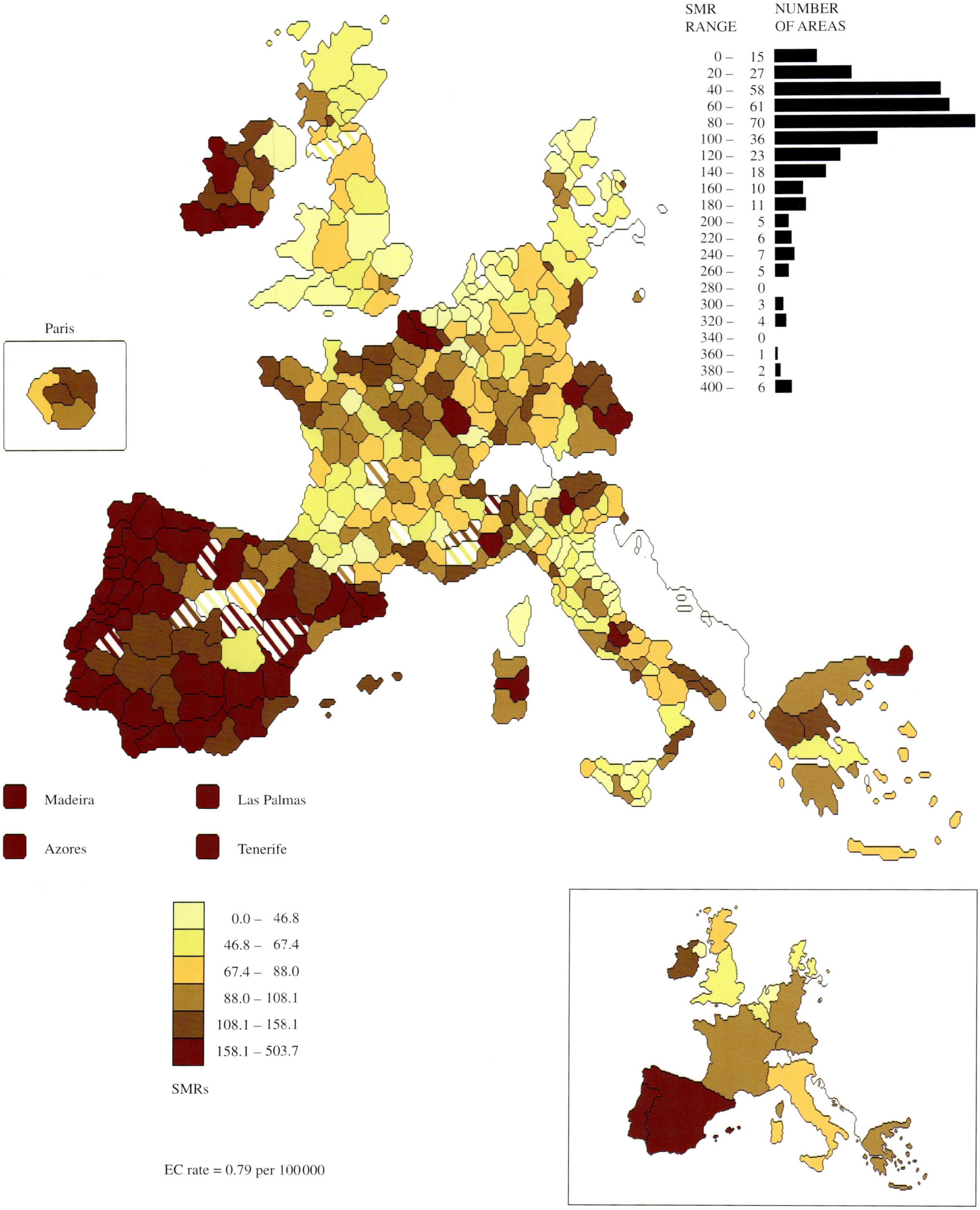

EC rate = 0.79 per 100 000

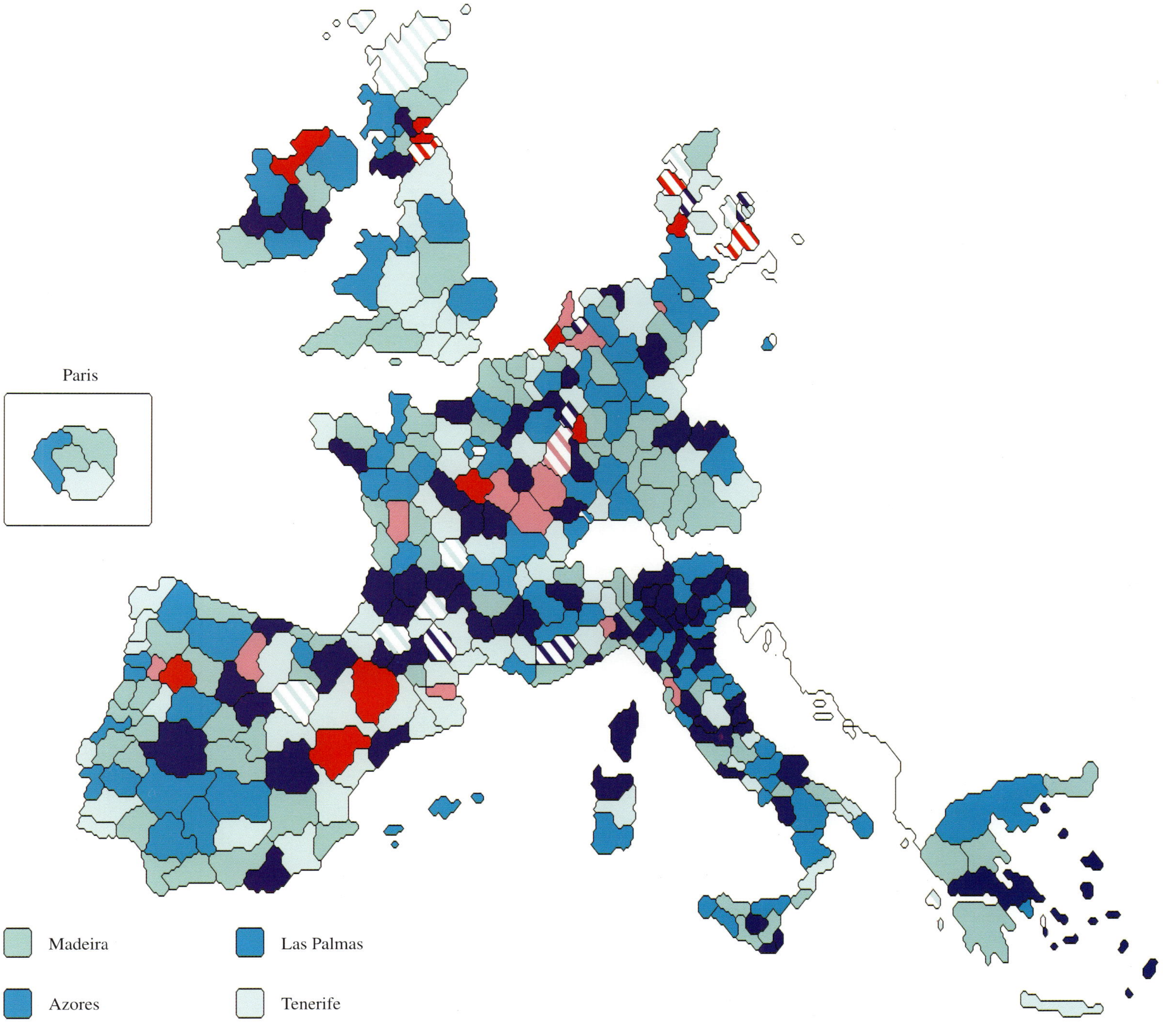

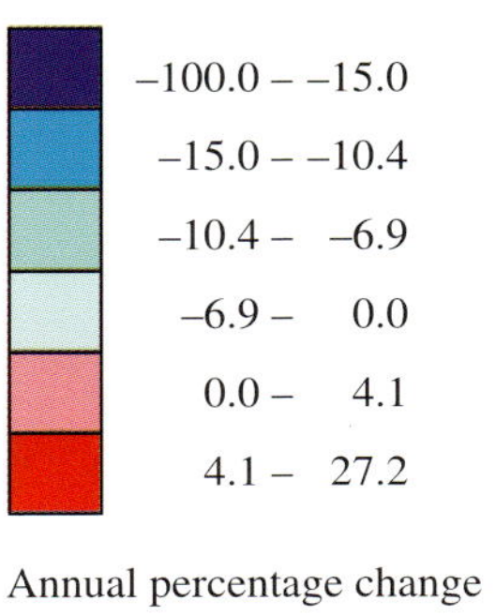

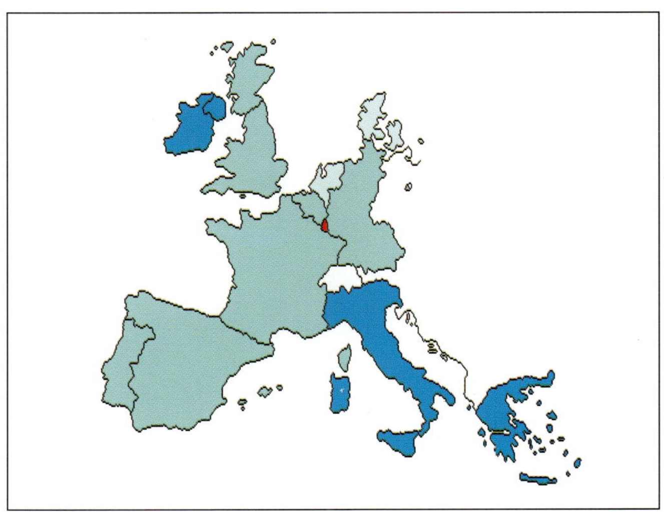

EC annual percentage change = –9.4%

MALIGNANT NEOPLASM OF CERVIX UTERI MORTALITY AGES 15–64: 1985–89

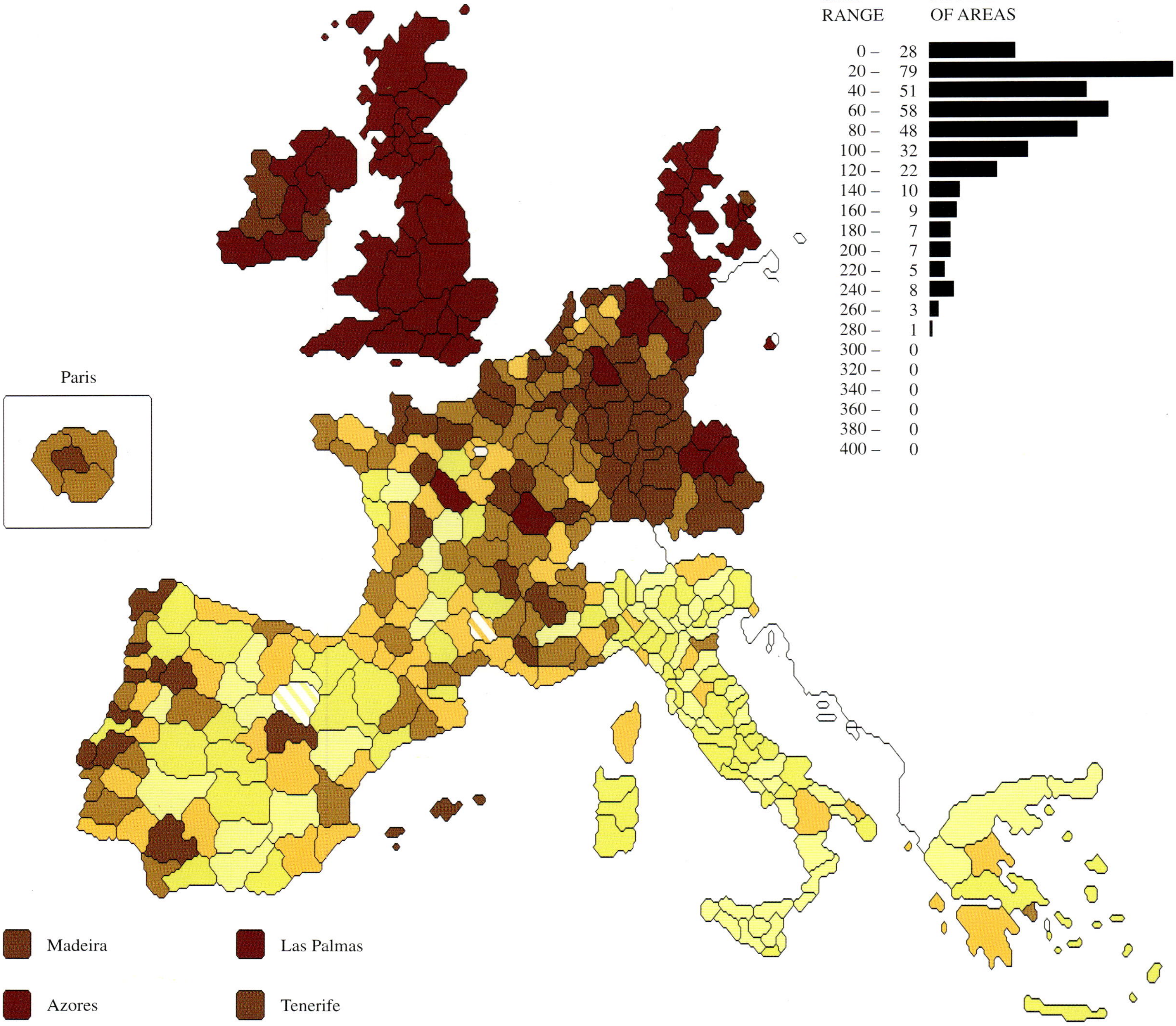

SMR RANGE	NUMBER OF AREAS
0 –	28
20 –	79
40 –	51
60 –	58
80 –	48
100 –	32
120 –	22
140 –	10
160 –	9
180 –	7
200 –	7
220 –	5
240 –	8
260 –	3
280 –	1
300 –	0
320 –	0
340 –	0
360 –	0
380 –	0
400 –	0

Paris

Madeira

Las Palmas

Azores

Tenerife

0.0 – 31.1

31.1 – 46.4

46.4 – 69.1

69.1 – 89.8

89.8 – 127.5

127.5 – 288.9

SMRs

EC rate = 3.18 per 100 000

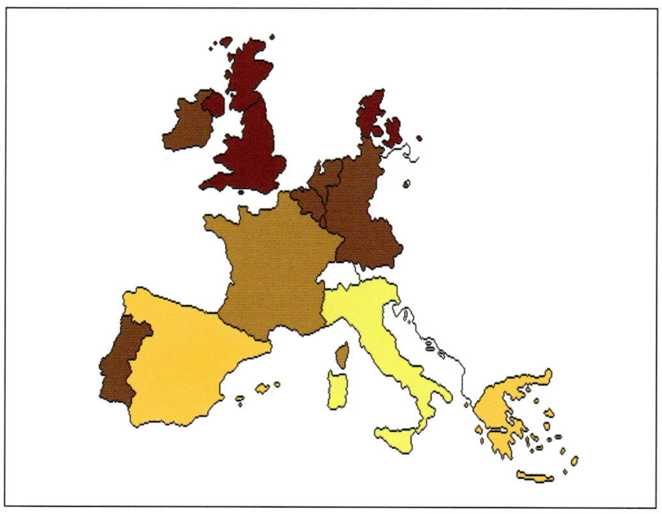

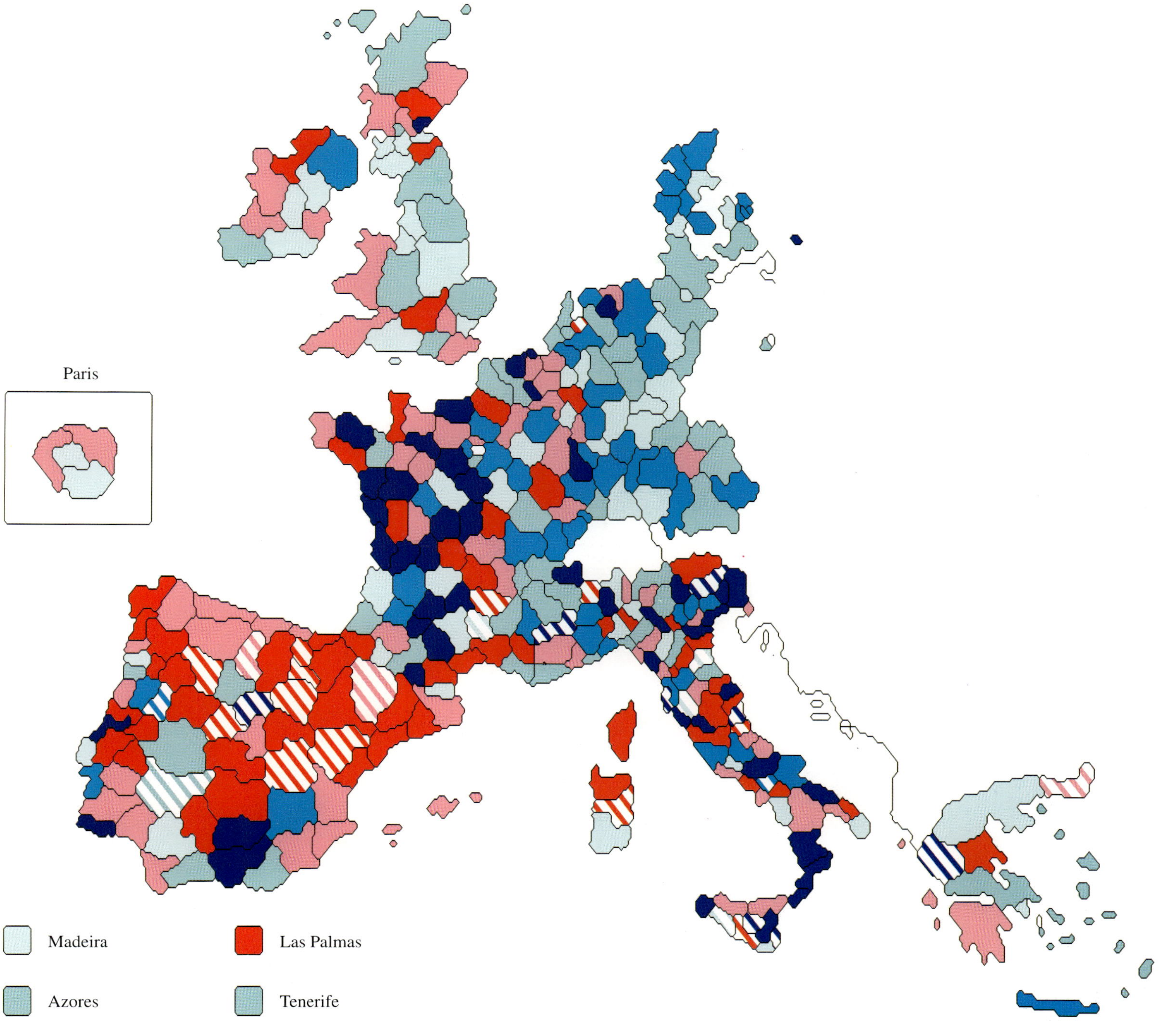

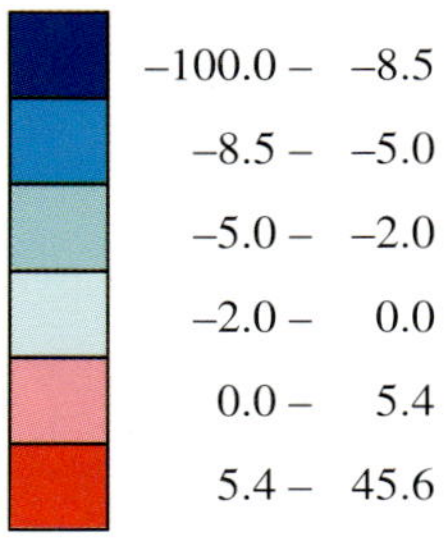

Annual percentage change

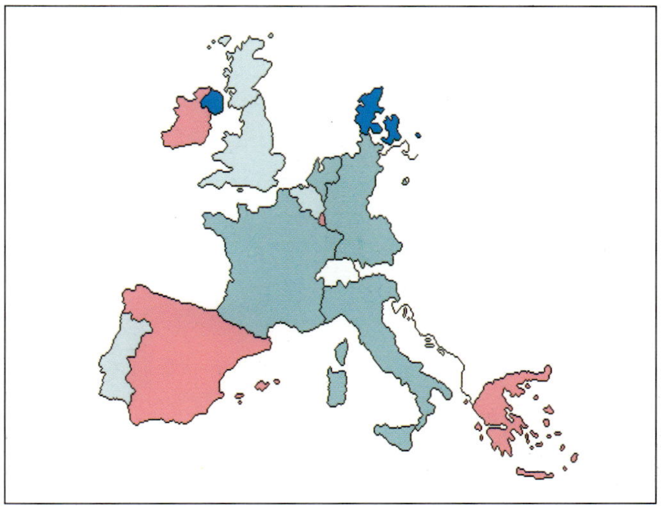

EC annual percentage change = –1.9%

MALIGNANT NEOPLASM OF CERVIX AND BODY OF UTERUS MORTALITY AGES 15–54: 1985–89

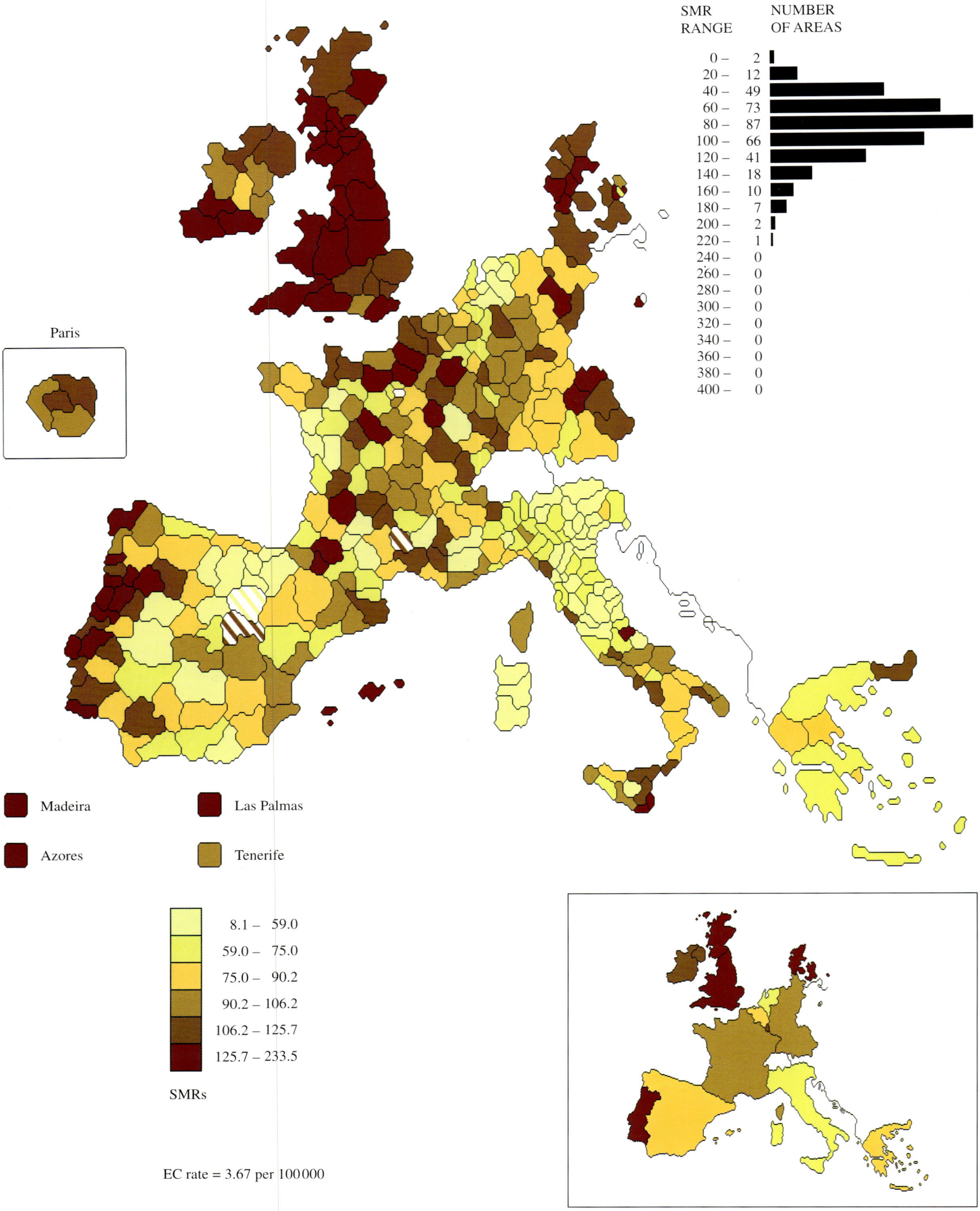

EC rate = 3.67 per 100 000

MALIGNANT NEOPLASM OF CERVIX AND BODY OF UTERUS MORTALITY AGES 15–54: ANNUAL PERCENTAGE CHANGE 1980–84 TO 1985–89

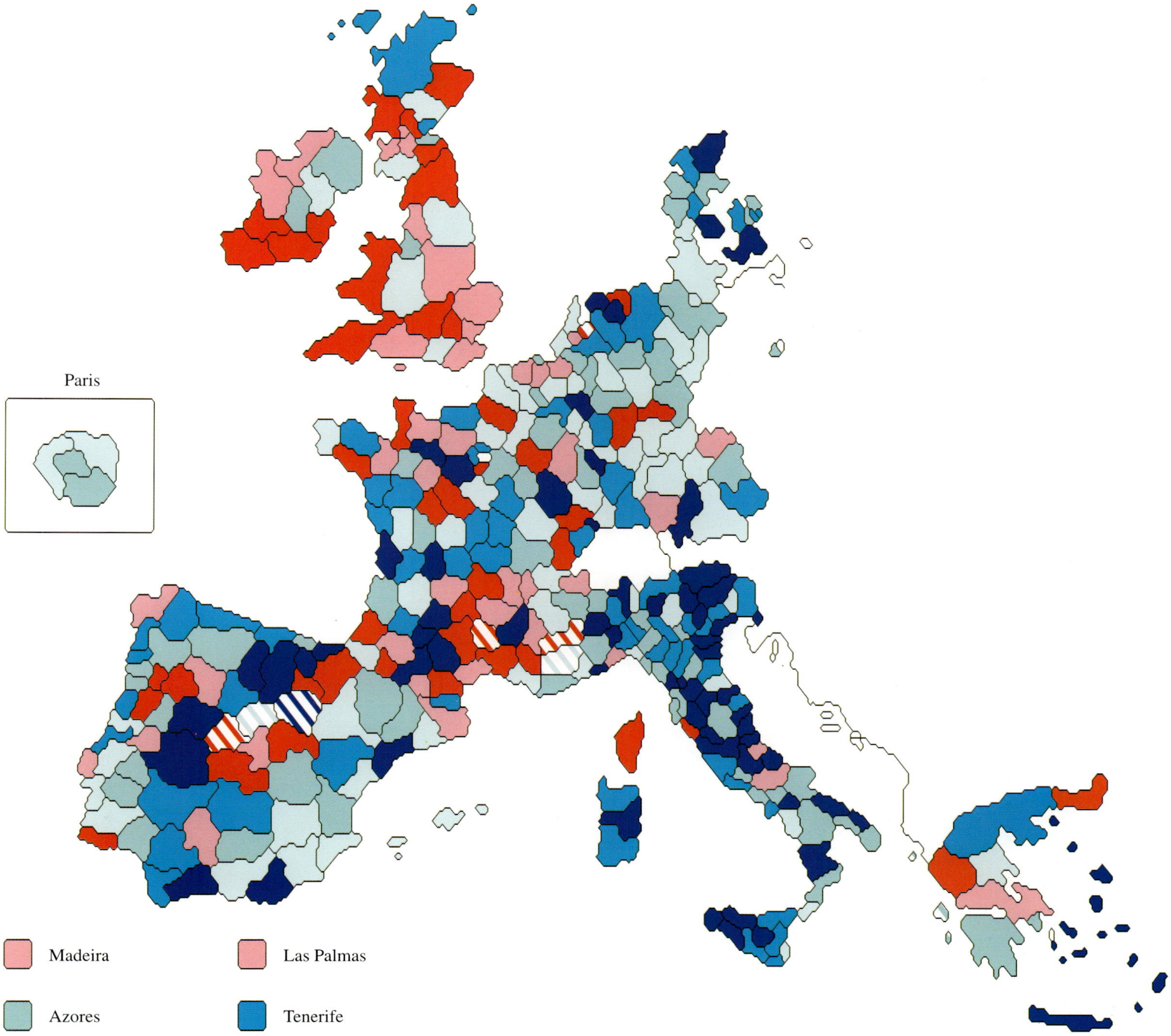

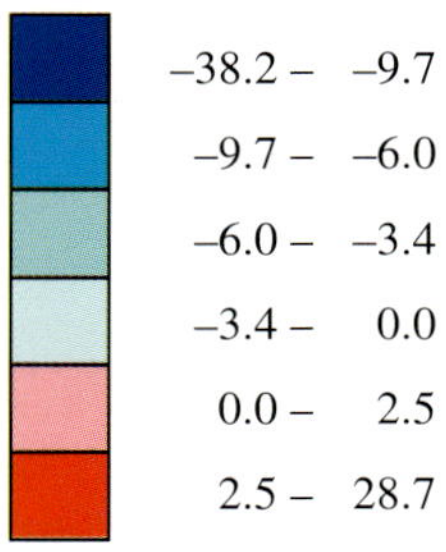

Annual percentage change

EC annual percentage change = –2.8%

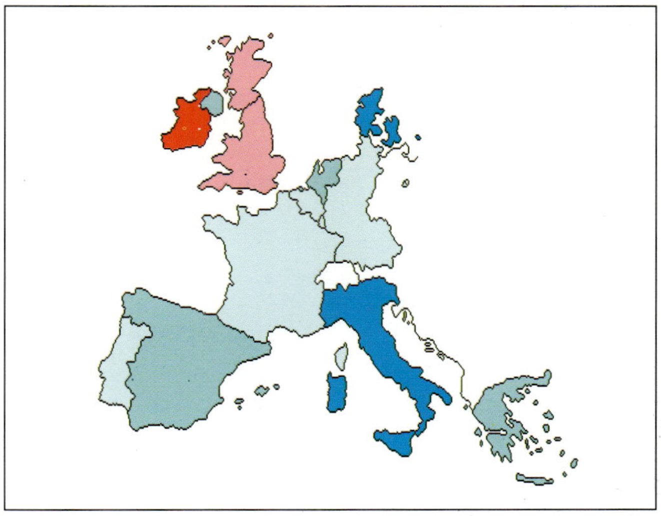

SMR RANGE	NUMBER OF AREAS
0 –	5
20 –	10
40 –	33
60 –	63
80 –	90
100 –	74
120 –	43
140 –	31
160 –	11
180 –	5
200 –	3
220 –	0
240 –	0
260 –	0
280 –	0
300 –	0
320 –	0
340 –	0
360 –	0
380 –	0
400 –	0

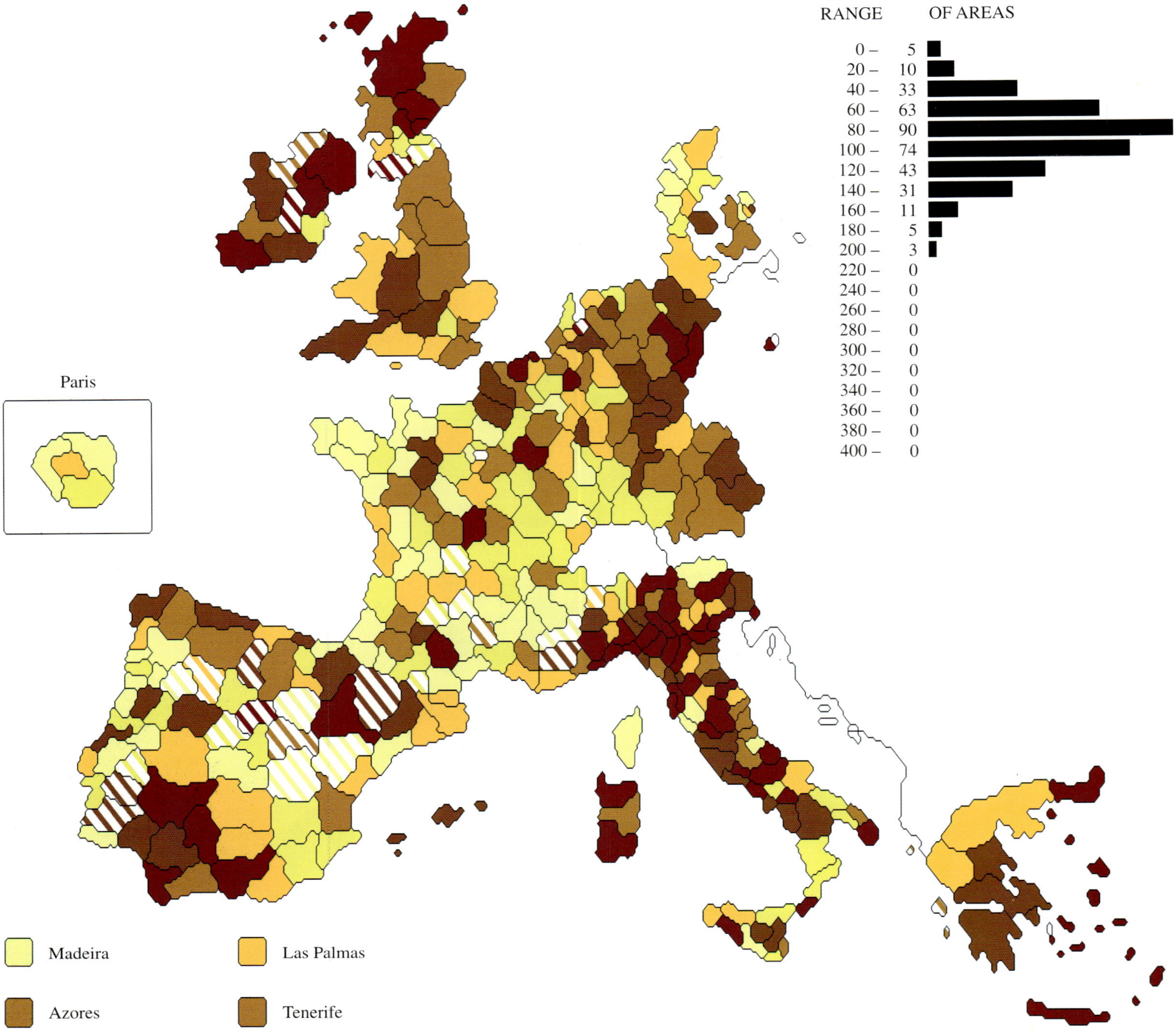

0.0 – 65.8
65.8 – 81.5
81.5 – 96.6
96.6 – 108.3
108.3 – 133.5
133.5 – 219.1

SMRs

EC rate = 0.71 per 100000

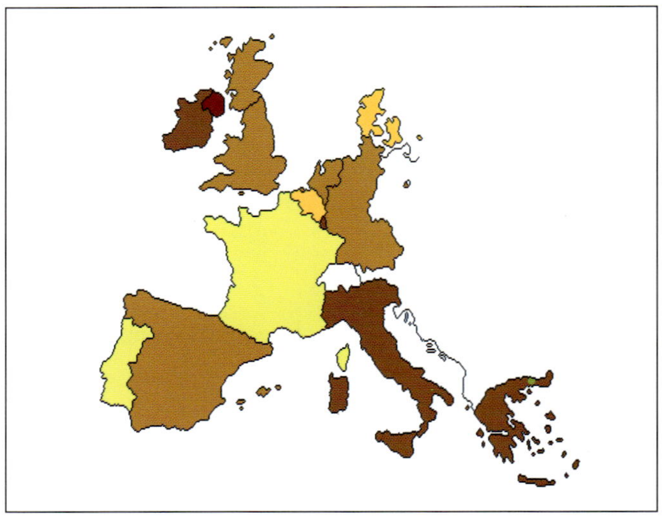

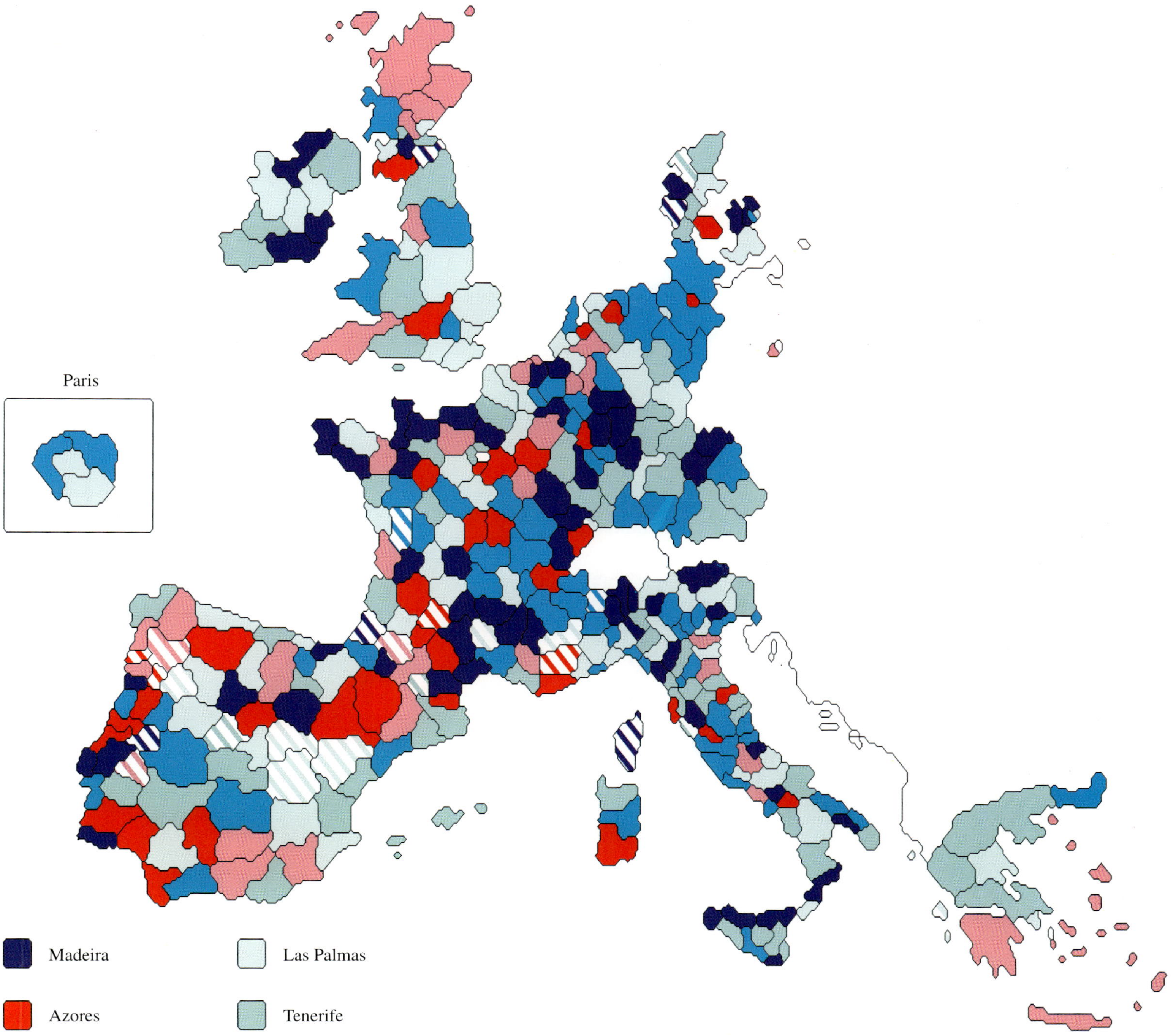

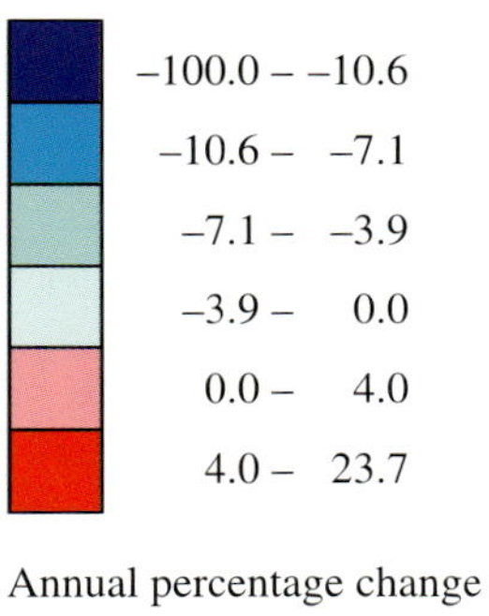

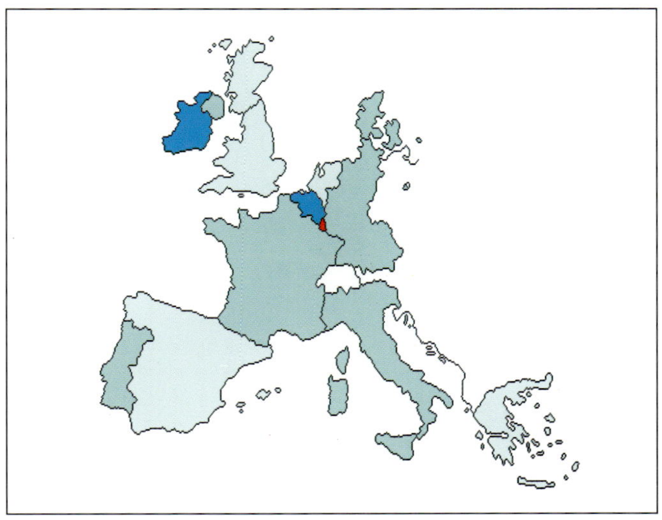

EC annual percentage change = –5.3%

CHRONIC RHEUMATIC HEART DISEASE MORTALITY AGES 5–44: 1985–89

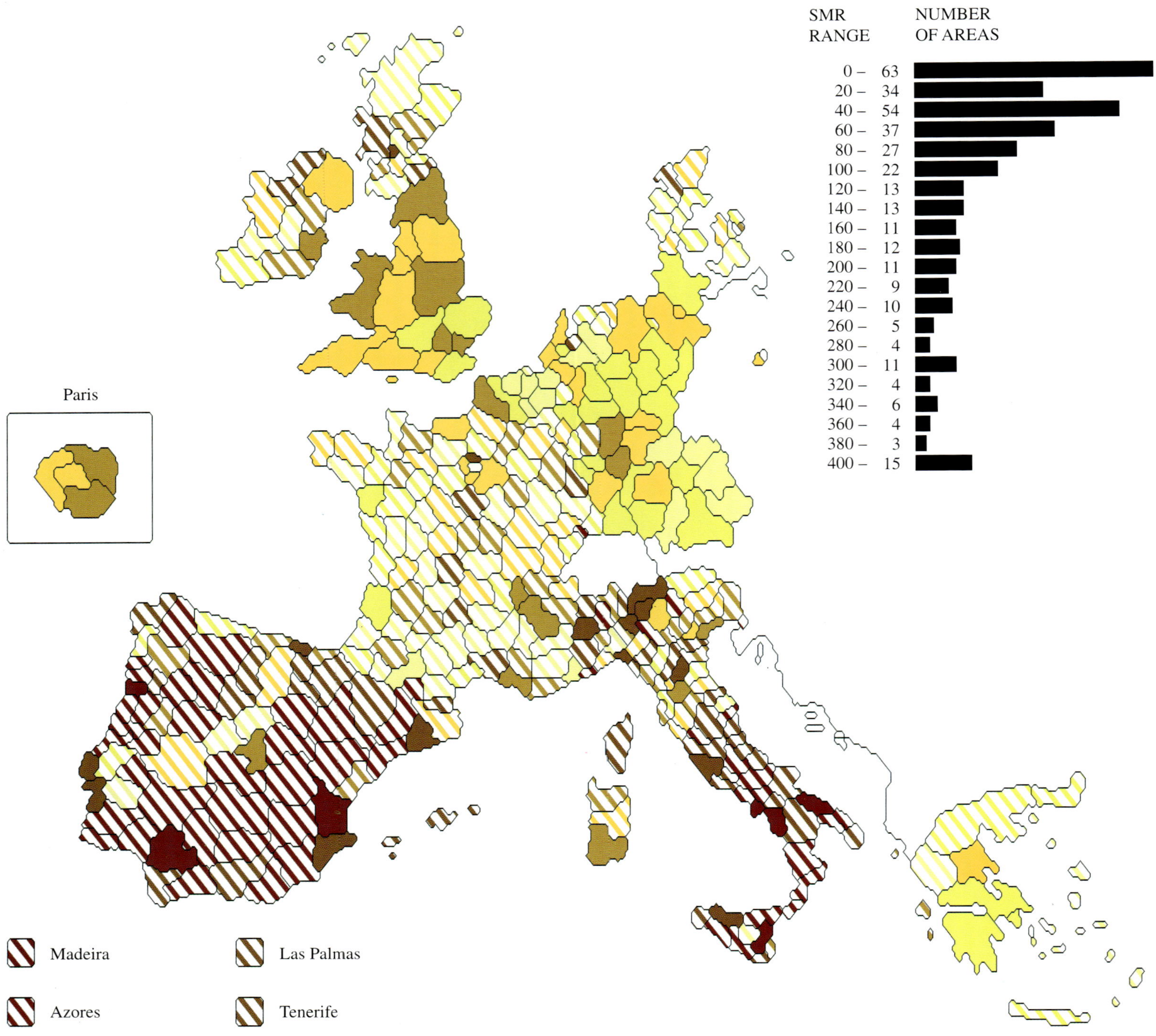

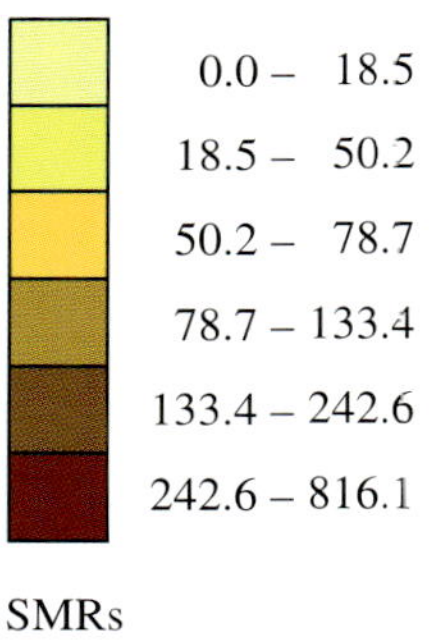

EC rate = 0.21 per 100 000

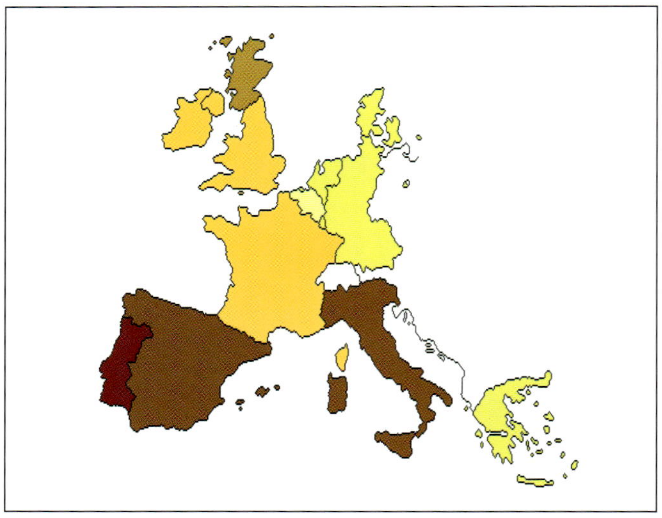

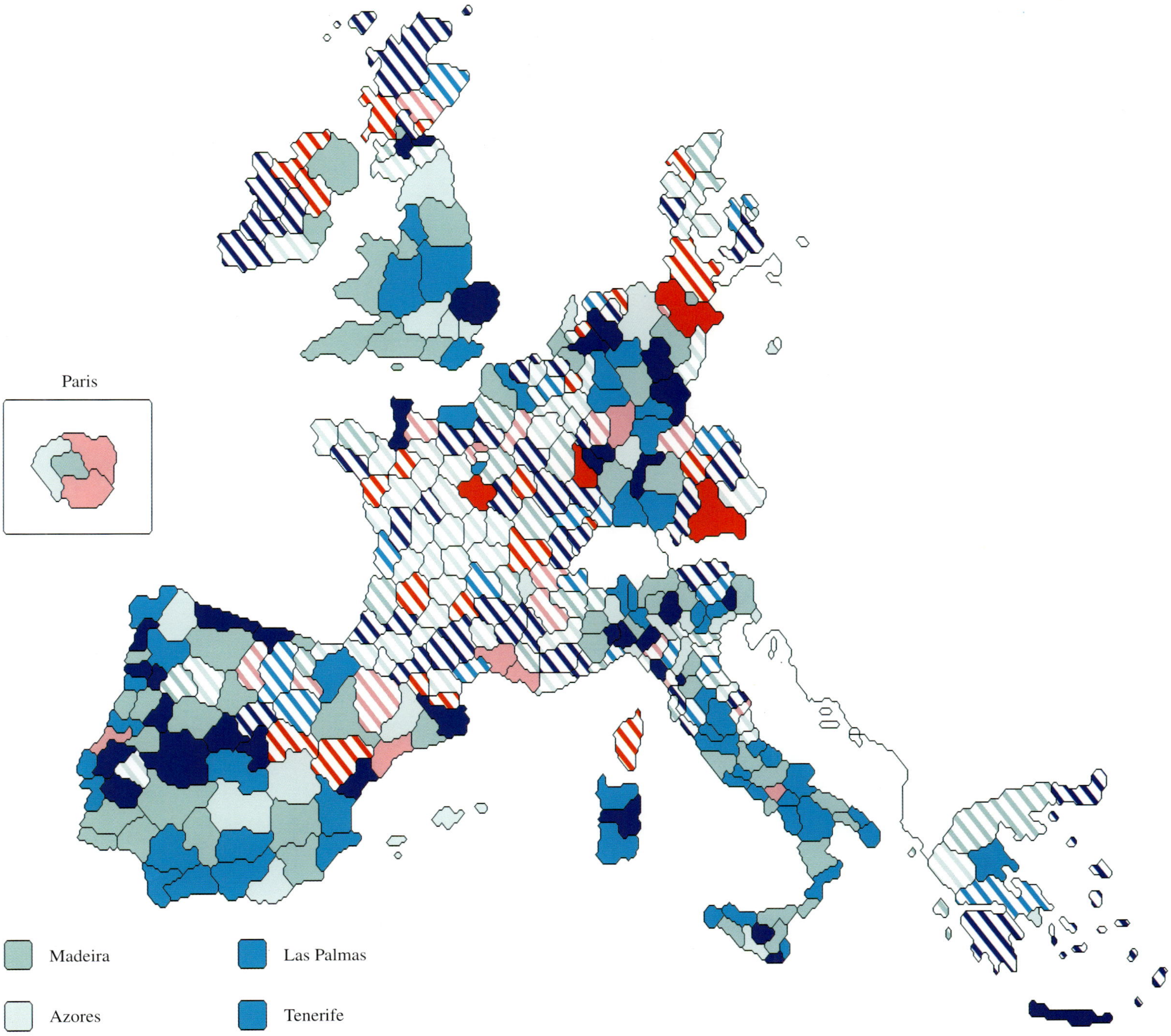

	−100.0 – −21.6
	−21.6 – −14.3
	−14.3 – −6.9
	−6.9 – 0.0
	0.0 – 11.5
	11.5 – 45.6

Annual percentage change

EC annual percentage change = −12.9%

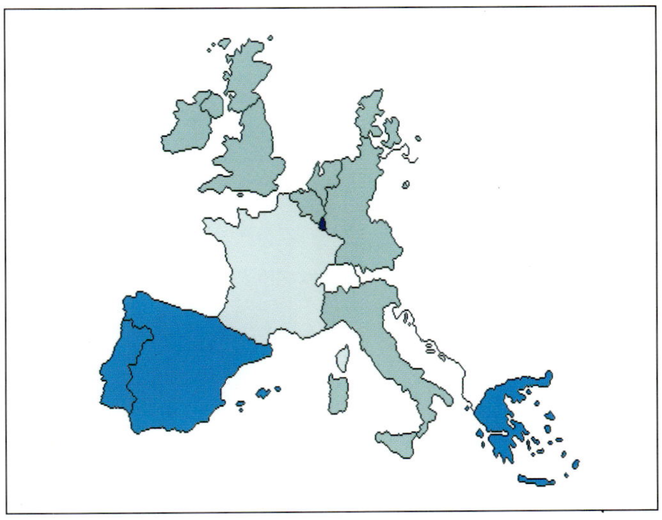

ALL RESPIRATORY DISEASES MORTALITY AGES 1–14: 1985–89

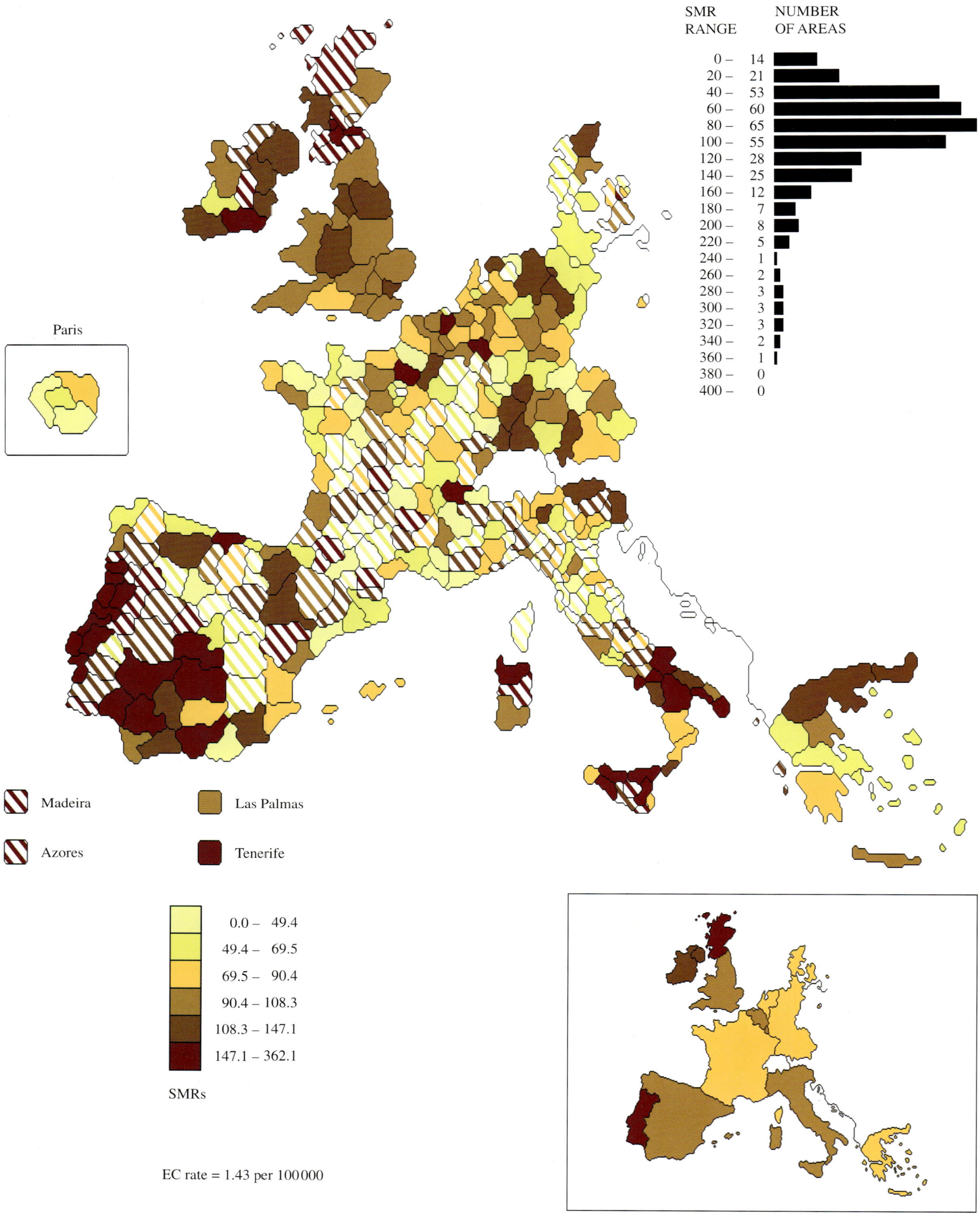

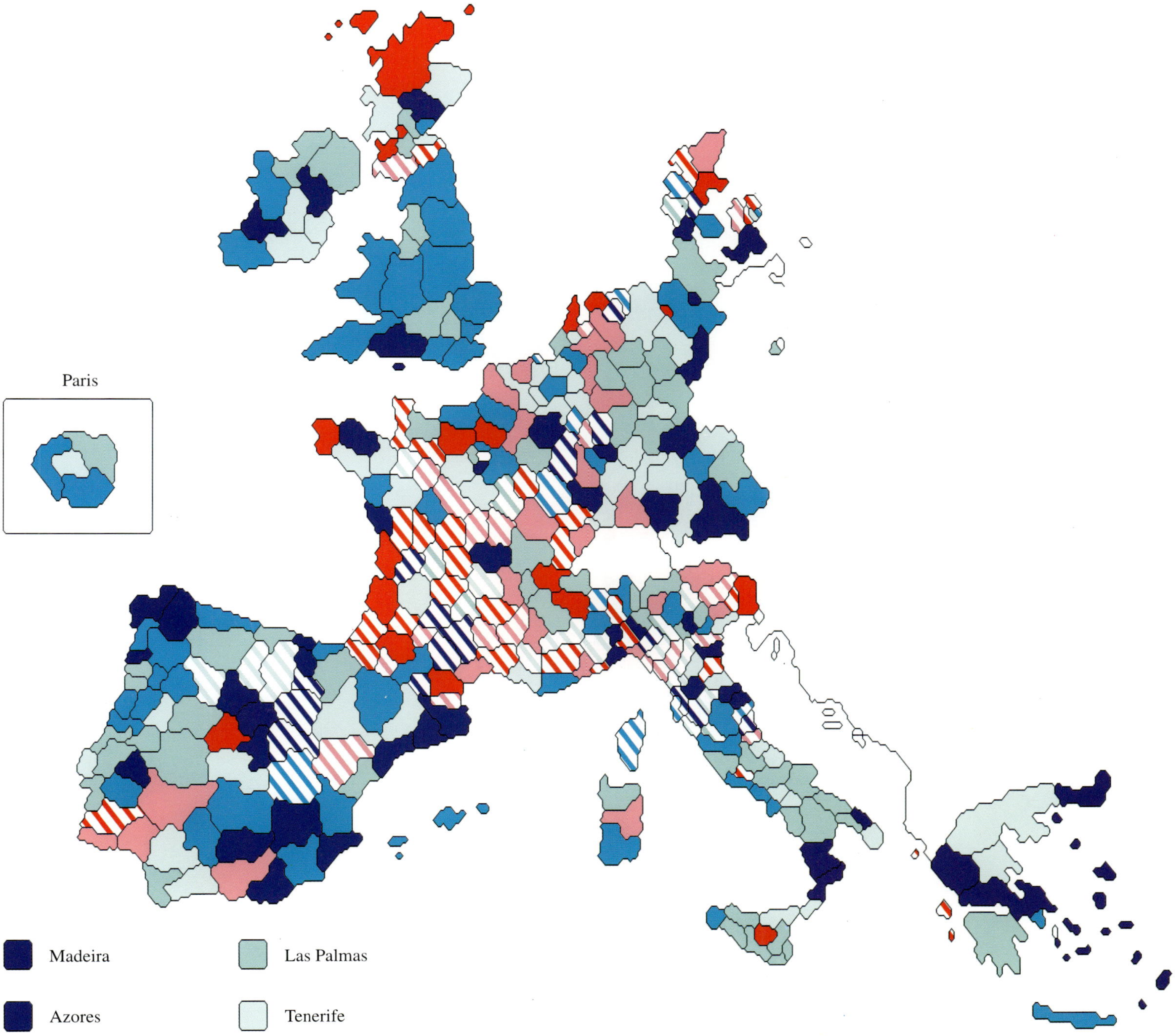

−100.0 – −14.7
−14.7 – −10.3
−10.3– −5.7
−5.7 – 0.0
0.0 – 4.7
4.7 – 53.8

Annual percentage change

EC annual percentage change = −8.0%

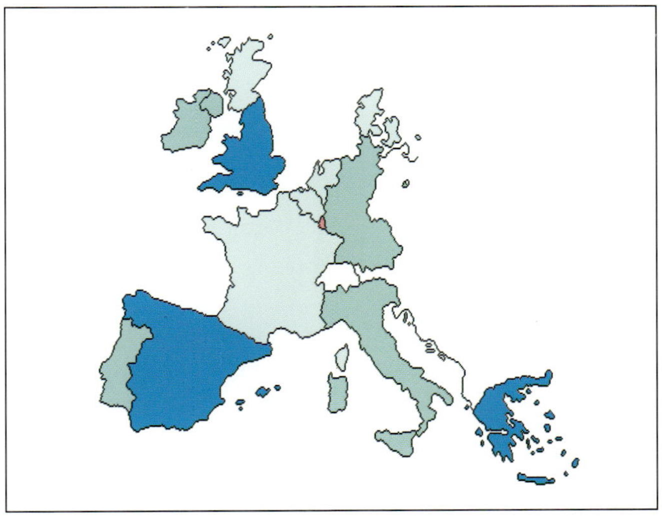

ASTHMA MORTALITY AGES 5–44: 1985–89

SMR RANGE	NUMBER OF AREAS
0 –	54
20 –	49
40 –	53
60 –	42
80 –	35
100 –	36
120 –	31
140 –	27
160 –	23
180 –	6
200 –	2
220 –	7
240 –	2
260 –	0
280 –	0
300 –	0
320 –	1
340 –	0
360 –	0
380 –	0
400 –	0

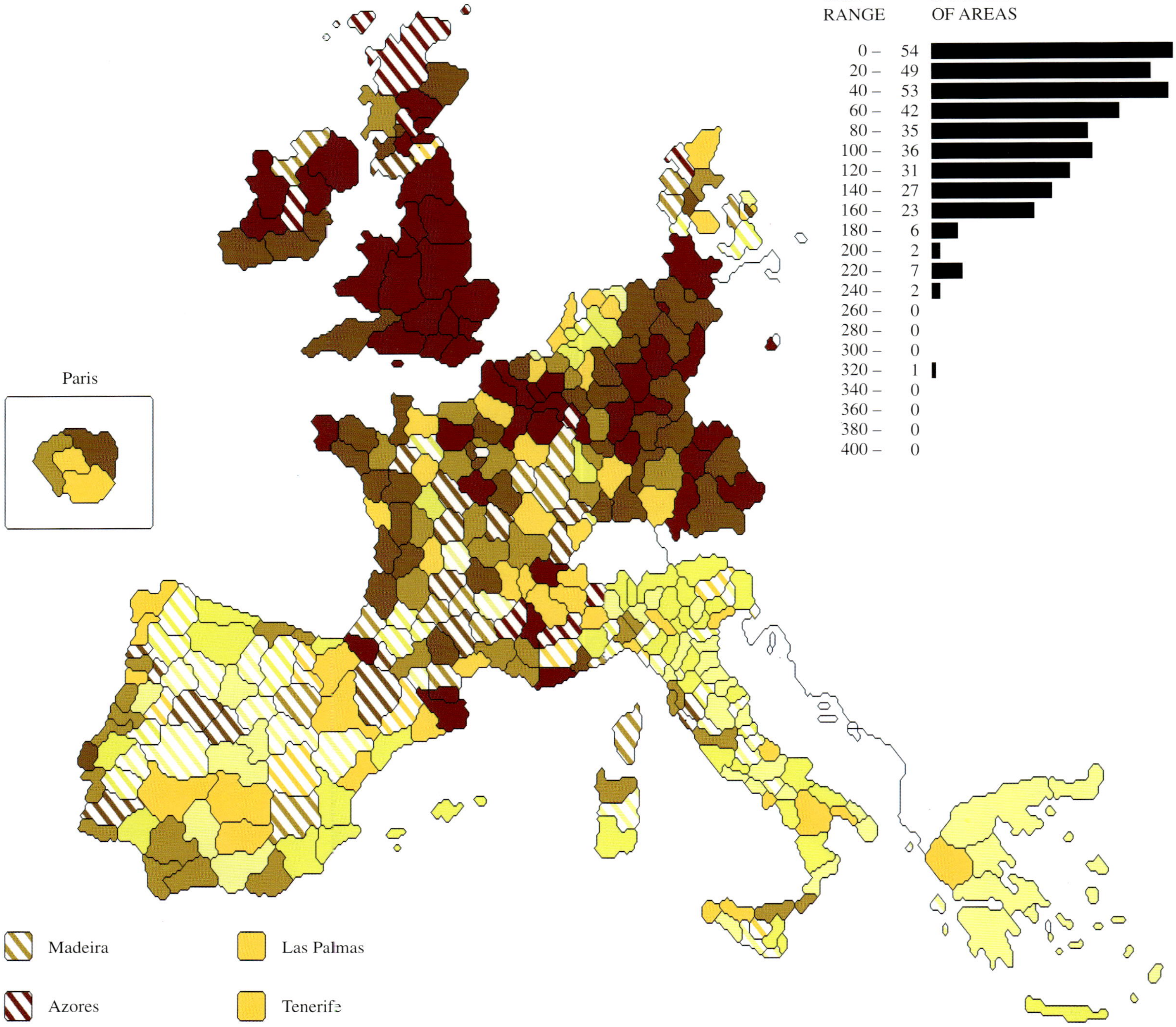

SMRs
0.0 – 21.9
21.9 – 45.5
46.5 – 74.3
74.3 – 106.5
106.5 – 144.9
144.9 – 324.7

EC rate = 0.59 per 100000

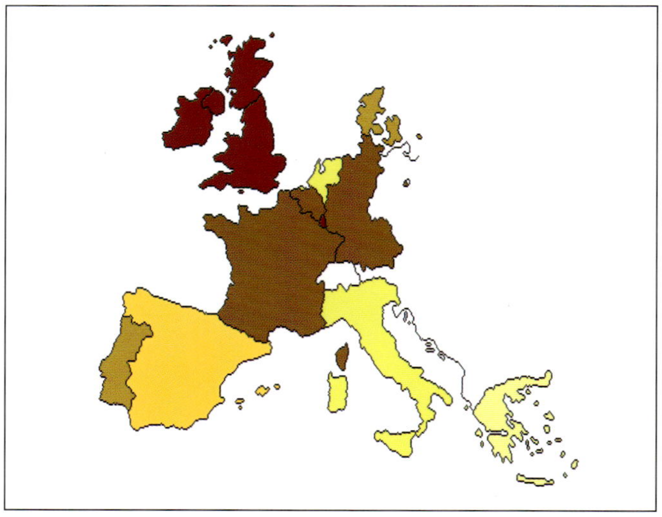

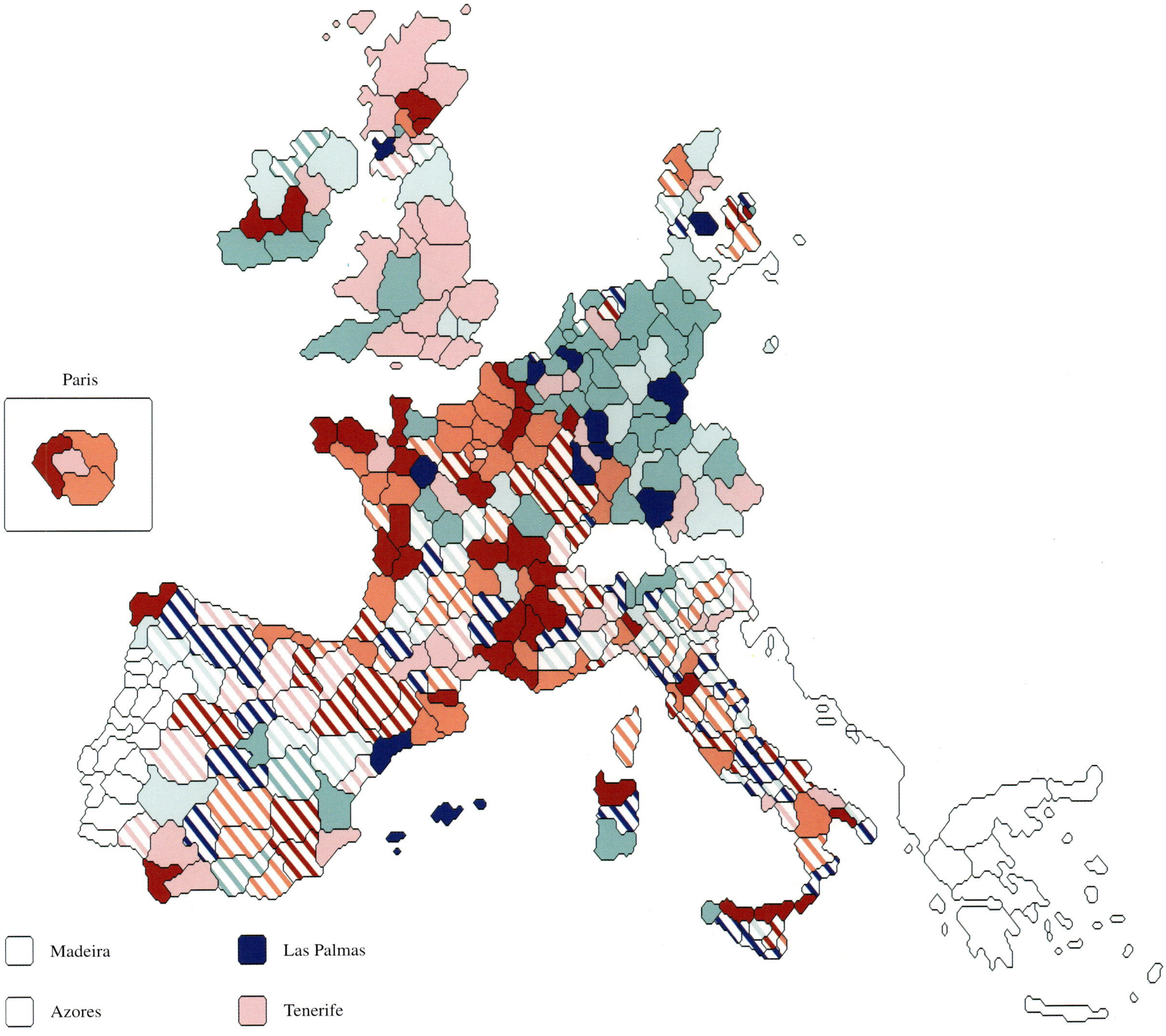

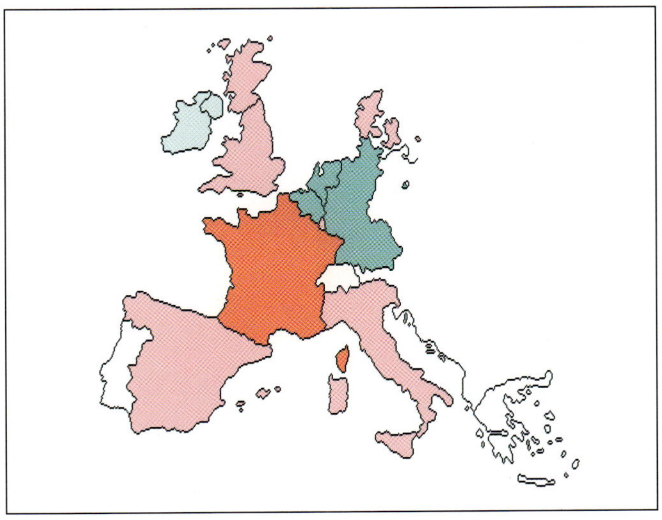

EC annual percentage change = +1.6%

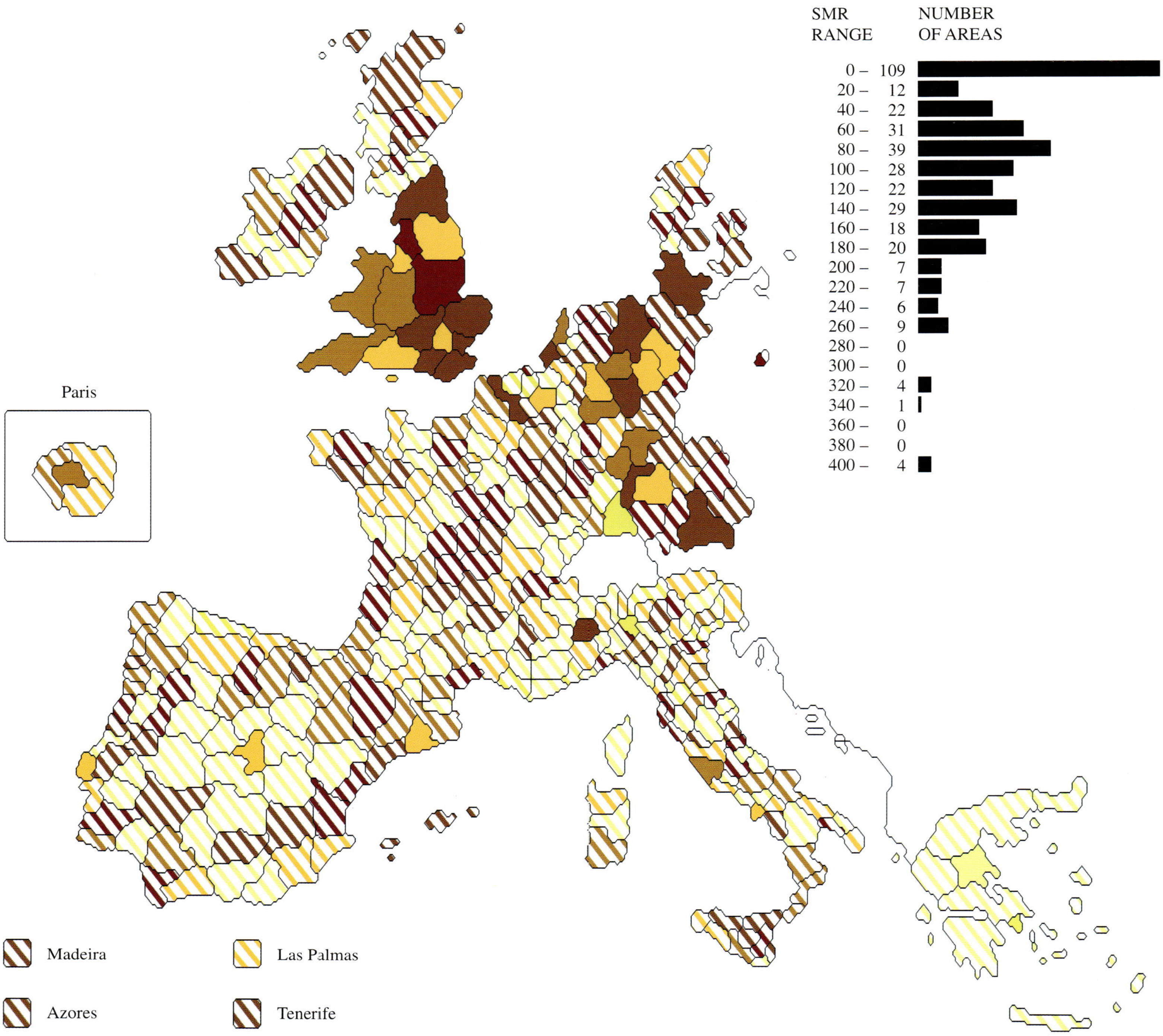

0.0
0.0 – 40.6
40.6 – 83.7
83.7 – 122.6
122.6 – 174.4
174.4 – 504.6

SMRs

EC rate = 0.07 per 100000

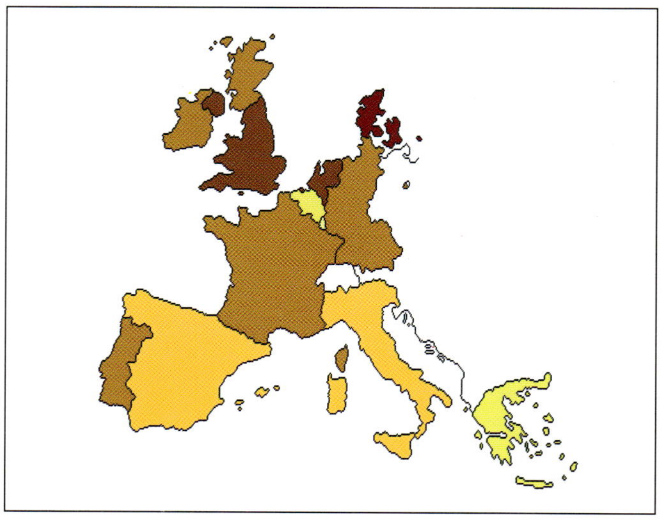

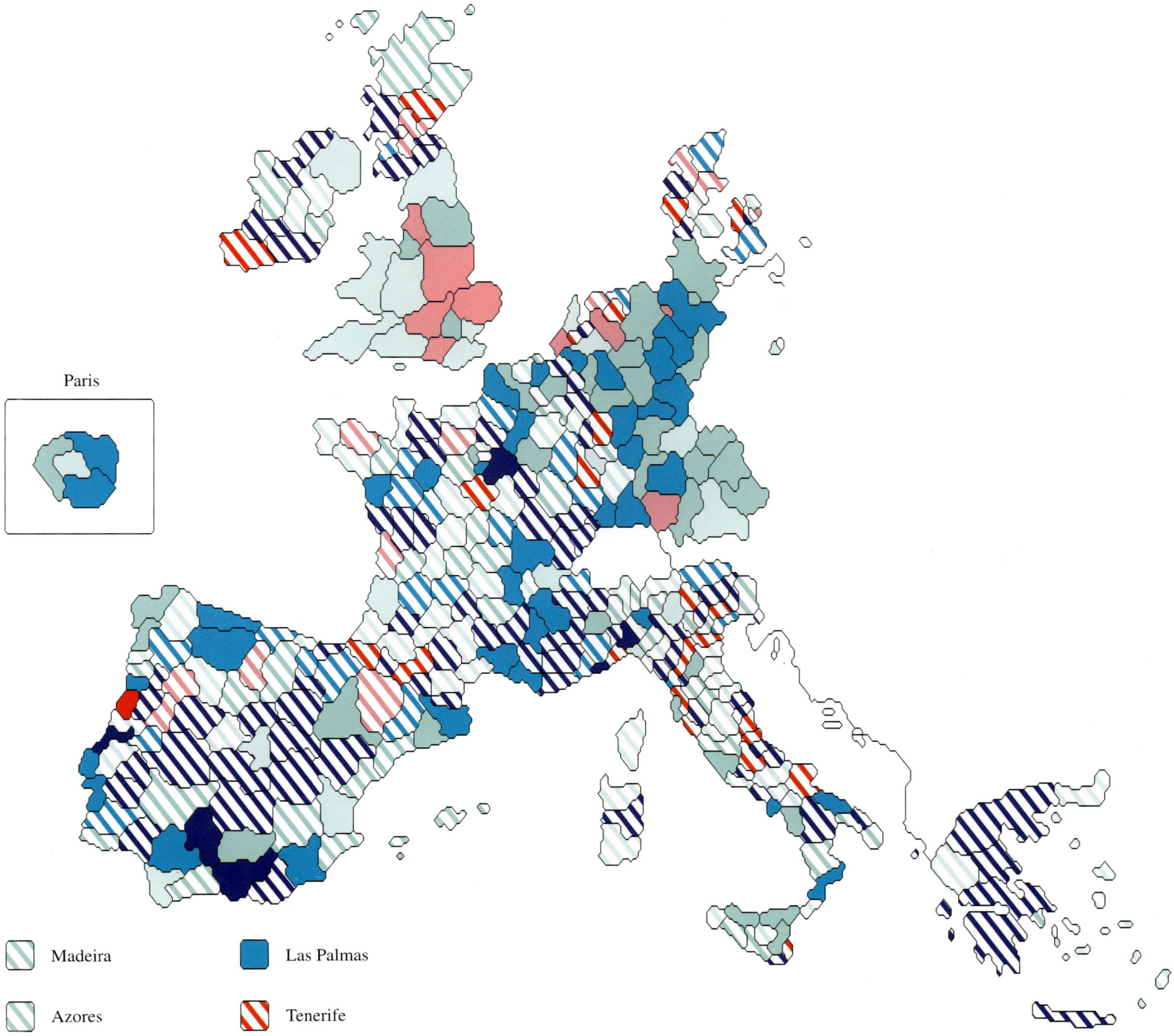

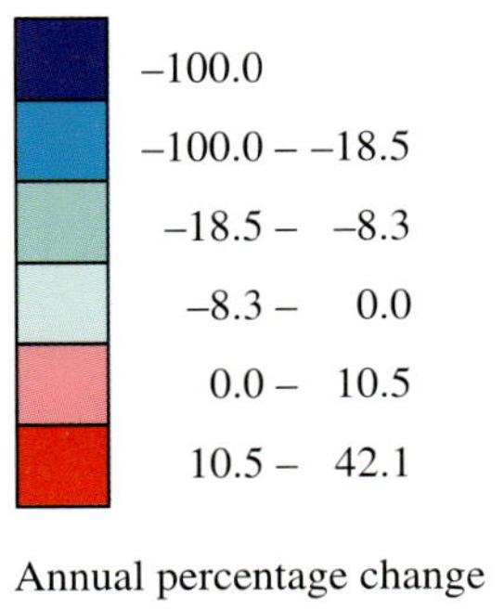

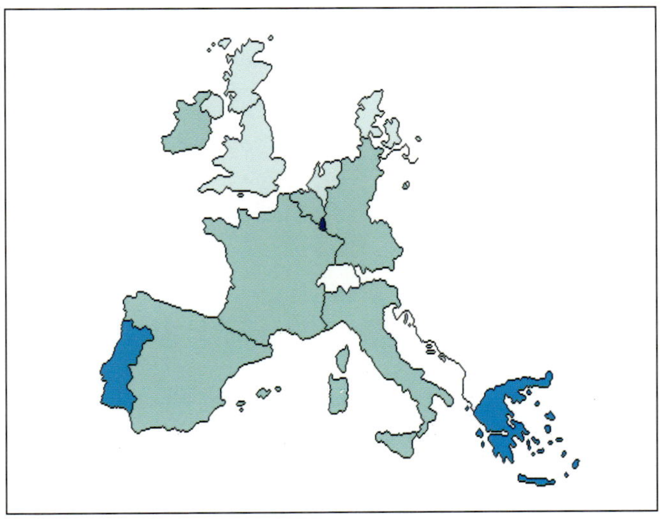

EC annual percentage change = –11.6%

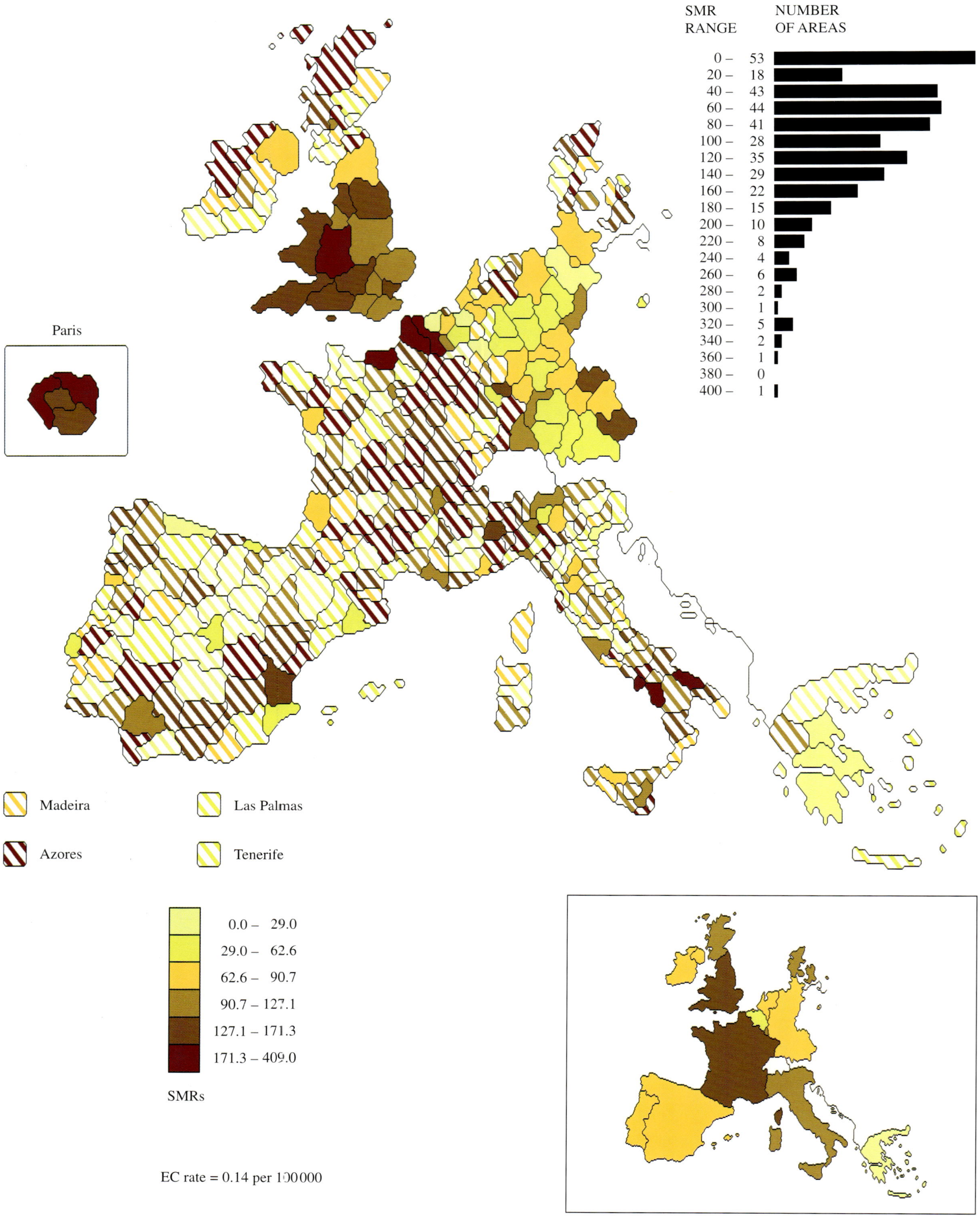
SMR RANGE
NUMBER OF AREAS
0 – 53
20 – 18
40 – 43
60 – 44
80 – 41
100 – 28
120 – 35
140 – 29
160 – 22
180 – 15
200 – 10
220 – 8
240 – 4
260 – 6
280 – 2
300 – 1
320 – 5
340 – 2
360 – 1
380 – 0
400 – 1
Paris
Madeira
Las Palmas
Azores
Tenerife
0.0 – 29.0
29.0 – 62.6
62.6 – 90.7
90.7 – 127.1
127.1 – 171.3
171.3 – 409.0
SMRs
EC rate = 0.14 per 100 000

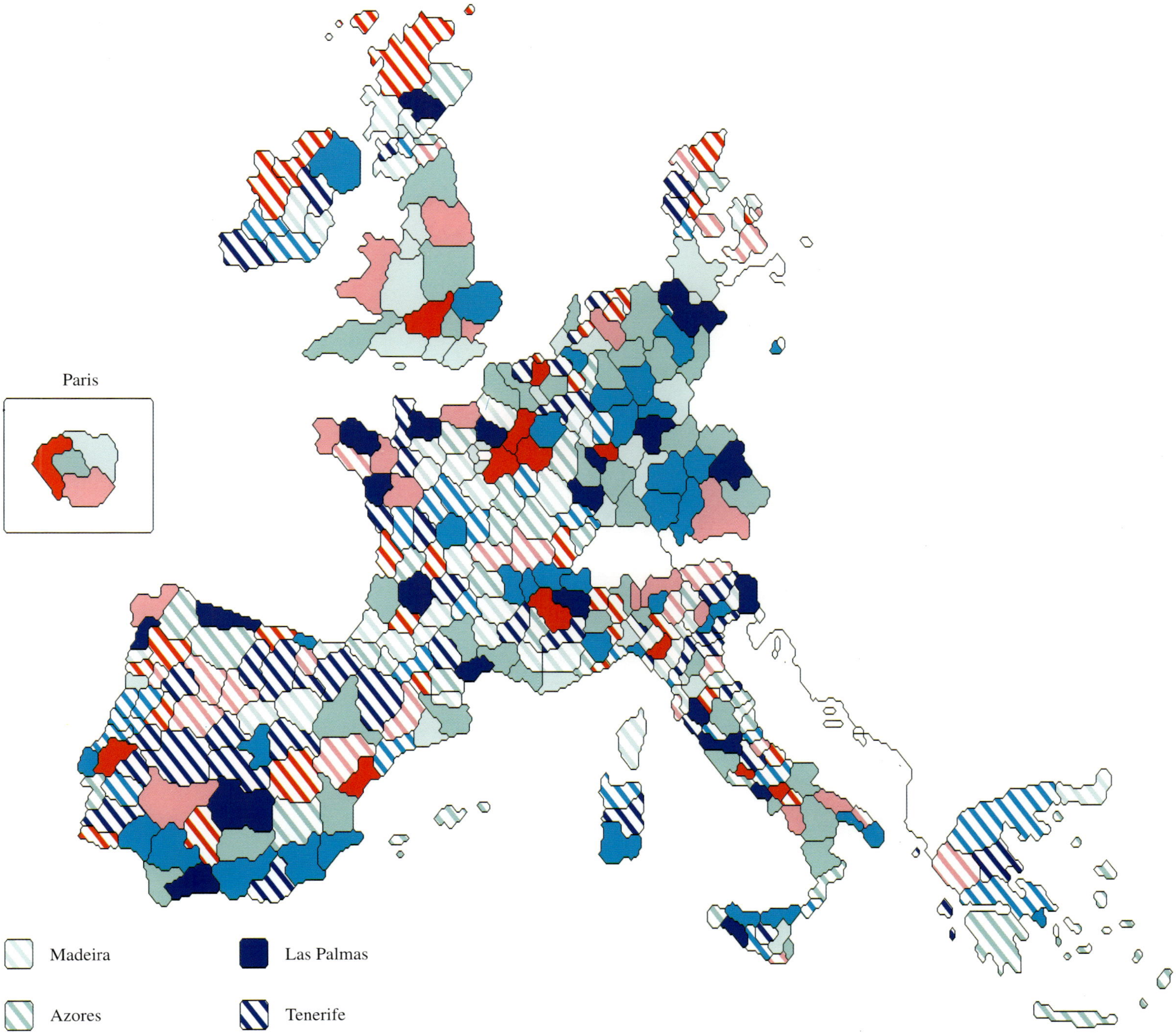

Paris

Madeira

Las Palmas

Azores

Tenerife

Annual percentage change
−100.0 – −19.6
−19.6 – −11.5
−11.5 – −4.8
−4.8 – 0.0
0.0 – 5.6
5.6 – 43.2

Annual percentage change

EC annual percentage change = −7.0%

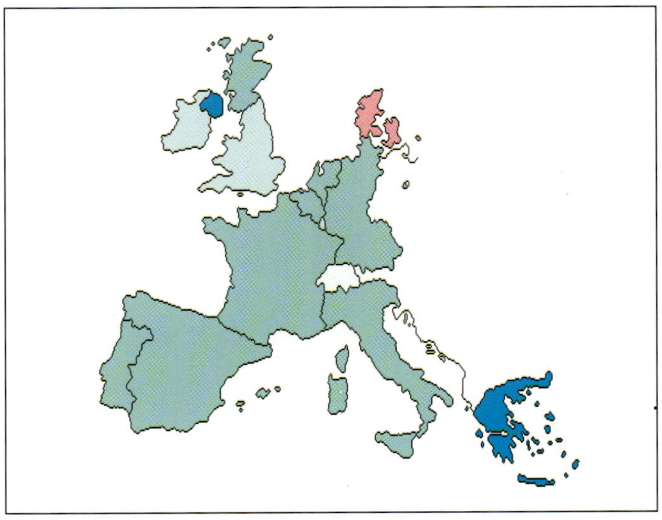

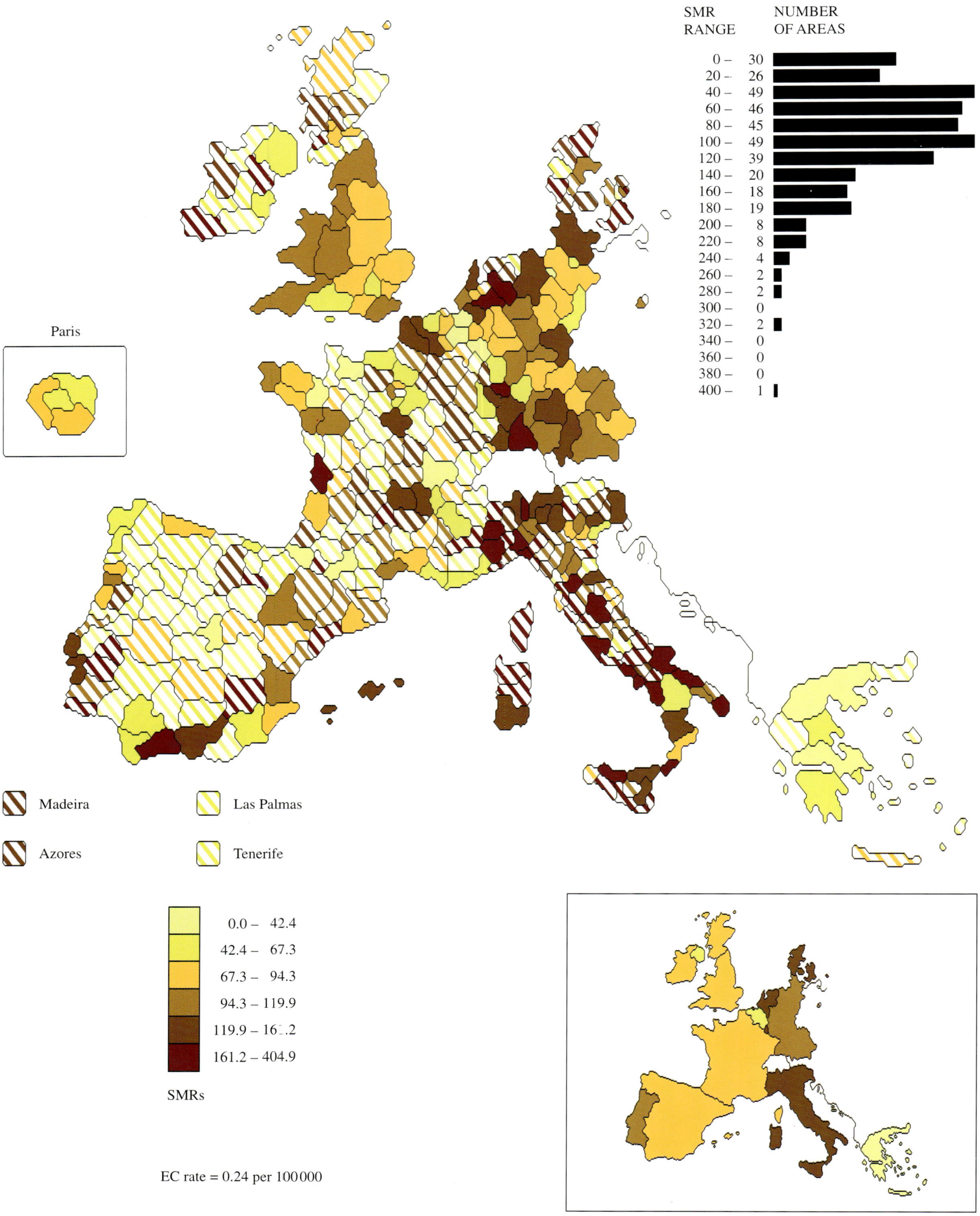
SMR RANGE
NUMBER OF AREAS
0 – 30
20 – 26
40 – 49
60 – 46
80 – 45
100 – 49
120 – 39
140 – 20
160 – 18
180 – 19
200 – 8
220 – 8
240 – 4
260 – 2
280 – 2
300 – 0
320 – 2
340 – 0
360 – 0
380 – 0
400 – 1
Paris
Madeira
Las Palmas
Azores
Tenerife
0.0 – 42.4
42.4 – 67.3
67.3 – 94.3
94.3 – 119.9
119.9 – 161.2
161.2 – 404.9
SMRs
EC rate = 0.24 per 100000

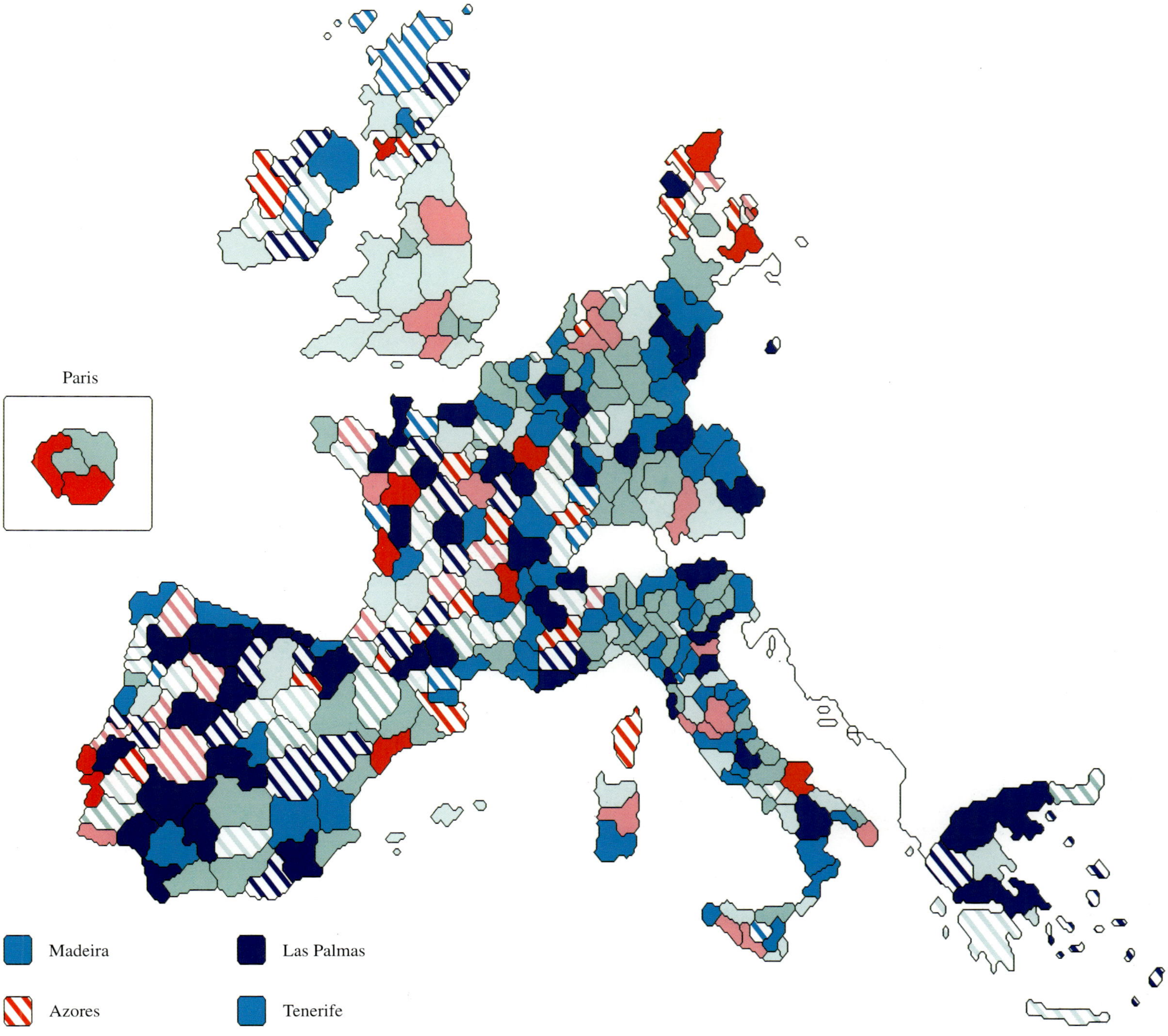

EC annual percentage change = –9.4%

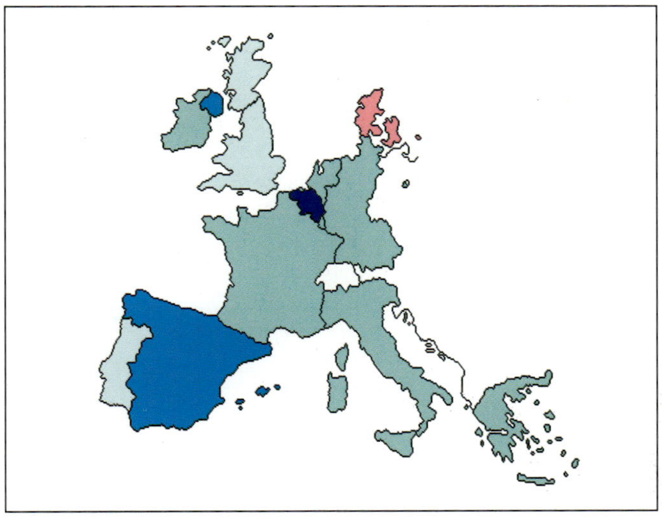

SMR RANGE	NUMBER OF AREAS
0 –	0
20 –	0
40 –	5
60 –	80
80 –	129
100 –	81
120 –	32
140 –	18
160 –	6
180 –	6
200 –	5
220 –	2
240 –	2
260 –	1
280 –	1
300 –	0
320 –	0
340 –	0
360 –	0
380 –	0
400 –	0

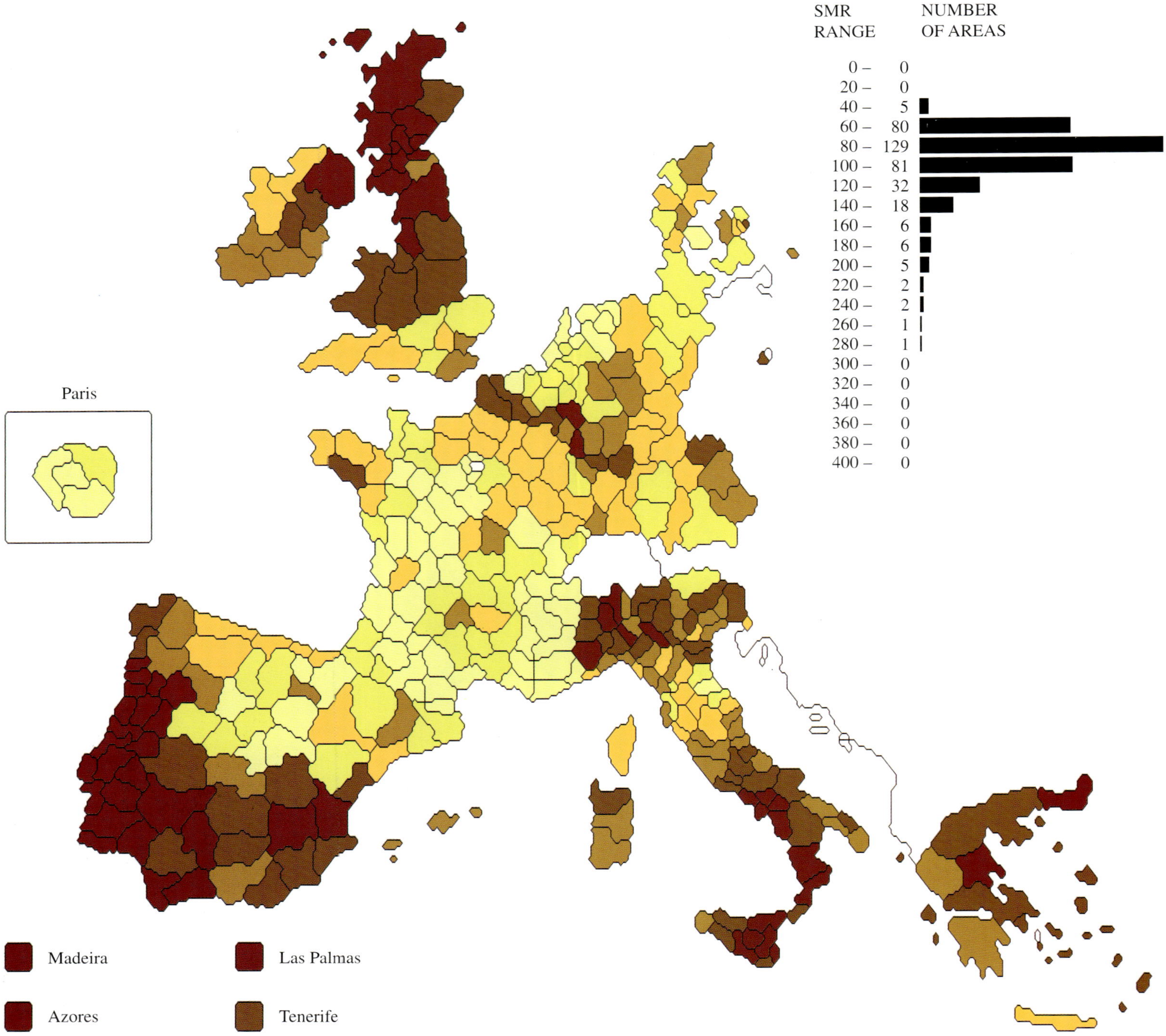

Paris

Madeira

Las Palmas

Azores

Tenerife

56.1 – 74.1

74.1 – 84.1

84.1 – 92.1

92.1 – 108.8

108.8 – 124.4

124.4 – 293.7

SMRs

EC rate = 34.72 per 100000

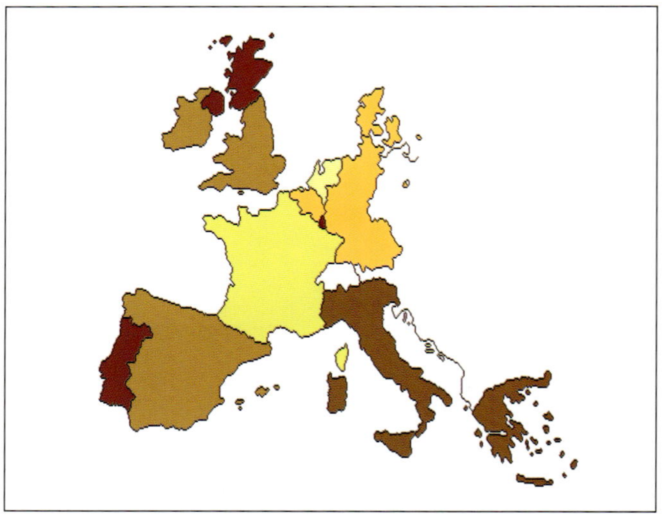

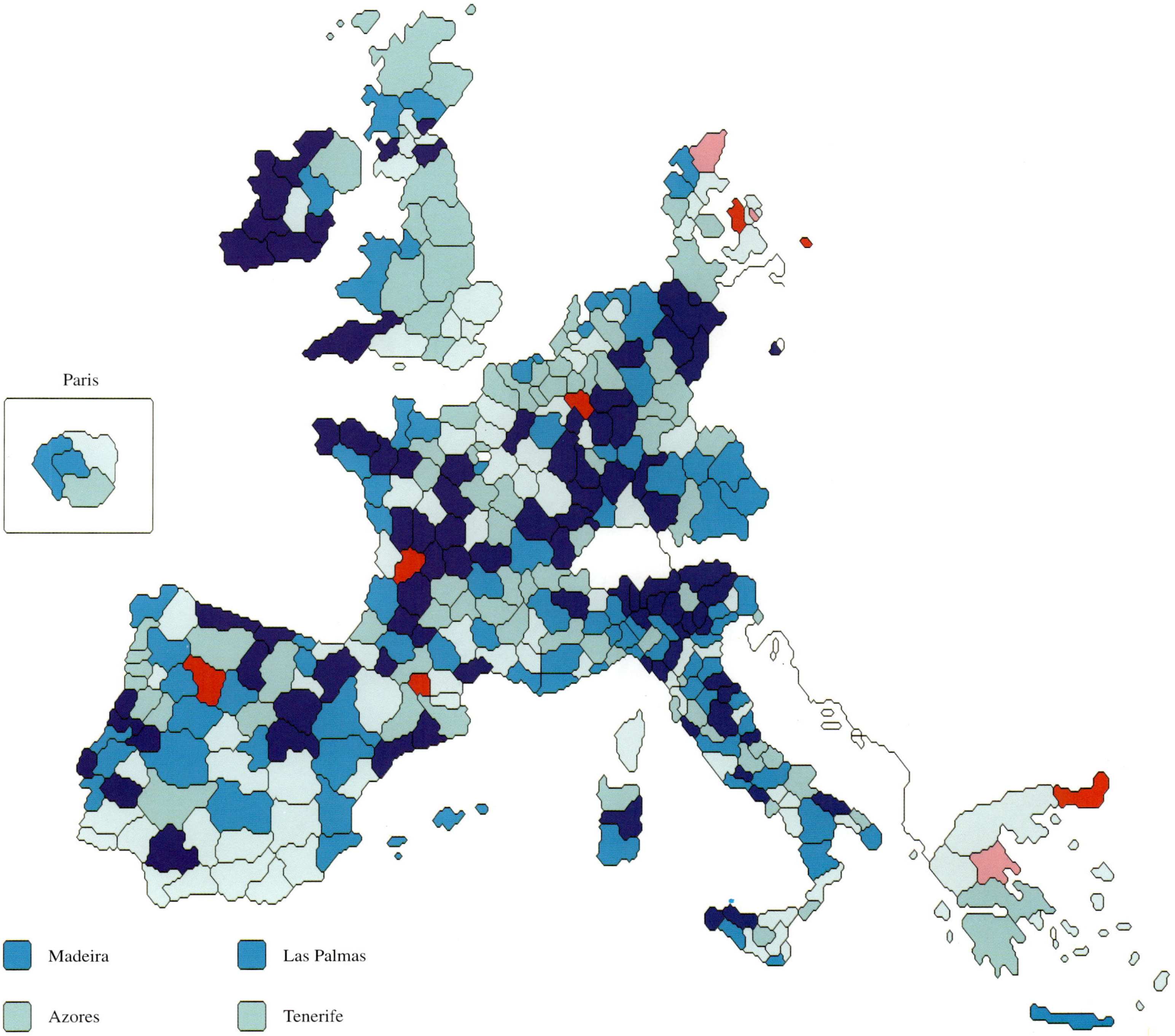

Paris

Madeira

Las Palmas

Azores

Tenerife

–13.3 –	–5.5
–5.5 –	–4.4
–4.4 –	–3.3
–3.3 –	0.0
0.0 –	0.4
0.4 –	5.1

Annual percentage change

EC annual percentage change = –4.3%

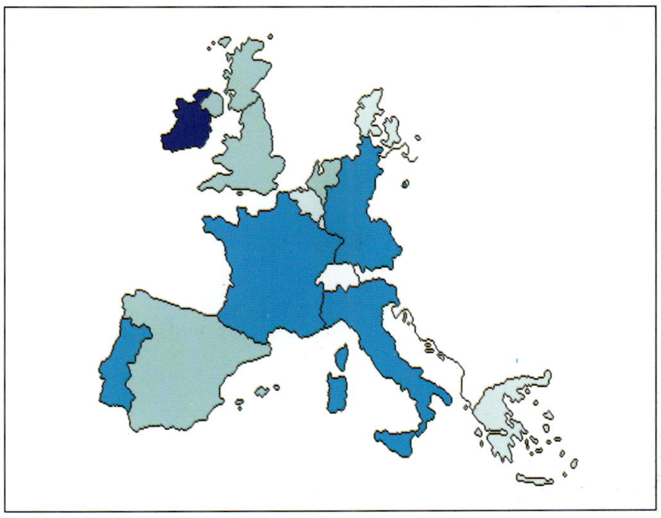

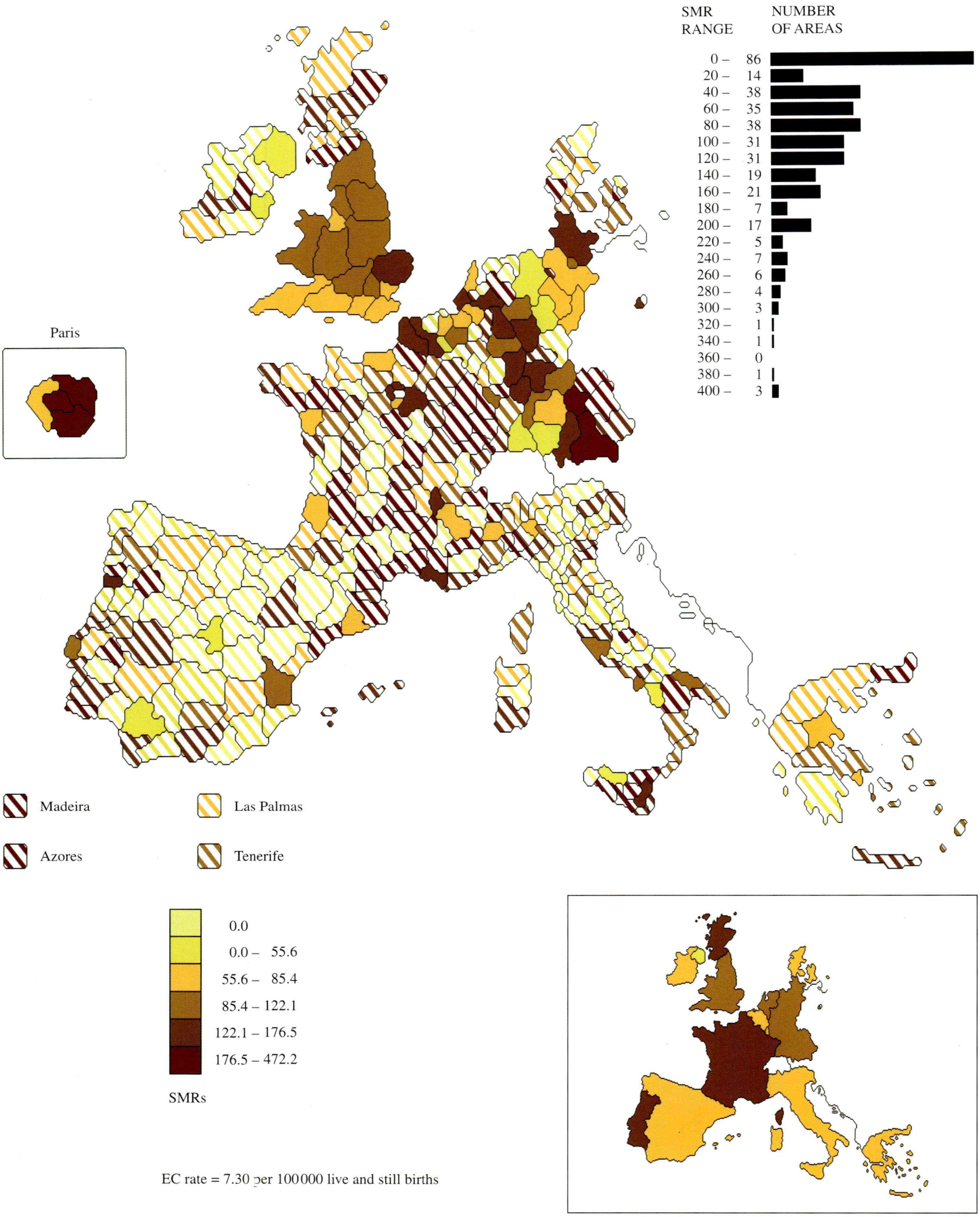

EC rate = 7.30 per 100000 live and still births

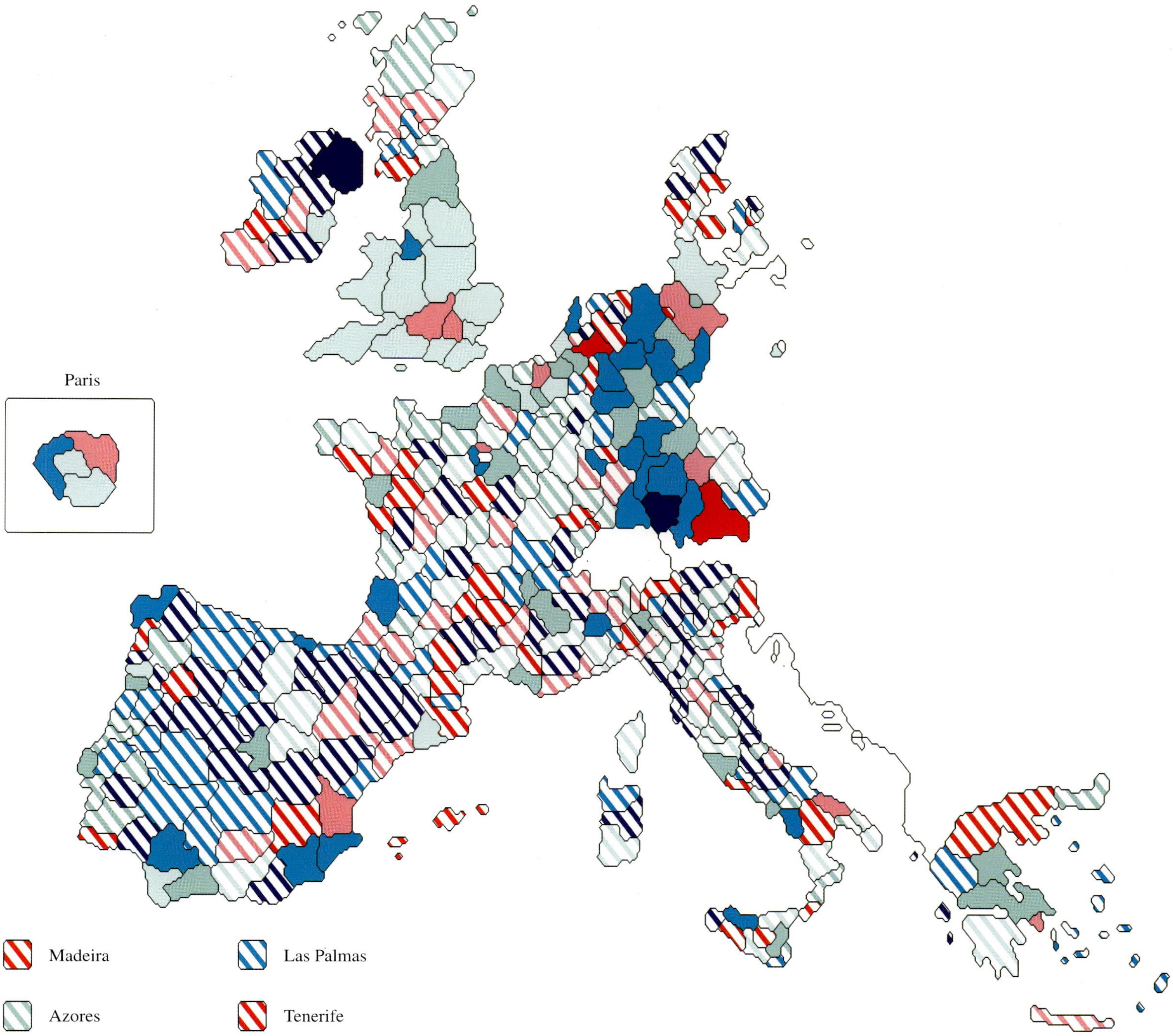

Paris

Madeira

Las Palmas

Azores

Tenerife

Annual percentage change
–100.0 – –35.8
–35.8 – –14.7
–14.7 – –6.9
–6.9 – 0.0
0.0 – 4.9
4.9 – 47.8

Annual percentage change

EC annual percentage change = –8.17%

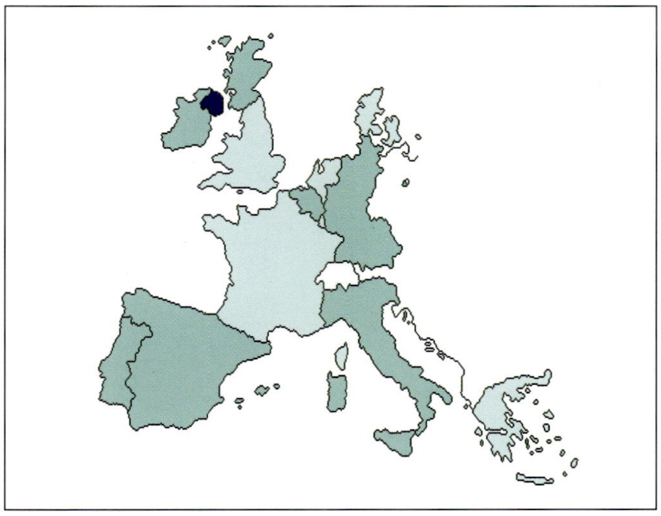

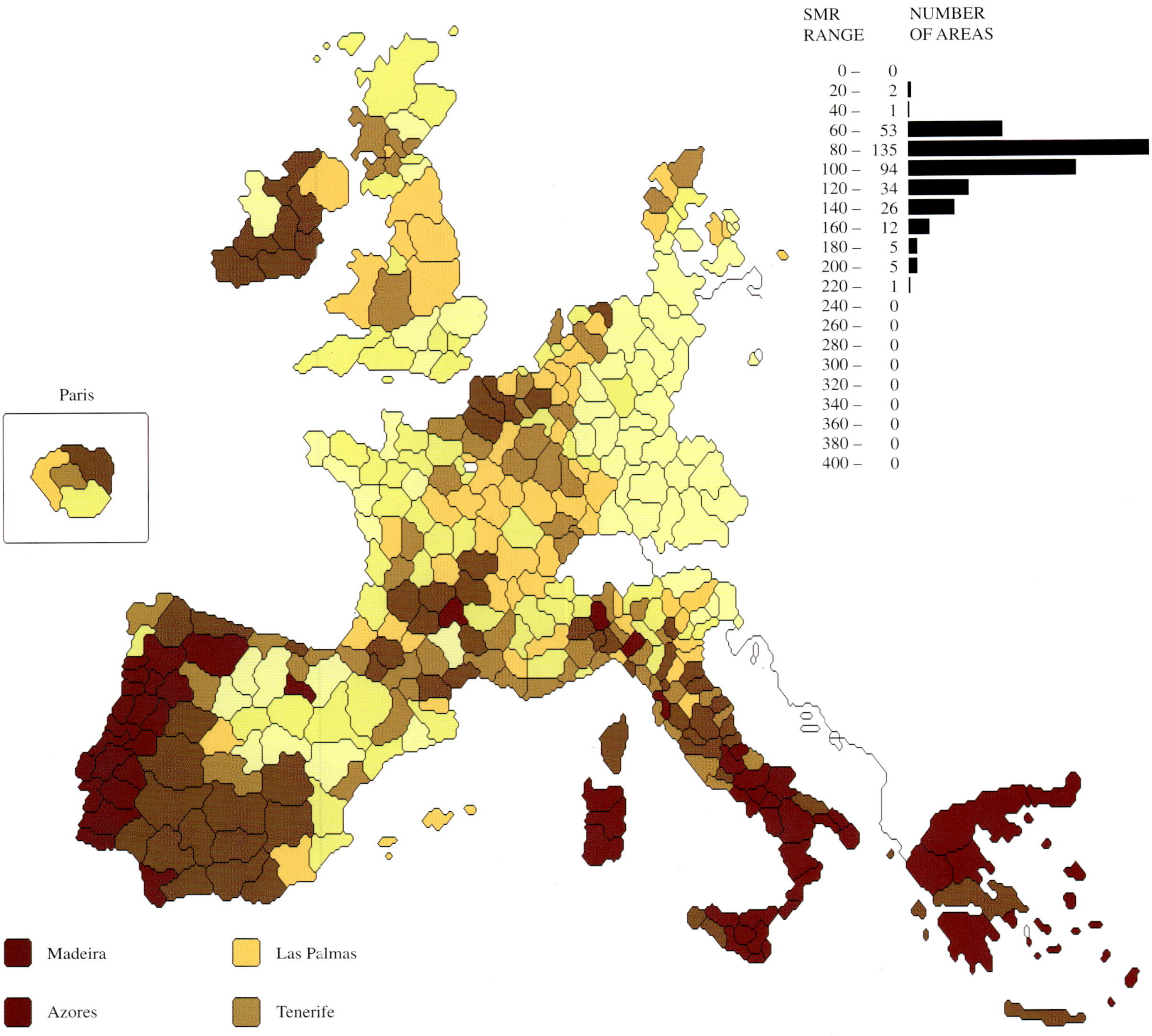

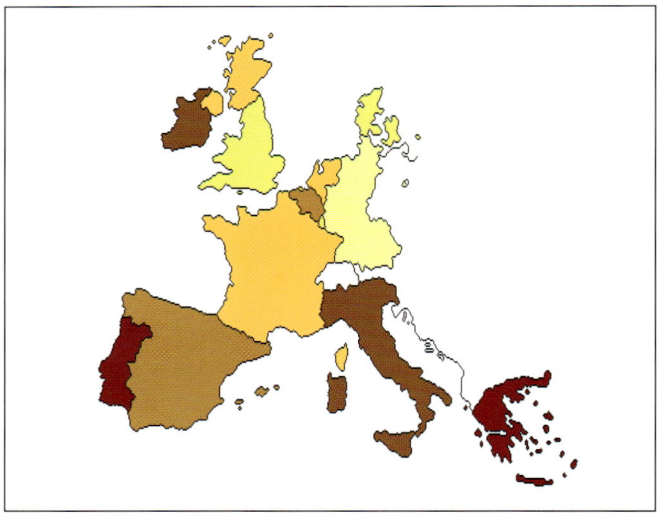

EC rate = 9.98 per 1000 live and still births

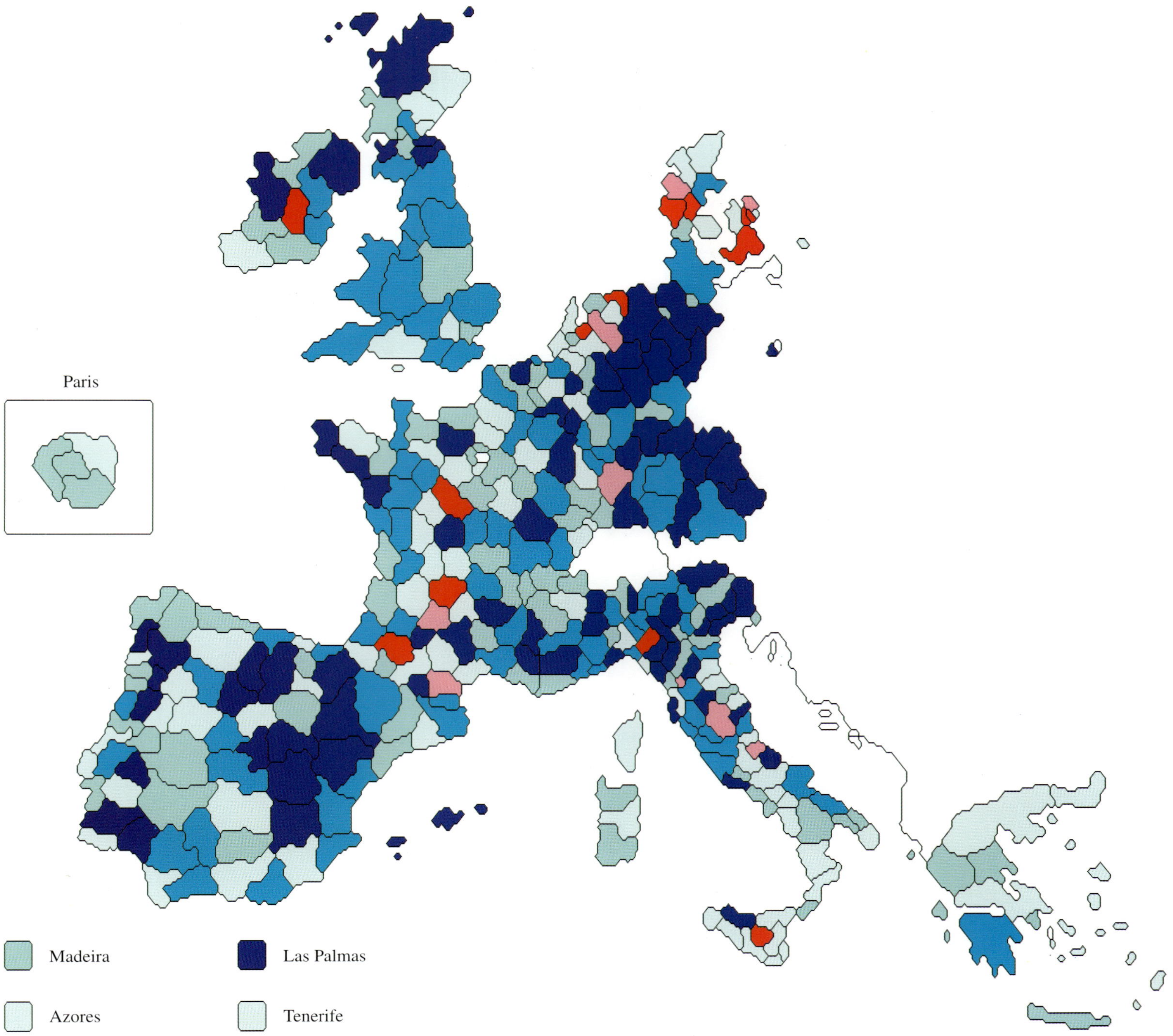

- –19.3 – –6.0
- –6.0 – –4.6
- –4.6 – –3.1
- –3.1 – 0.0
- 0.0 – 0.8
- 0.8 – 3.6

Annual percentage change

EC annual percentage change = –4.37%

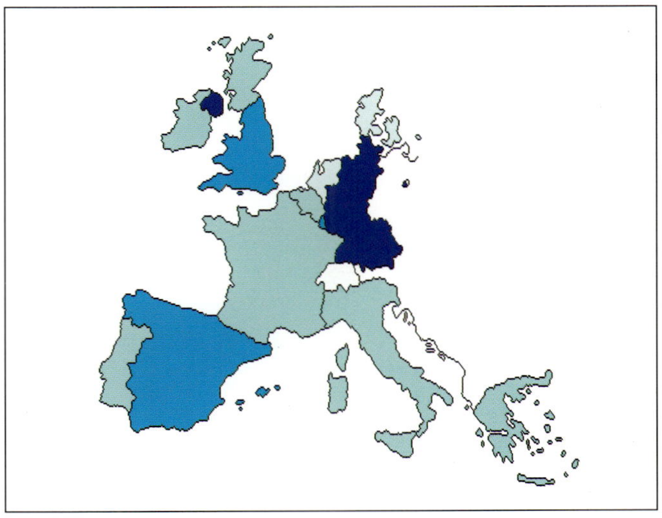

CANCER OF THE BREAST MORTALITY AGES 25–64: 1985–89

SMR RANGE	NUMBER OF AREAS
0 –	0
20 –	0
40 –	14
60 –	106
80 –	136
100 –	64
120 –	43
140 –	5
160 –	0
180 –	0
200 –	0
220 –	0
240 –	0
260 –	0
280 –	0
300 –	0
320 –	0
340 –	0
360 –	0
380 –	0
400 –	0

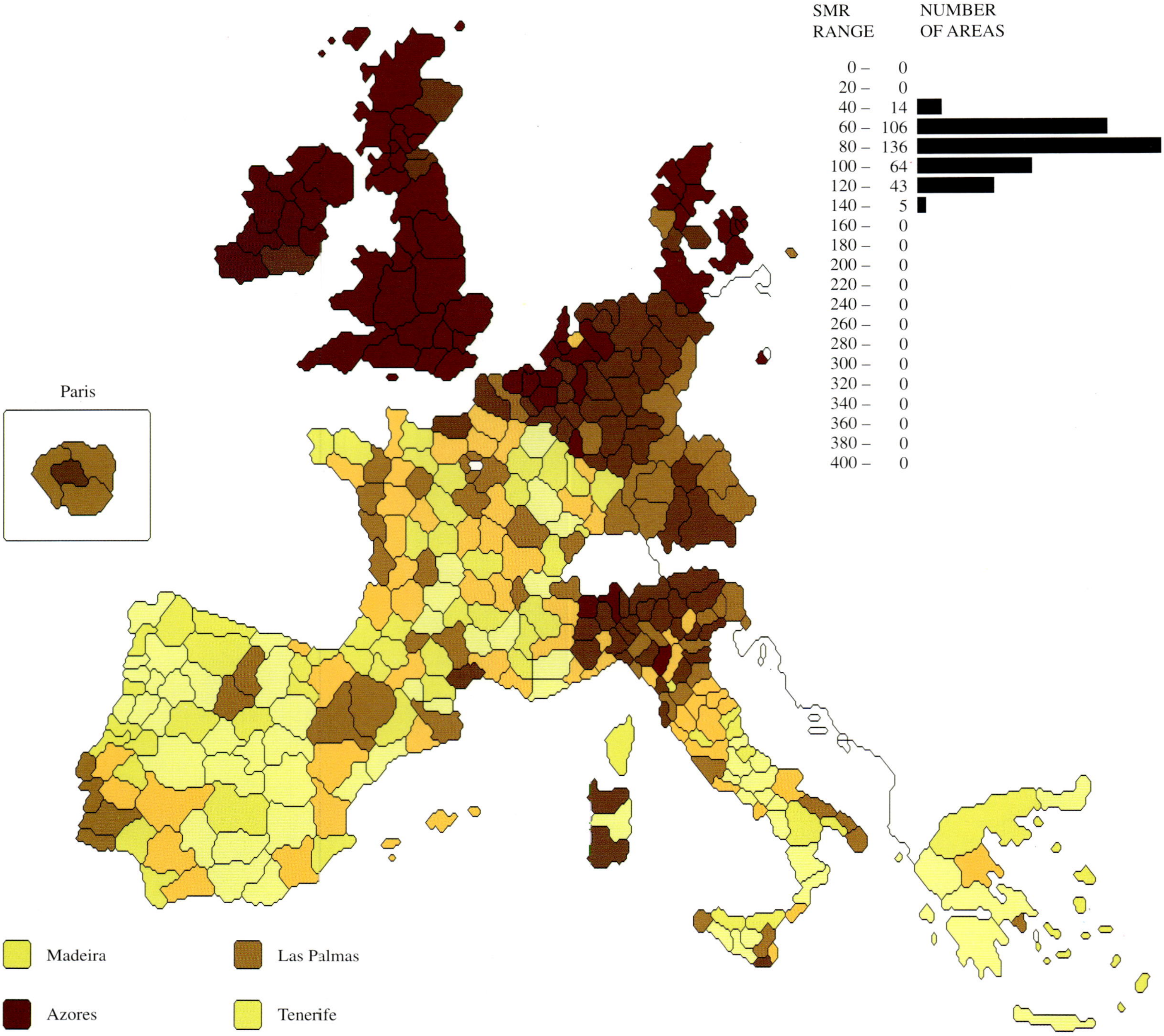

SMRs

- 41.8 – 71.8
- 71.8 – 80.1
- 80.1 – 89.1
- 89.1 – 98.7
- 98.7 – 112.4
- 112.4 – 159.2

EC rate = 34.10 per 100000

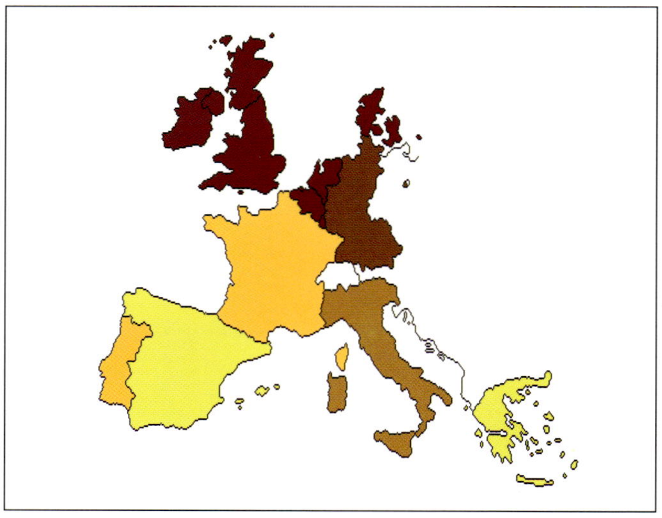

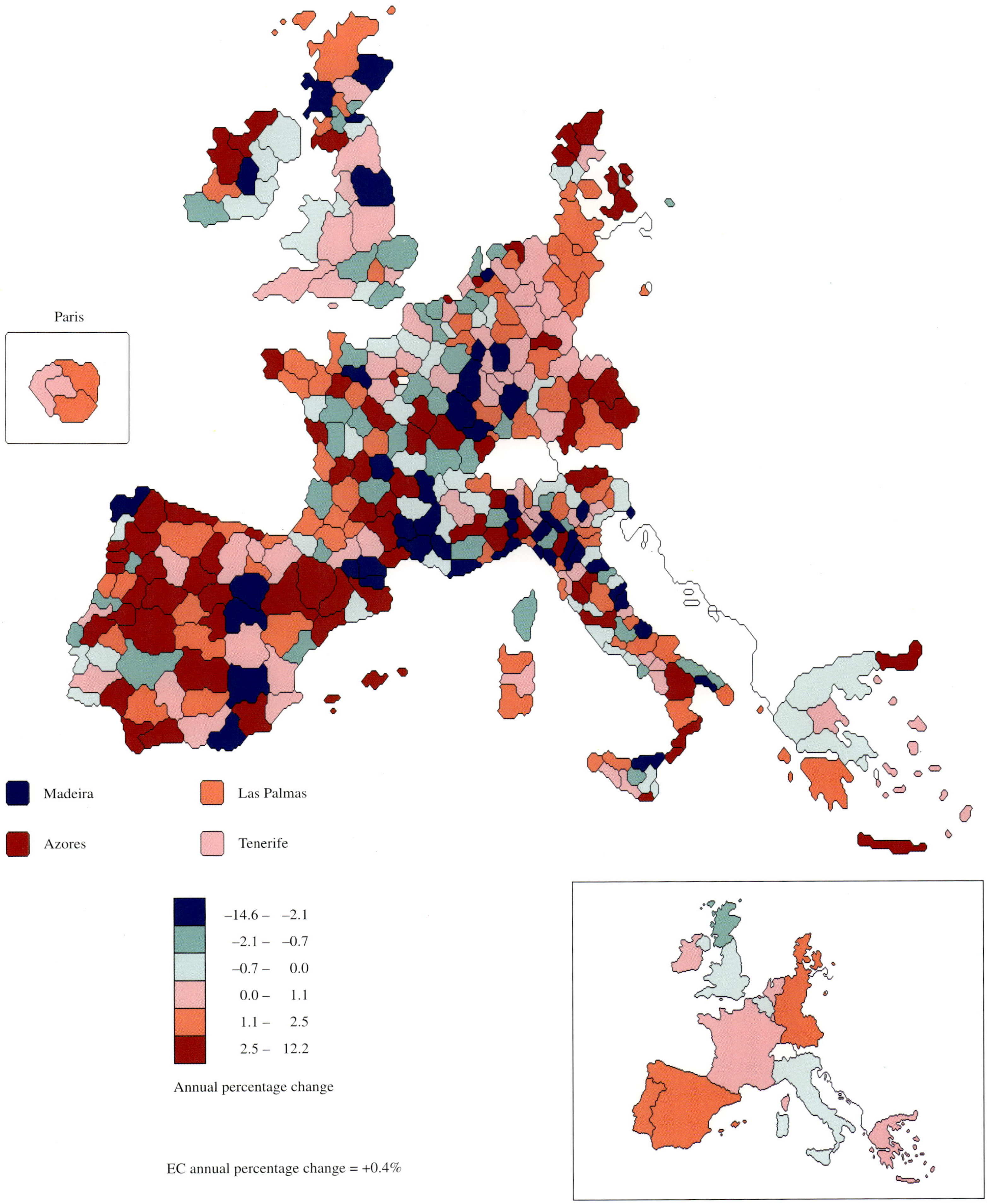
Paris
Madeira
Las Palmas
Azores
Tenerife
–14.6 – –2.1
–2.1 – –0.7
–0.7 – 0.0
0.0 – 1.1
1.1 – 2.5
2.5 – 12.2
Annual percentage change
EC annual percentage change = +0.4%

SMR RANGE	NUMBER OF AREAS
0 –	0
20 –	14
40 –	124
60 –	101
80 –	38
100 –	31
120 –	12
140 –	17
160 –	2
180 –	7
200 –	9
220 –	8
240 –	1
260 –	3
280 –	1
300 –	0
320 –	0
340 –	0
360 –	0
380 –	0
400 –	0

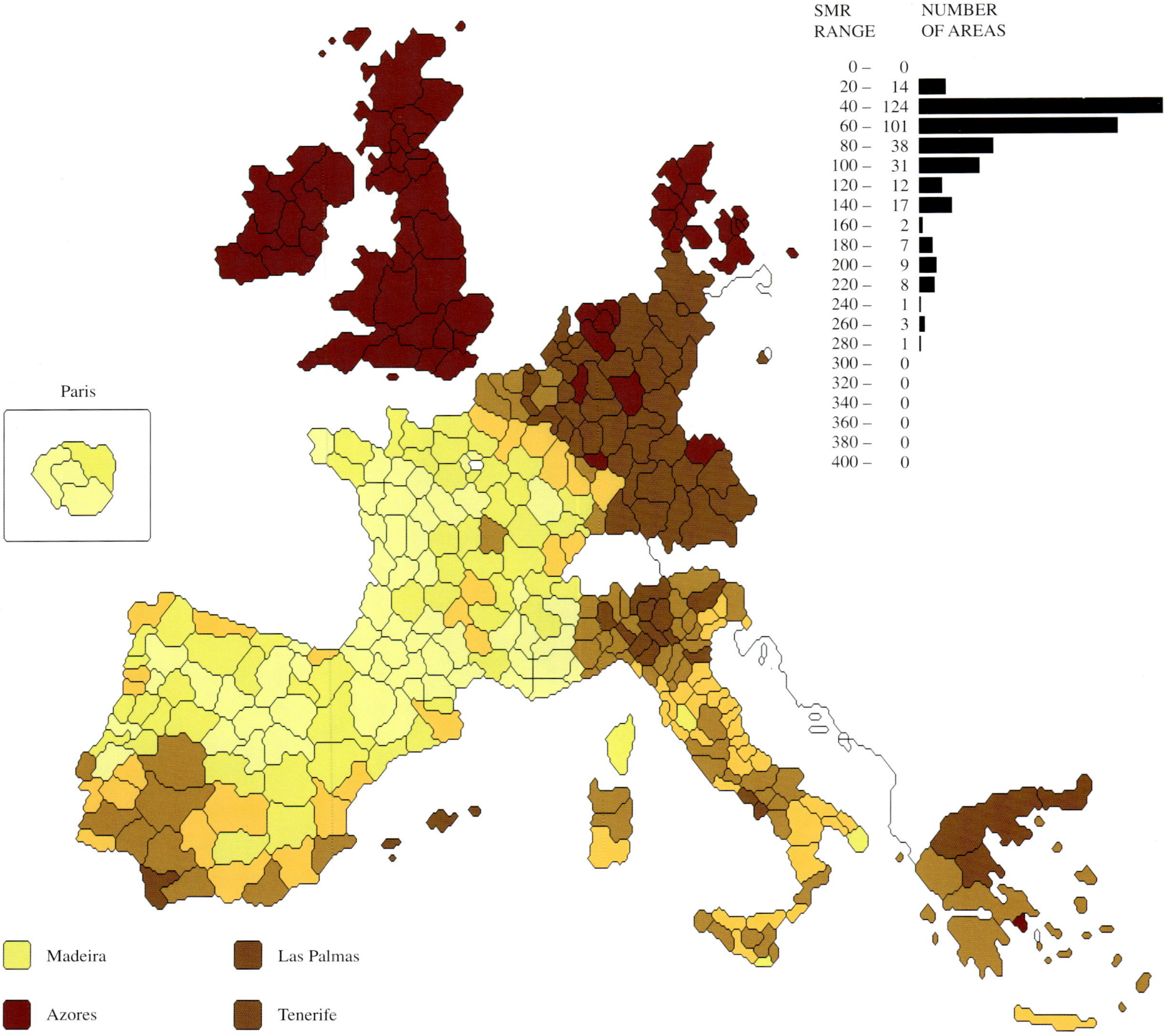

SMRs
35.6 – 48.1
48.1 – 58.0
58.0 – 67.4
67.4 – 81.6
81.6 – 116.7
116.7 – 288.0

EC rate = 88.51 per 100000

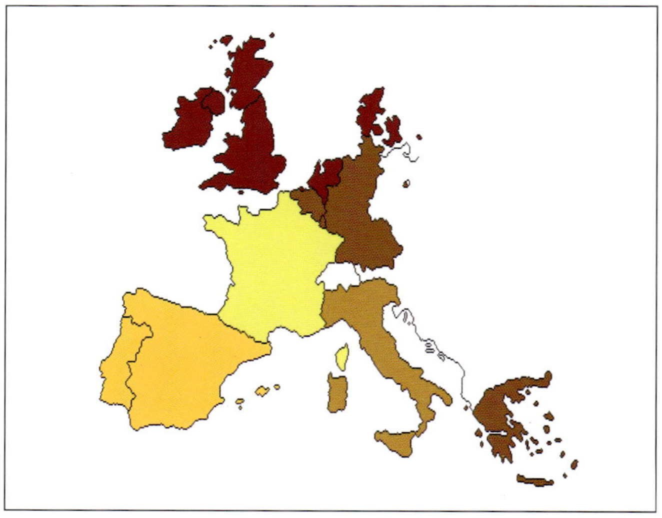

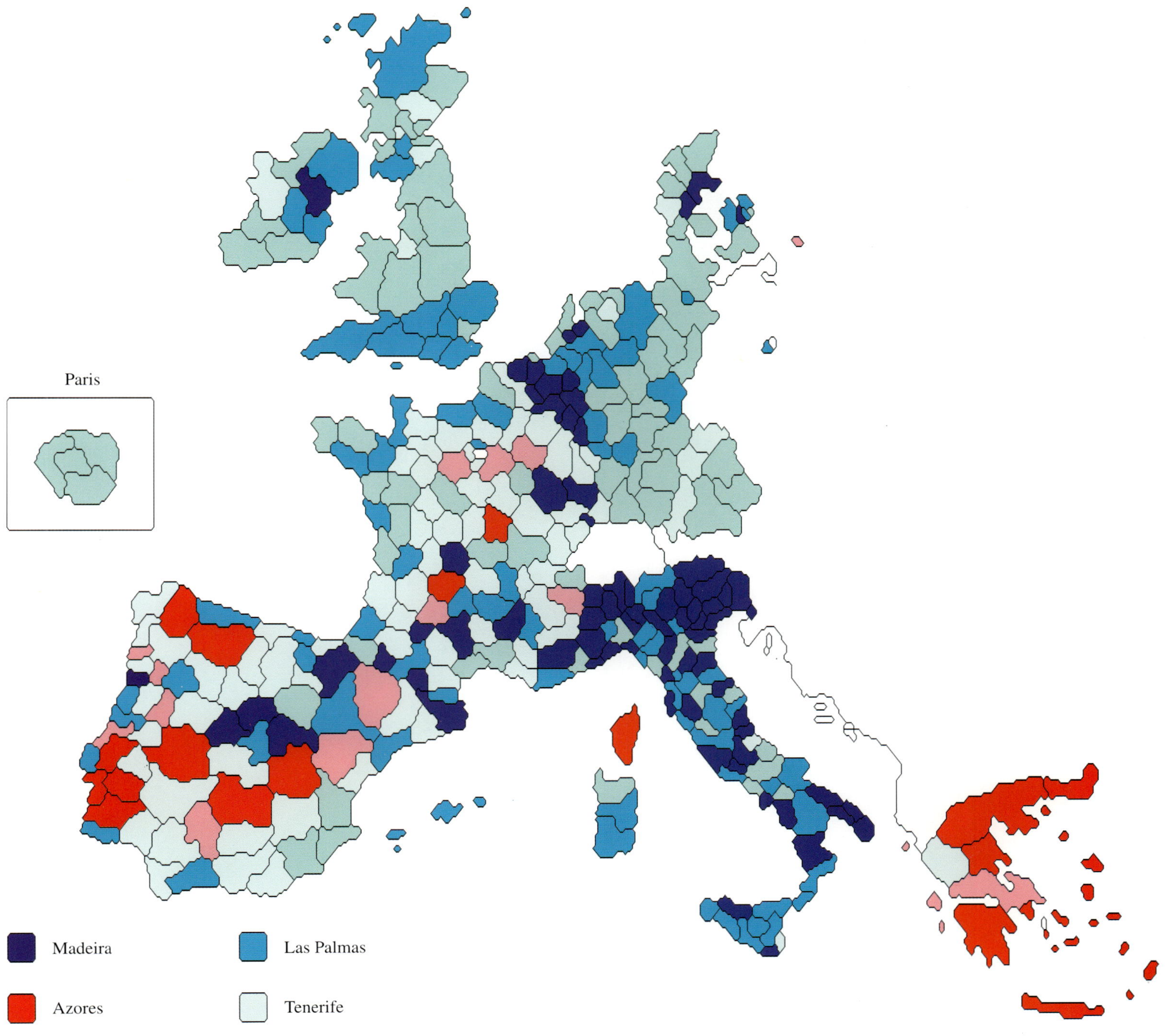

EC annual percentage change = –2.8%

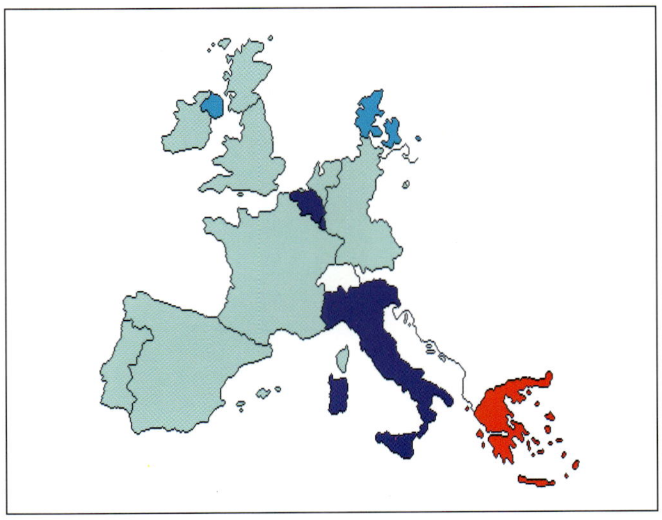

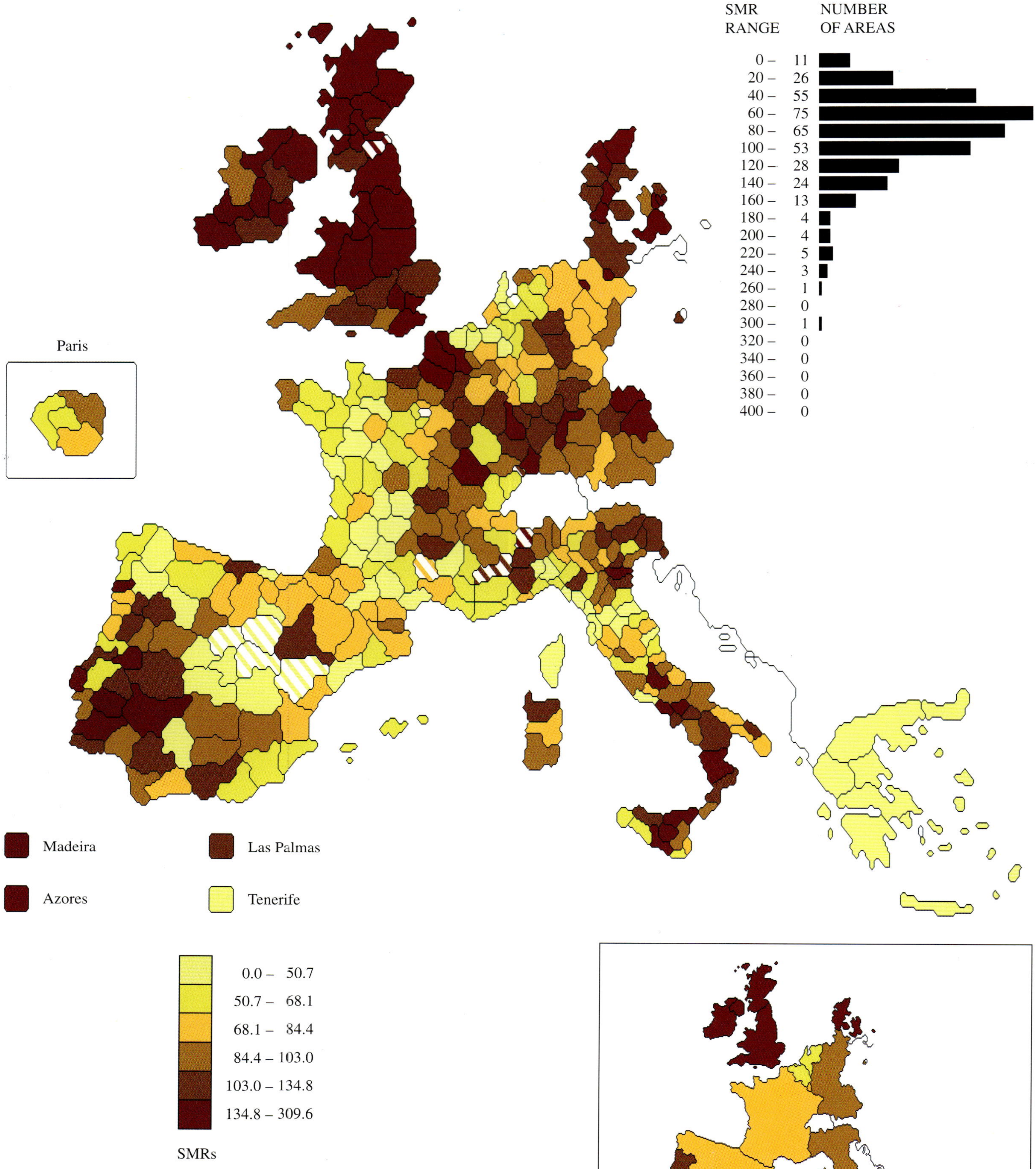

EC rate = 1.45 per 100000

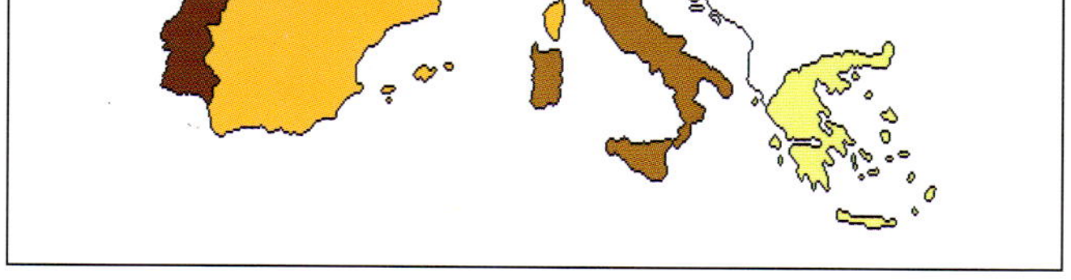

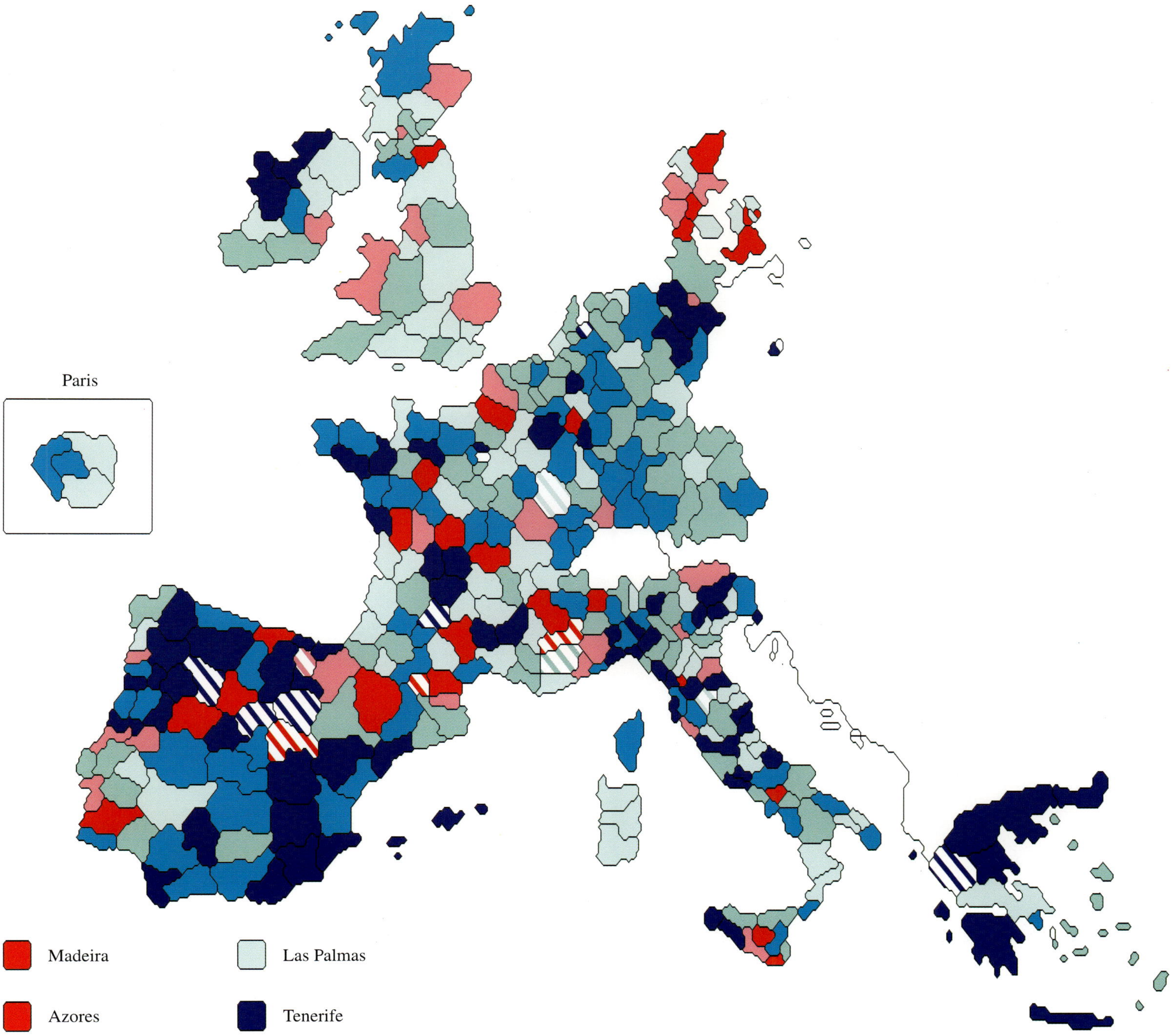

–100.0 – –13.5
–13.5 – –8.8
–8.8 – –5.4
–5.4 – 0.0
0.0 – 2.3
2.3 – 31.2

Annual percentage change

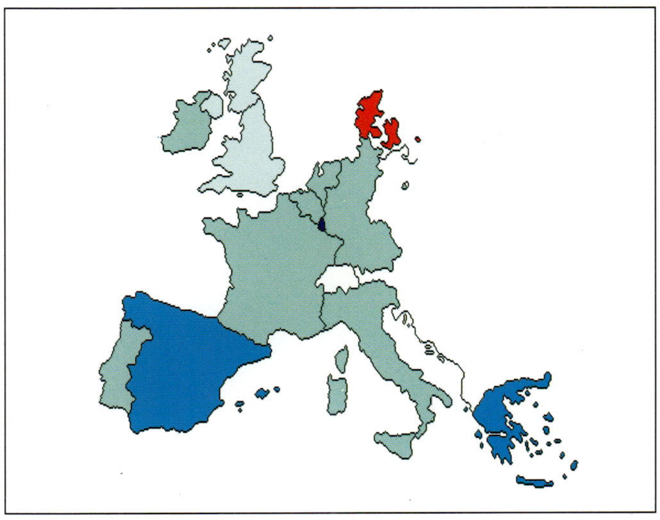

EC annual percentage change = –5.9%

SMR RANGE	NUMBER OF AREAS
0 –	0
20 –	0
40 –	0
60 –	27
80 –	179
100 –	134
120 –	24
140 –	3
160 –	1
180 –	0
200 –	0
220 –	0
240 –	0
260 –	0
280 –	0
300 –	0
320 –	0
340 –	0
360 –	0
380 –	0
400 –	0

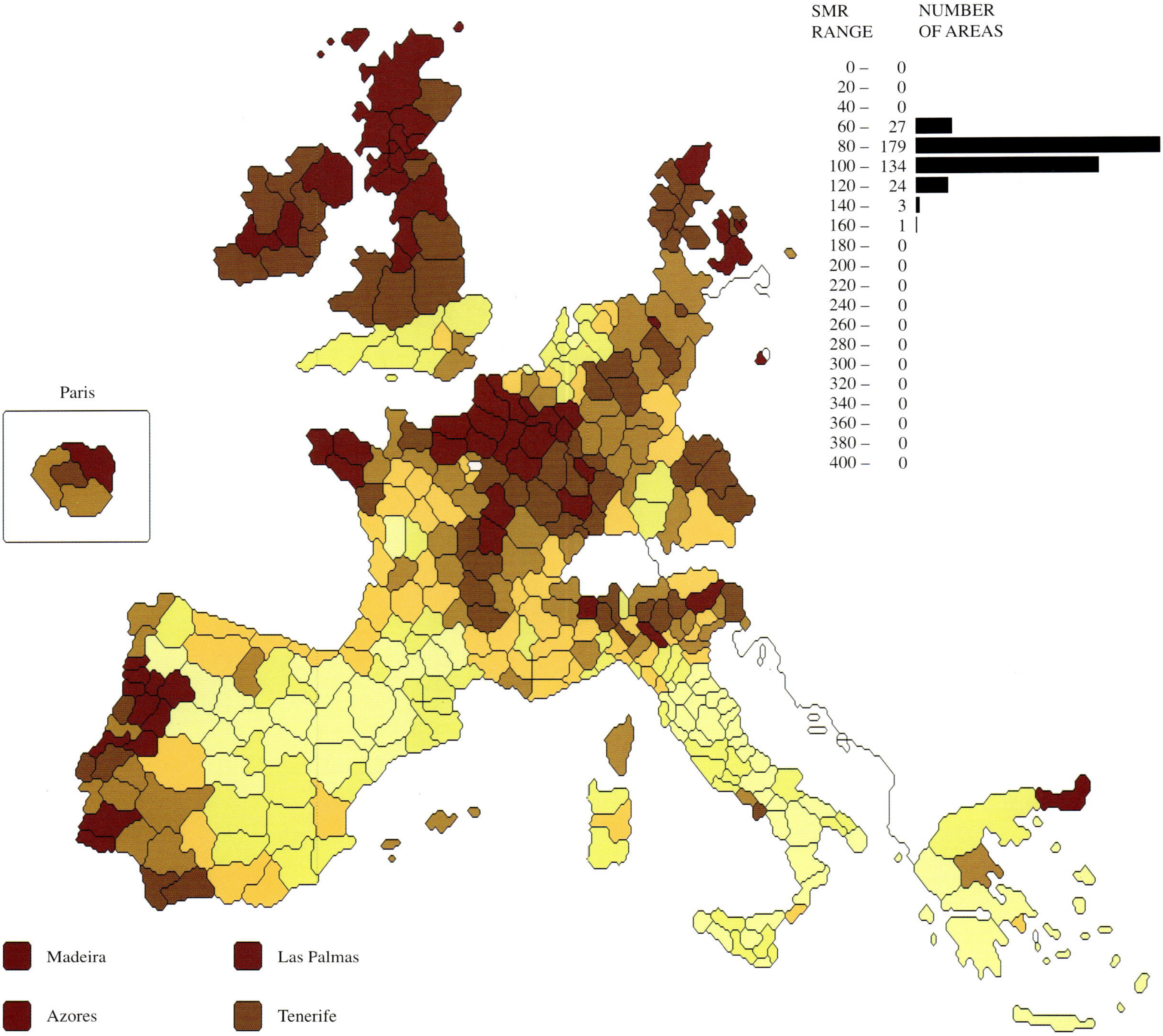

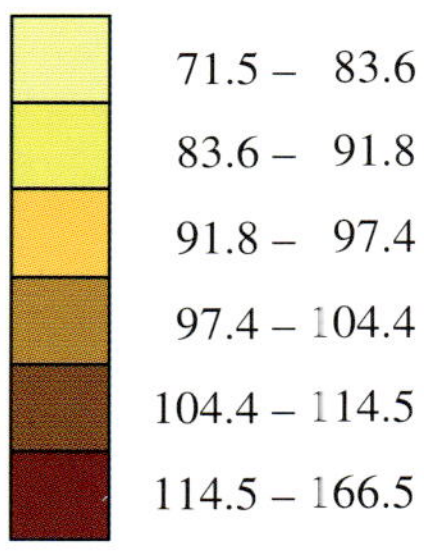

SMRs

EC rate = 271 per 100000

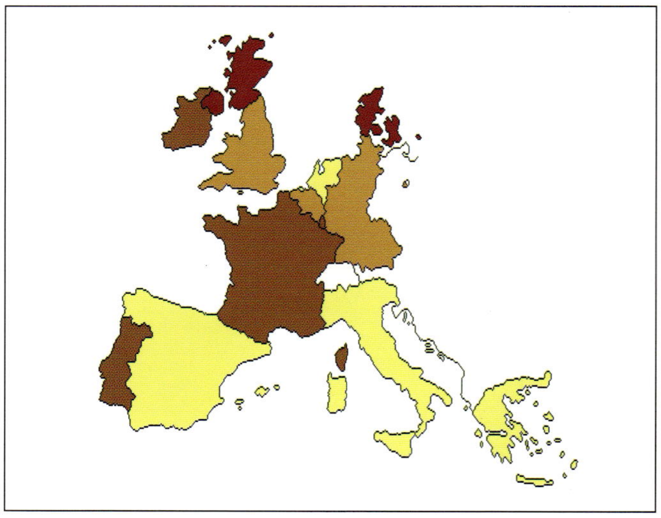

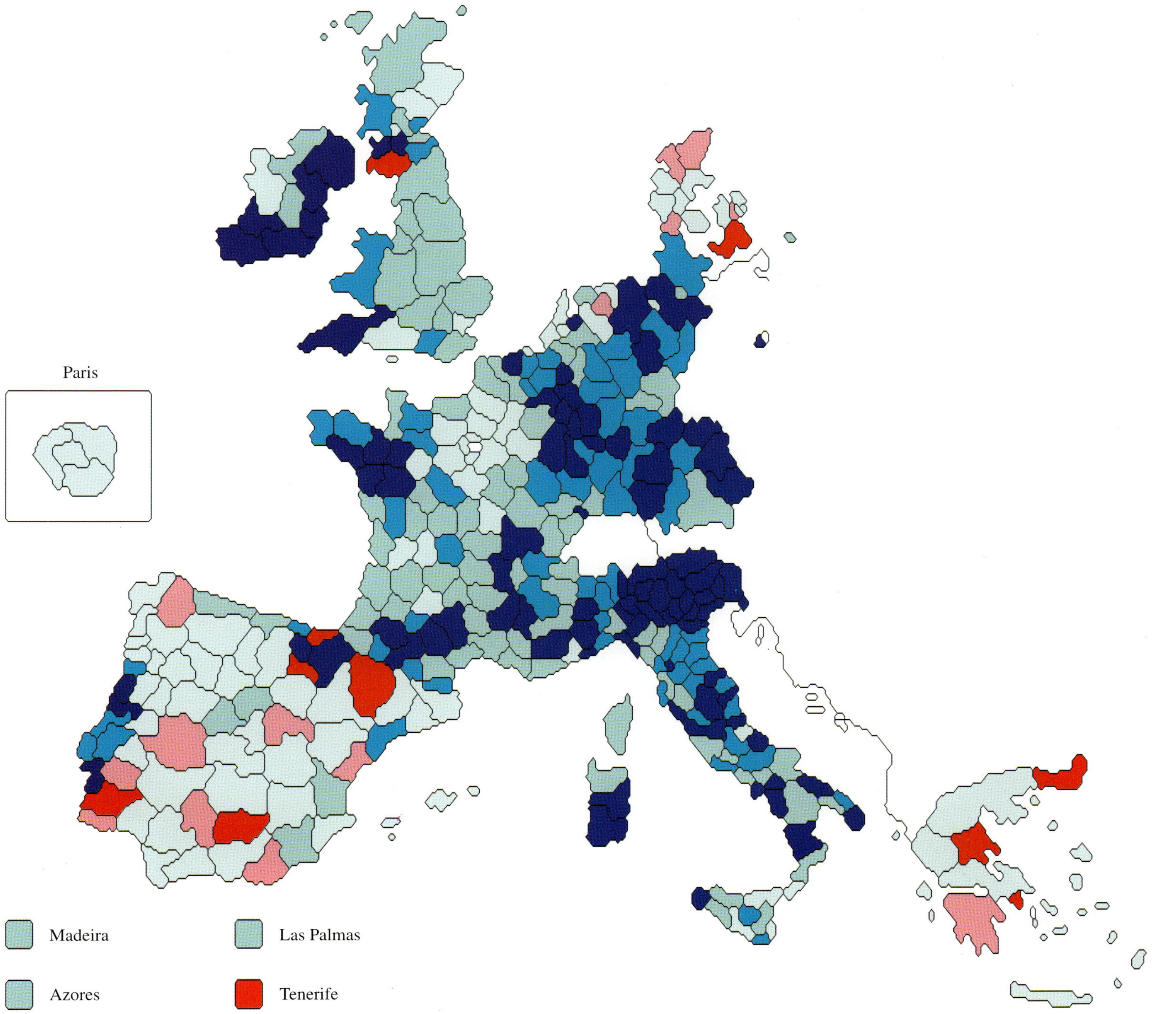

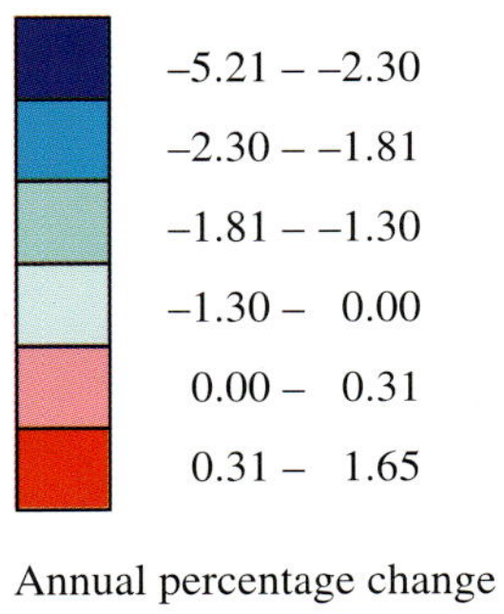

EC annual percentage change = –1.7%

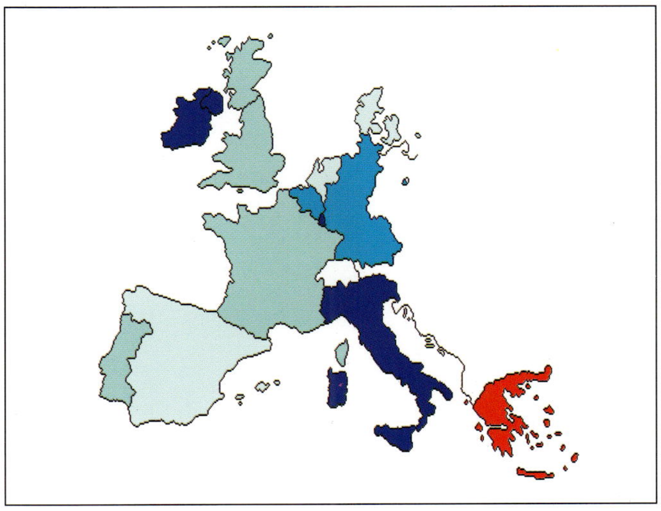

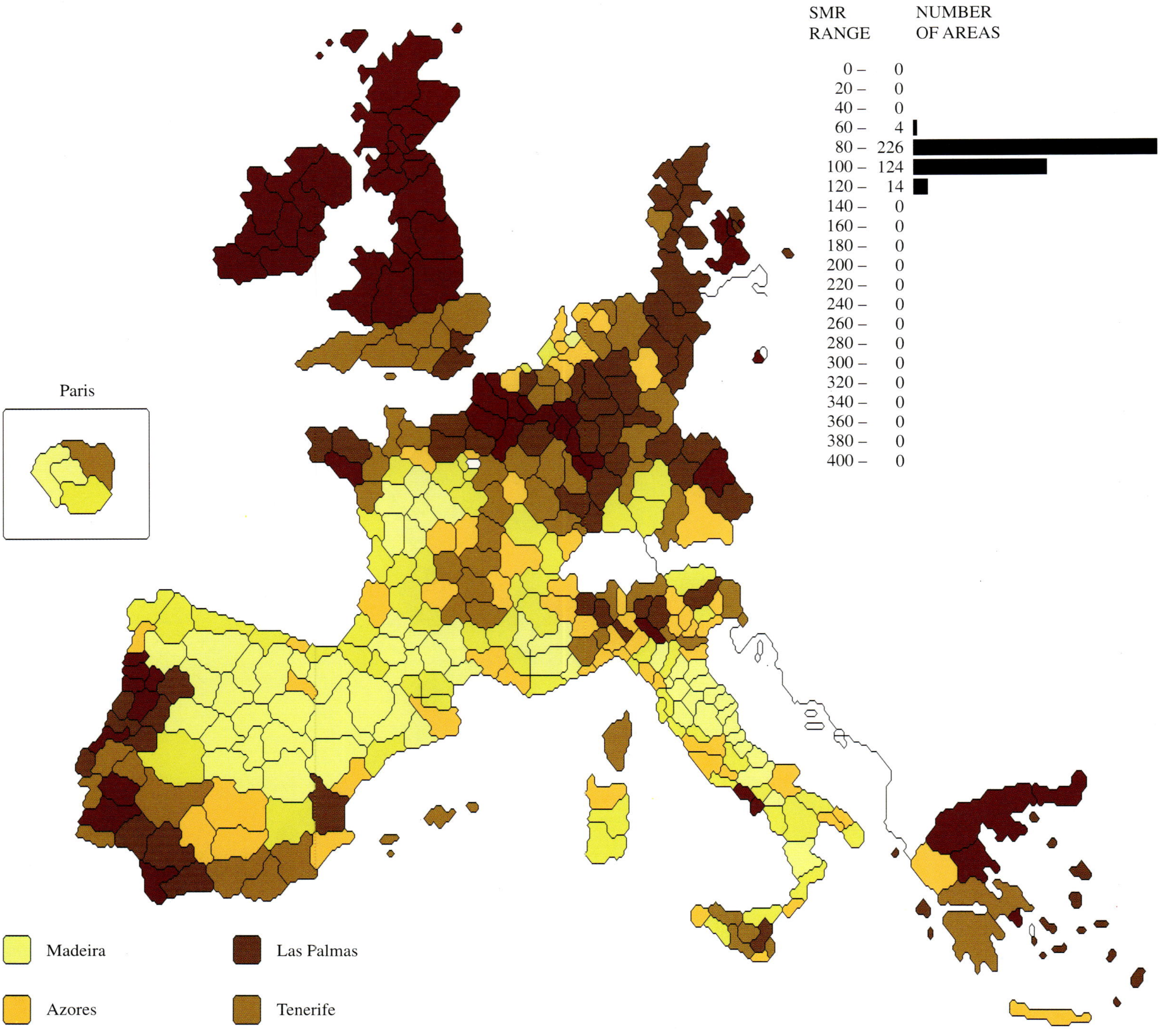

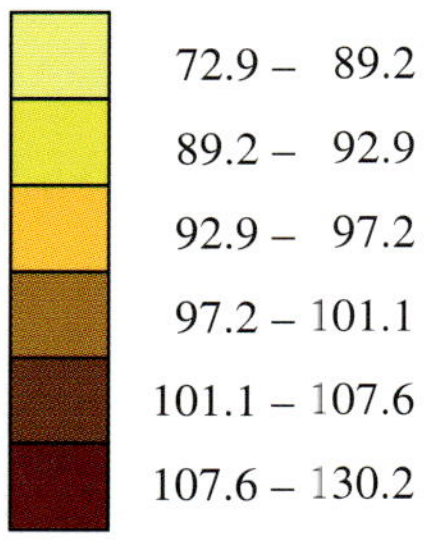

SMRs

EC rate = 1006 per 100000

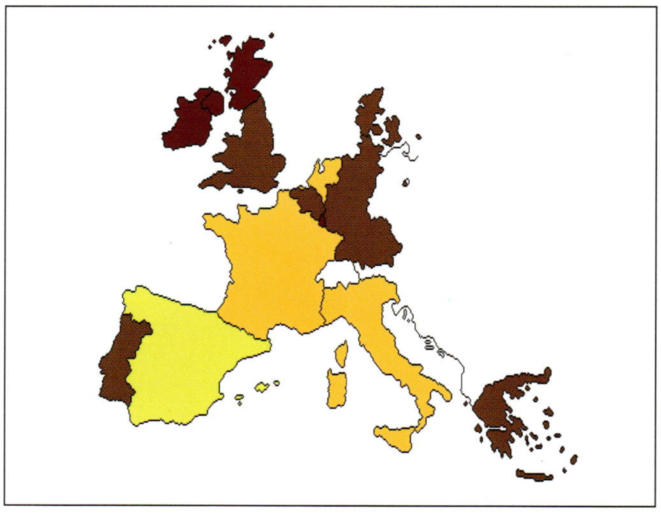

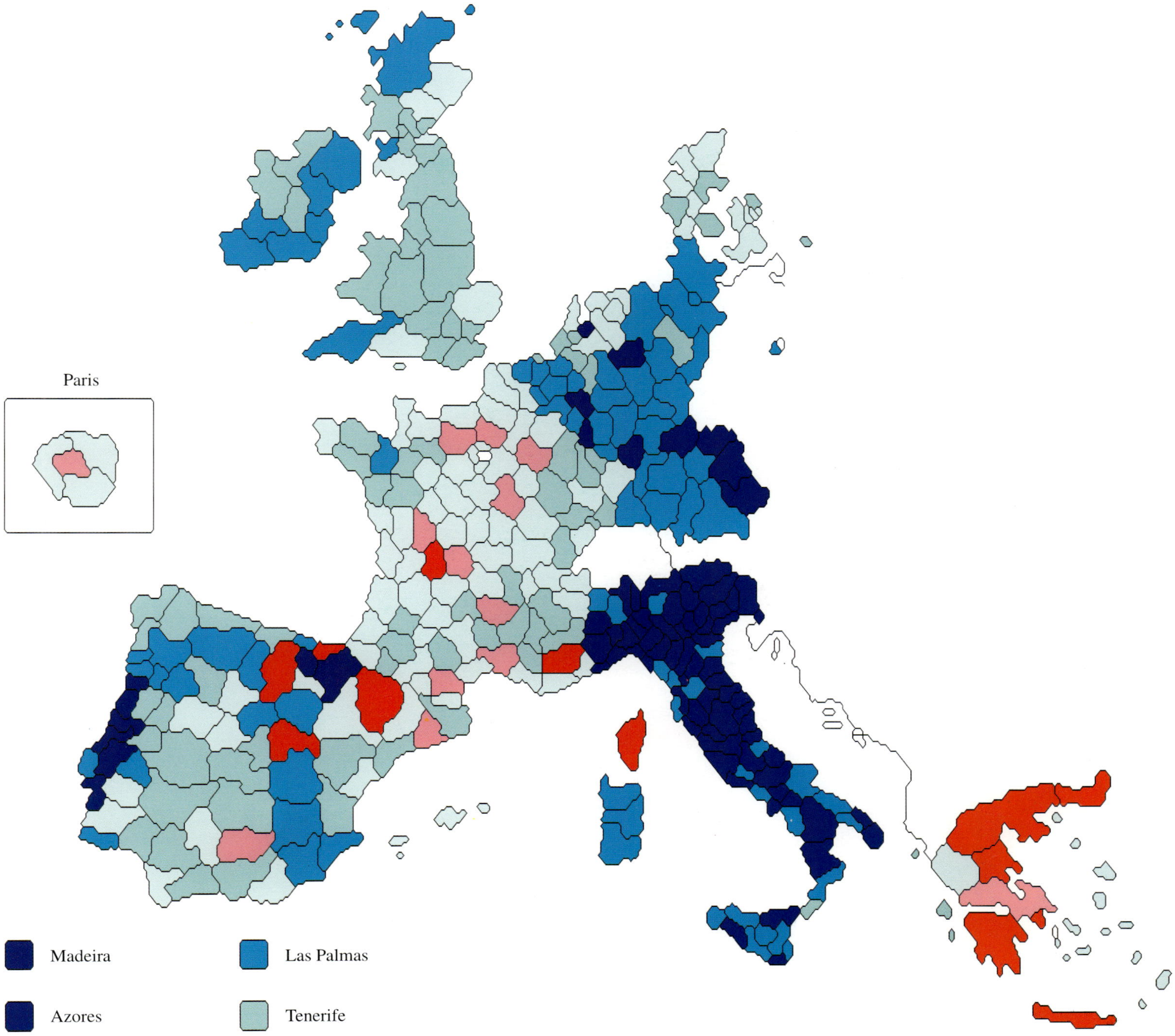

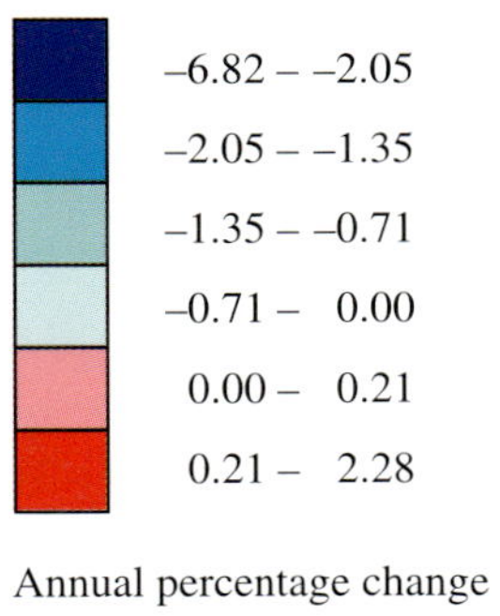

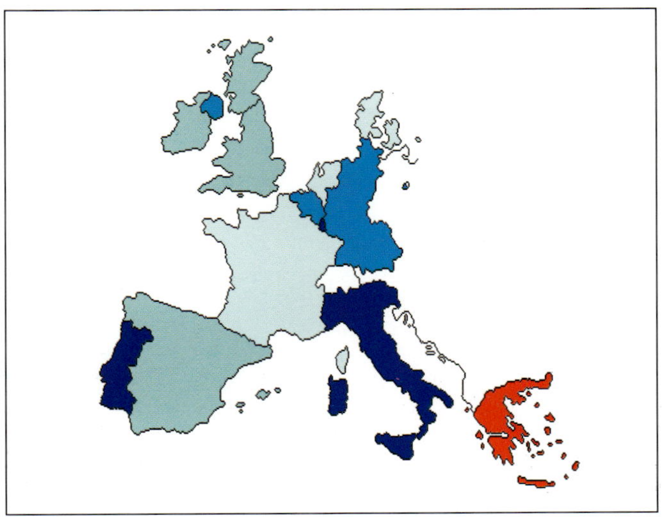

EC annual percentage change = –1.28%

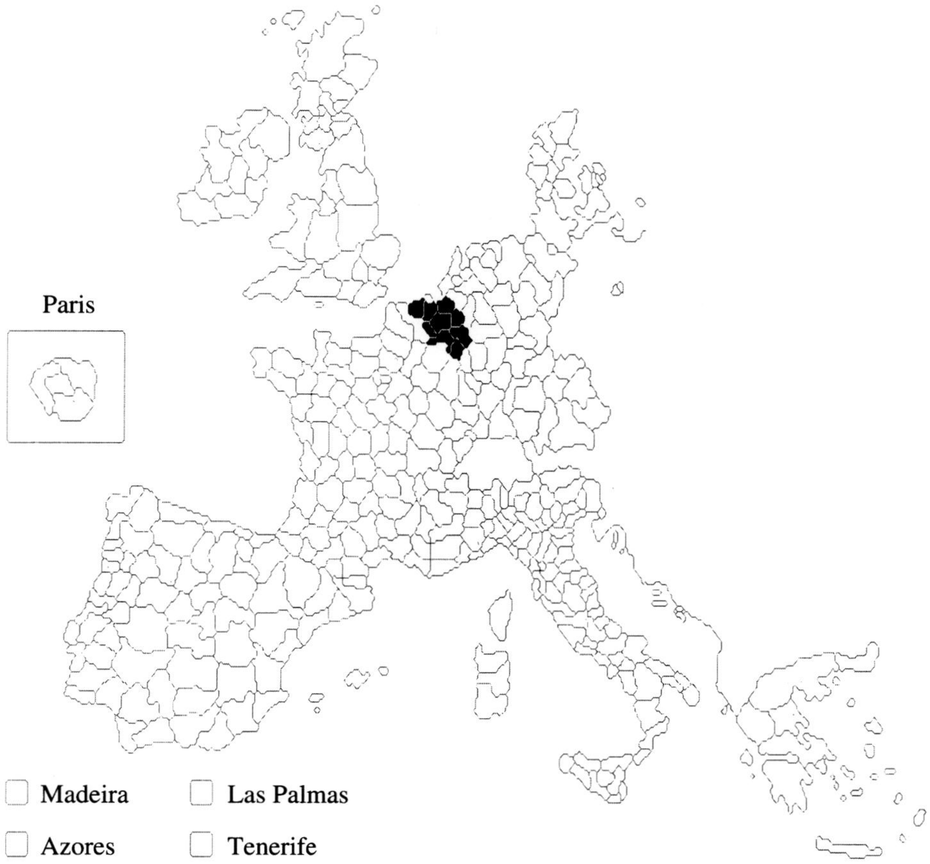

KEY MAP: BELGIUM

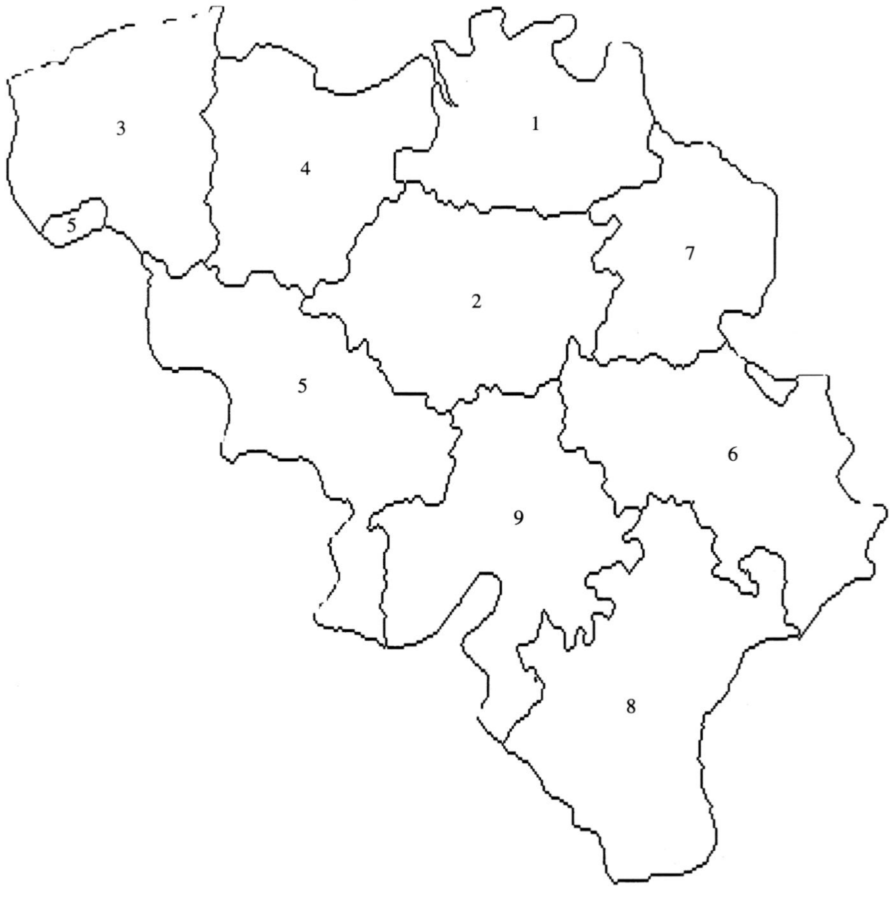

TUBERCULOSIS MORTALITY AGES 5–64: 1985–89

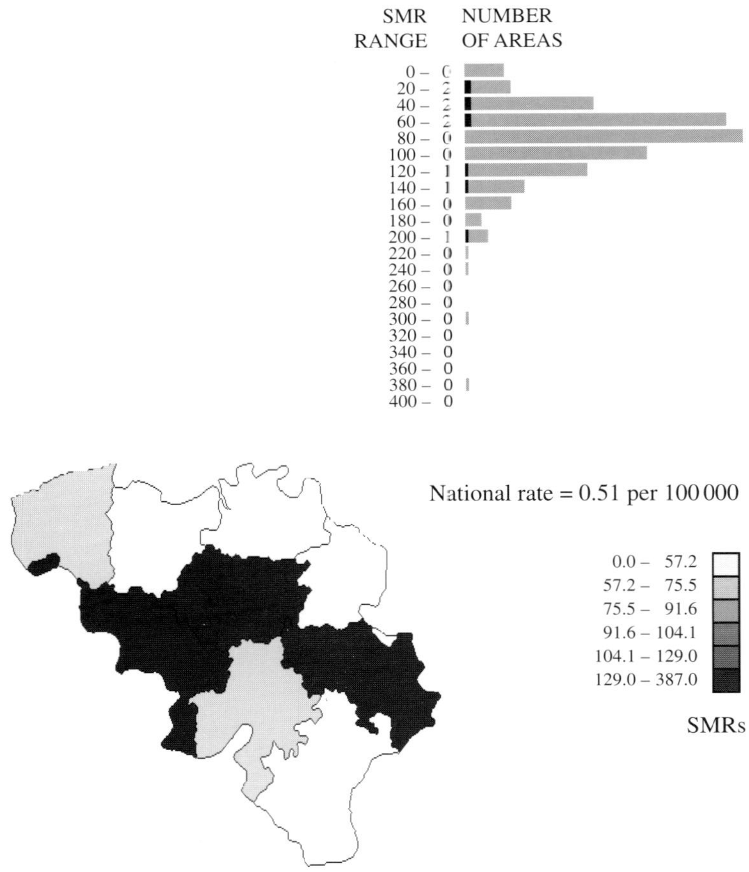

MALIGNANT NEOPLASM OF CERVIX UTERI MORTALITY AGES 15–64: 1985–89

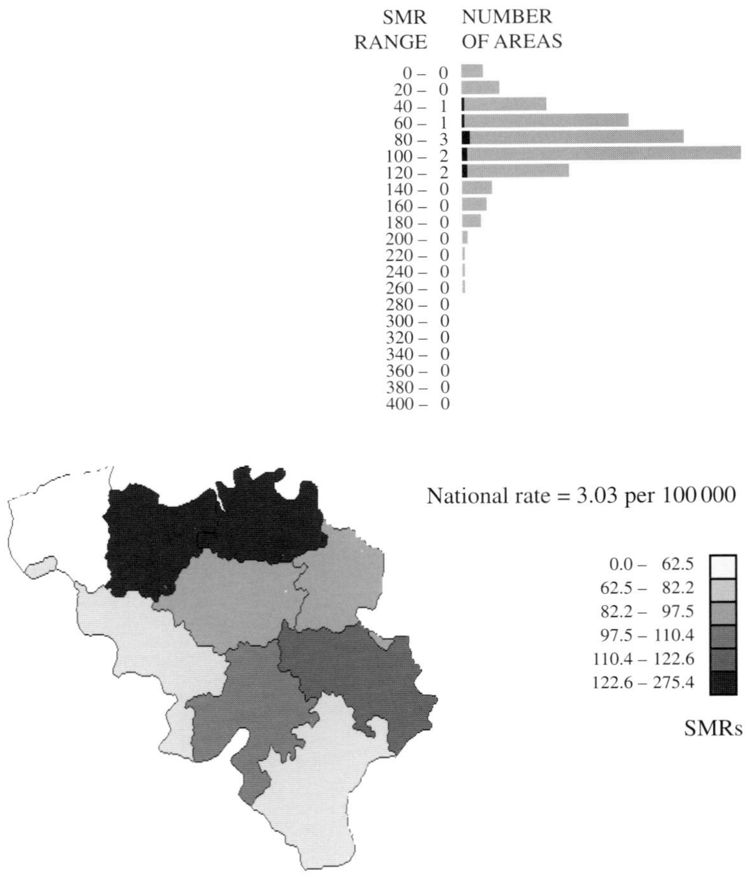

MALIGNANT NEOPLASM OF CERVIX AND BODY OF UTERUS MORTALITY AGES 15–54: 1985–89

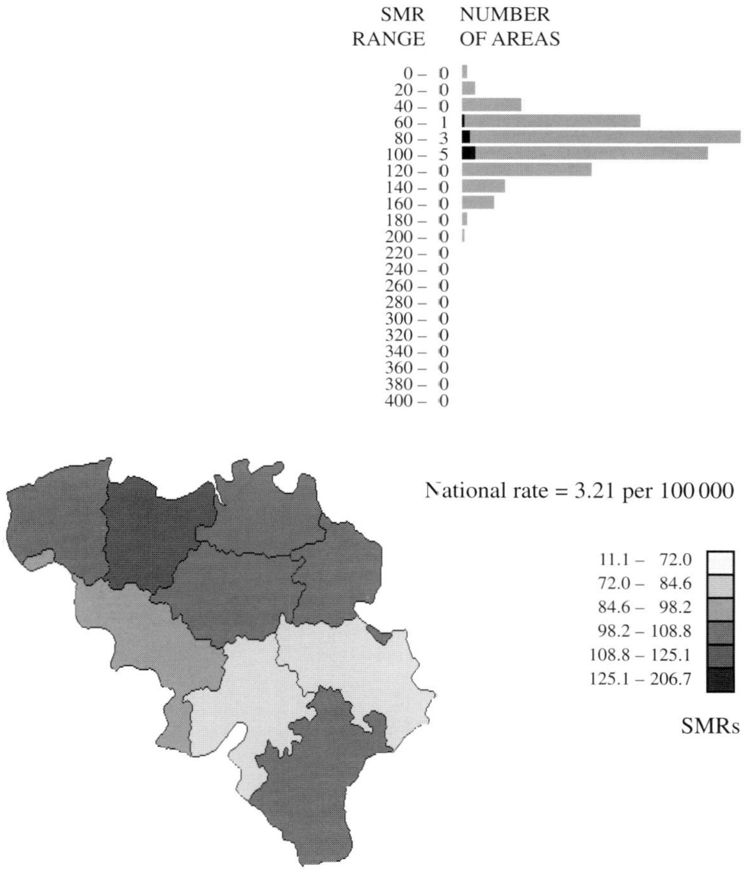

HODGKIN'S DISEASE MORTALITY AGES 5–64: 1985–89

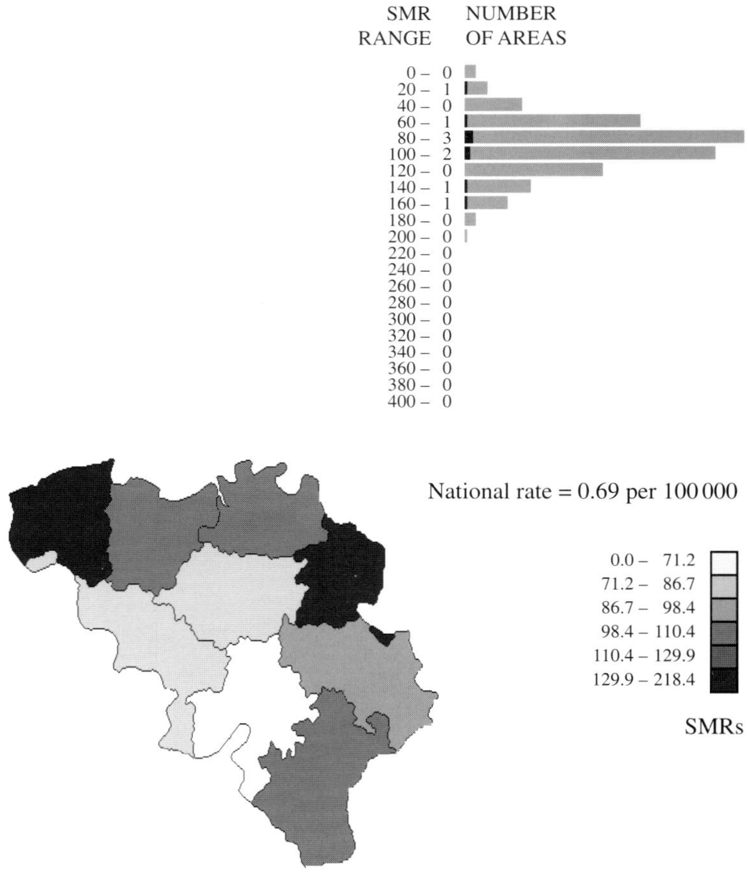

CHRONIC RHEUMATIC HEART DISEASE MORTALITY AGES 5–44: 1985–89

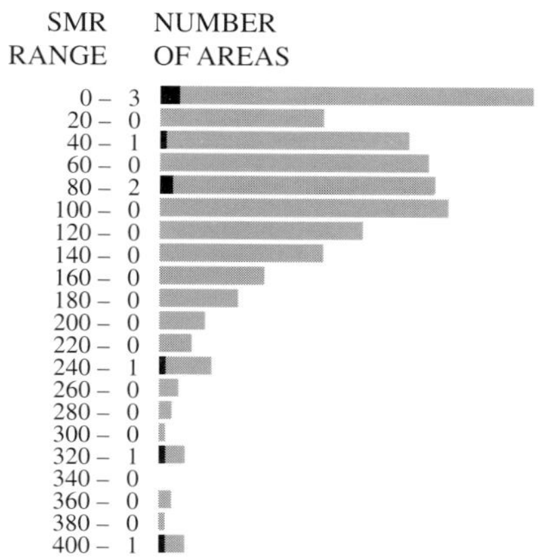

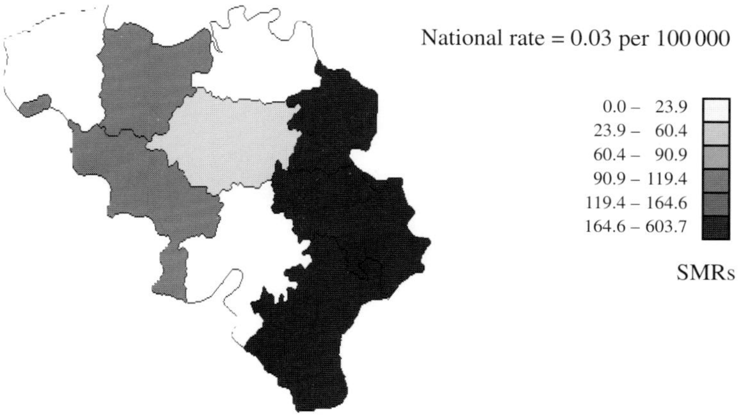

ALL RESPIRATORY DISEASES MORTALITY AGES 1–14: 1985–89

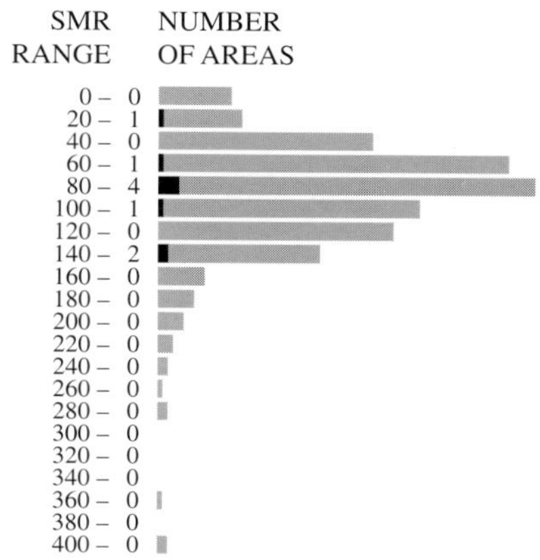

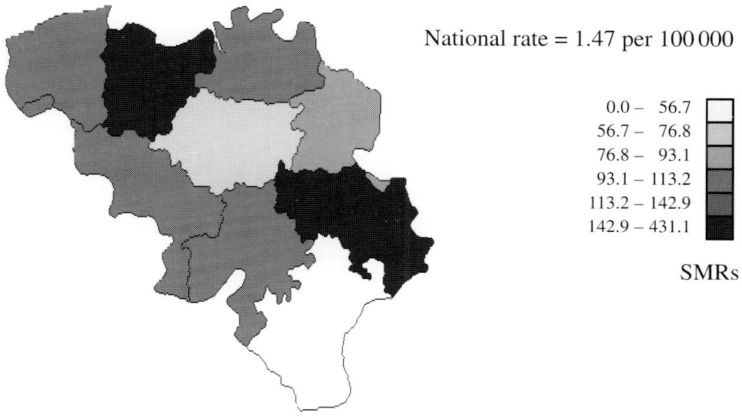

ASTHMA MORTALITY AGES 5–44: 1985–89

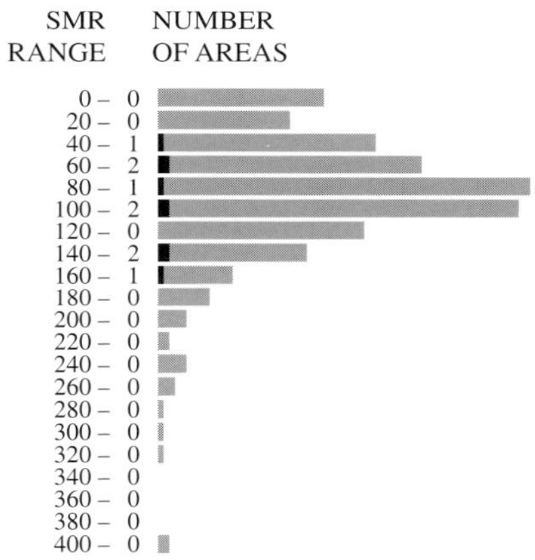

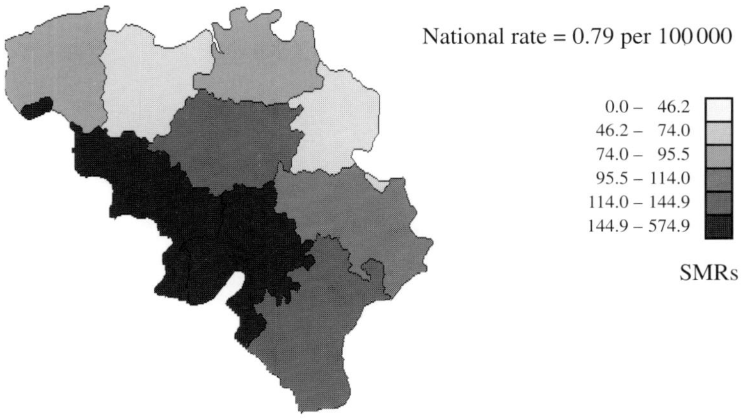

APPENDICITIS MORTALITY AGES 5–64: 1985–89

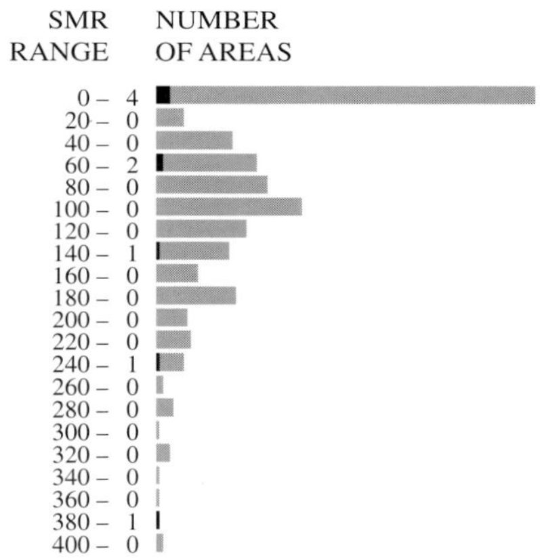

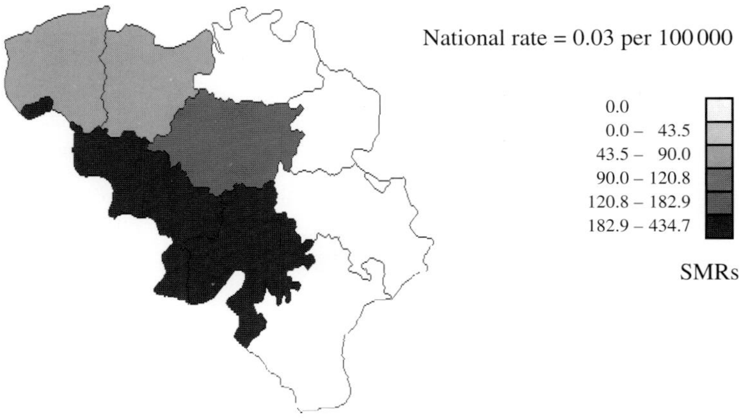

ABDOMINAL HERNIA MORTALITY AGES 5–64: 1985–89

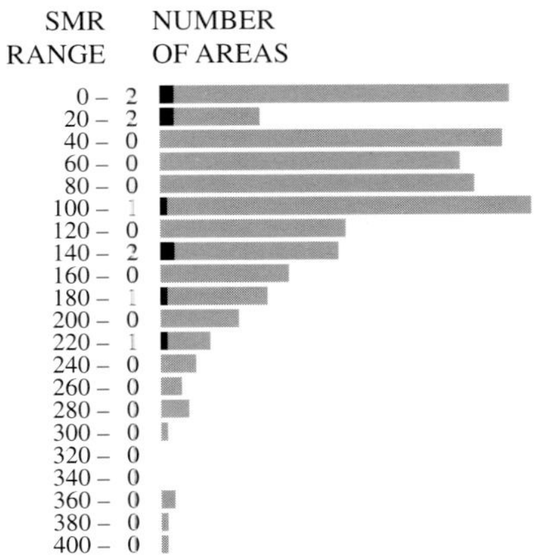

National rate = 0.07 per 100 000

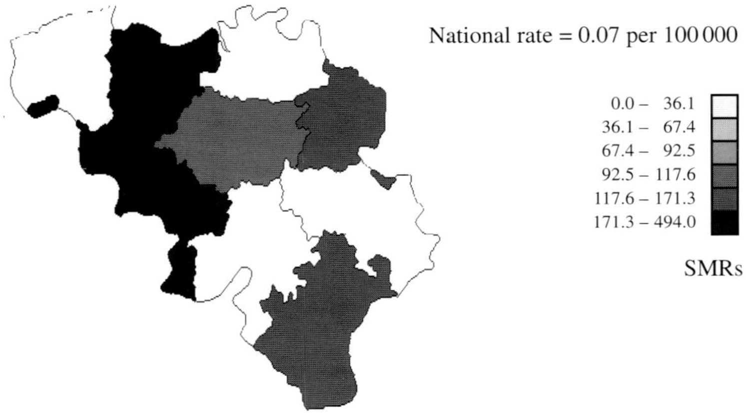

CHOLELITHIASIS AND CHOLECYSTITIS MORTALITY AGES 5–64: 1985–89

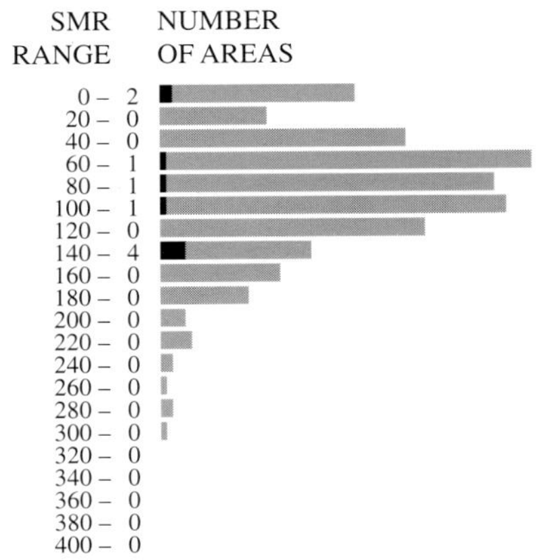

National rate = 0.12 per 100 000

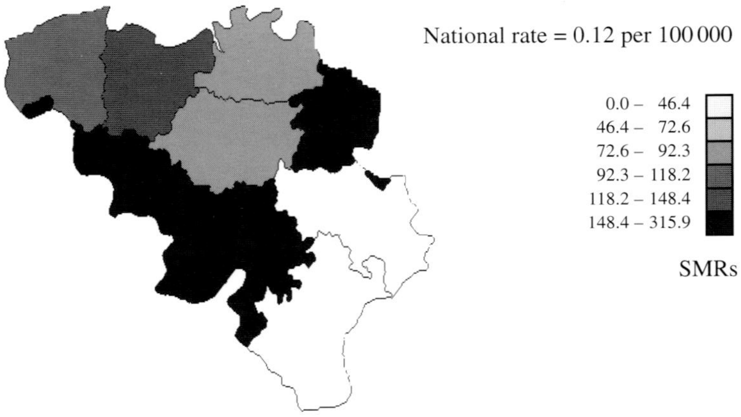

HYPERTENSIVE AND CEREBROVASCULAR DISEASES MORTALITY AGES 35–64: 1985–89

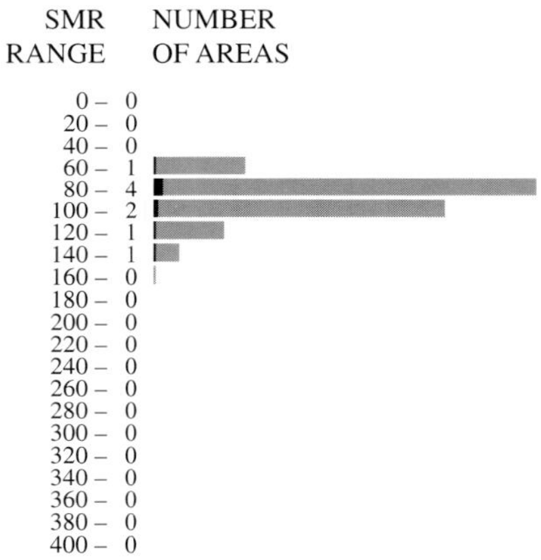

National rate = 31.80 per 100 000

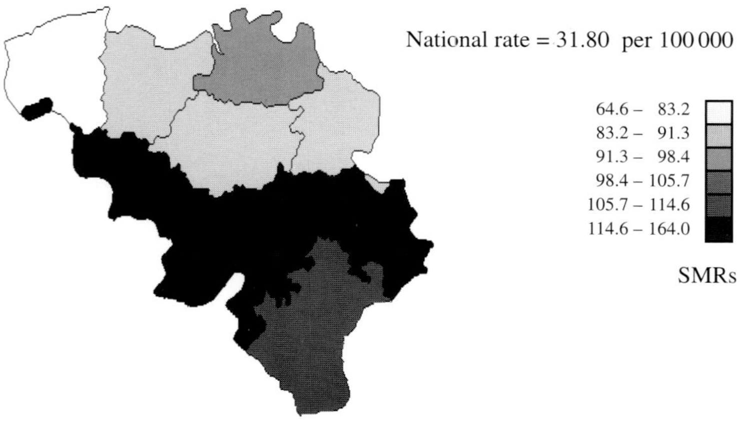

MATERNAL MORTALITY ALL AGES: 1985–89

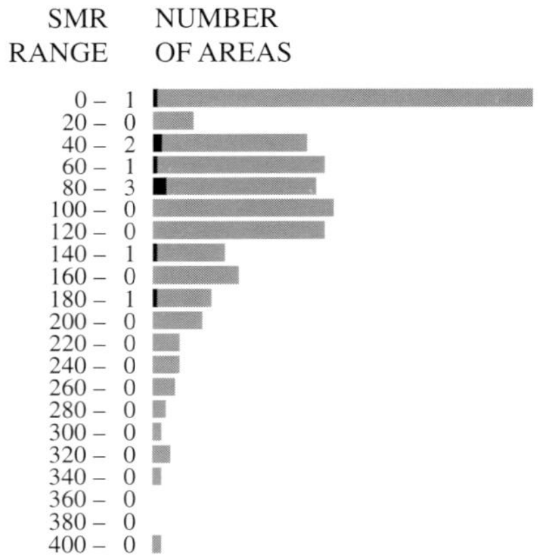

National rate = 4.55 per 100 000 live and still births

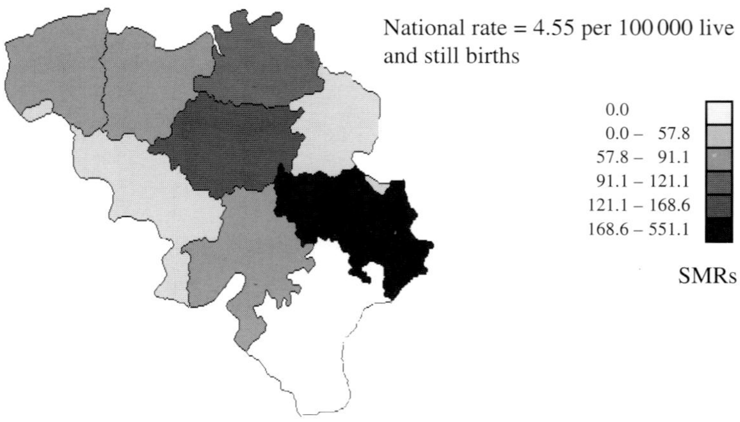

PERINATAL MORTALITY: 1985–89

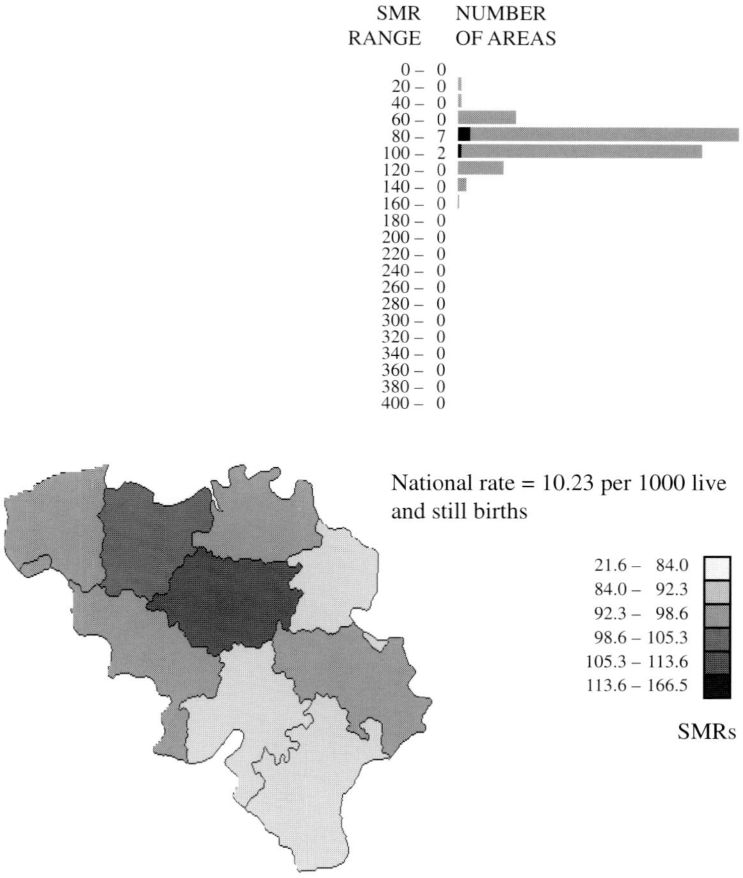

CANCER OF THE BREAST MORTALITY AGES 25–64: 1985–89

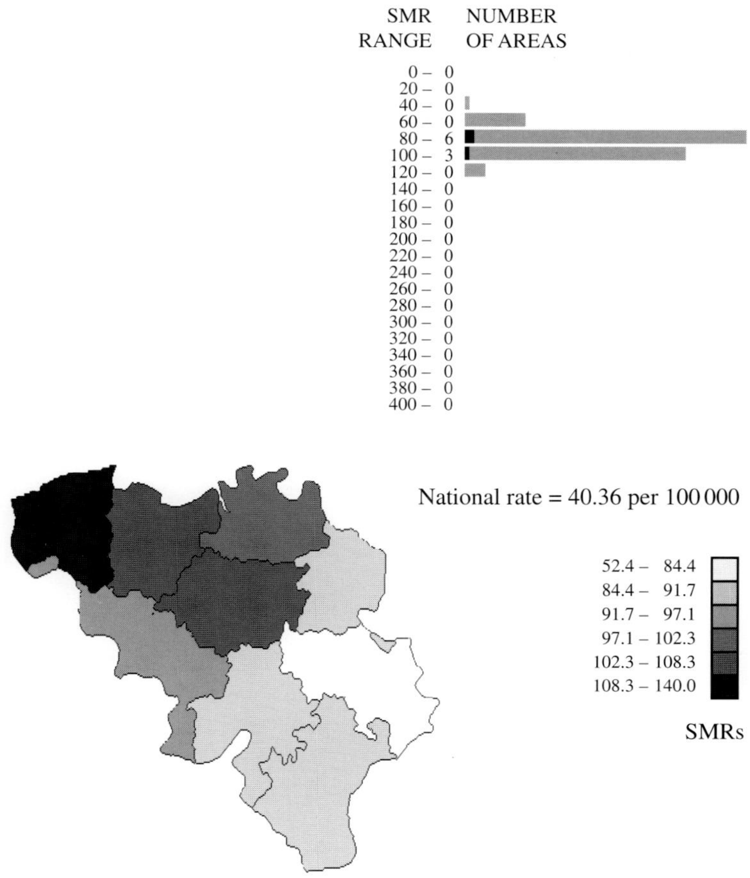

ISCHAEMIC HEART DISEASE MORTALITY AGES 35–64: 1985–89

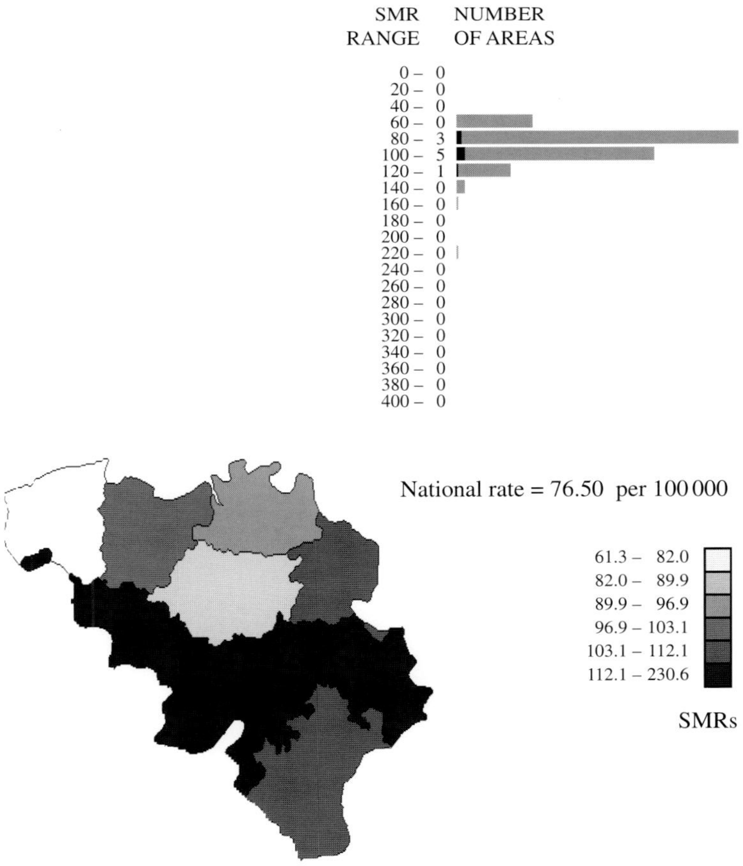

PEPTIC ULCERS MORTALITY AGES 25–64: 1985–89

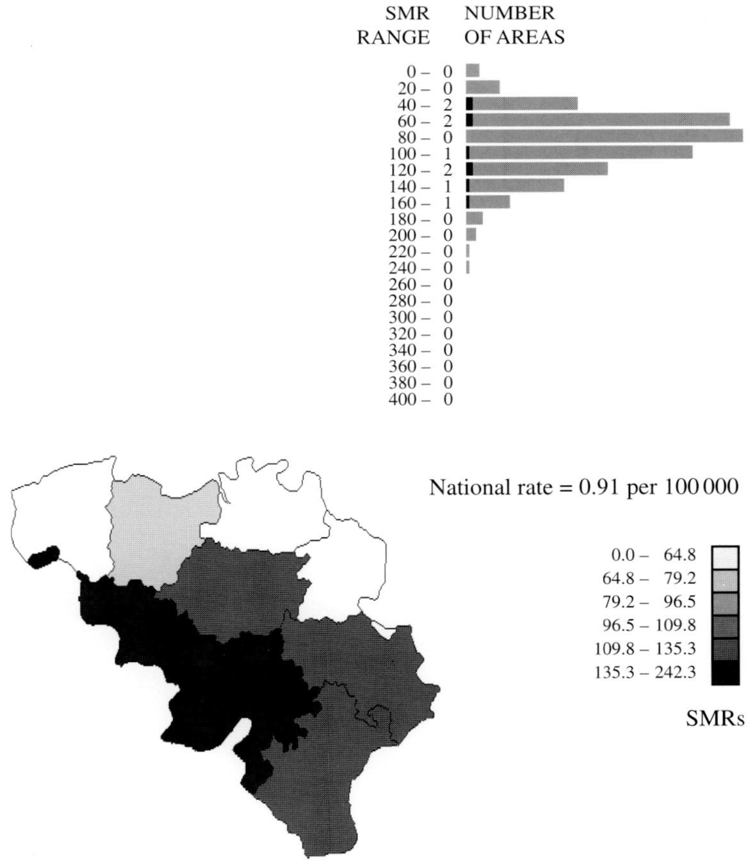

ALL CAUSES MORTALITY AGES 5–64: 1985–89

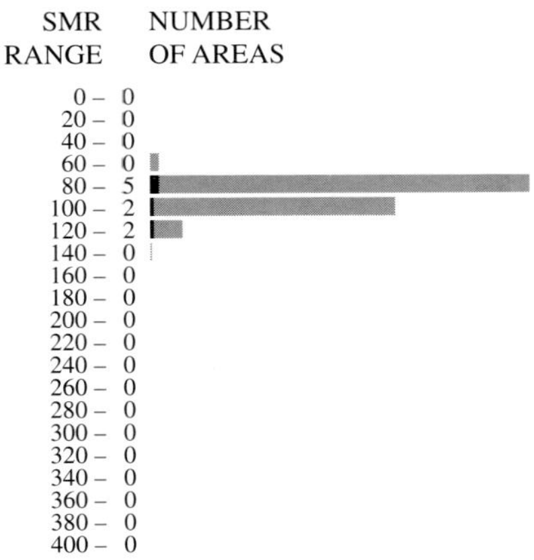

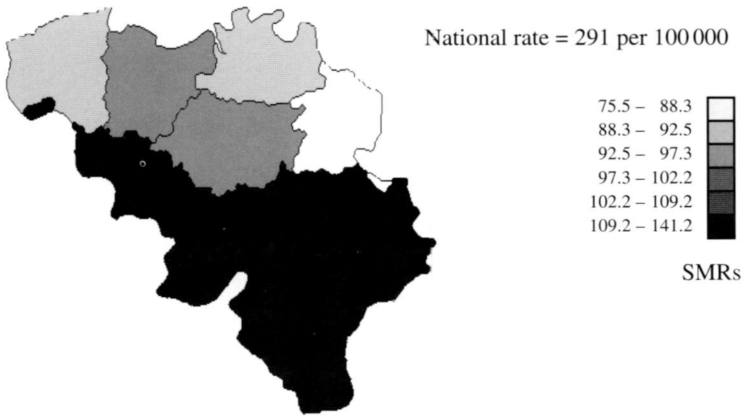

ALL CAUSES MORTALITY ALL AGES: 1985–89

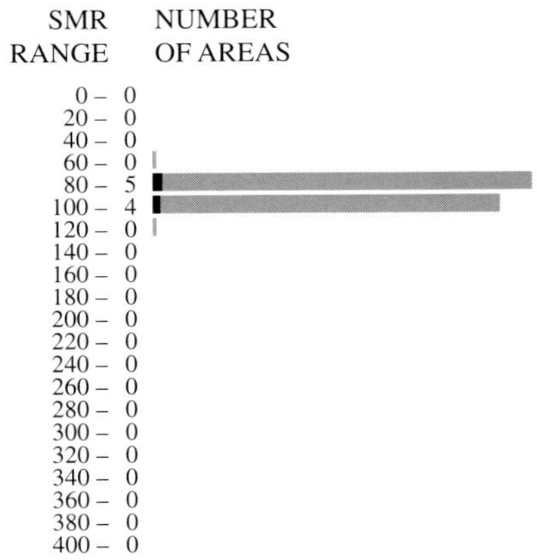

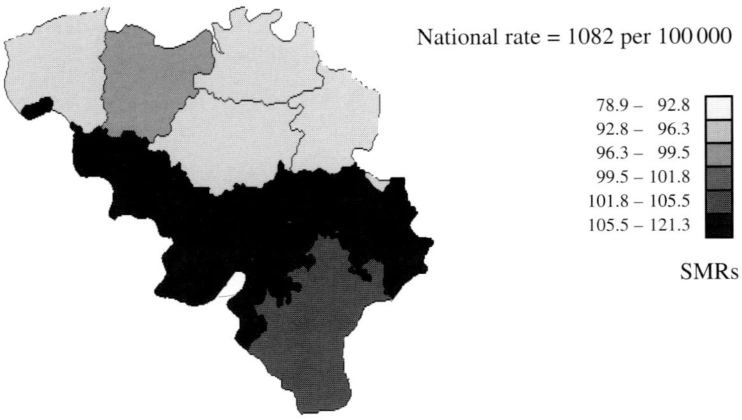

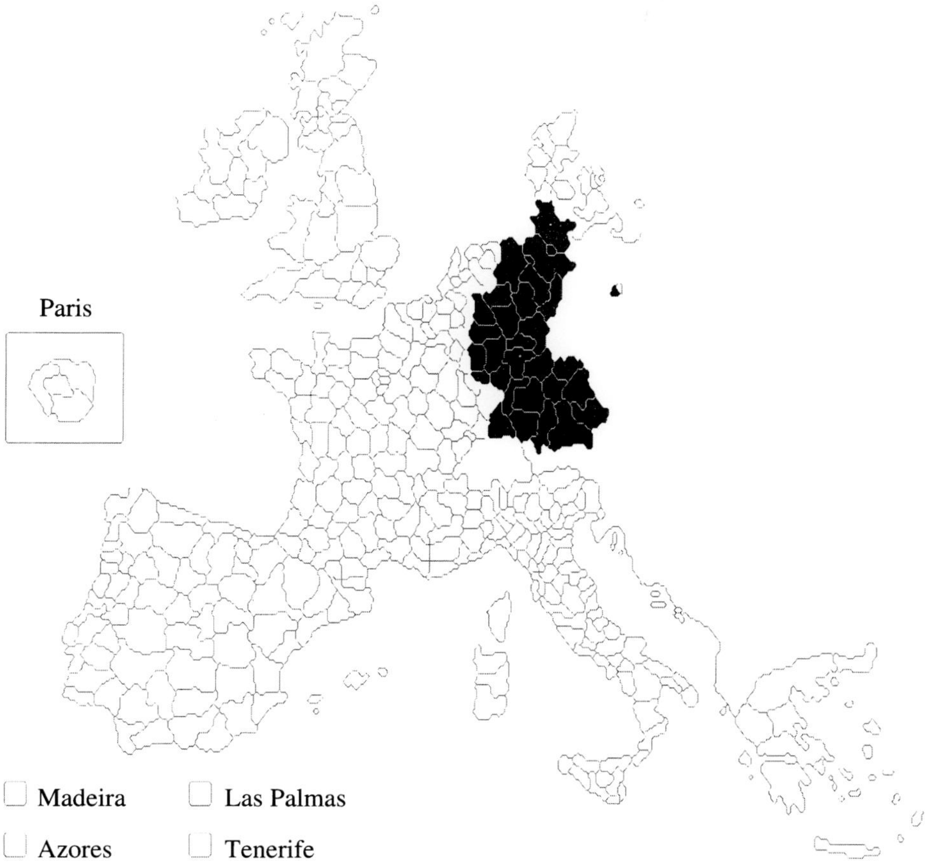

KEY MAP: FEDERAL REPUBLIC OF GERMANY

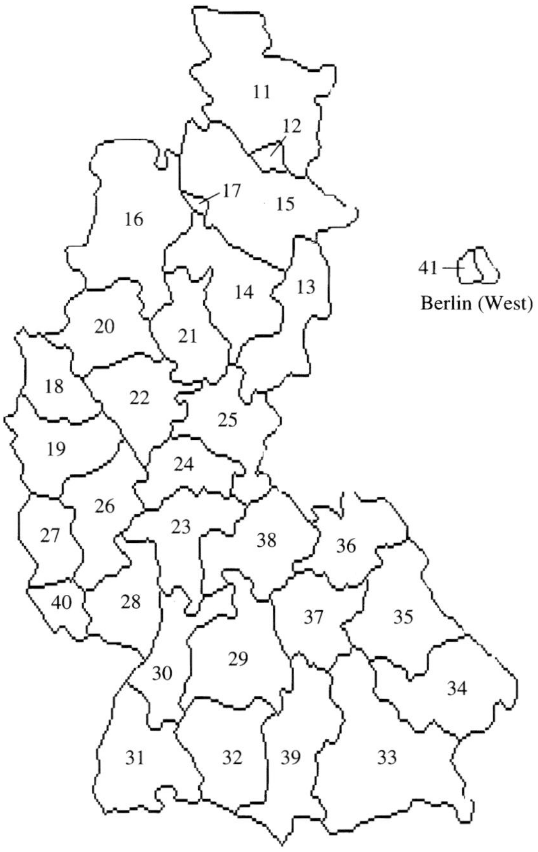

TUBERCULOSIS MORTALITY AGES 5–64: 1985–89

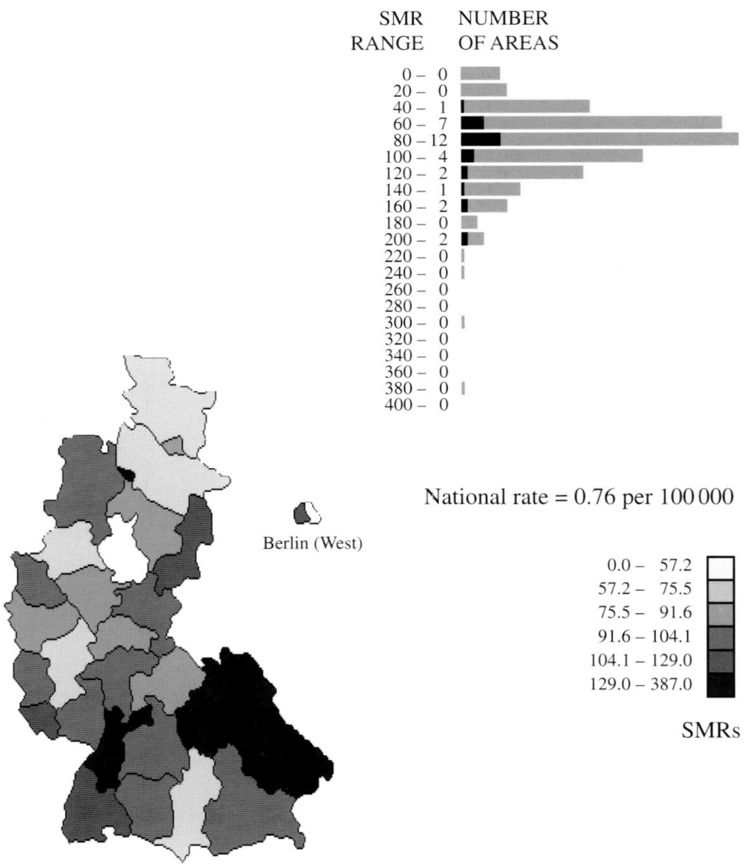

MALIGNANT NEOPLASM OF CERVIX UTERI MORTALITY AGES 15–64: 1985–89

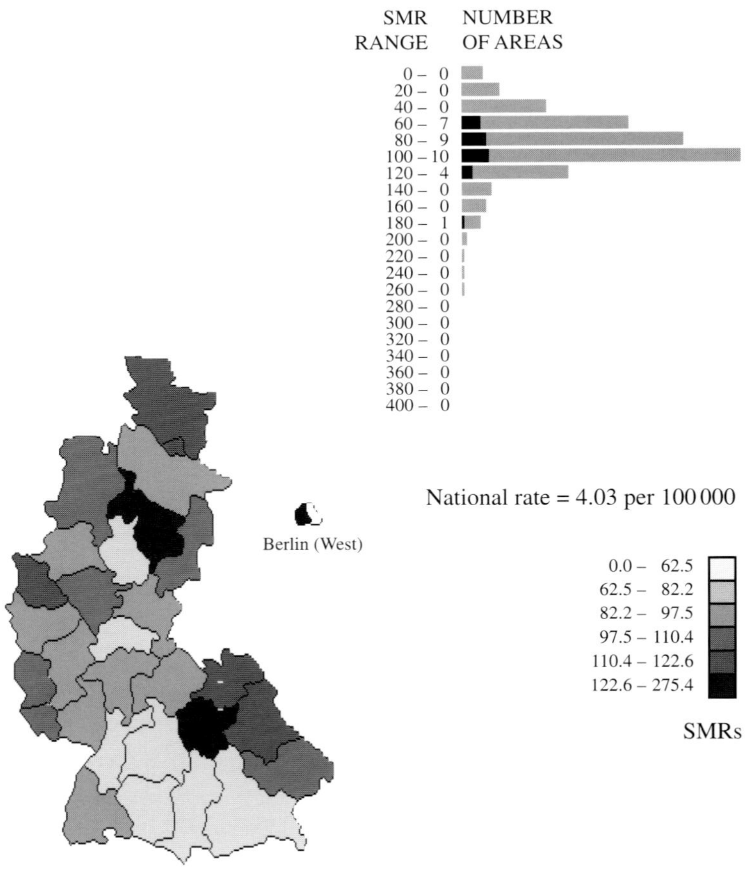

MALIGNANT NEOPLASM OF CERVIX AND BODY OF UTERUS MORTALITY AGES 15–54: 1985–89

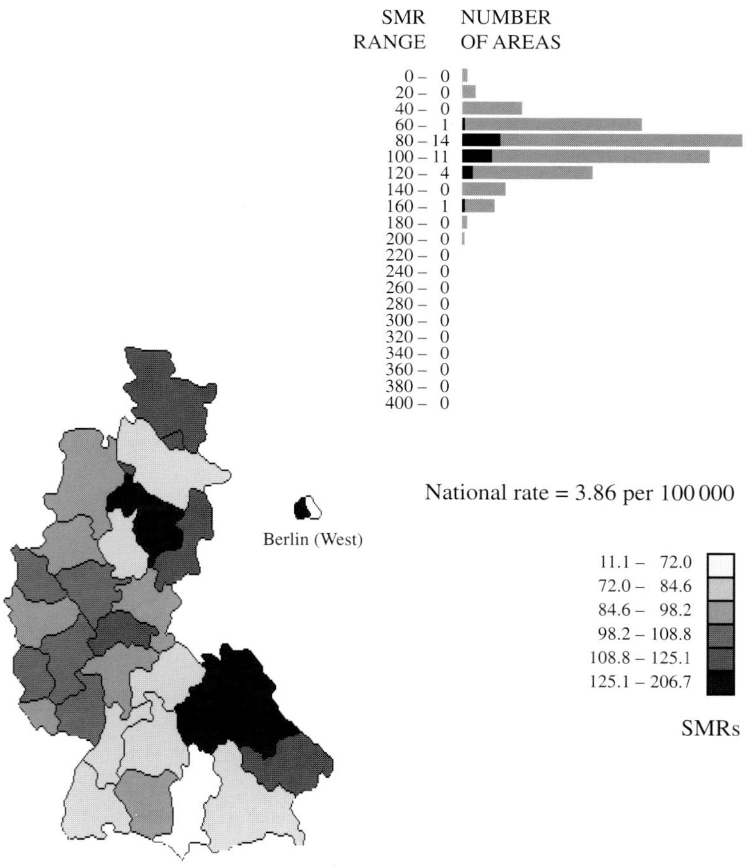

HODGKIN'S DISEASE MORTALITY AGES 5–64: 1985–89

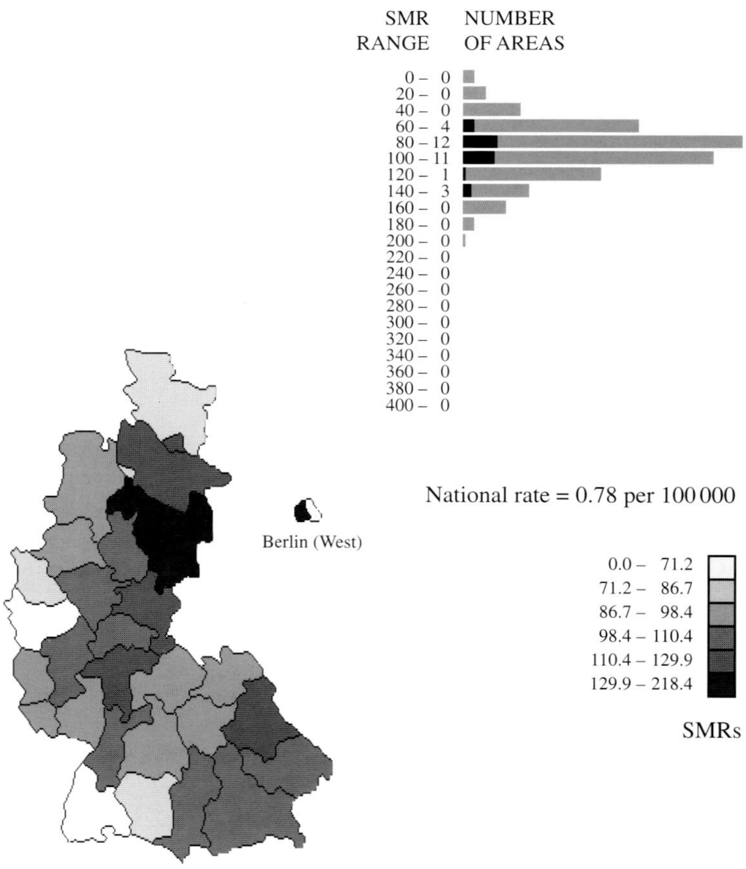

CHRONIC RHEUMATIC HEART DISEASE MORTALITY AGES 5–44: 1985–89

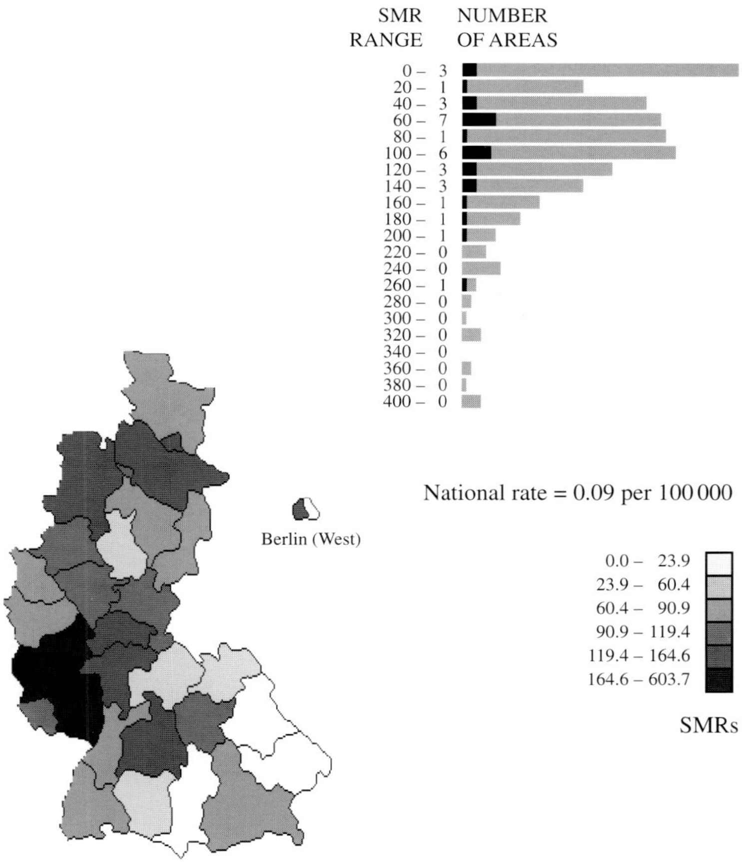

ALL RESPIRATORY DISEASES MORTALITY AGES 1–14: 1985–89

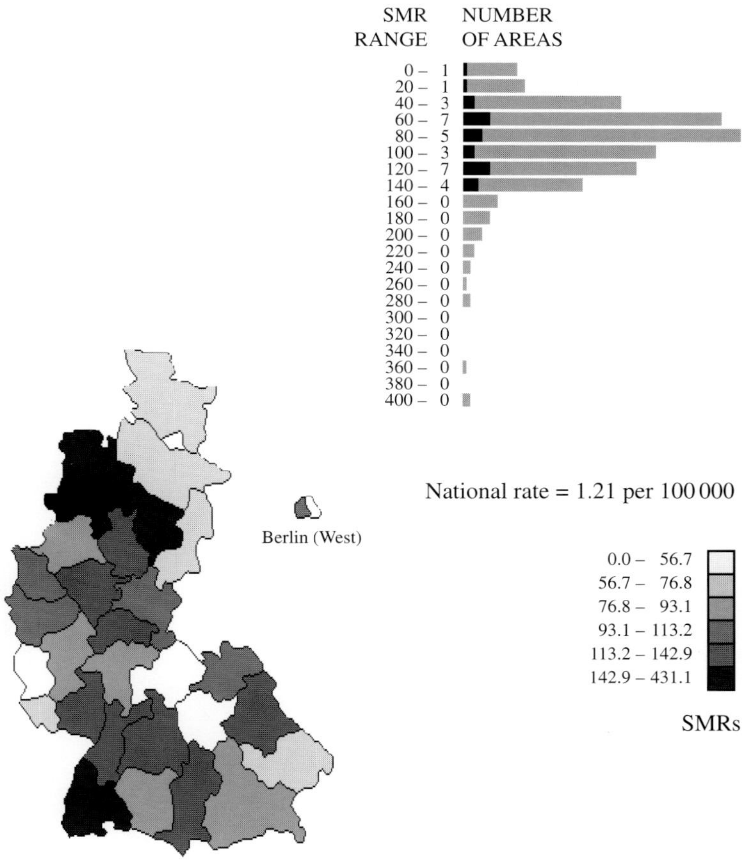

ASTHMA MORTALITY AGES 5–44: 1985–89

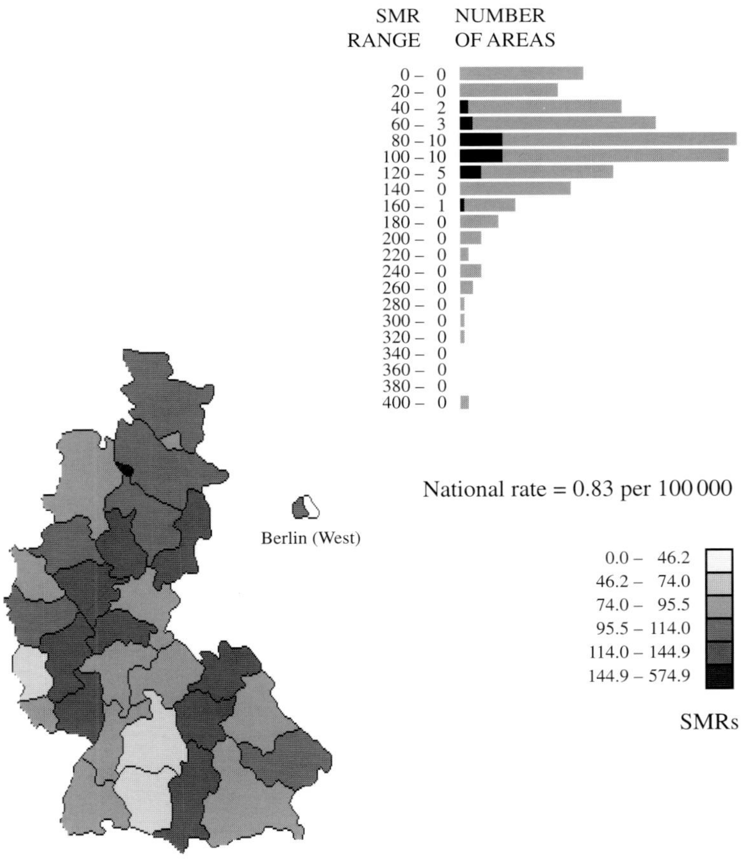

APPENDICITIS MORTALITY AGES 5–64: 1985–89

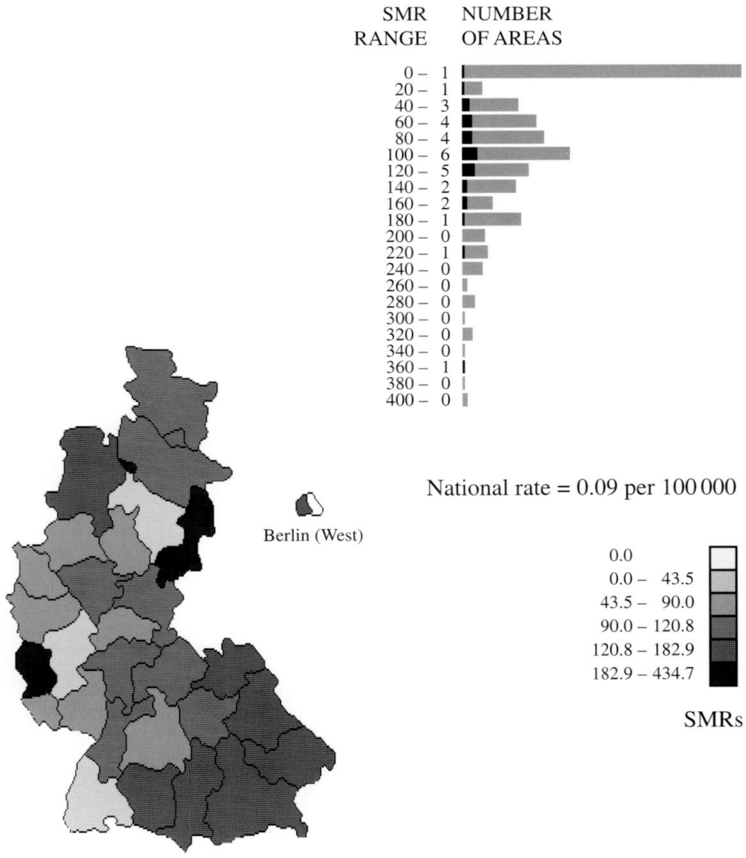

ABDOMINAL HERNIA MORTALITY AGES 5–64: 1985–89

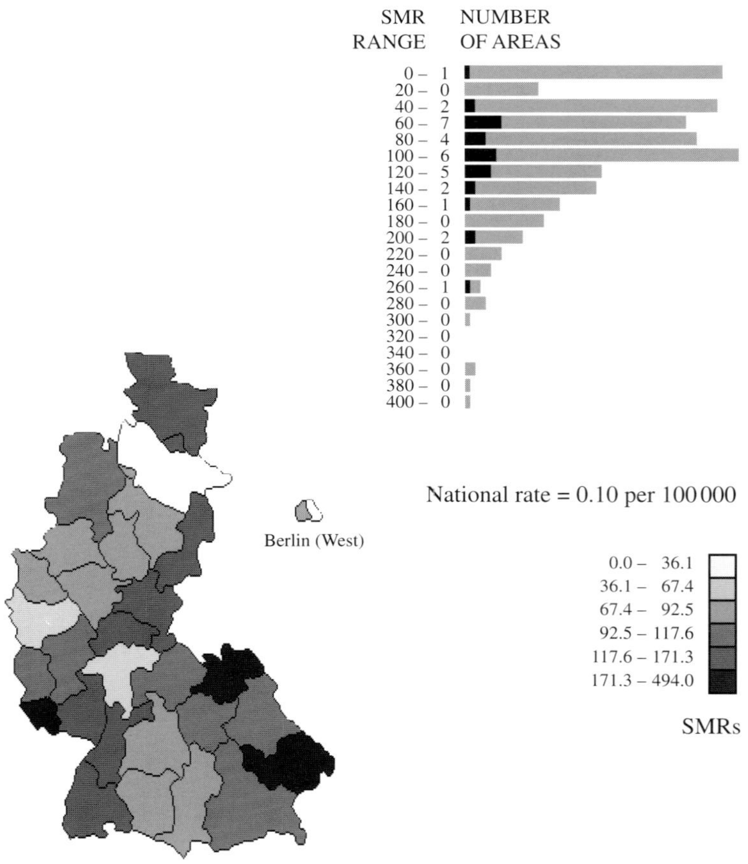

CHOLELITHIASIS AND CHOLECYSTITIS MORTALITY AGES 5–64: 1985–89

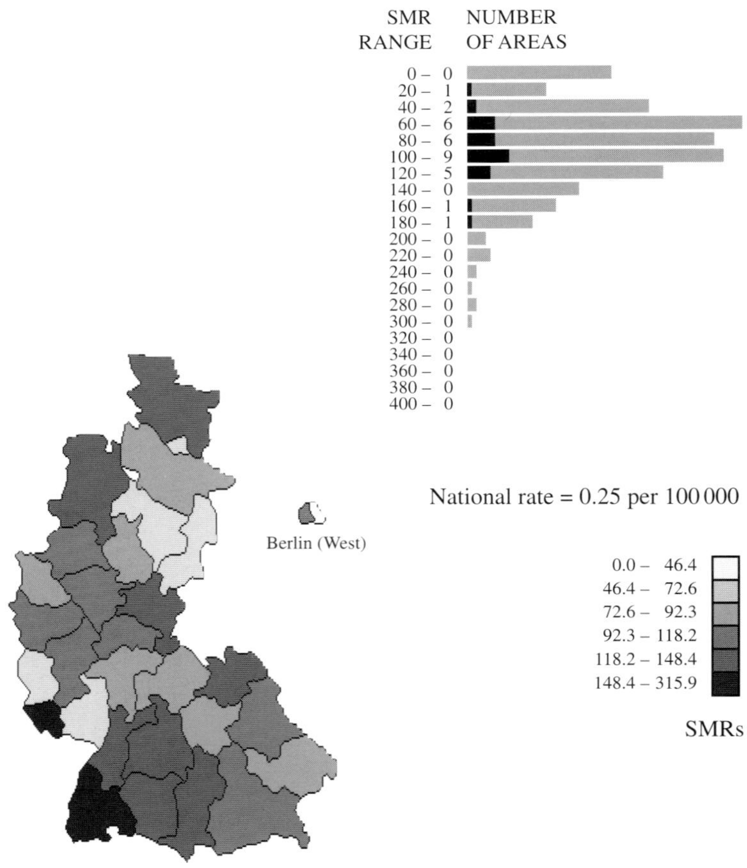

HYPERTENSIVE AND CEREBROVASCULAR DISEASES MORTALITY AGES 35–64: 1985–89

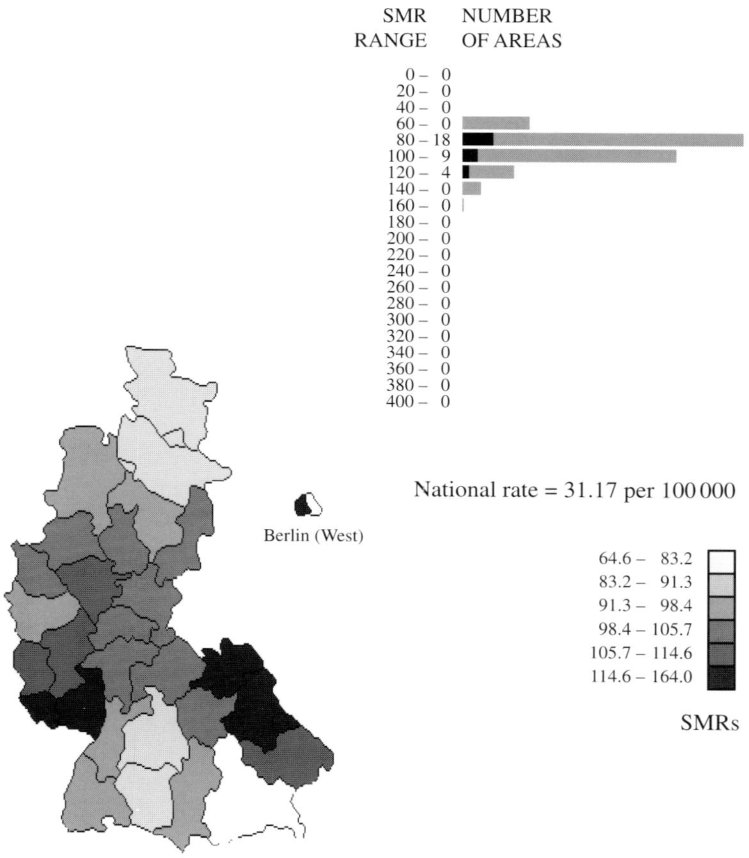

MATERNAL MORTALITY ALL AGES: 1985–89

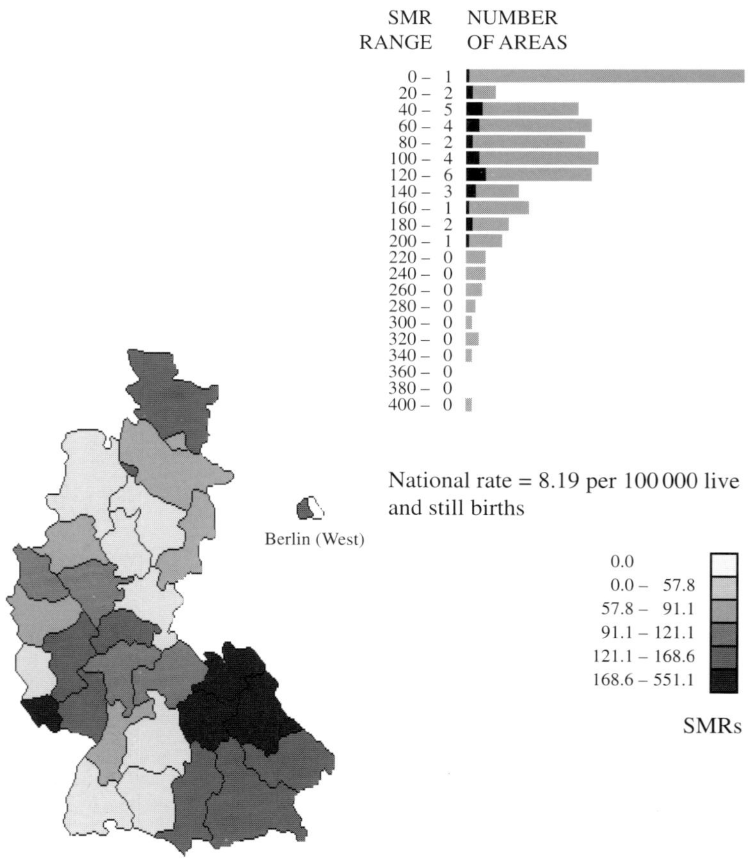

PERINATAL MORTALITY: 1985–89

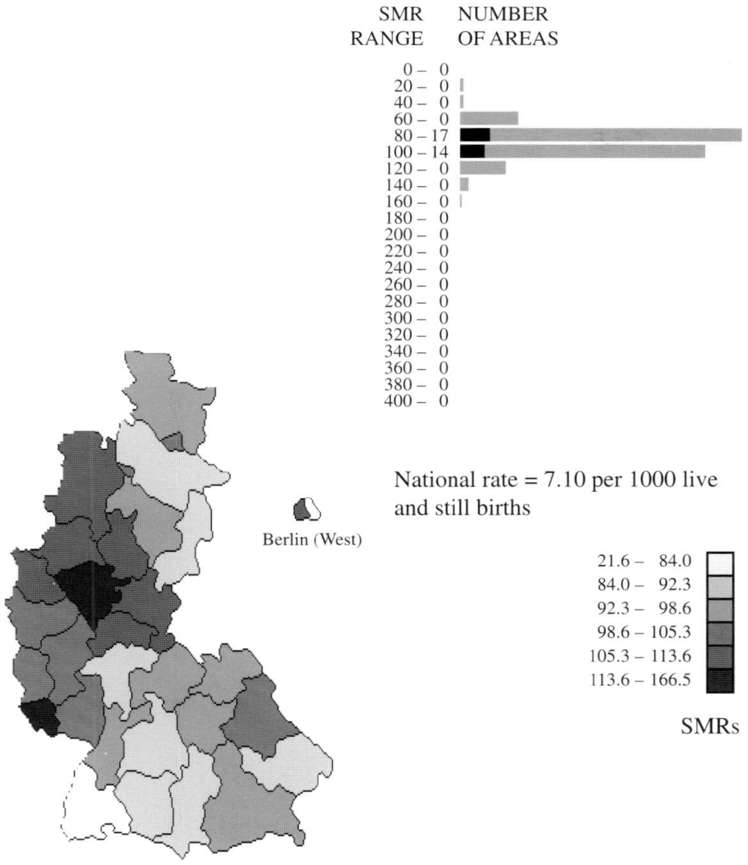

CANCER OF THE BREAST MORTALITY AGES 25–64: 1985–89

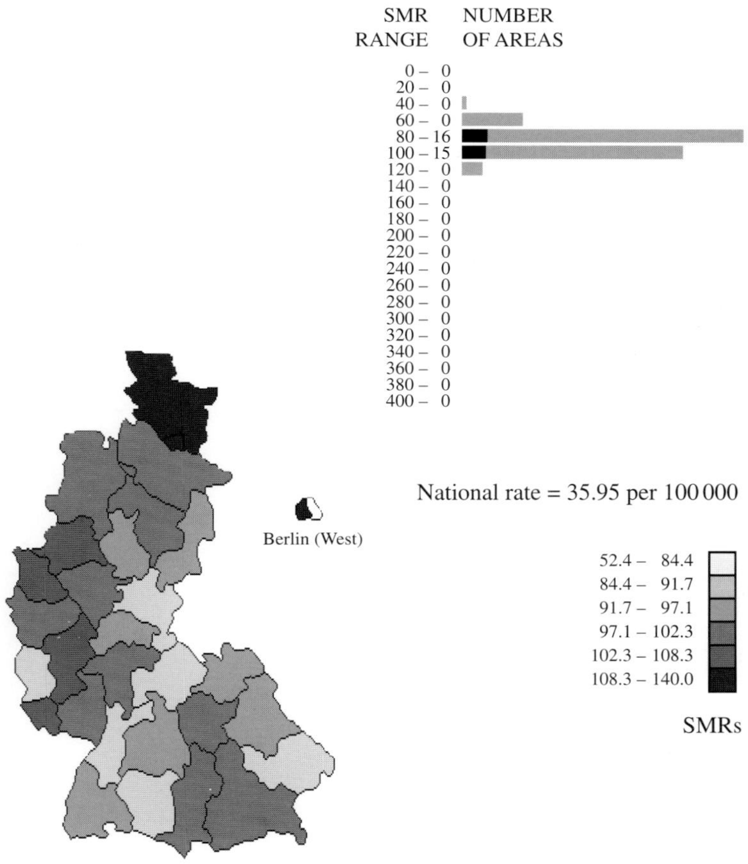

ISCHAEMIC HEART DISEASE MORTALITY AGES 35–64: 1985–89

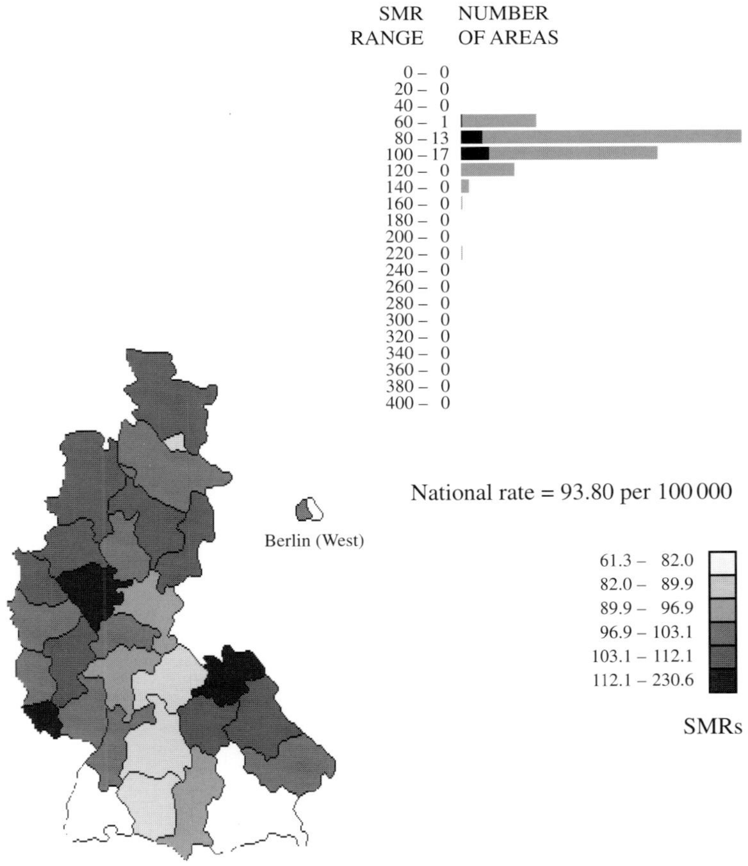

PEPTIC ULCERS MORTALITY AGES 25–64: 1985–89

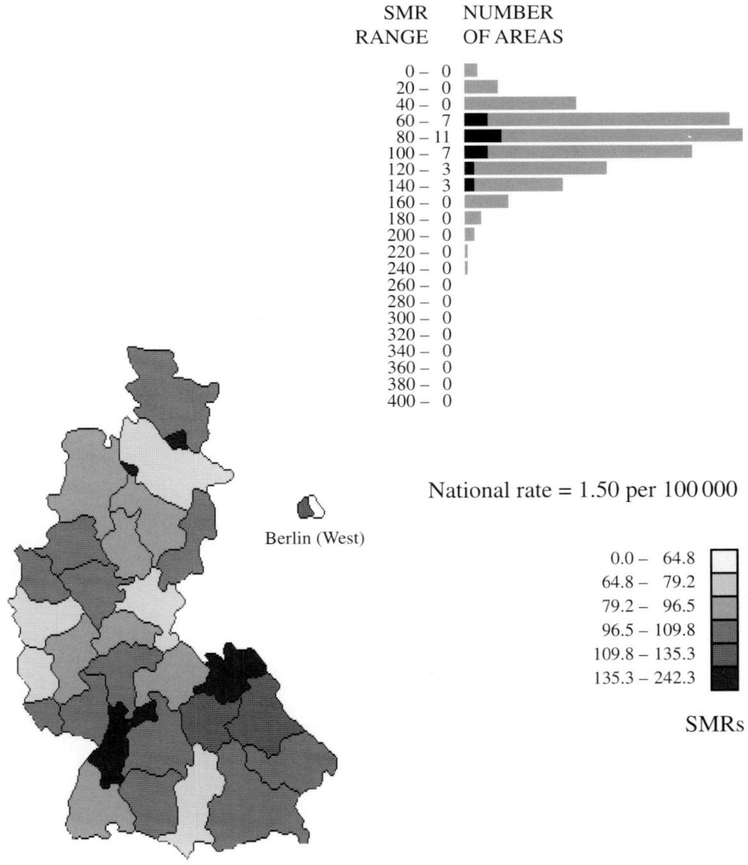

ALL CAUSES MORTALITY AGES 5–64: 1985–89

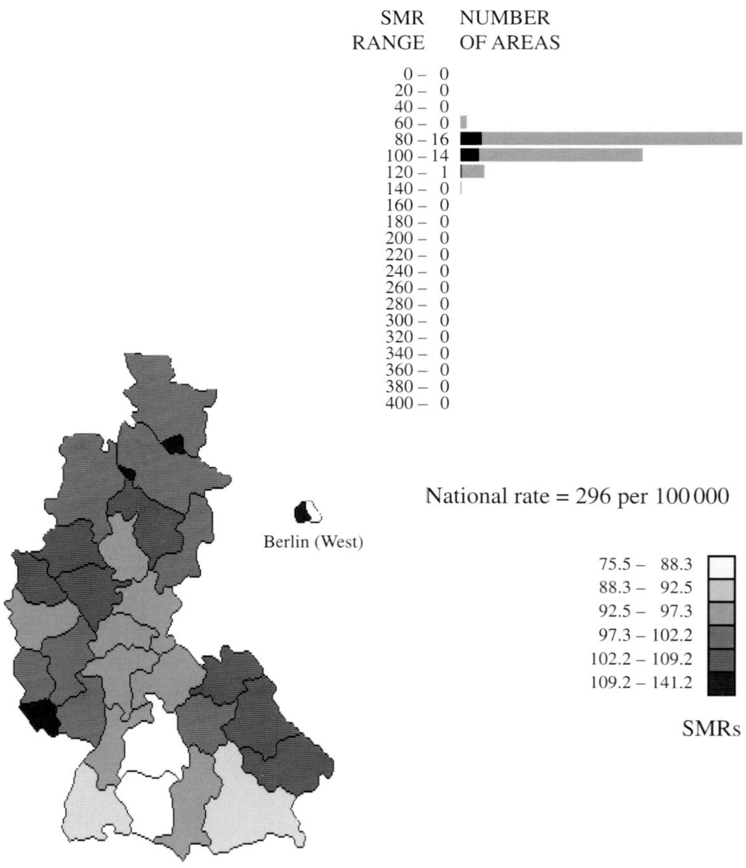

ALL CAUSES MORTALITY ALL AGES: 1985–89

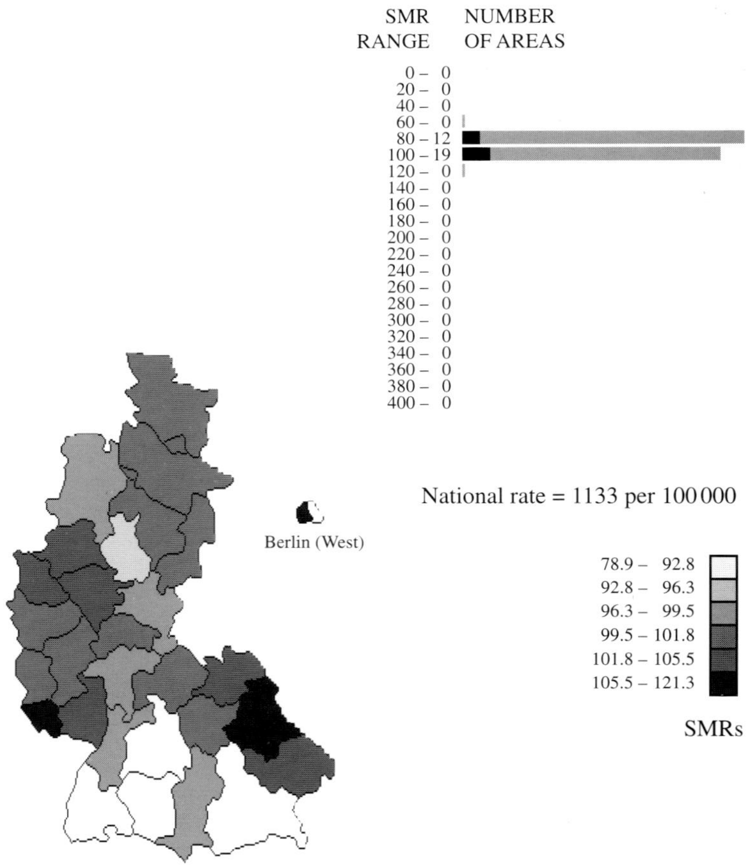

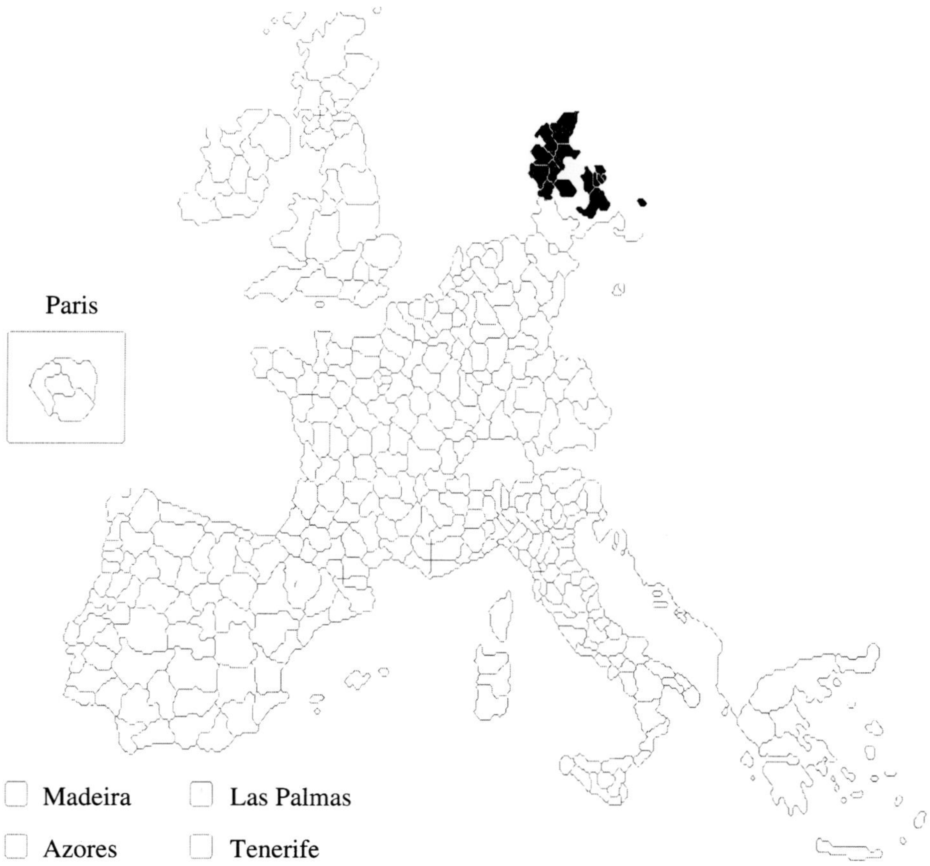

KEY MAP: DENMARK

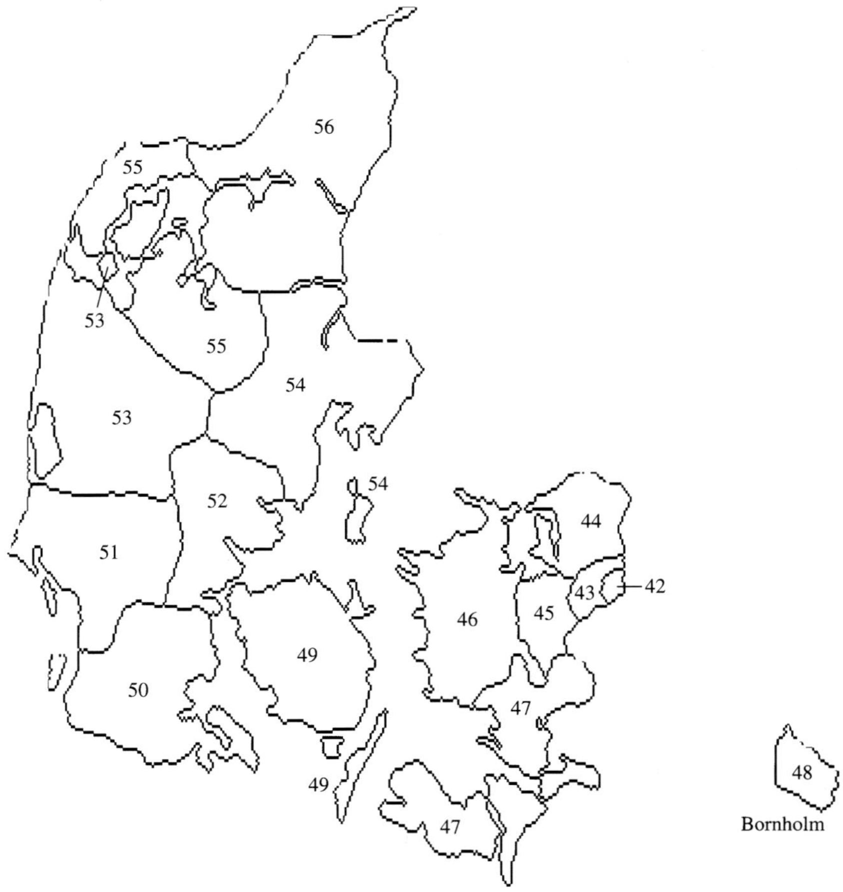

TUBERCULOSIS MORTALITY AGES 5–64: 1985–89

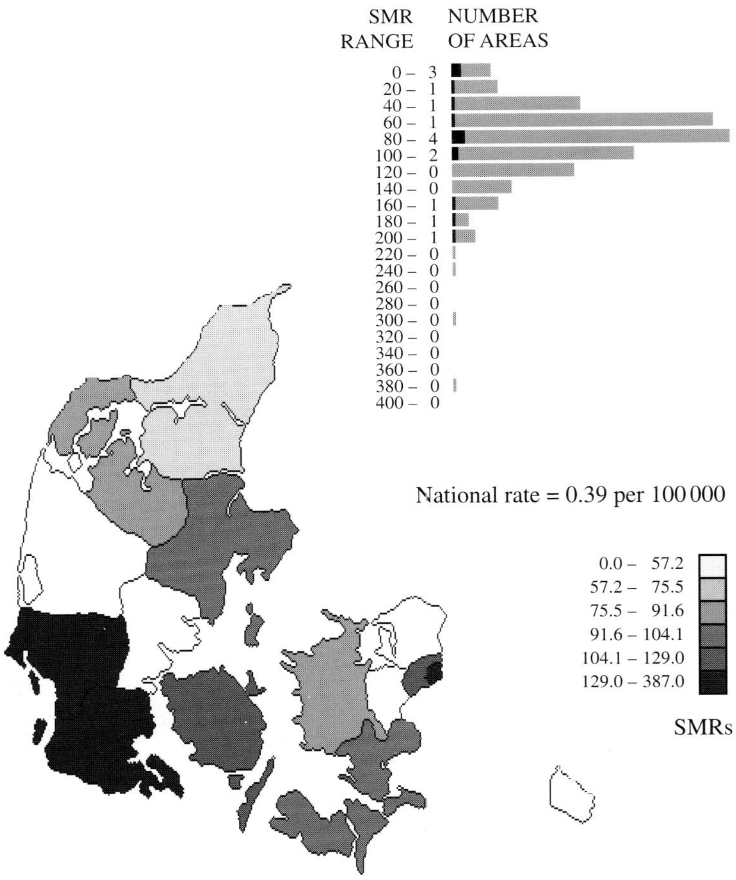

MALIGNANT NEOPLASM OF CERVIX UTERI MORTALITY AGES 15–64: 1985–89

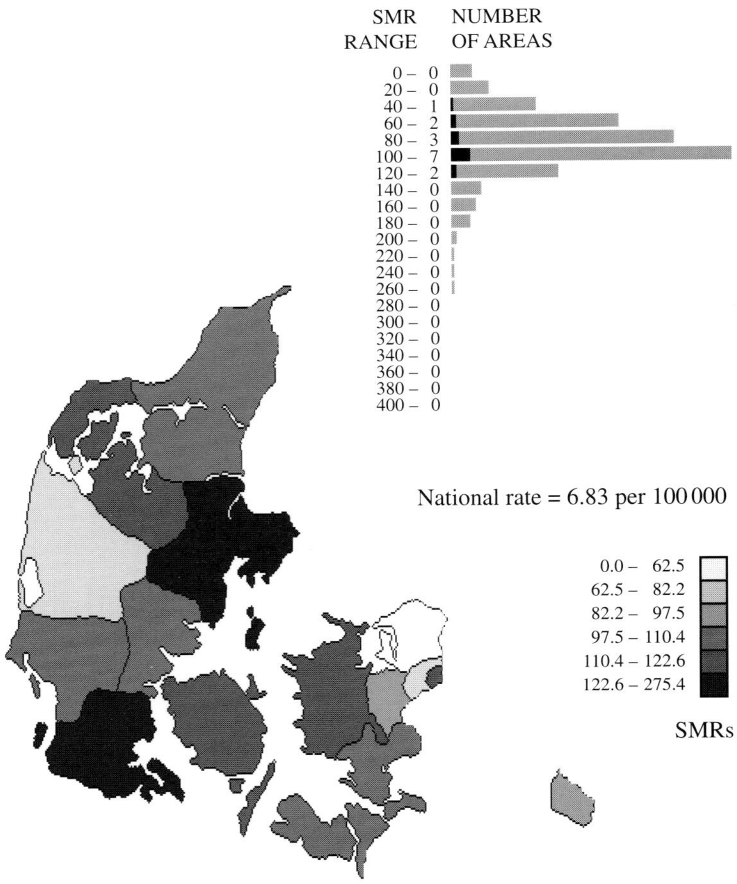

MALIGNANT NEOPLASM OF CERVIX AND BODY OF UTERUS MORTALITY AGES 15–54: 1985–89

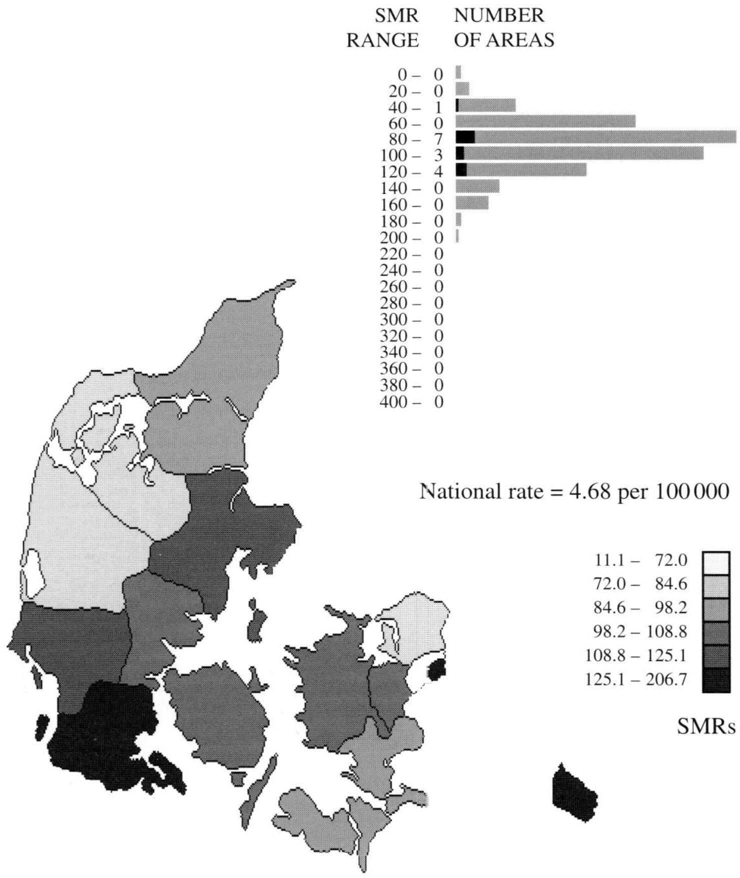

HODGKIN'S DISEASE MORTALITY AGES 5–64: 1985–89

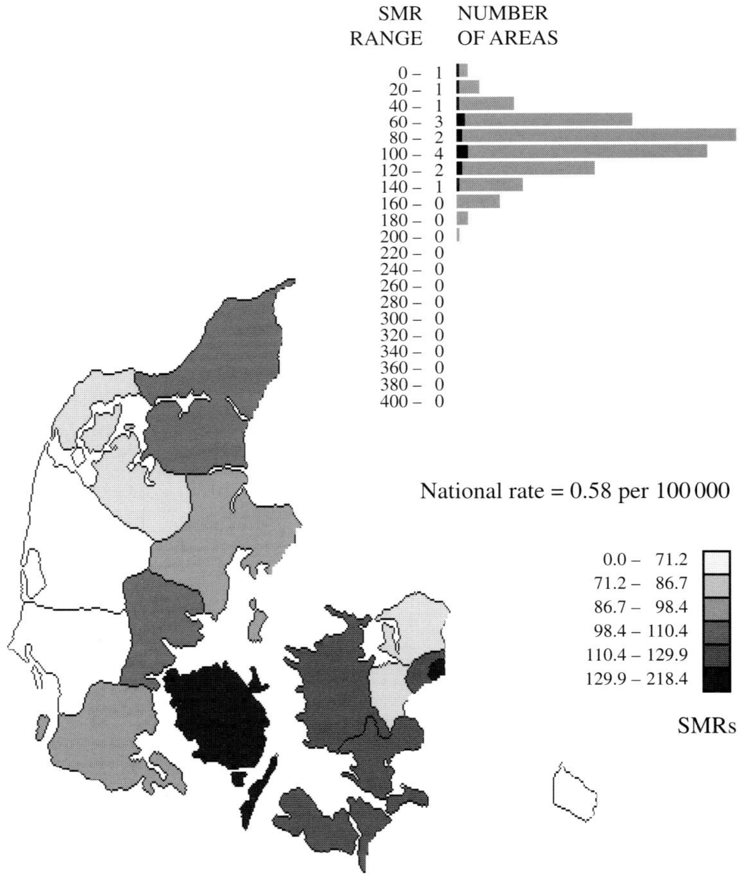

CHRONIC RHEUMATIC HEART DISEASE MORTALITY AGES 5–44: 1985–89

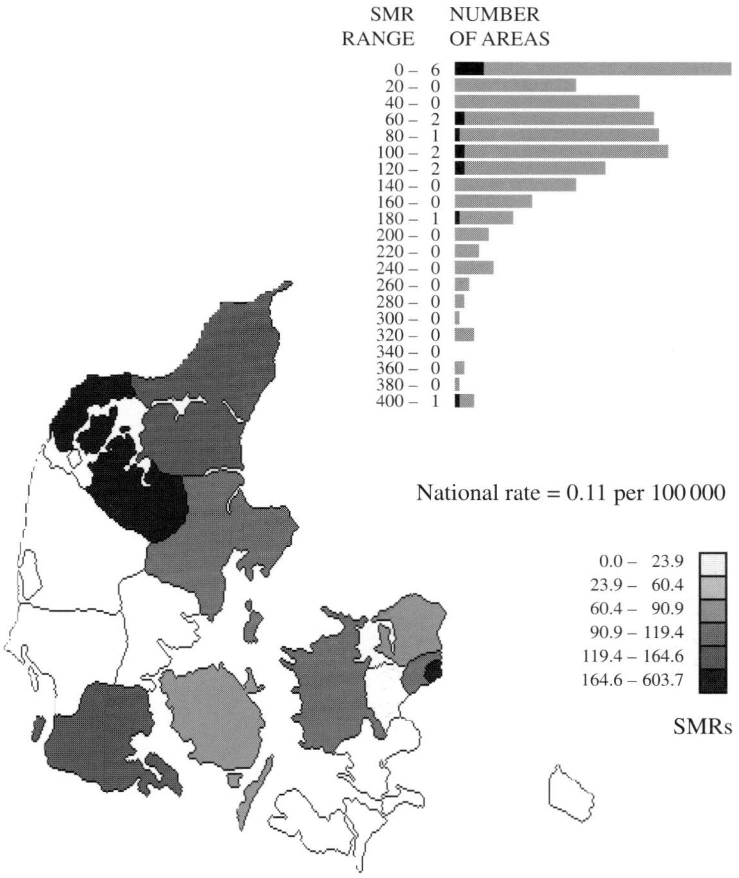

ALL RESPIRATORY DISEASES MORTALITY AGES 1–14: 1985–89

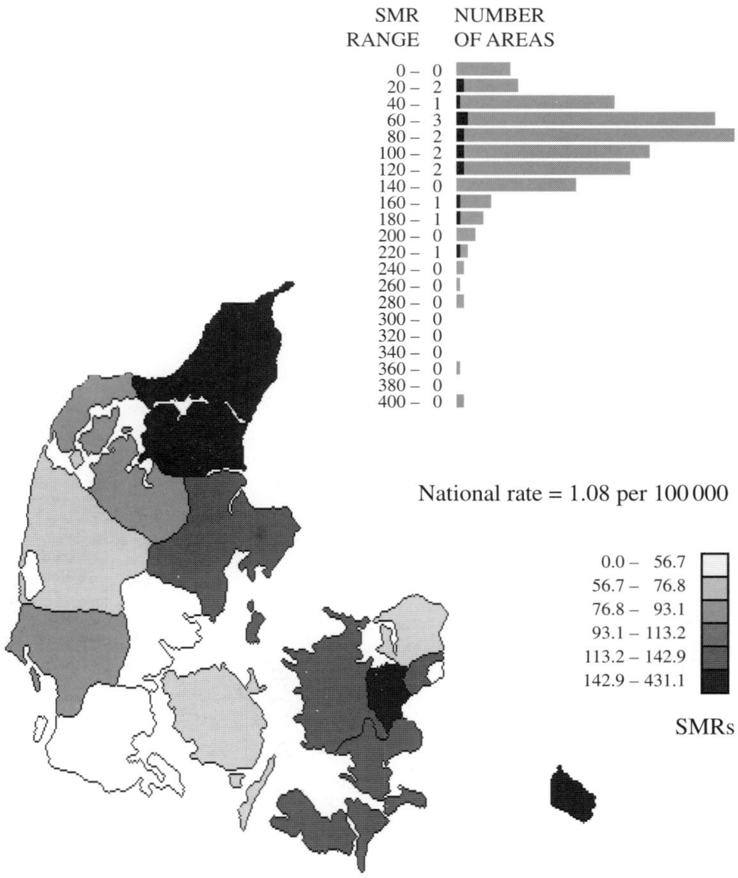

ASTHMA MORTALITY AGES 5–44: 1985–89

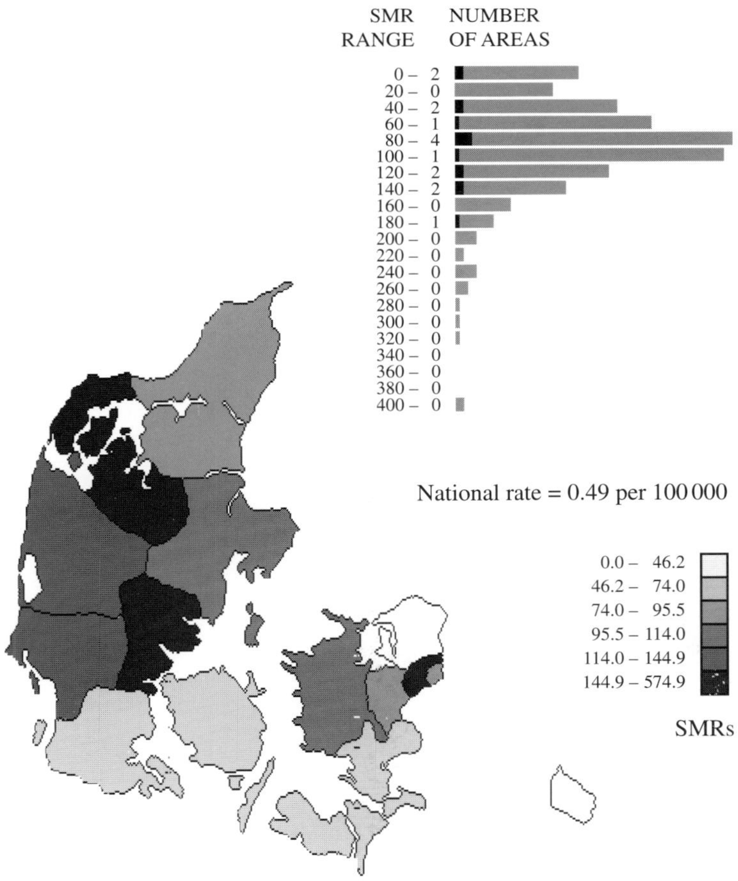

APPENDICITIS MORTALITY AGES 5–64: 1985–89

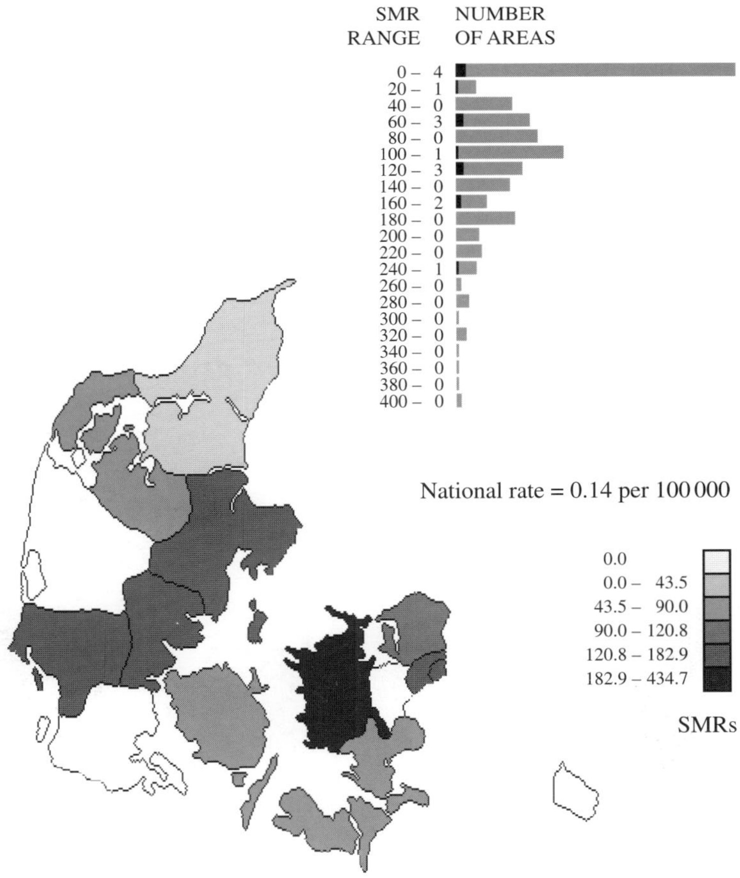

ABDOMINAL HERNIA MORTALITY AGES 5–64: 1985–89

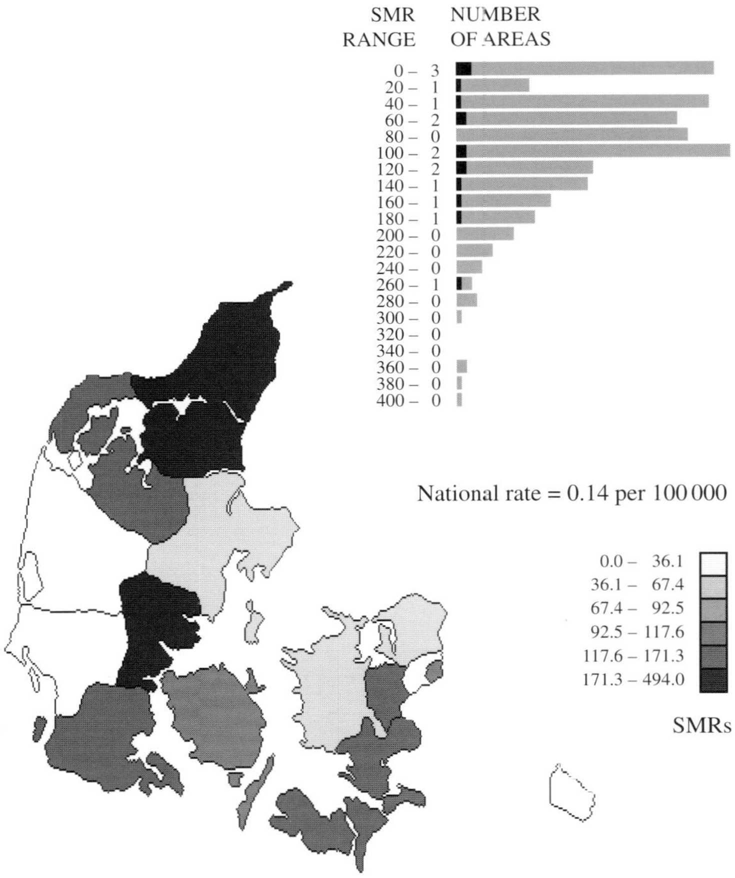

CHOLELITHIASIS AND CHOLECYSTITIS MORTALITY AGES 5–64: 1985–89

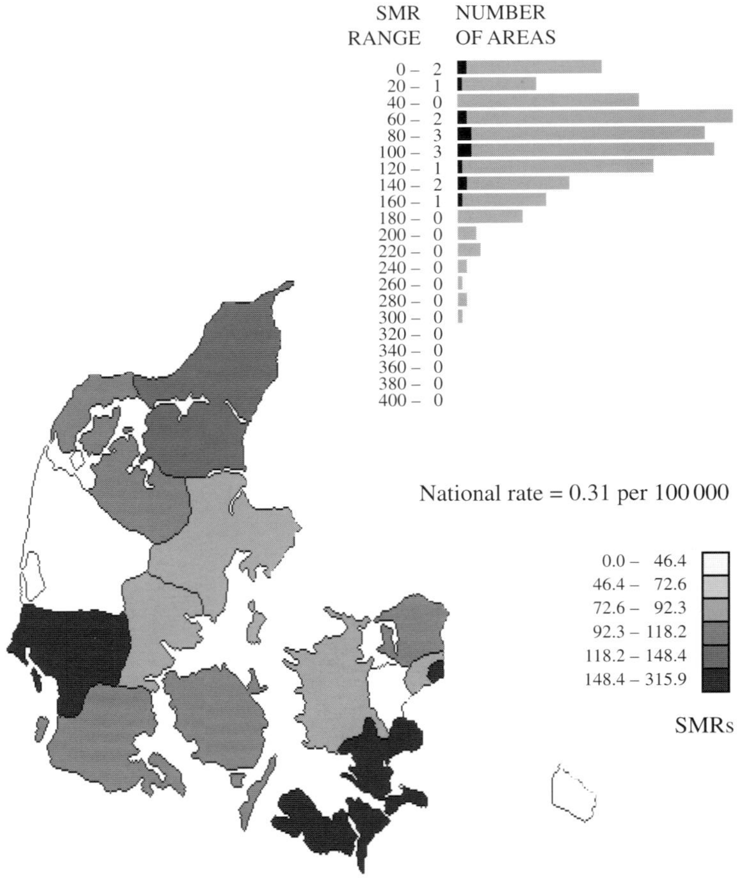

HYPERTENSIVE AND CEREBROVASCULAR DISEASES MORTALITY AGES 35–64: 1985–89

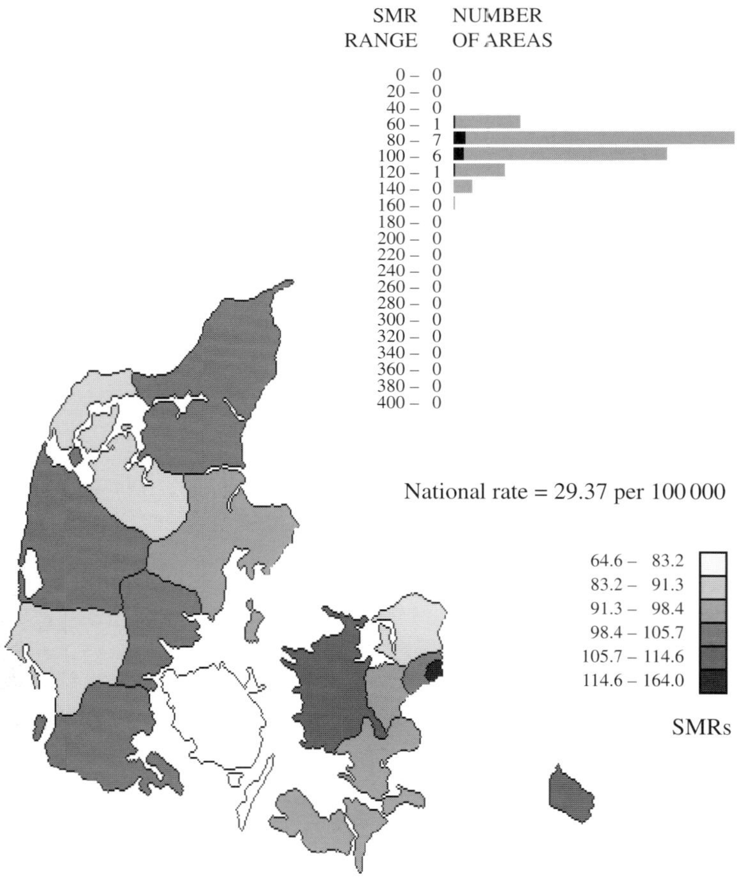

MATERNAL MORTALITY ALL AGES: 1985–89

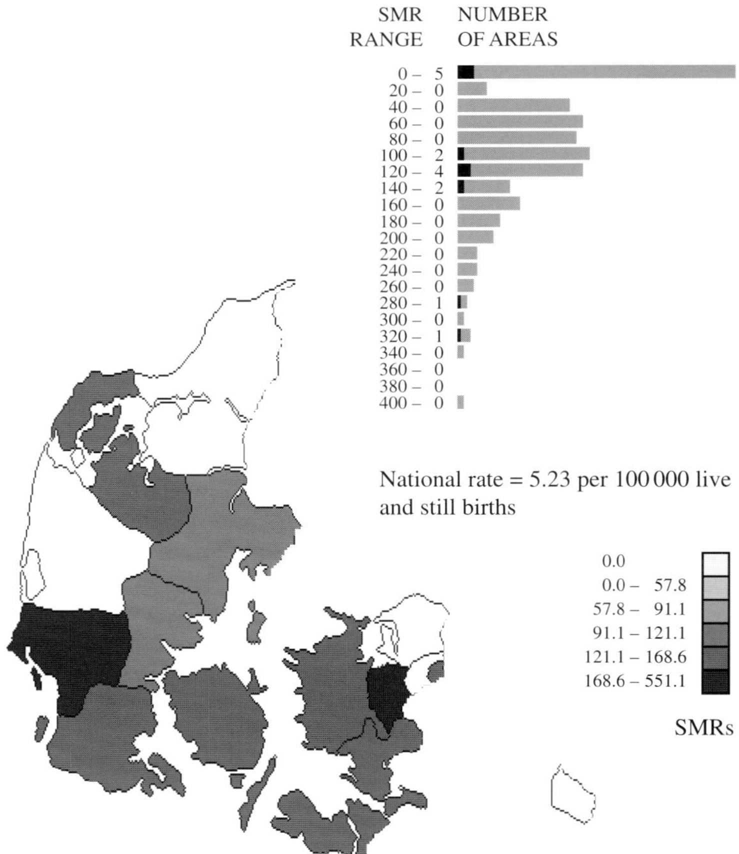

PERINATAL MORTALITY: 1985–89

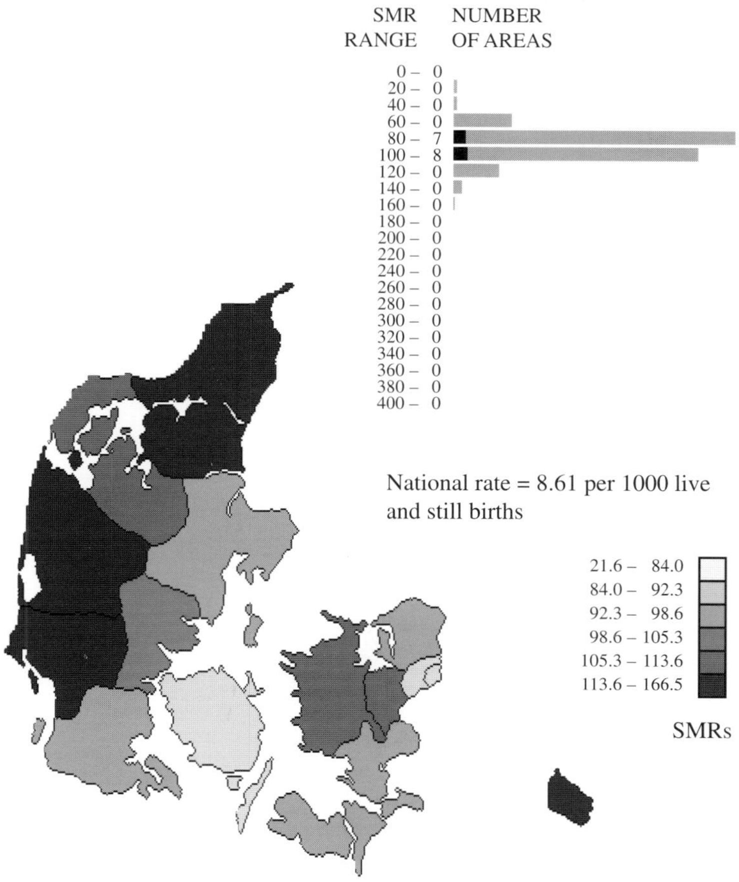

CANCER OF THE BREAST MORTALITY AGES 25–64: 1985–89

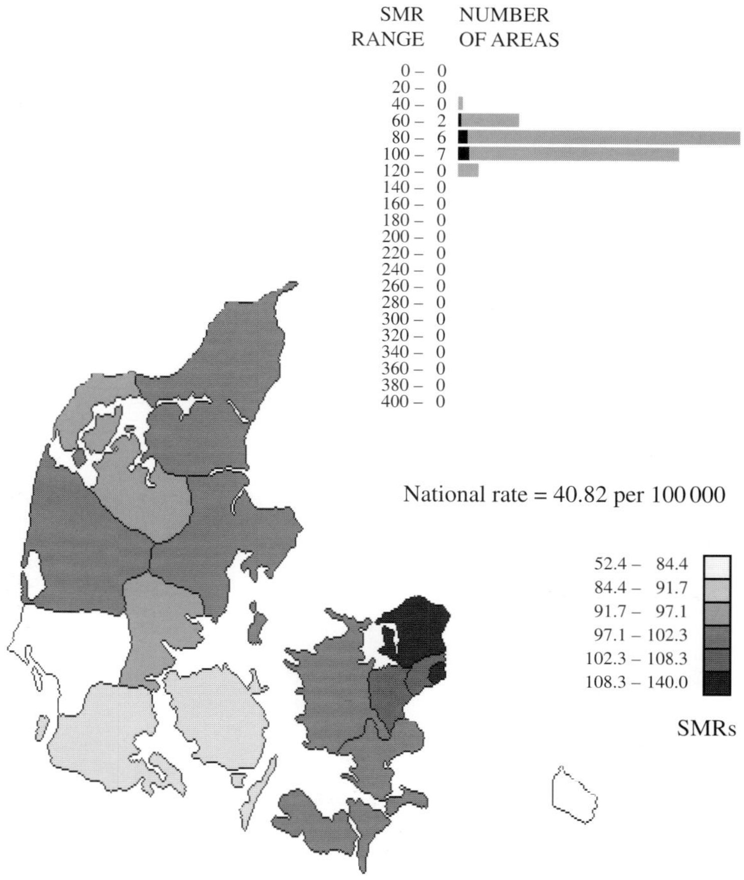

ISCHAEMIC HEART DISEASE MORTALITY AGES 35–64: 1985–89

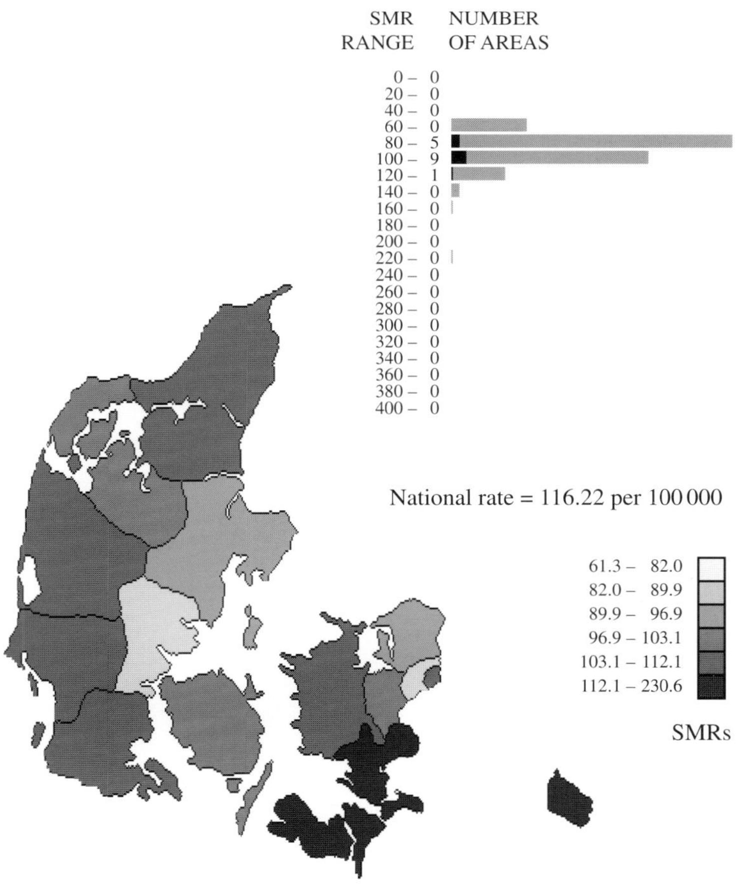

PEPTIC ULCERS MORTALITY AGES 25–64: 1985–89

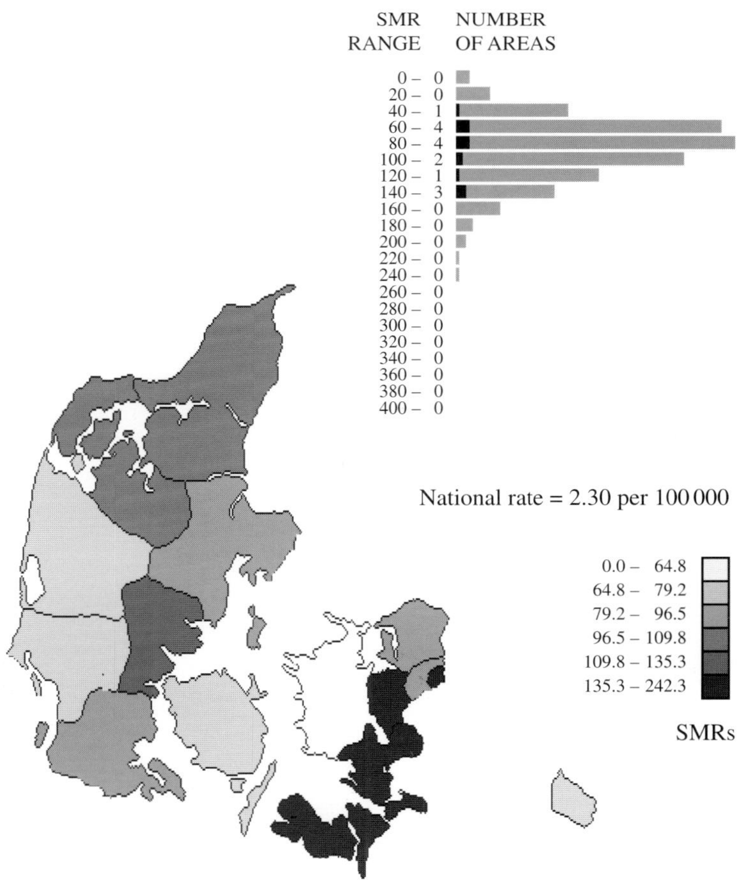

ALL CAUSES MORTALITY AGES 5–64: 1985–89

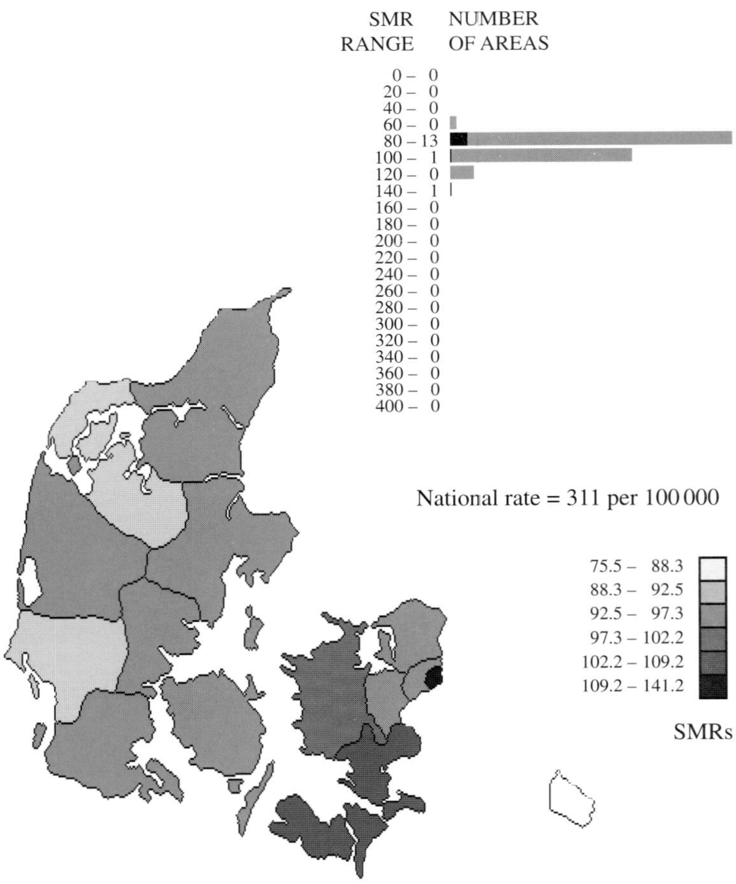

ALL CAUSES MORTALITY ALL AGES: 1985–89

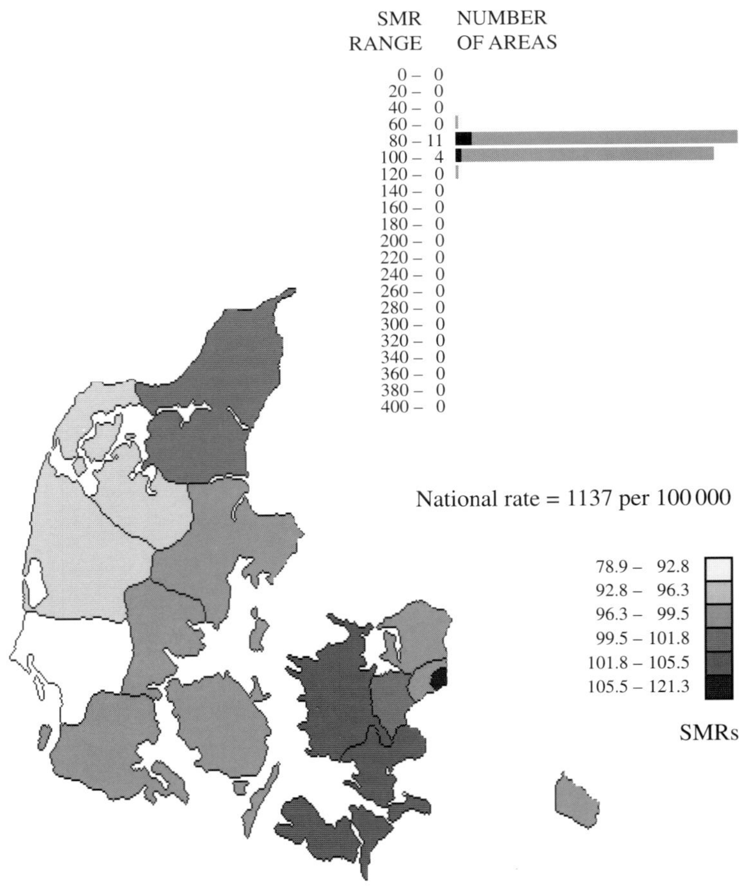

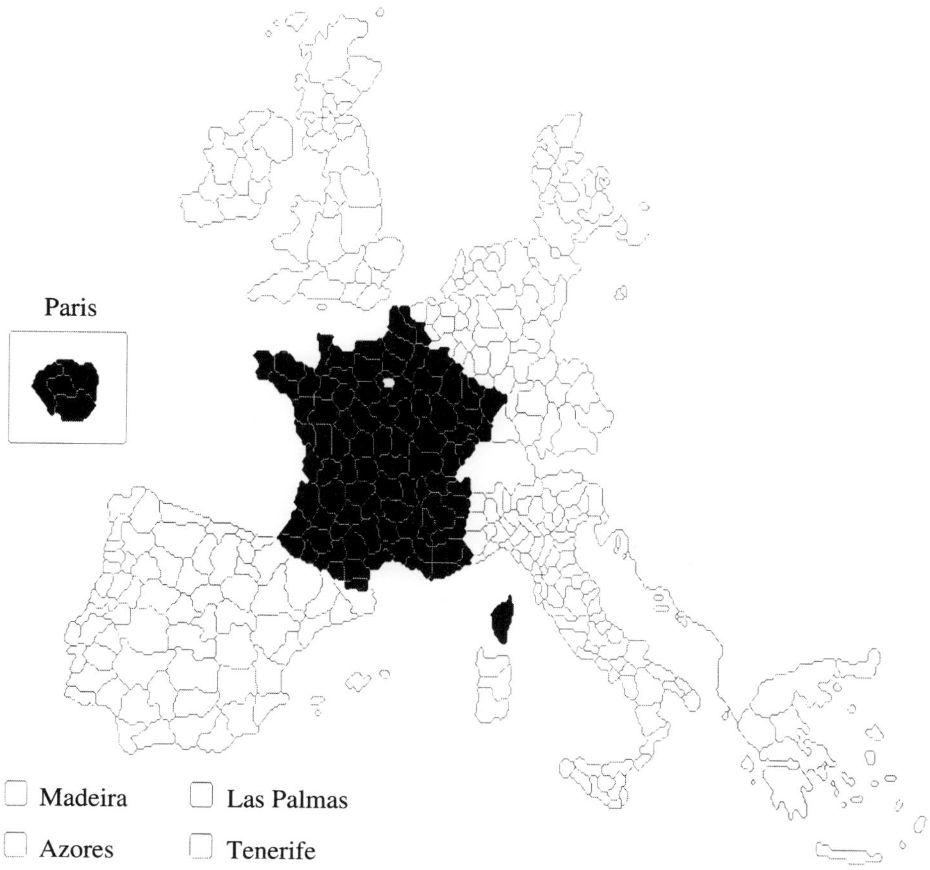

KEY MAP: FRANCE

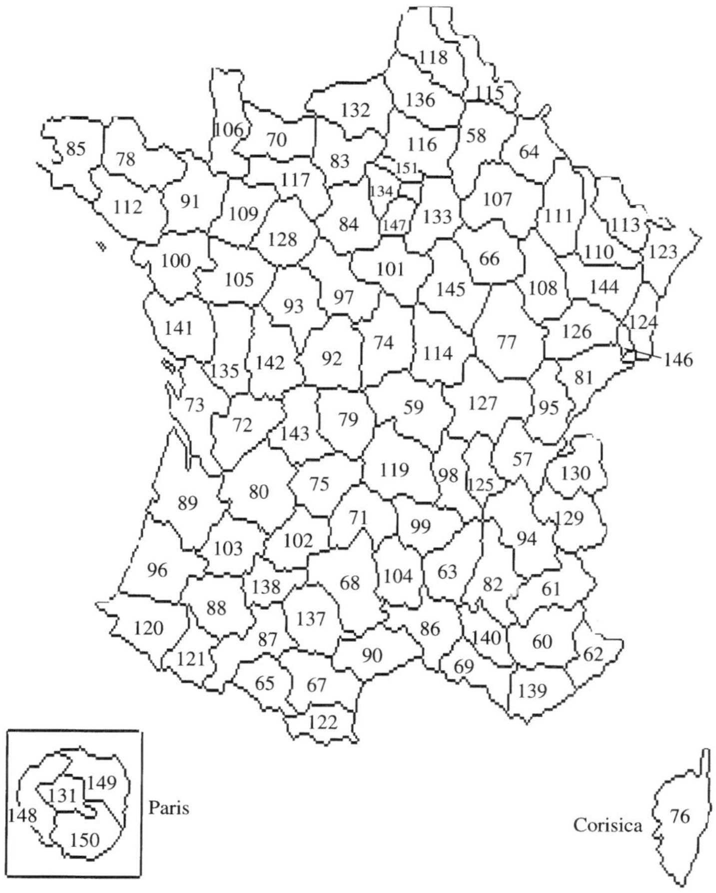

TUBERCULOSIS MORTALITY AGES 5–64: 1985–89

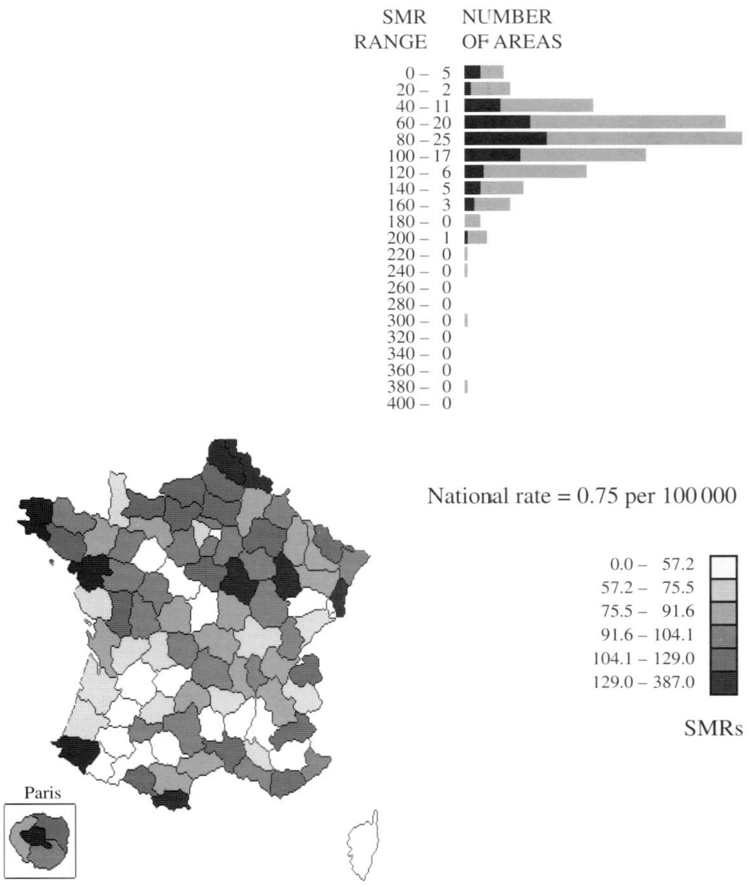

MALIGNANT NEOPLASM OF CERVIX UTERI MORTALITY AGES 15–64: 1985–89

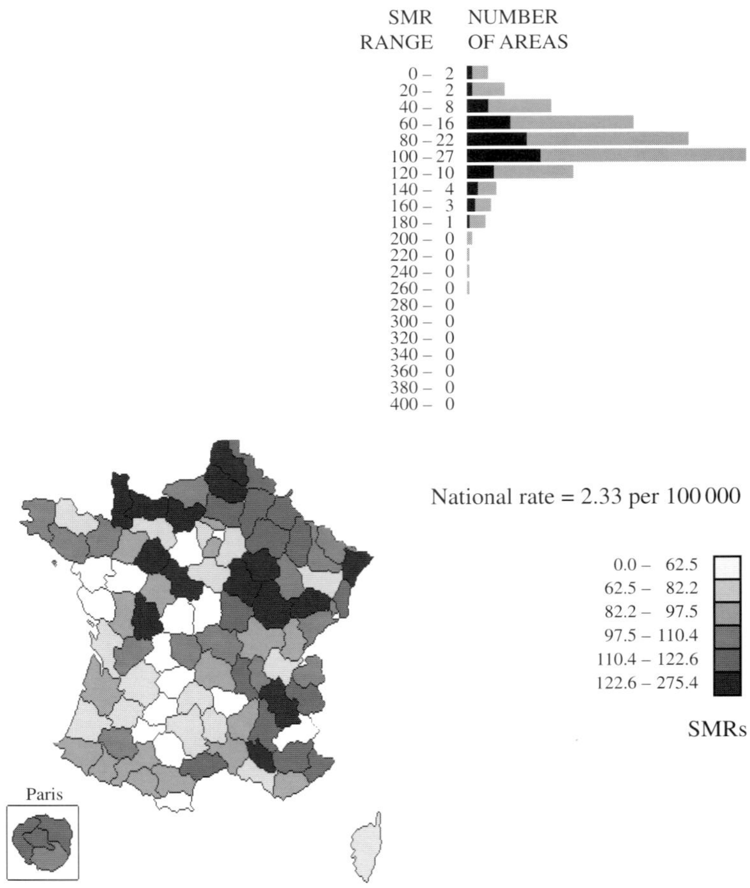

MALIGNANT NEOPLASM OF CERVIX AND BODY OF UTERUS MORTALITY AGES 15–54: 1985–89

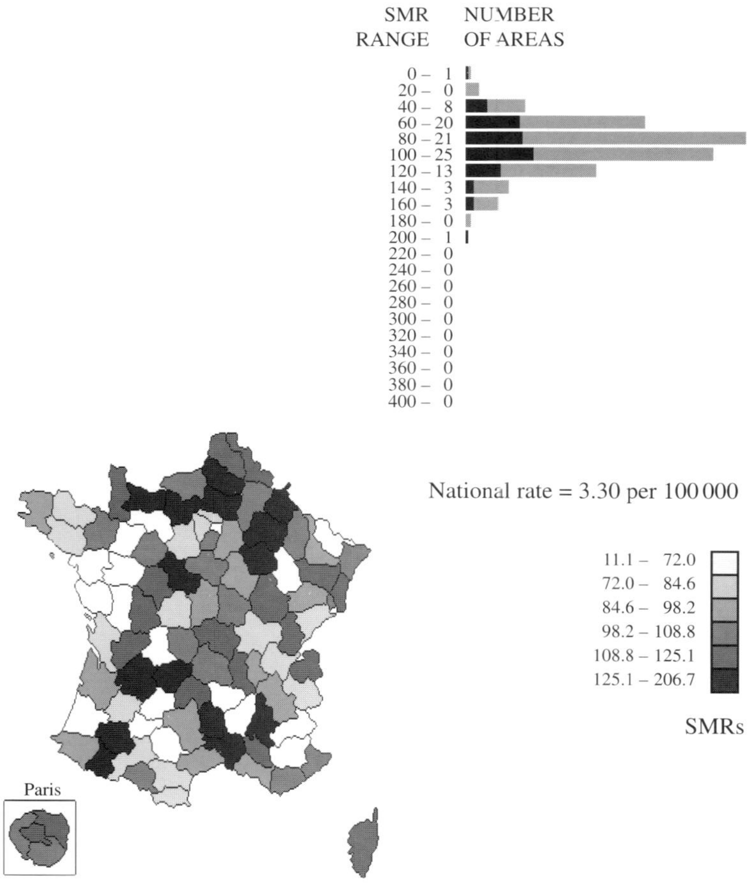

HODGKIN'S DISEASE MORTALITY AGES 5–64: 1985–89

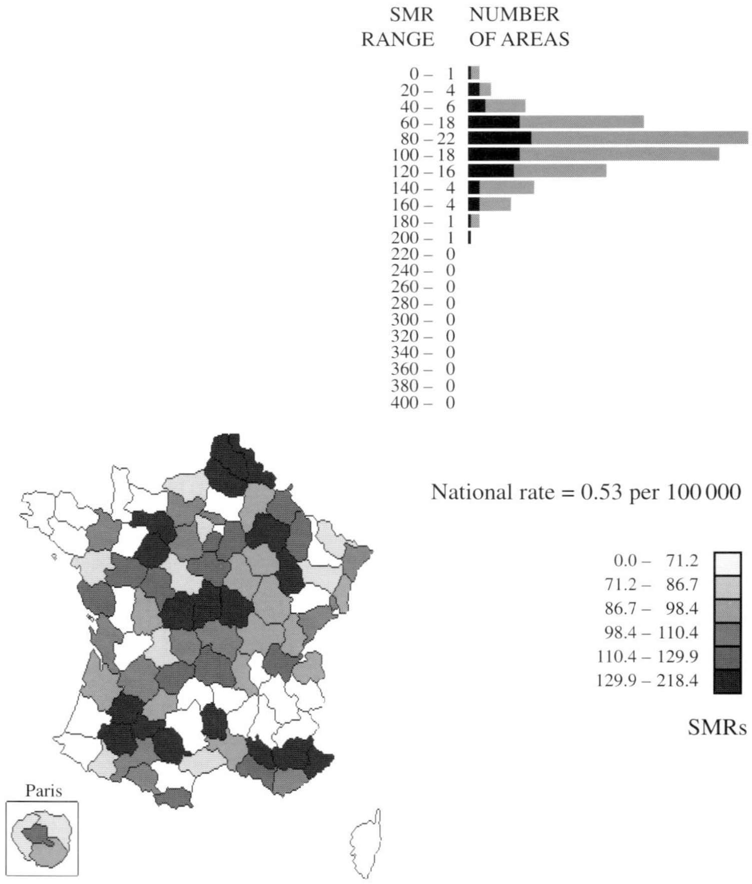

CHRONIC RHEUMATIC HEART DISEASE MORTALITY AGES 5–44: 1985–89

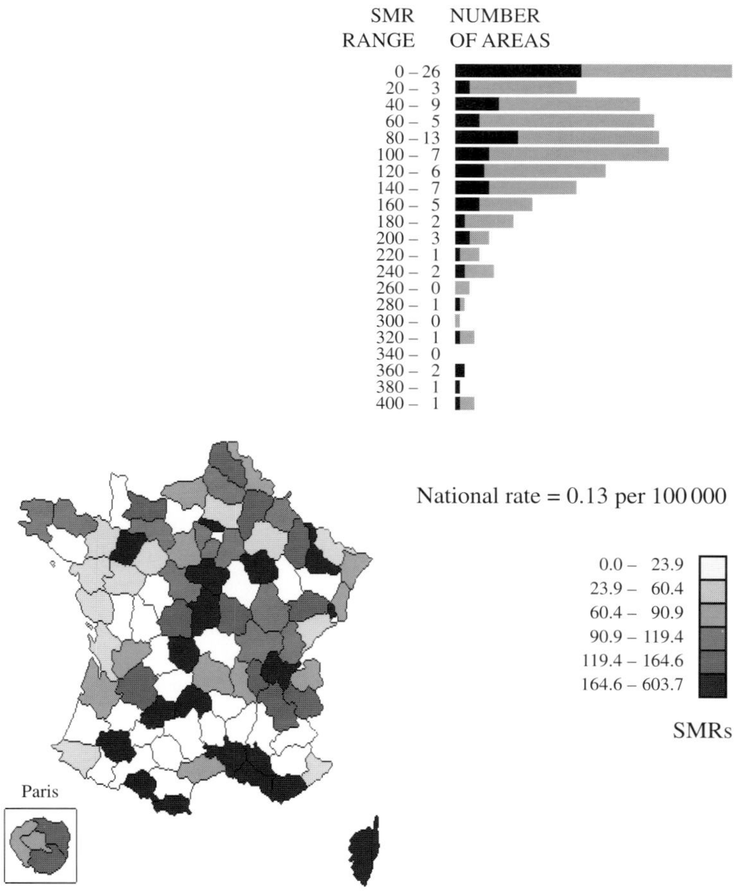

ALL RESPIRATORY DISEASES MORTALITY AGES 1–14: 1985–89

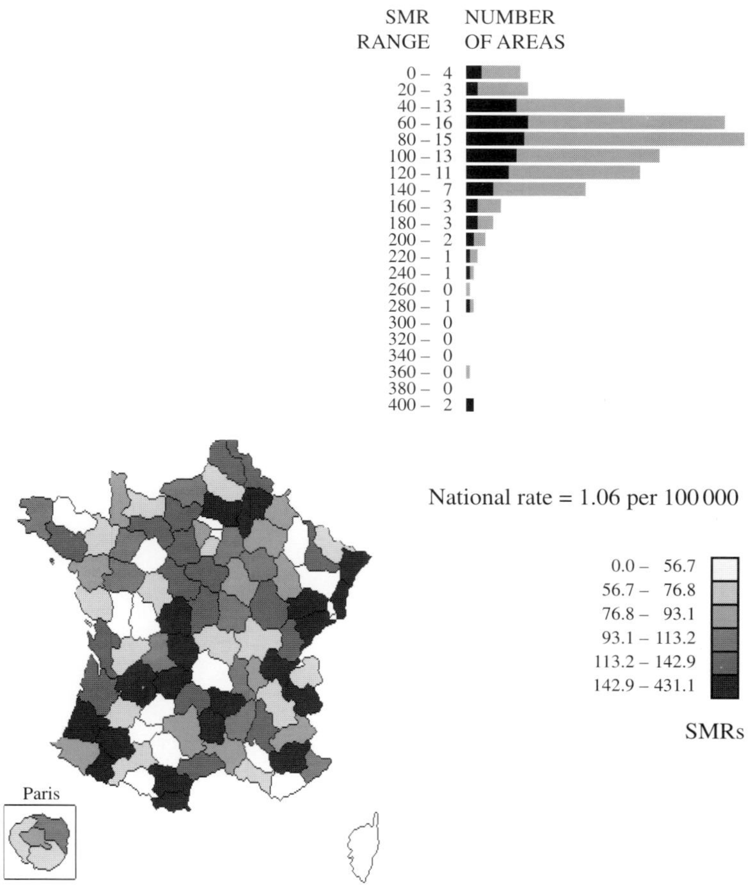

ASTHMA MORTALITY AGES 5–44: 1985–89

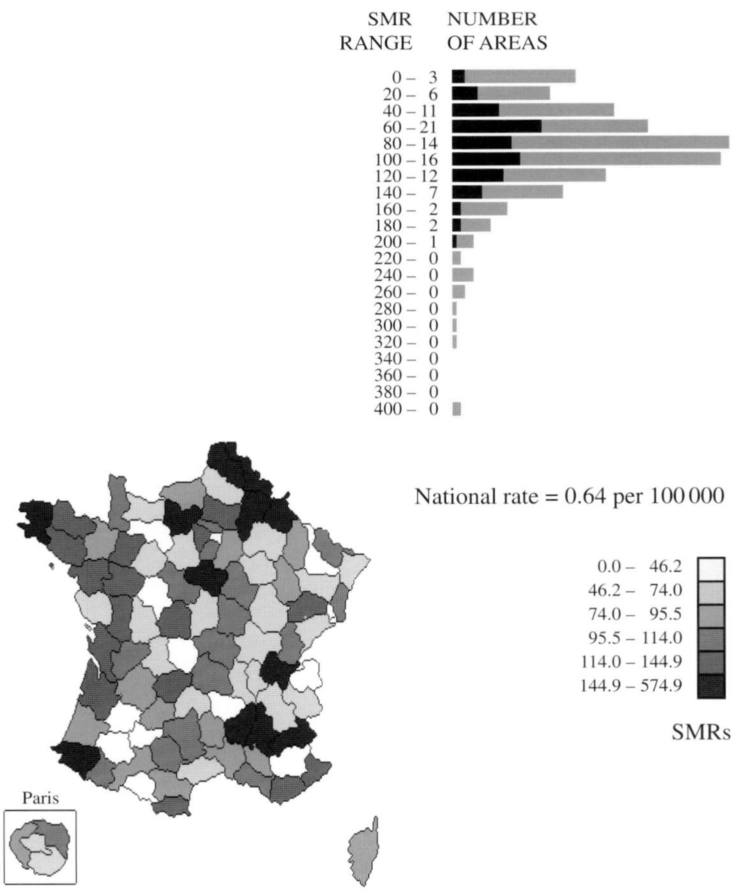

APPENDICITIS MORTALITY AGES 5–64: 1985–89

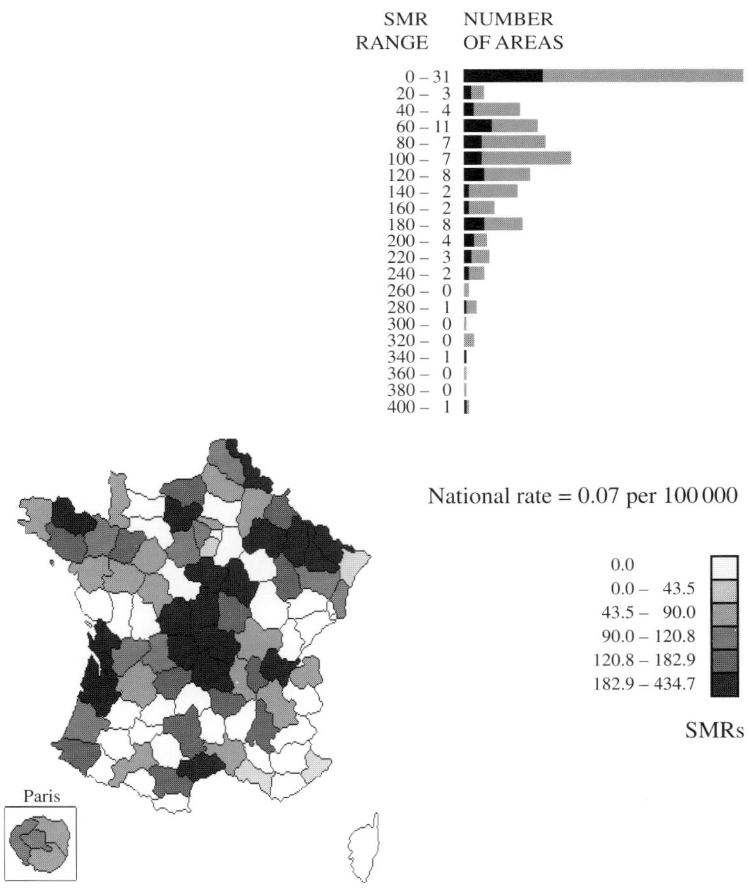

ABDOMINAL HERNIA MORTALITY AGES 5–64: 1985–89

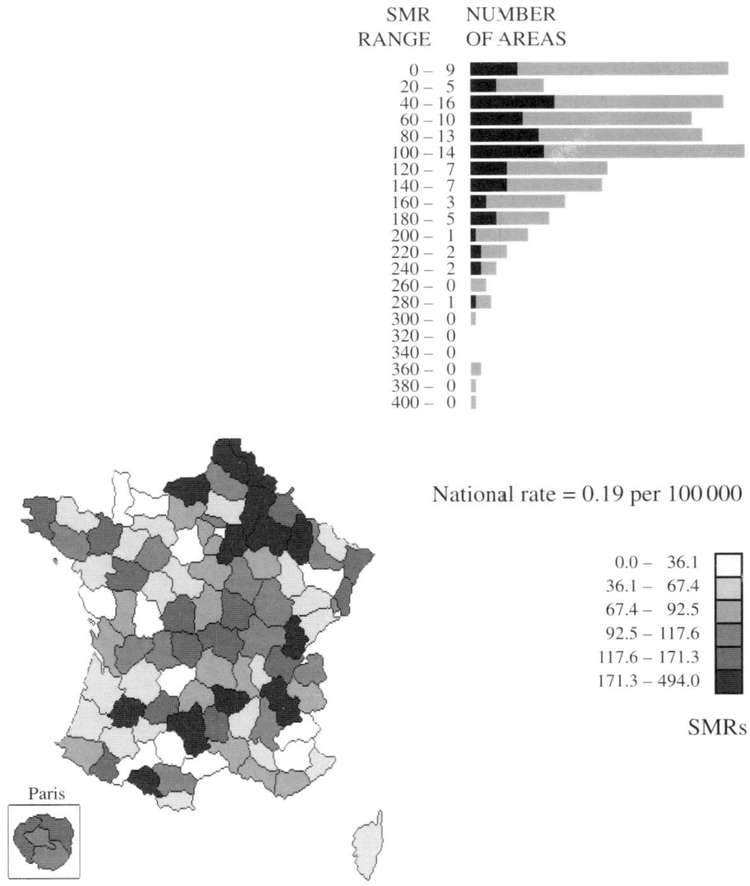

CHOLELITHIASIS AND CHOLECYSTITIS MORTALITY AGES 5–64: 1985–89

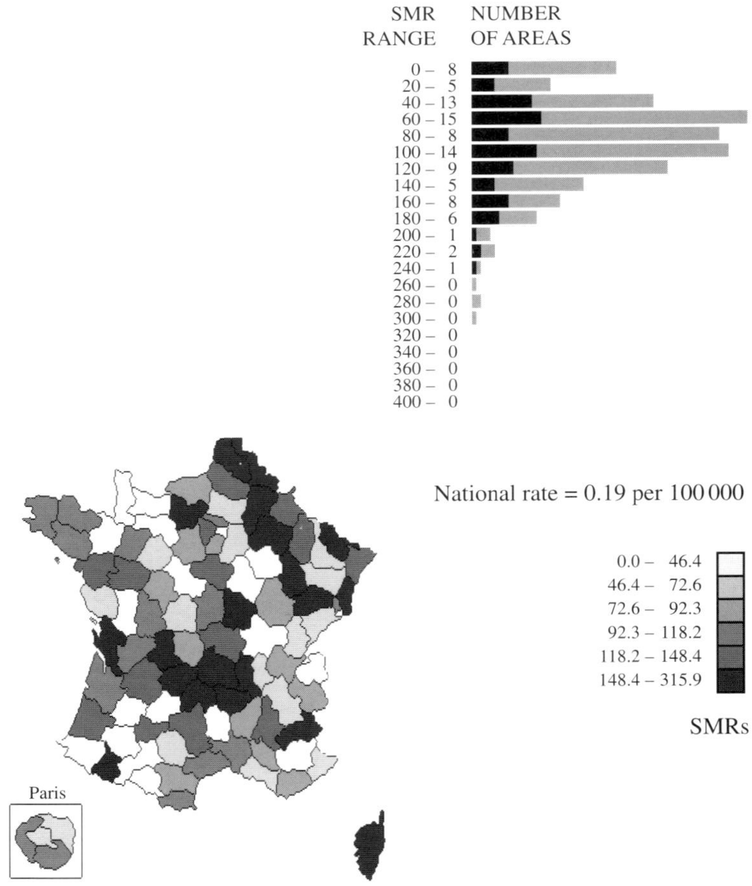

HYPERTENSIVE AND CEREBROVASCULAR DISEASES MORTALITY AGES 35–64: 1985–89

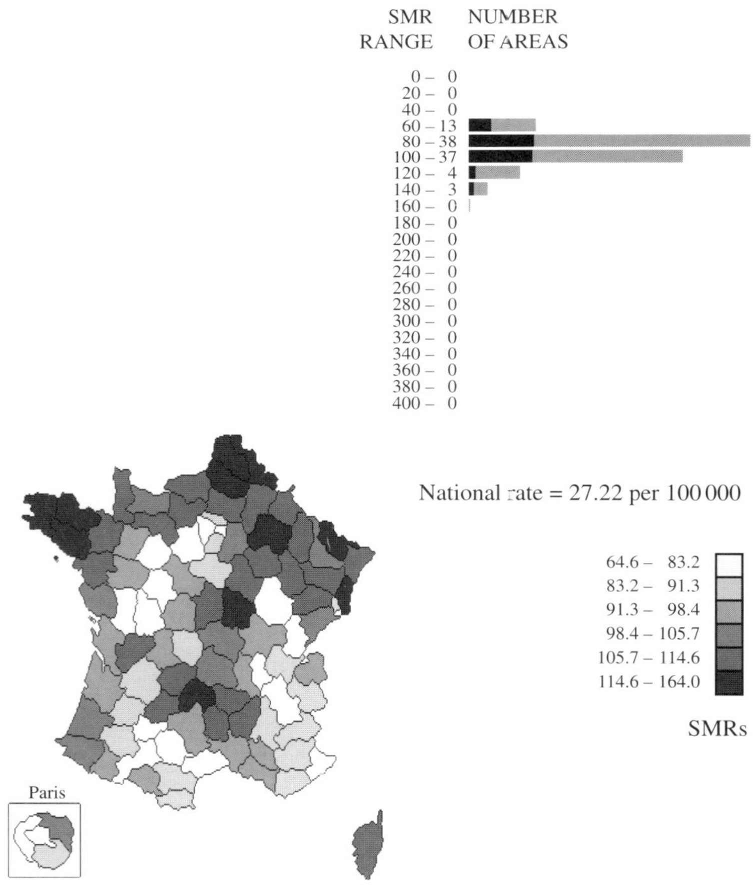

MATERNAL MORTALITY ALL AGES: 1985–89

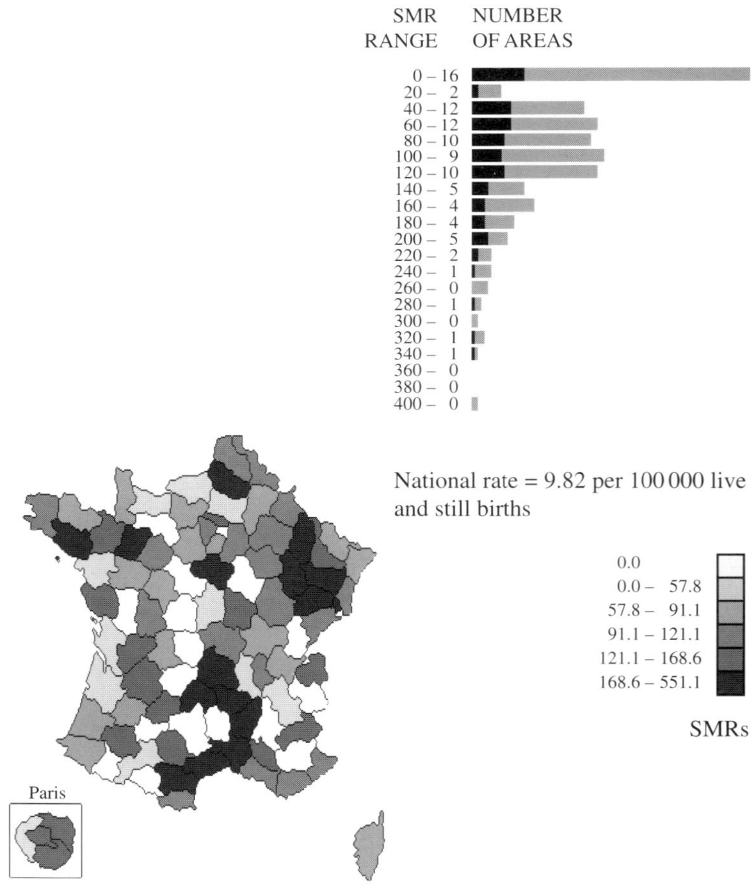

PERINATAL MORTALITY: 1985–89

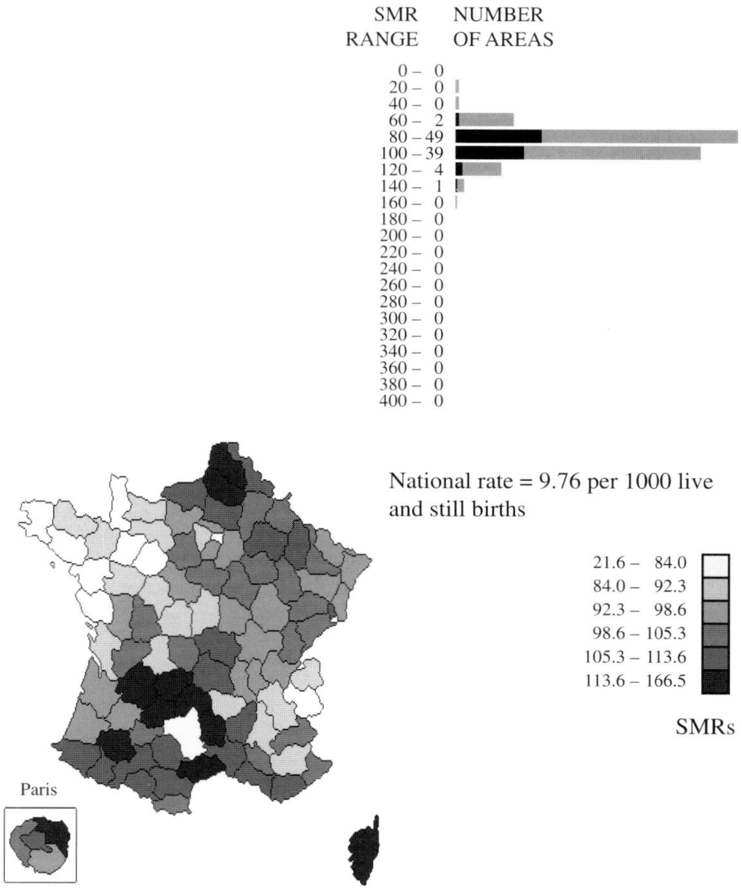

CANCER OF THE BREAST MORTALITY AGES 25–64: 1985–89

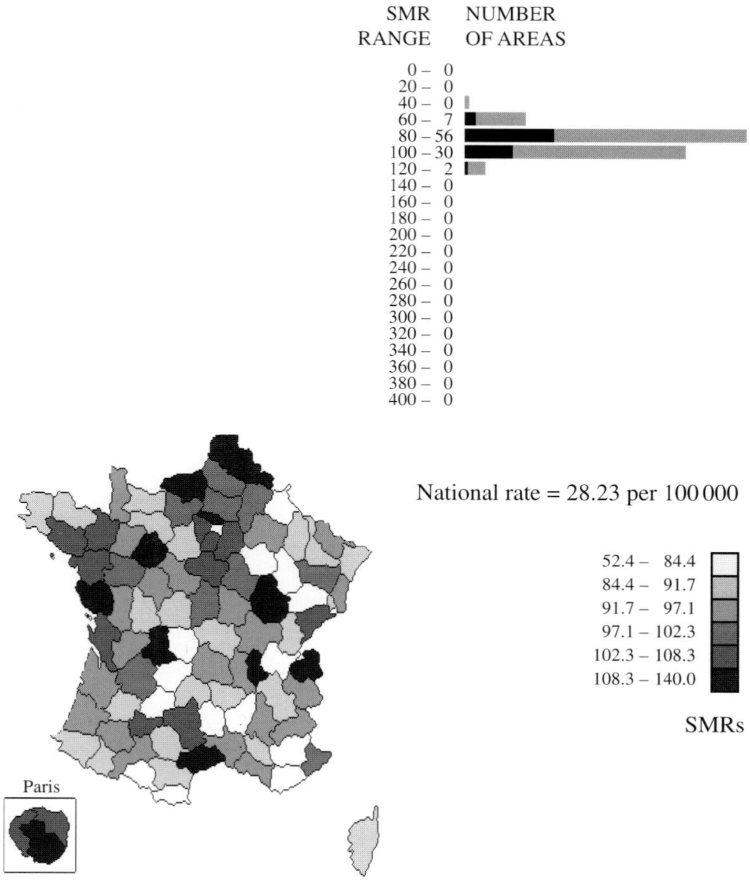

ISCHAEMIC HEART DISEASE MORTALITY AGES 35–64: 1985–89

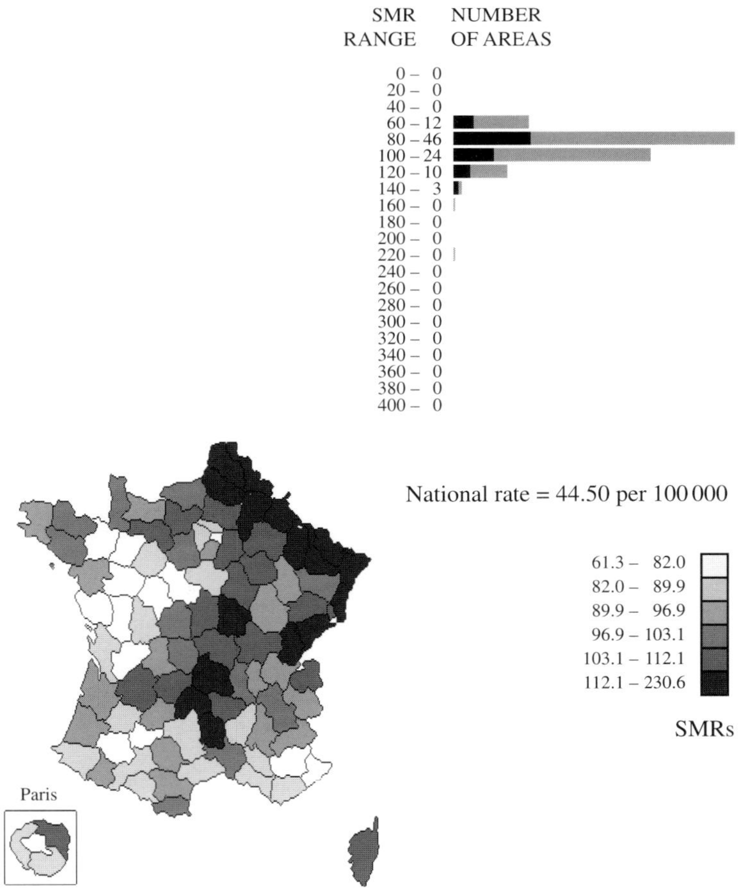

PEPTIC ULCERS MORTALITY AGES 25–64: 1985–89

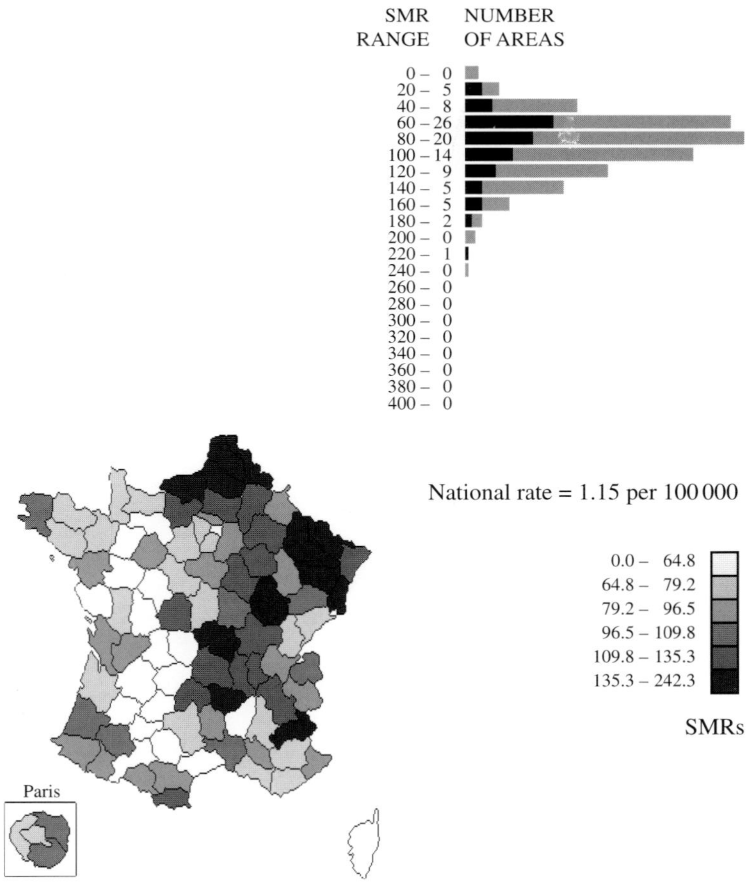

ALL CAUSES MORTALITY AGES 5–64: 1985–89

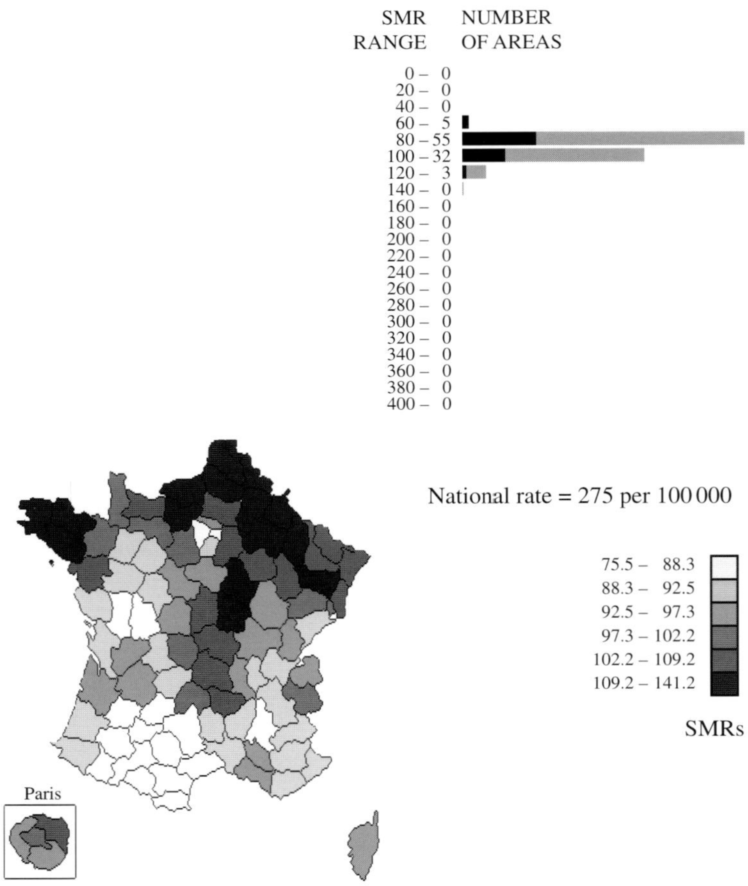

ALL CAUSES MORTALITY ALL AGES: 1985–89

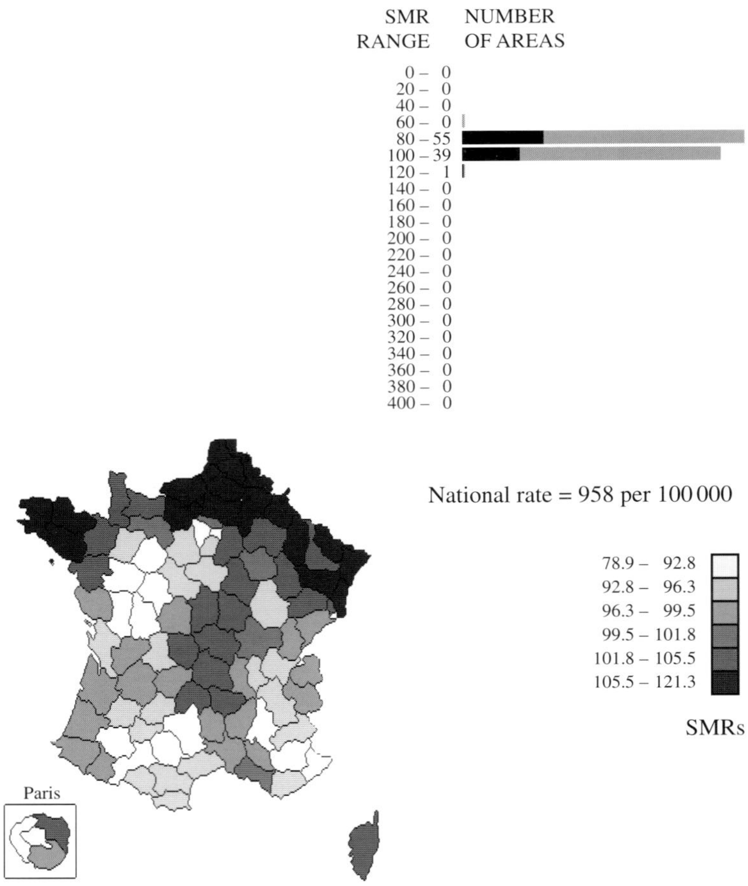

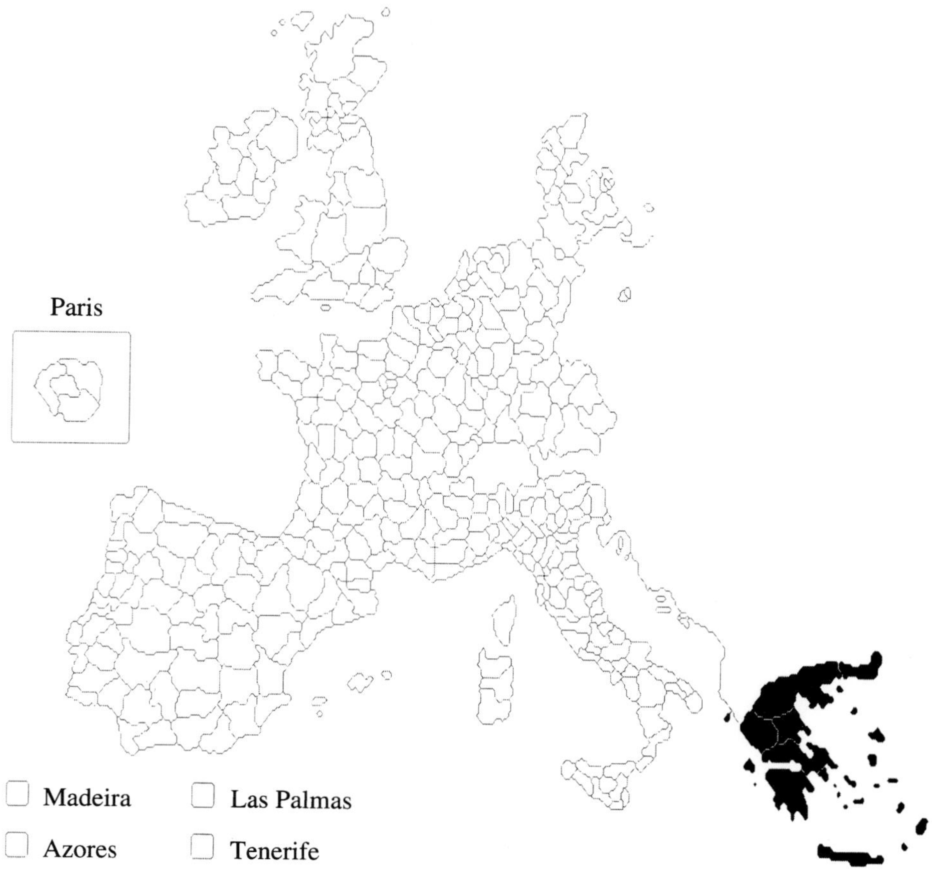

KEY MAP: GREECE

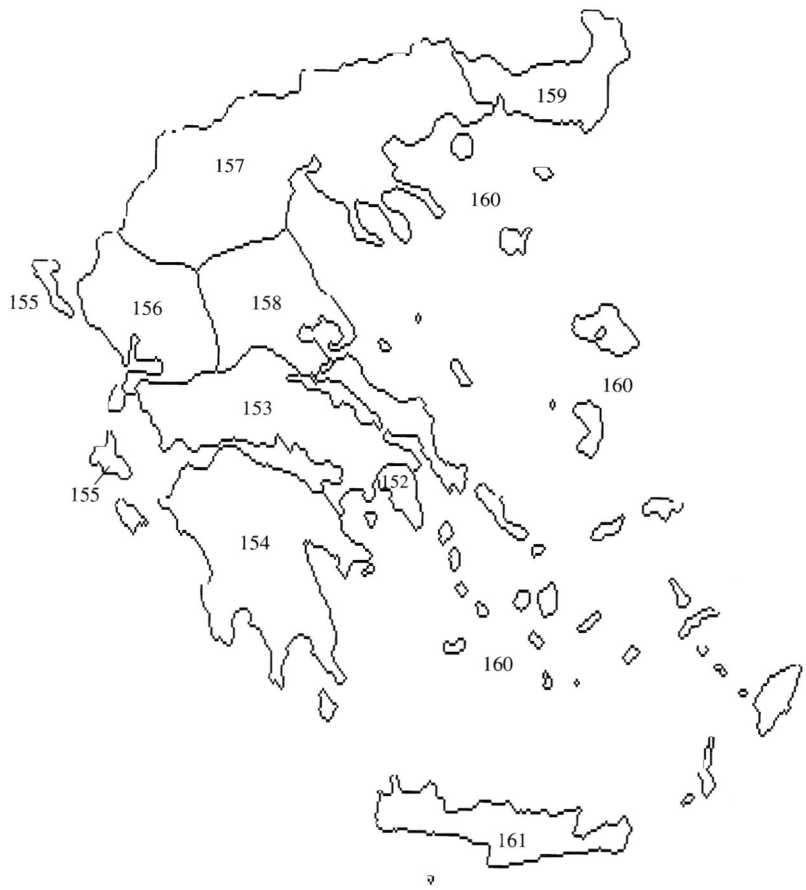

TUBERCULOSIS MORTALITY AGES 5–64: 1985–89

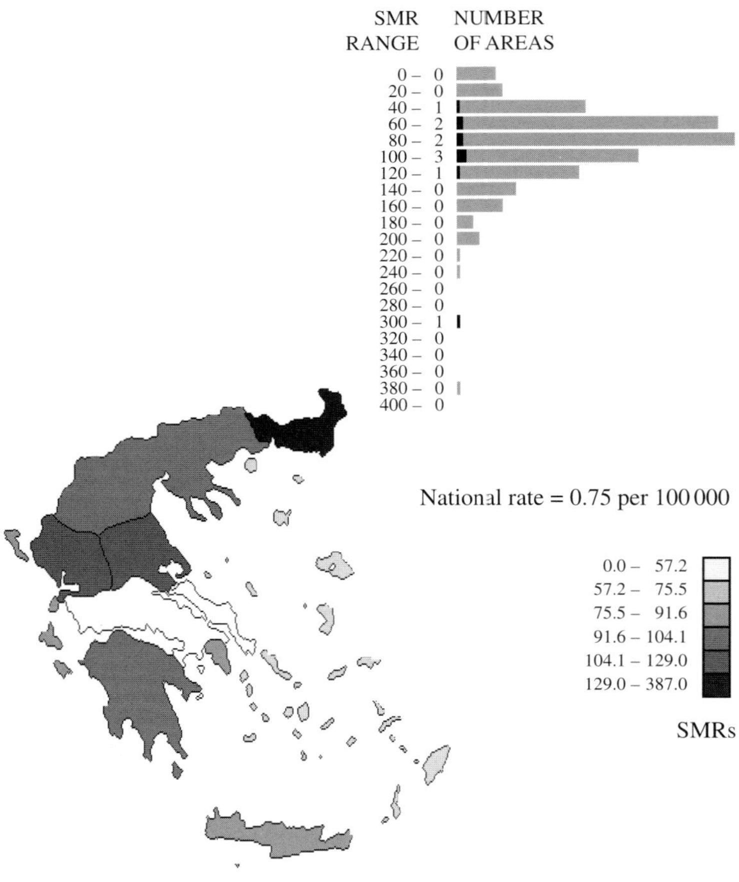

MALIGNANT NEOPLASM OF CERVIX UTERI MORTALITY AGES 15–64: 1985–89

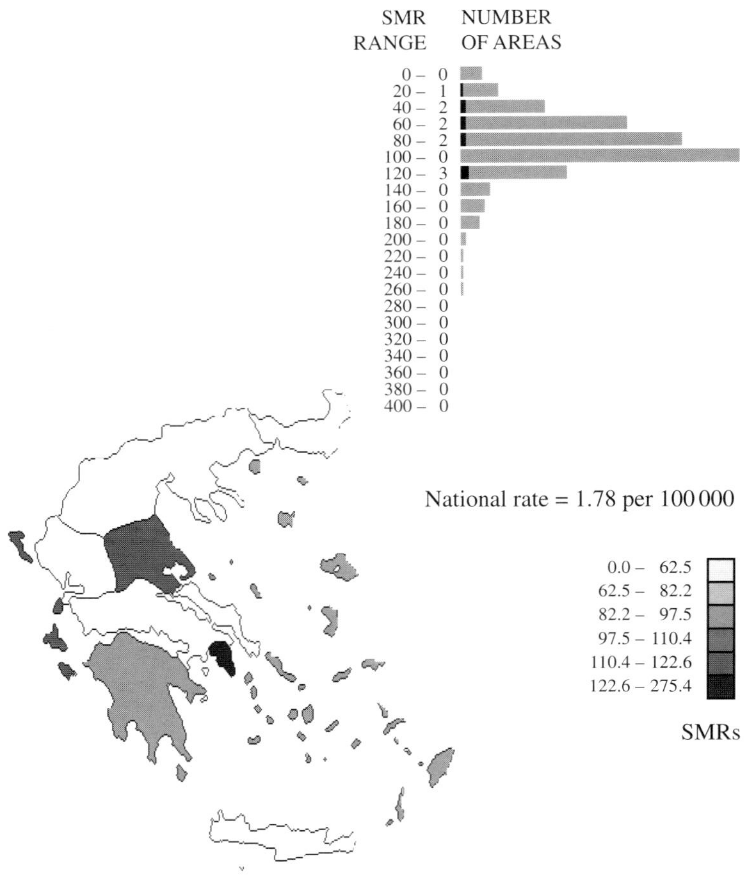

MALIGNANT NEOPLASM OF CERVIX AND BODY OF UTERUS MORTALITY AGES 15–54: 1985–89

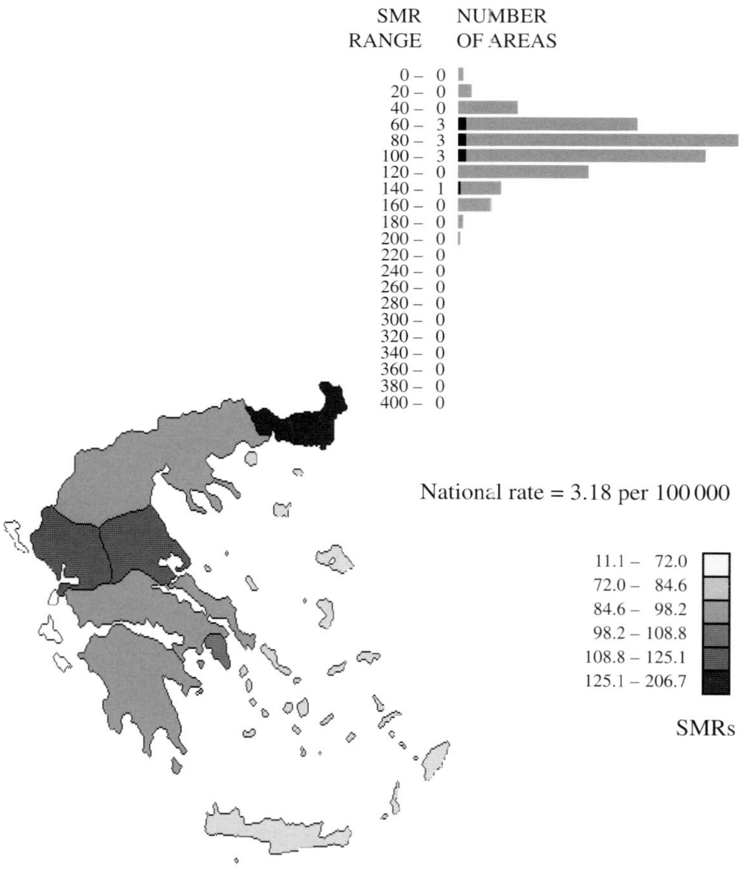

HODGKIN'S DISEASE MORTALITY AGES 5–64: 1985–89

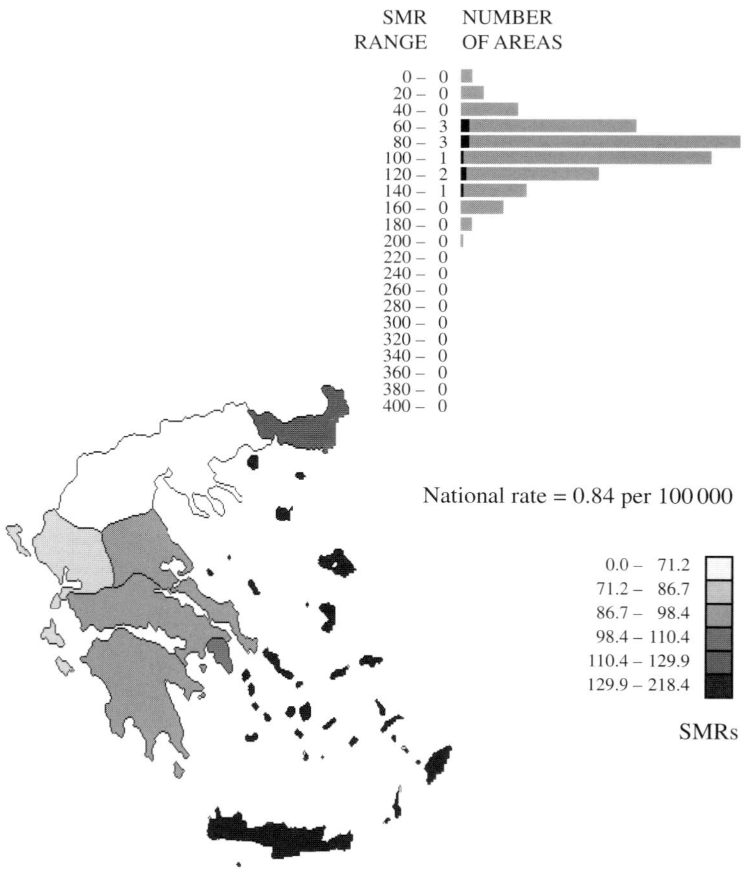

CHRONIC RHEUMATIC HEART DISEASE MORTALITY AGES 5–44: 1985–89

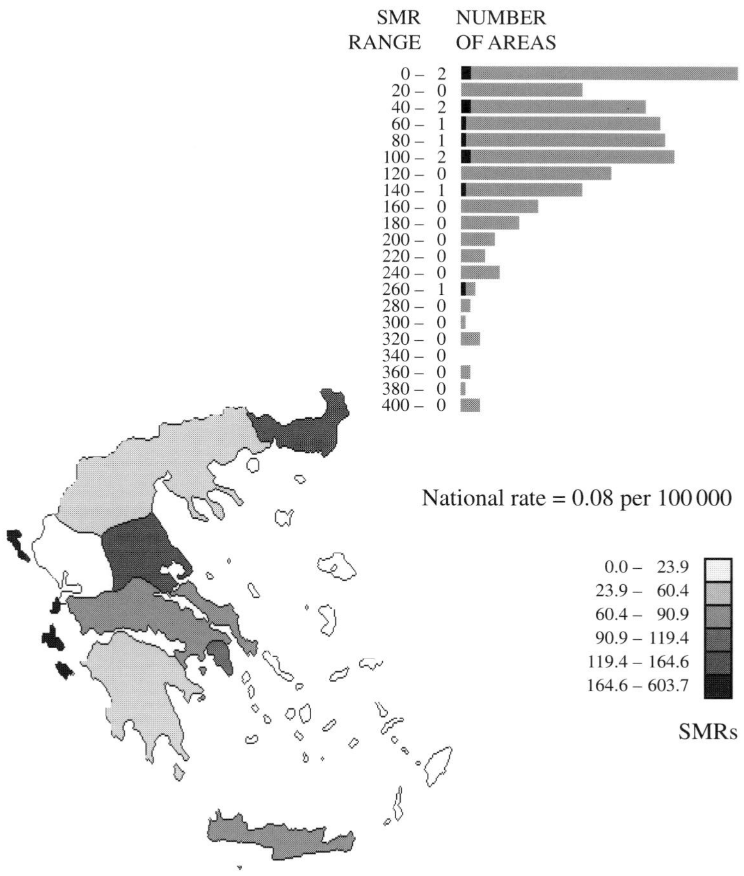

ALL RESPIRATORY DISEASES MORTALITY AGES 1–14: 1985–89

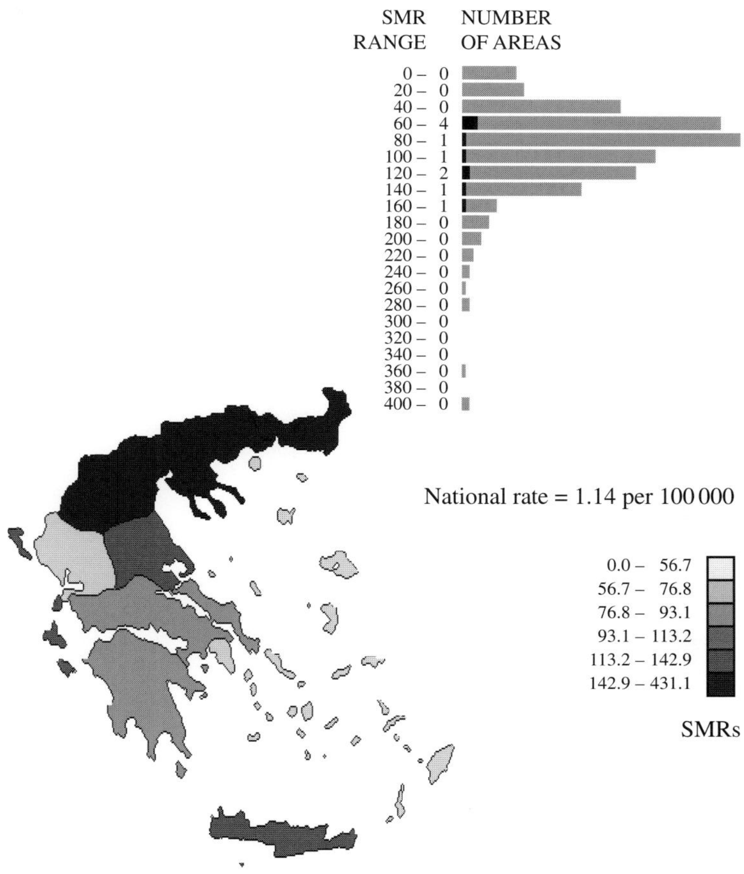

ASTHMA MORTALITY AGES 5–44: 1985–89

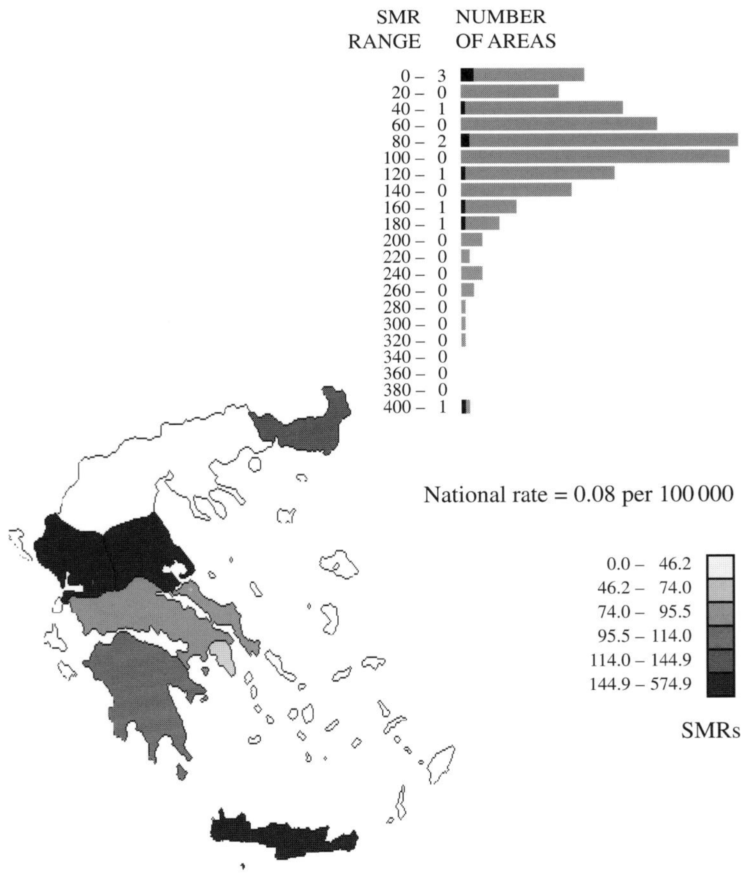

APPENDICITIS MORTALITY AGES 5–64: 1985–89

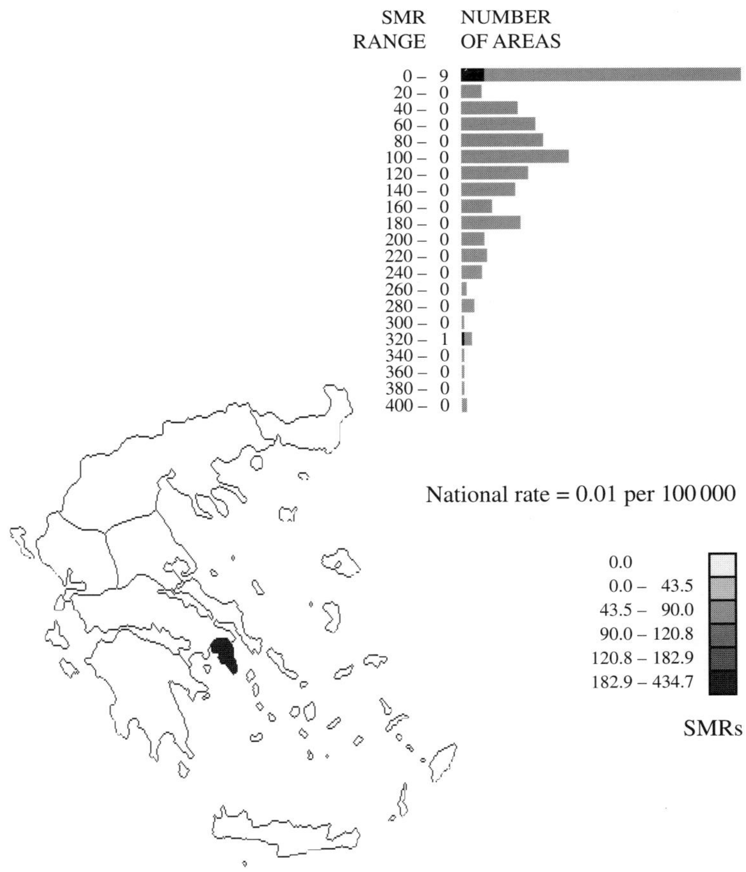

ABDOMINAL HERNIA MORTALITY AGES 5–64: 1985–89

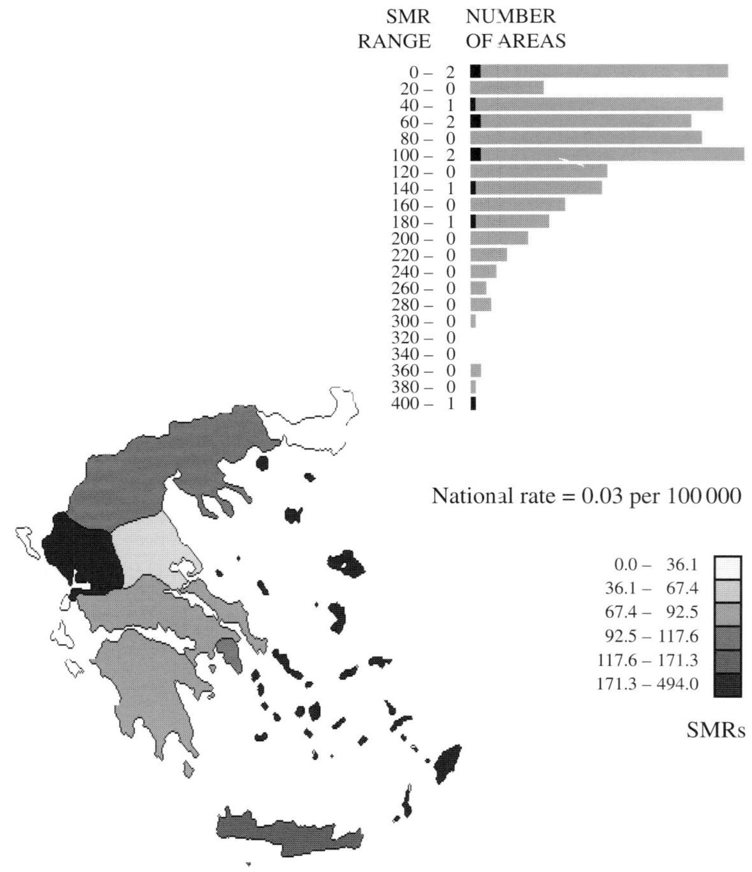

CHOLELITHIASIS AND CHOLECYSTITIS MORTALITY AGES 5–64: 1985–89

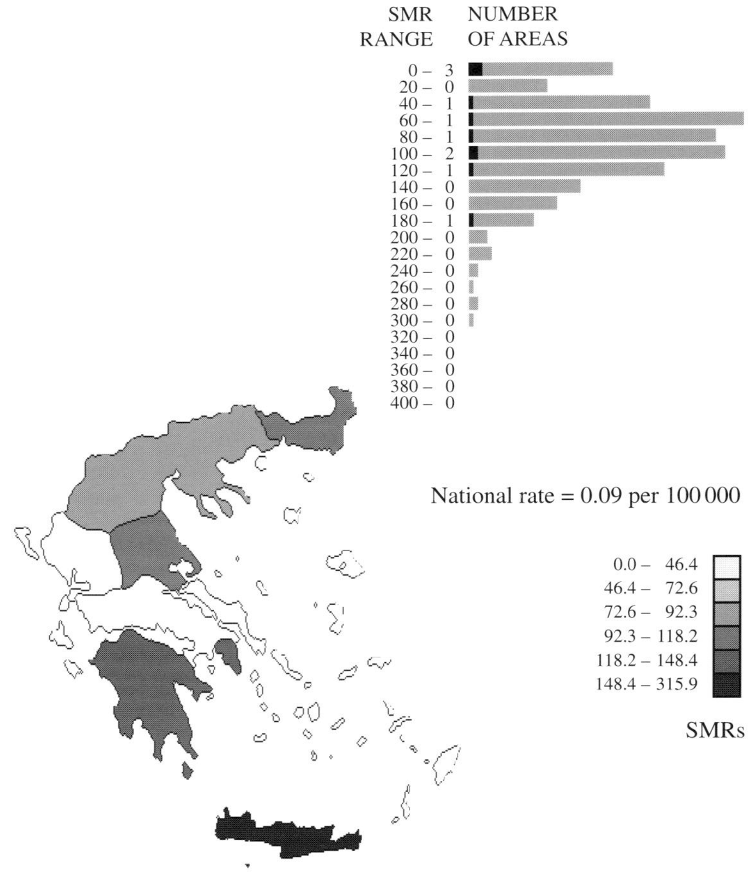

HYPERTENSIVE AND CEREBROVASCULAR DISEASES MORTALITY AGES 35–64: 1985–89

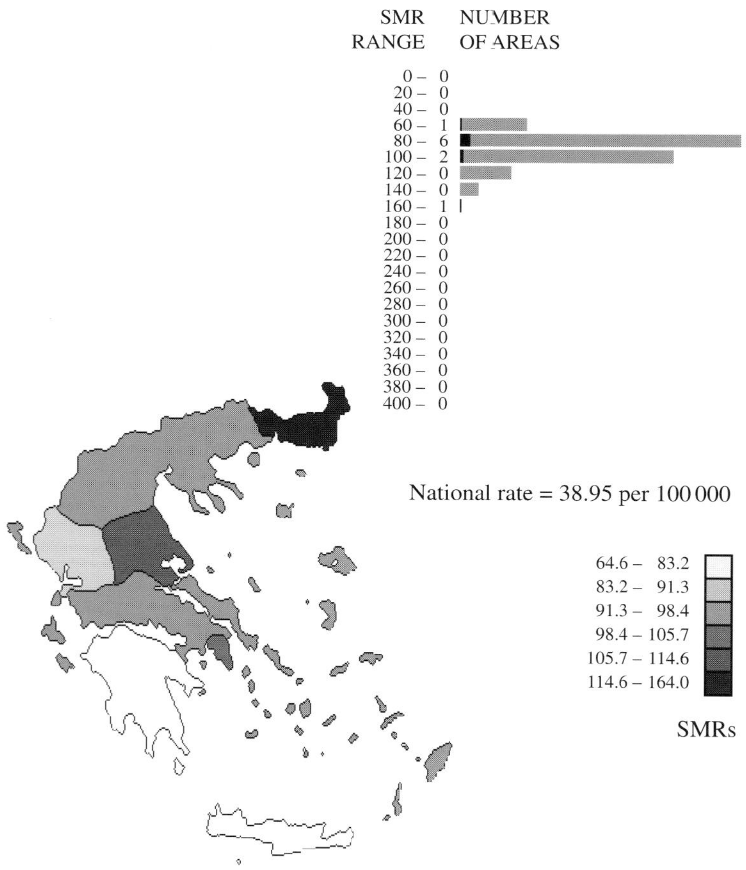

MATERNAL MORTALITY ALL AGES: 1985–89

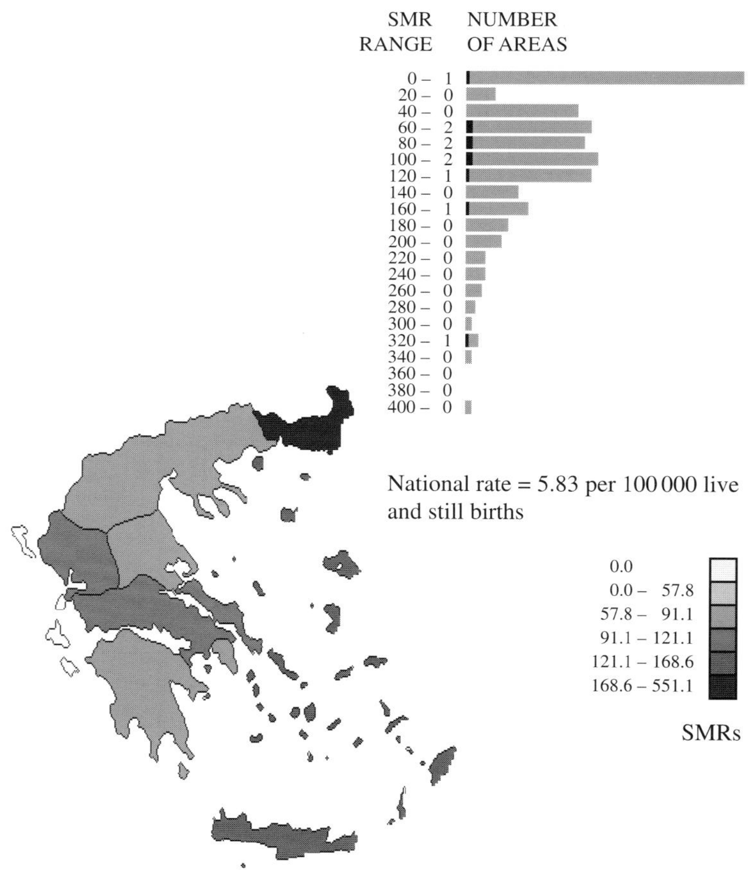

PERINATAL MORTALITY: 1985–89

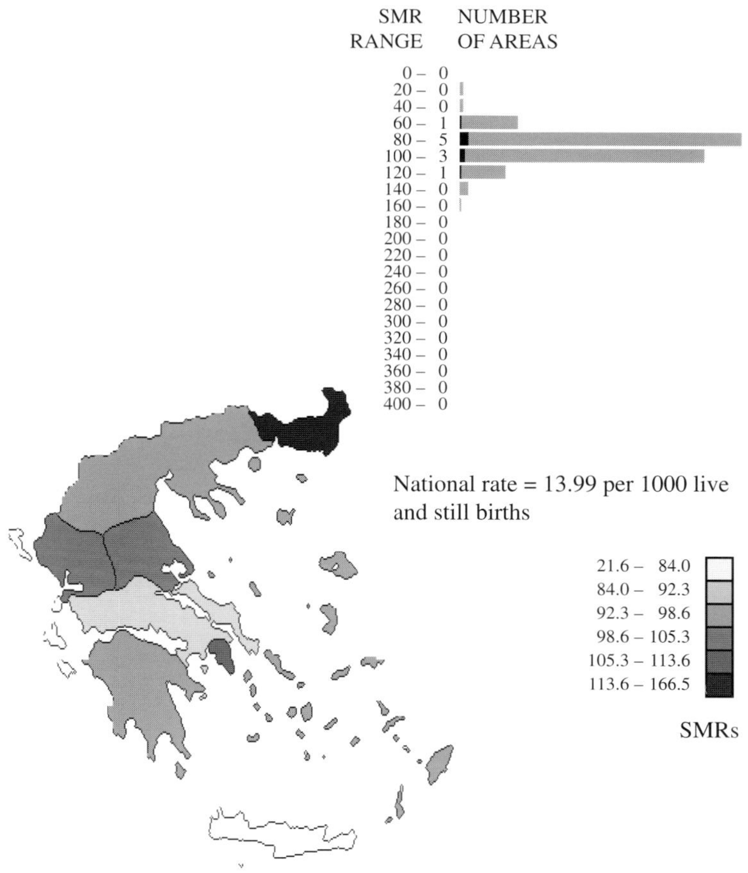

CANCER OF THE BREAST MORTALITY AGES 25–64: 1985–89

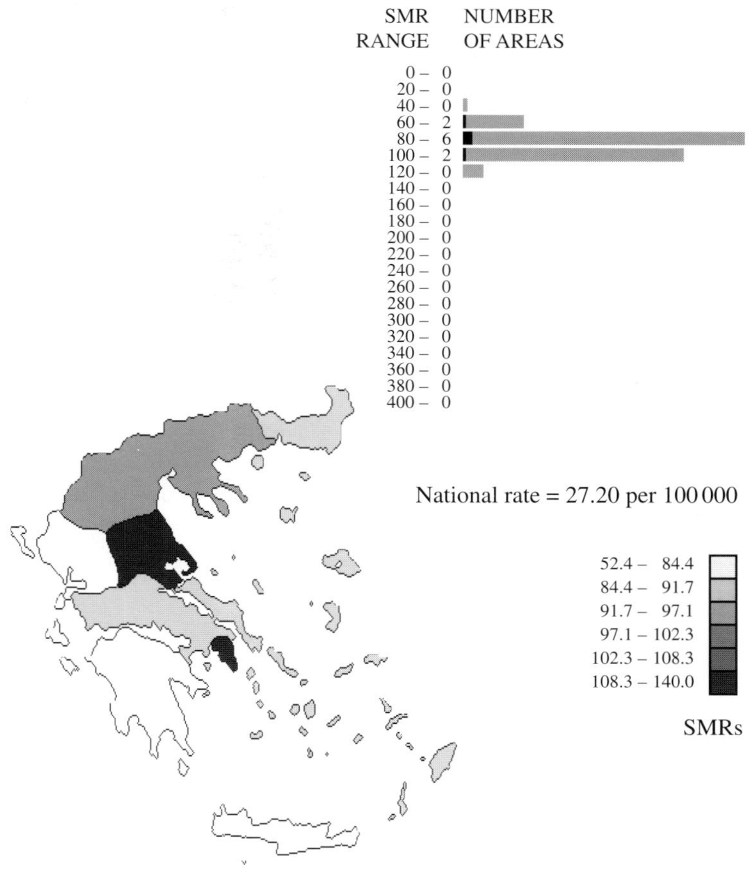

ISCHAEMIC HEART DISEASE MORTALITY AGES 35–64: 1985–89

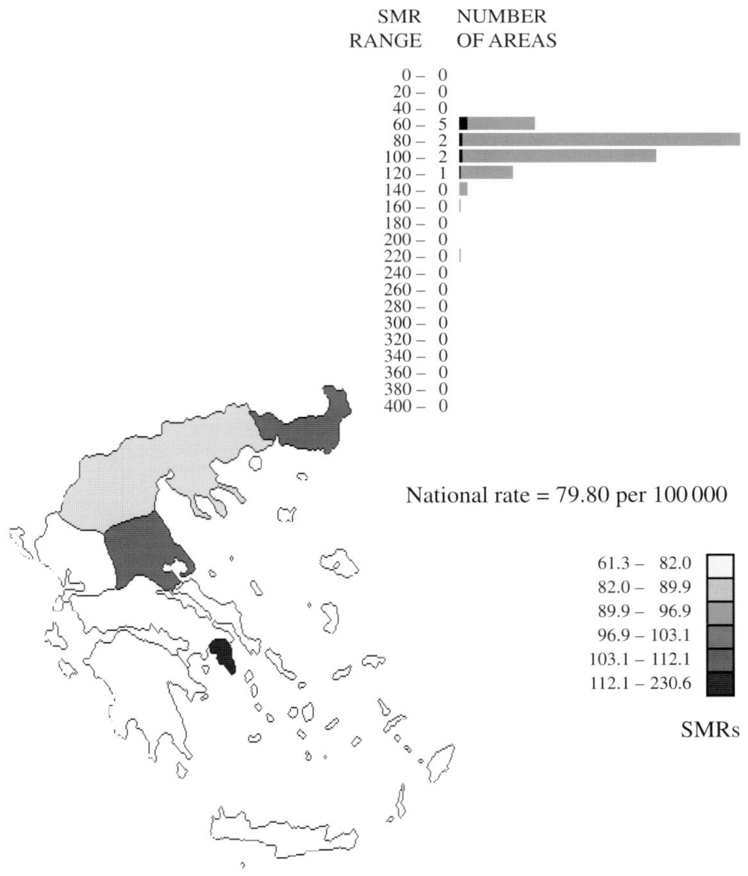

PEPTIC ULCERS MORTALITY AGES 25–64: 1985–89

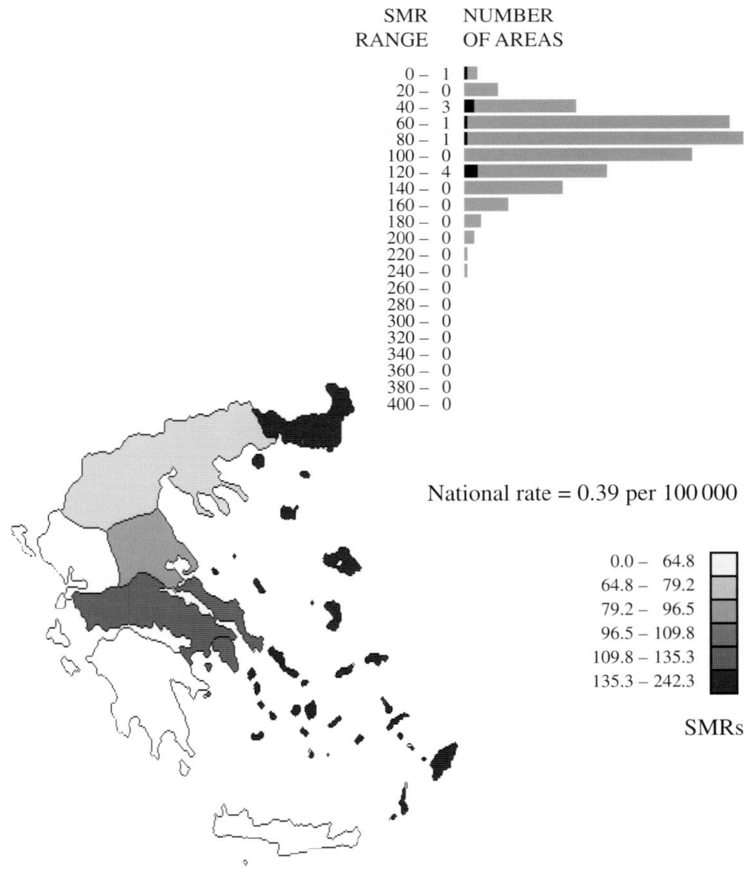

ALL CAUSES MORTALITY AGES 5–64: 1985–89

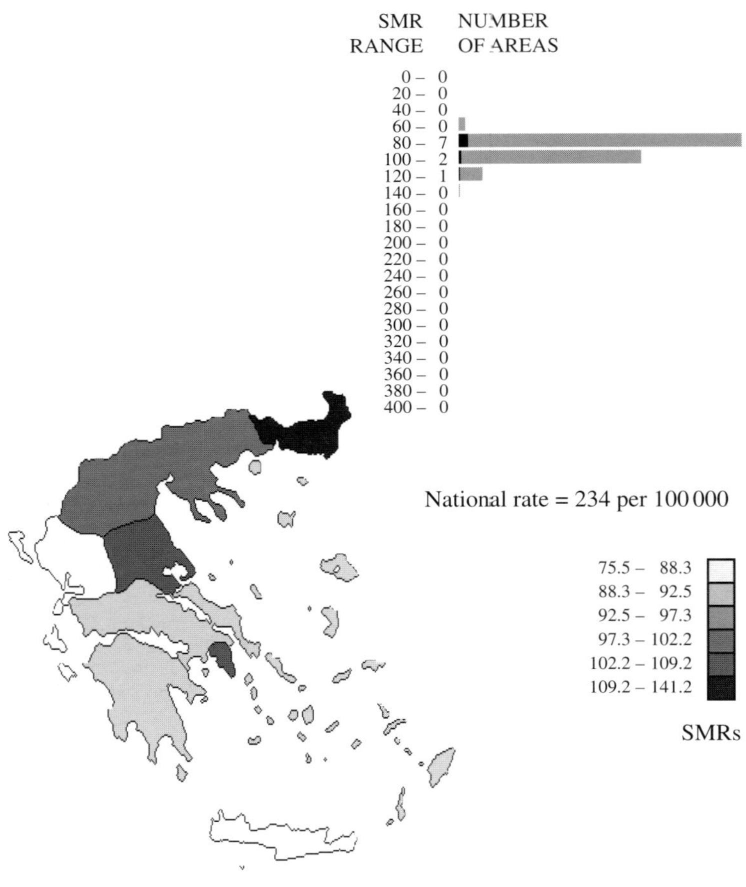

ALL CAUSES MORTALITY ALL AGES: 1985–89

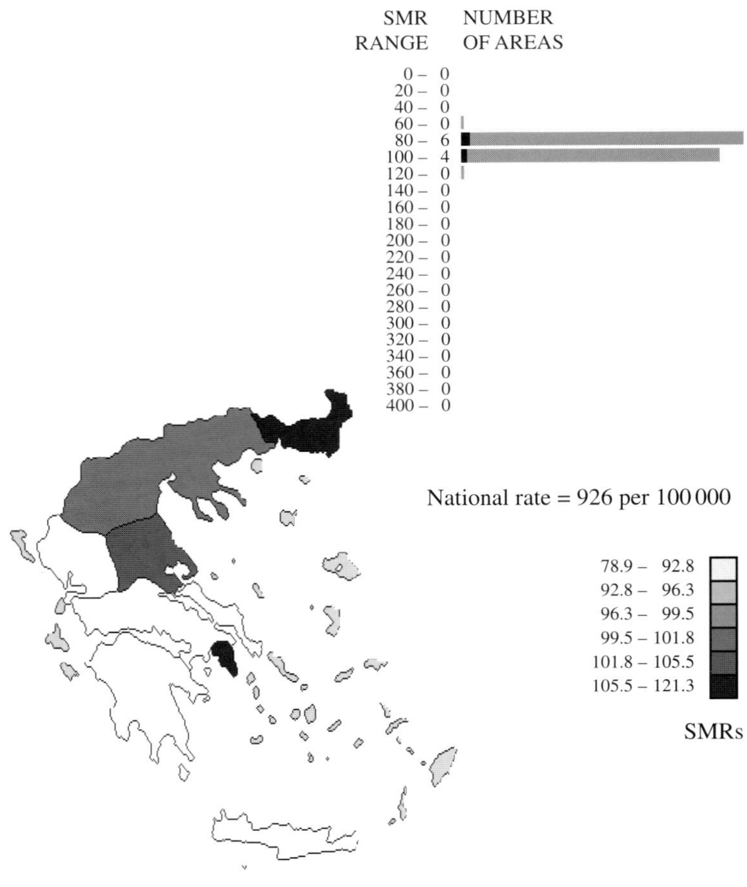

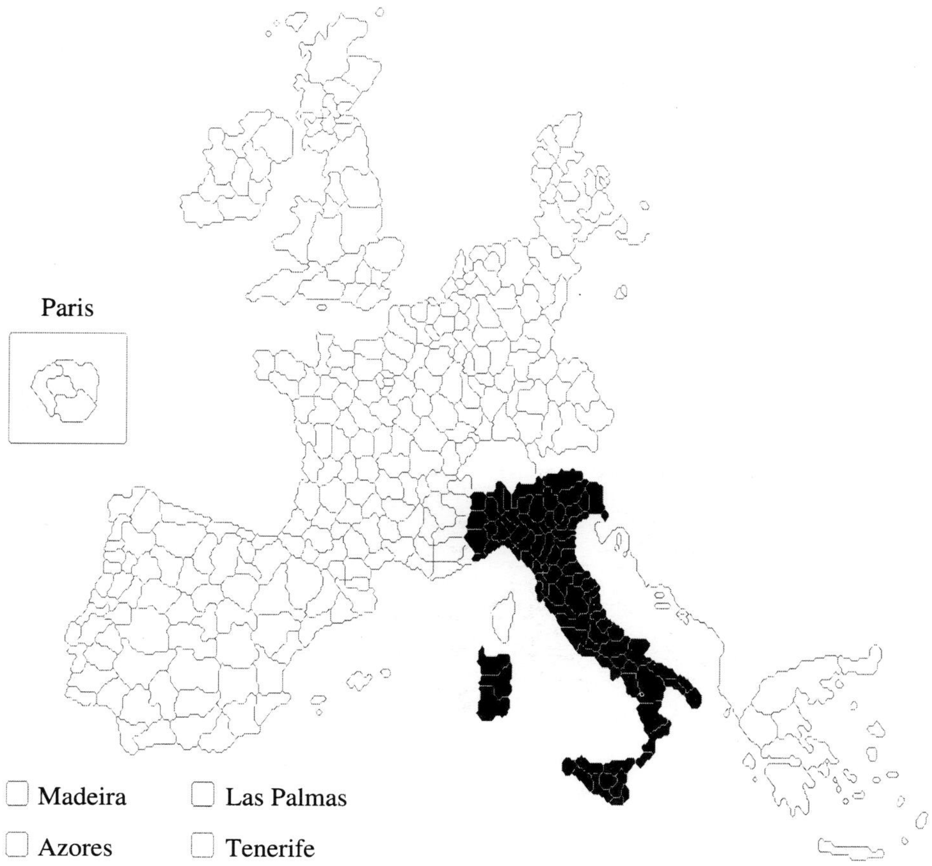

KEY MAP: ITALY

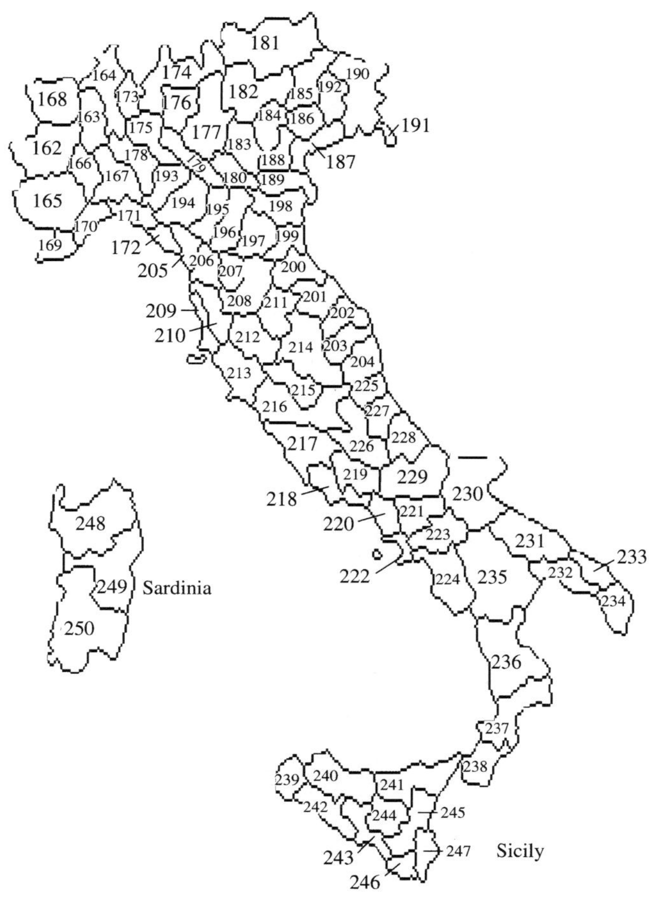

TUBERCULOSIS MORTALITY AGES 5–64: 1985–89

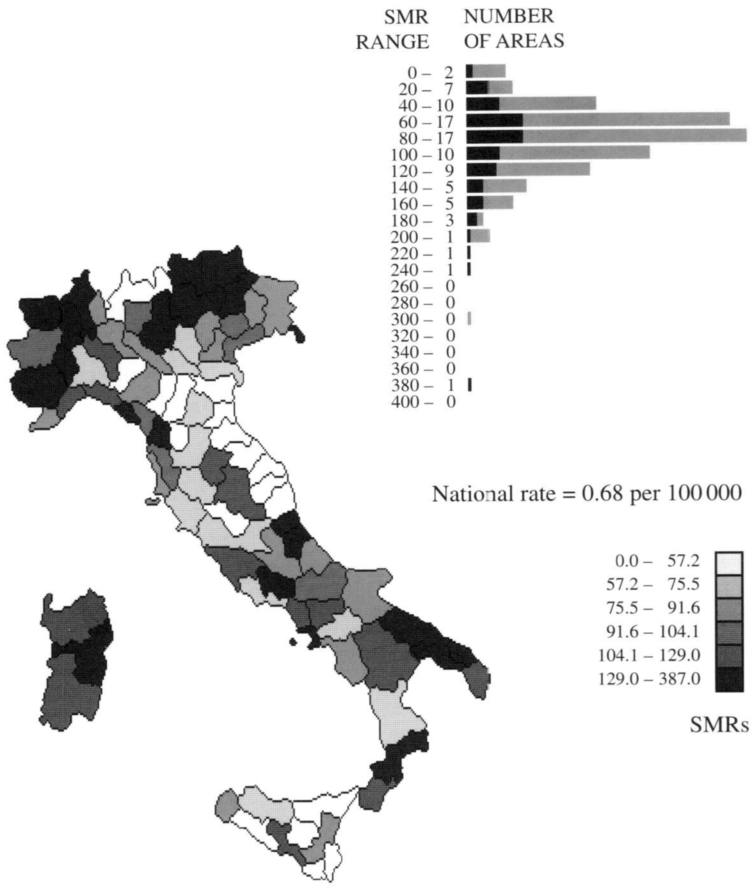

MALIGNANT NEOPLASM OF CERVIX UTERI MORTALITY AGES 15–64: 1985–89

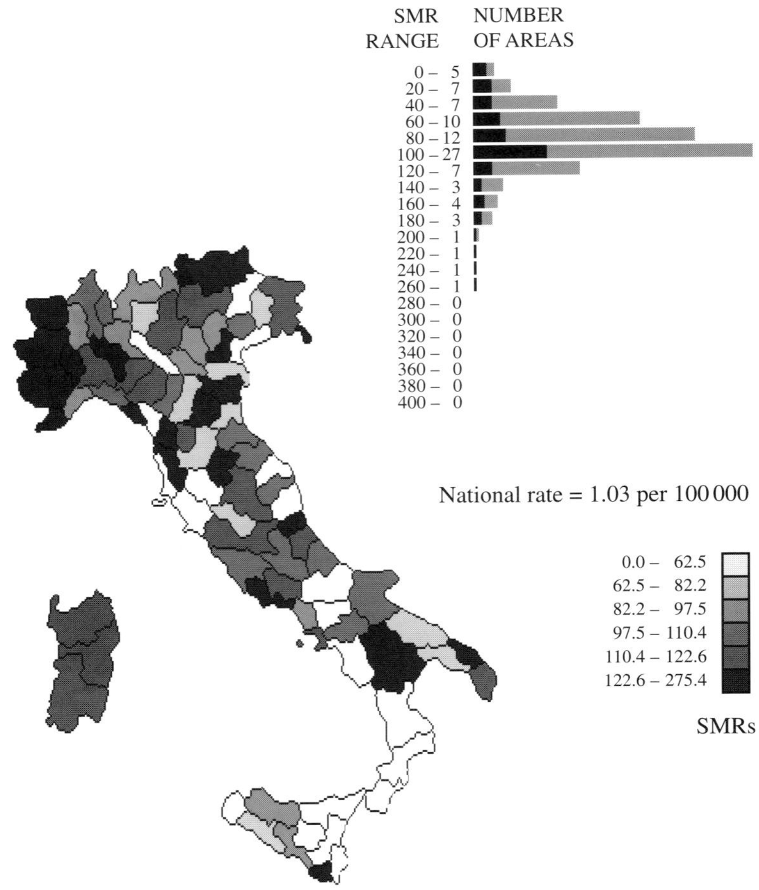

MALIGNANT NEOPLASM OF CERVIX AND BODY OF UTERUS MORTALITY AGES 15–54: 1985–89

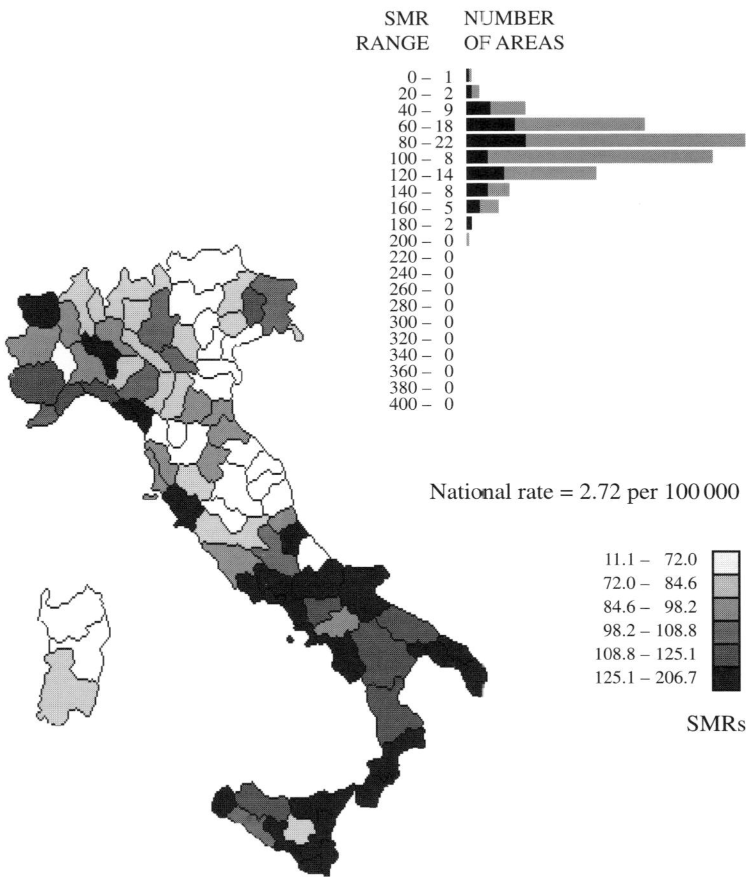

HODGKIN'S DISEASE MORTALITY AGES 5–64: 1985–89

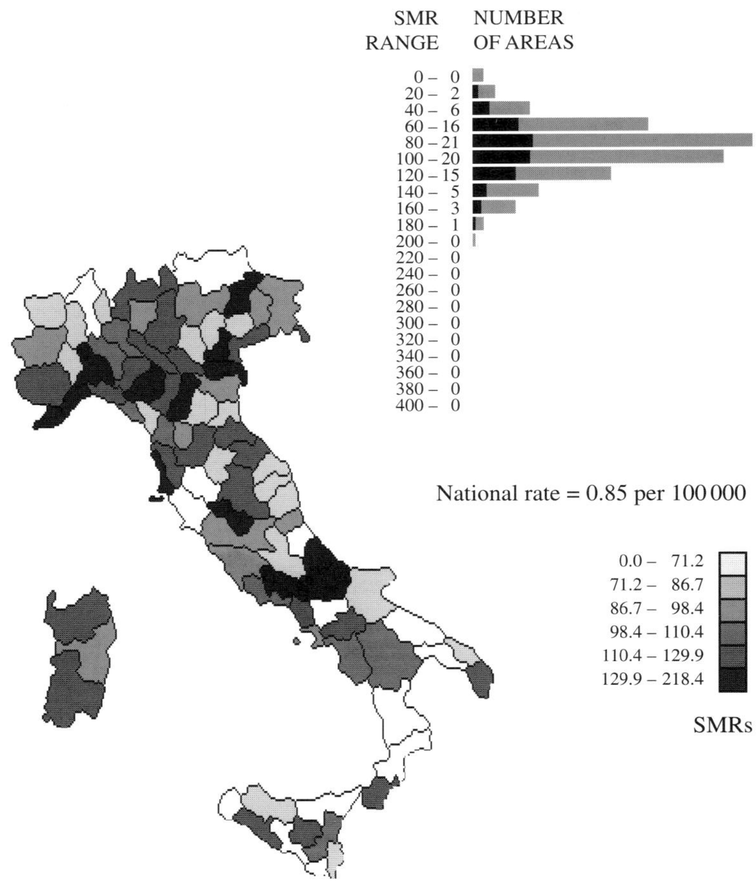

CHRONIC RHEUMATIC HEART DISEASE MORTALITY AGES 5–44: 1985–89

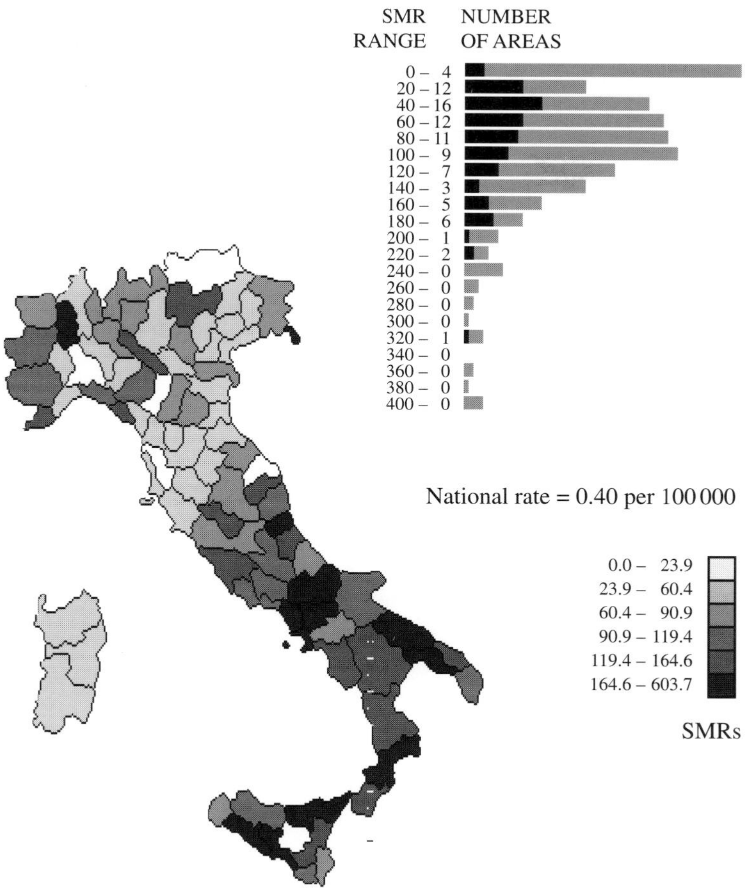

ALL RESPIRATORY DISEASES MORTALITY AGES 1–14: 1985–89

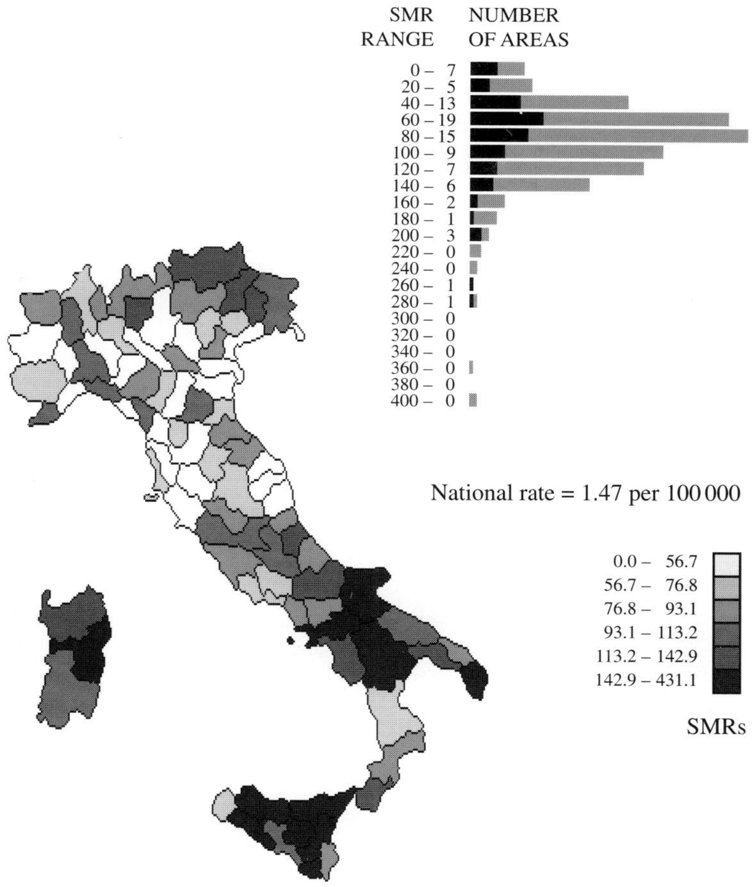

ASTHMA MORTALITY AGES 5–44: 1985–89

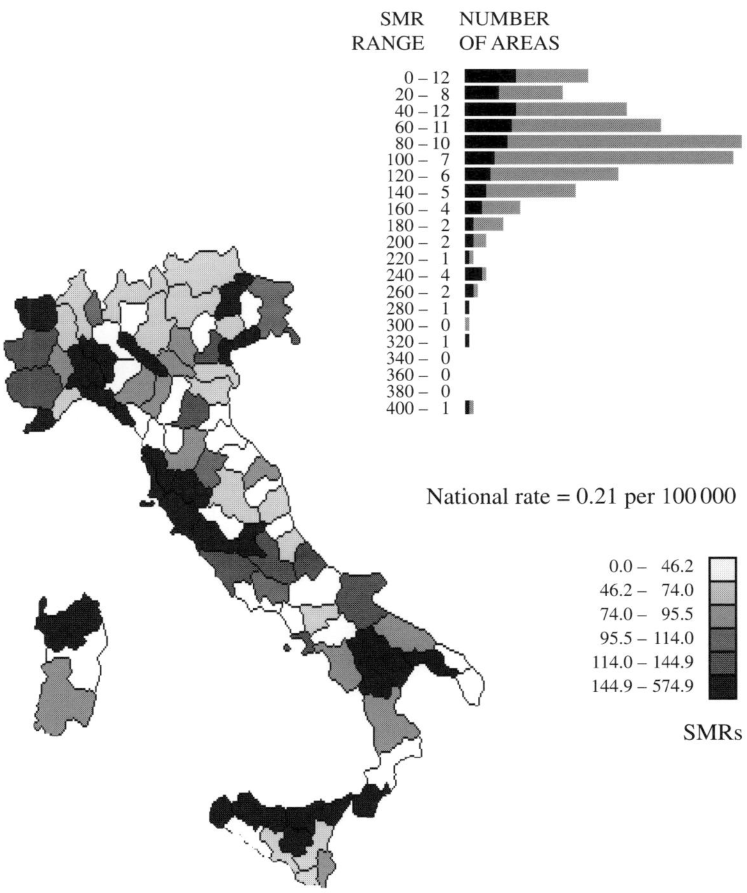

APPENDICITIS MORTALITY AGES 5–64: 1985–89

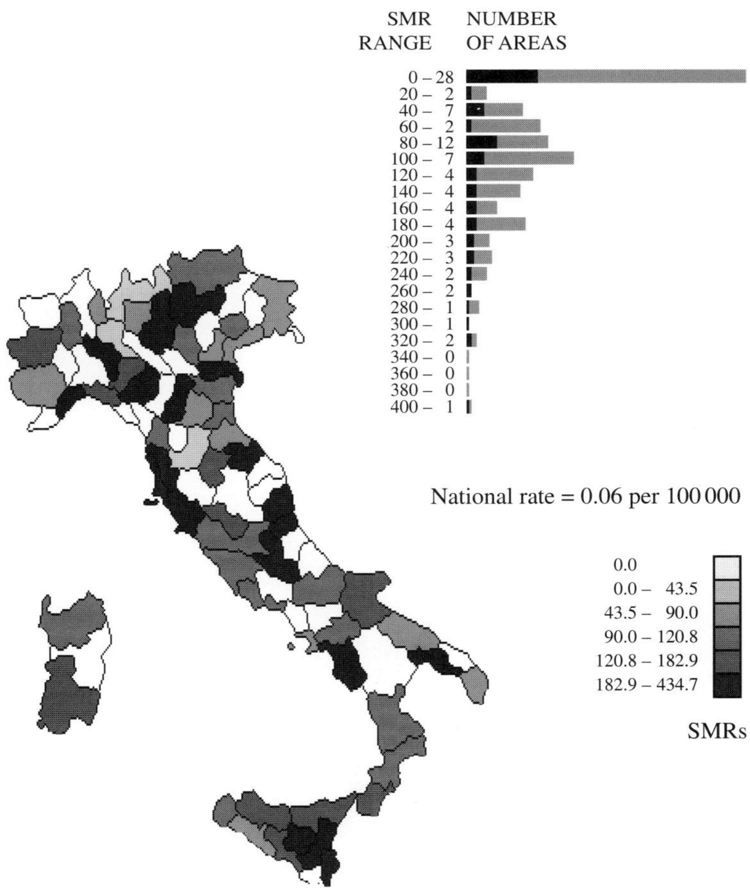

ABDOMINAL HERNIA MORTALITY AGES 5–64: 1985–89

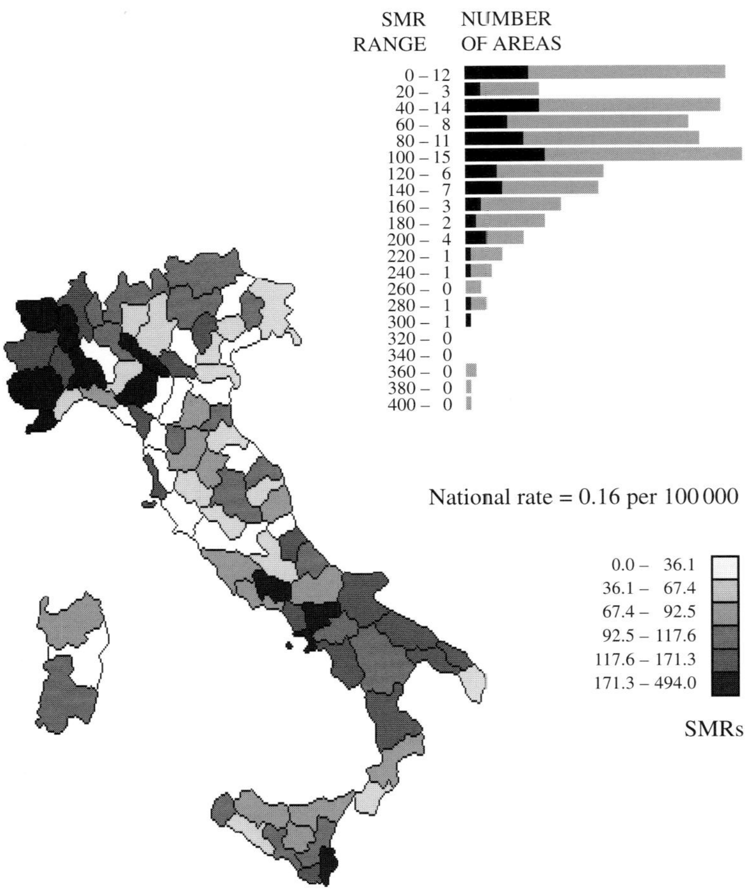

CHOLELITHIASIS AND CHOLECYSTITIS MORTALITY AGES 5–64: 1985–89

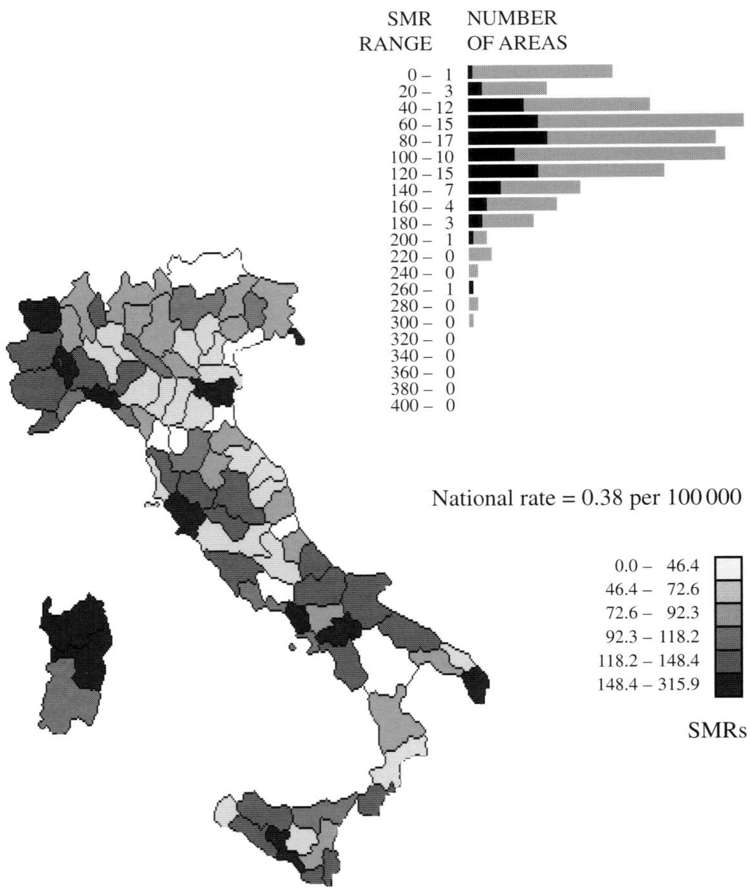

HYPERTENSIVE AND CEREBROVASCULAR DISEASES MORTALITY AGES 35–64: 1985–89

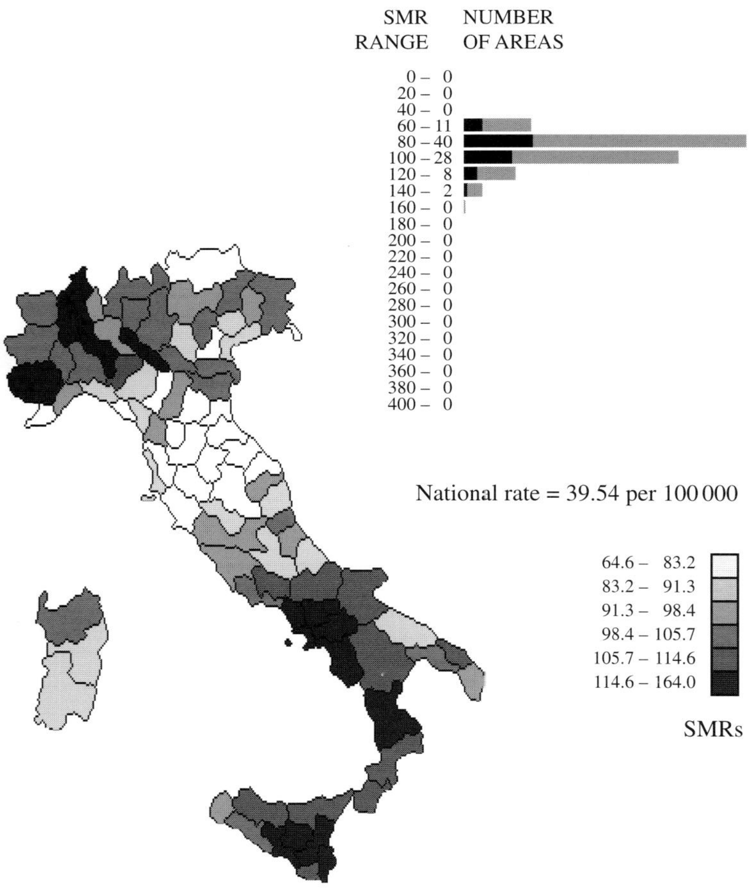

MATERNAL MORTALITY ALL AGES: 1985–89

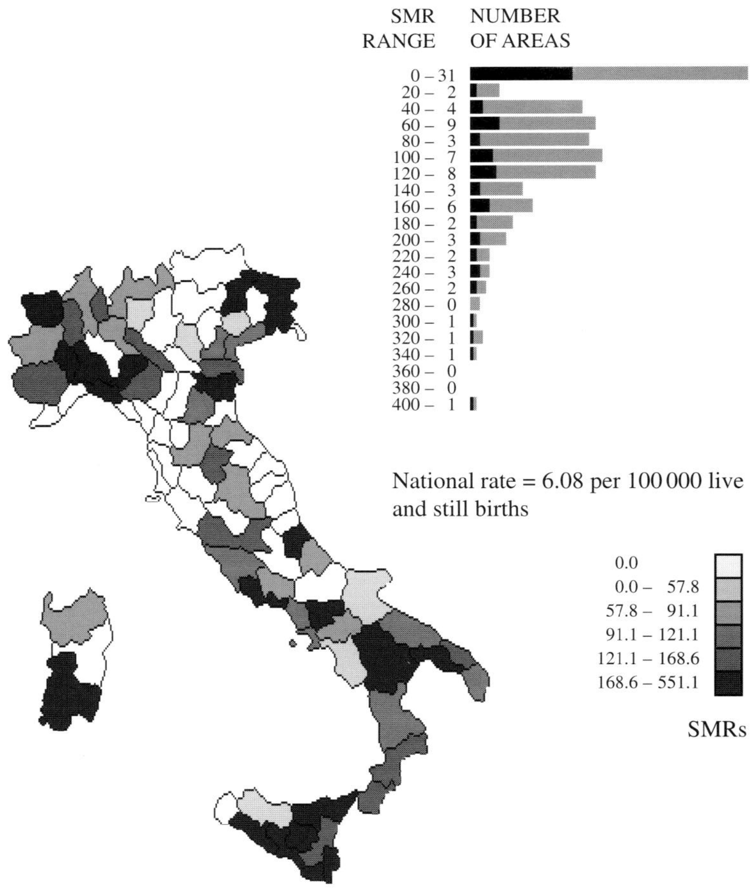

PERINATAL MORTALITY: 1985–89

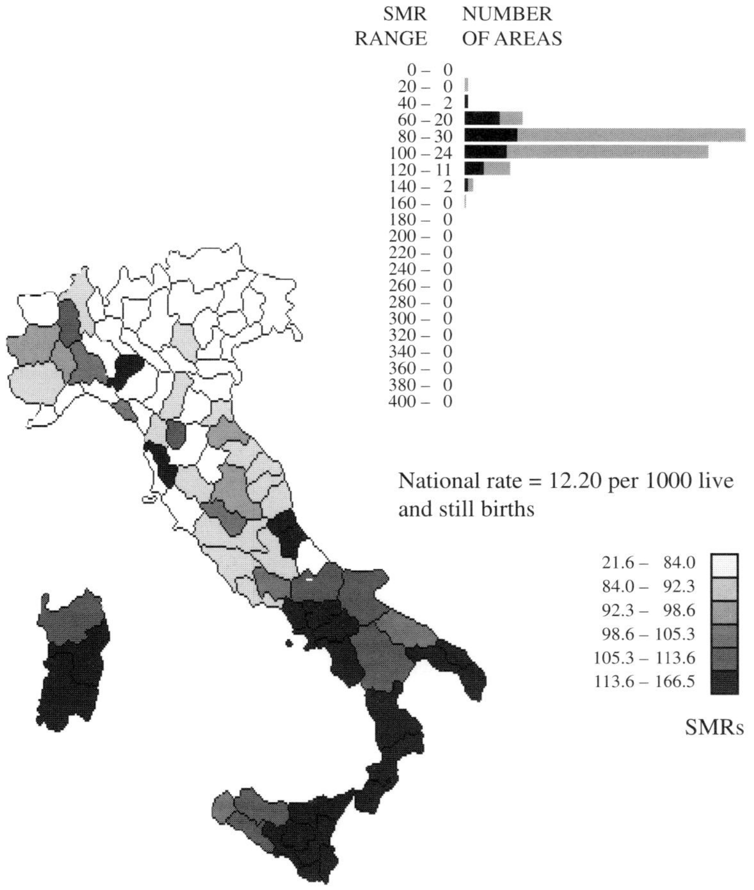

CANCER OF THE BREAST MORTALITY AGES 25–64: 1985–89

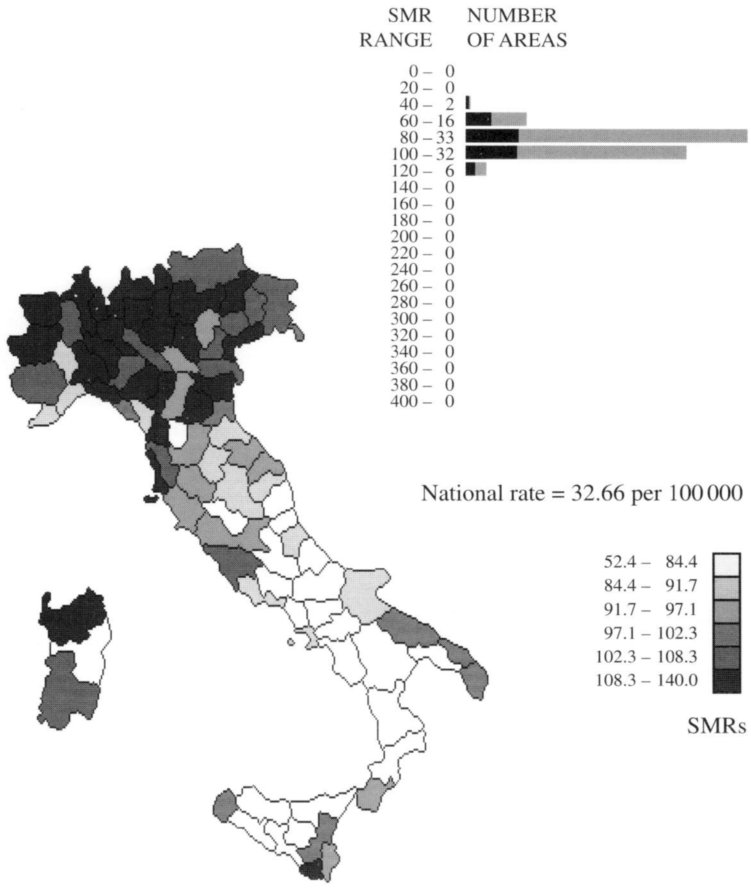

ISCHAEMIC HEART DISEASE MORTALITY AGES 35–64: 1985–89

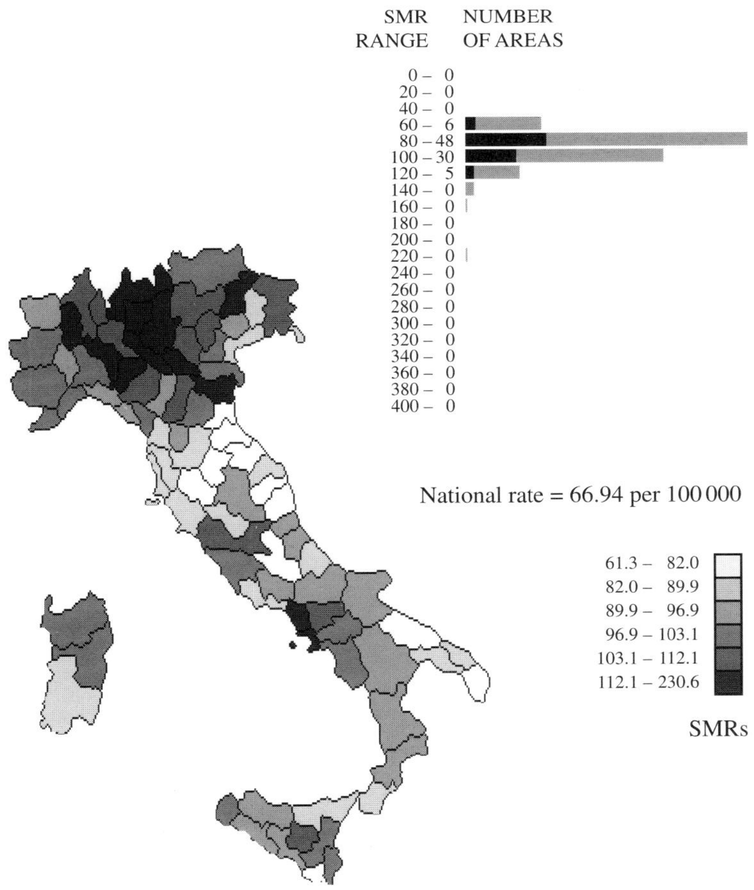

PEPTIC ULCERS MORTALITY AGES 25–64: 1985–89

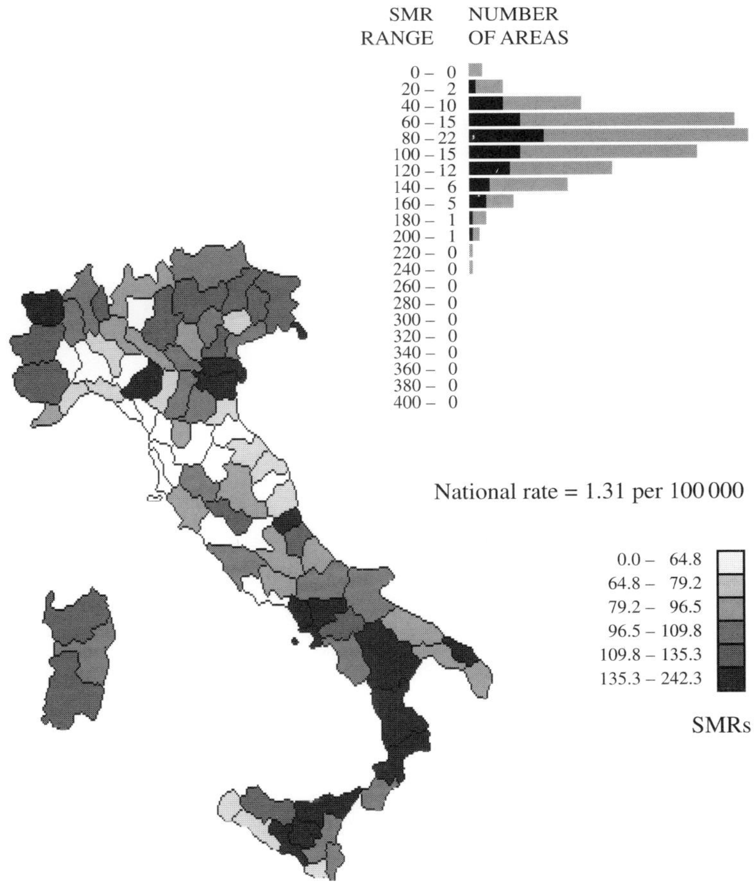

ALL CAUSES MORTALITY AGES 5–64: 1985–89

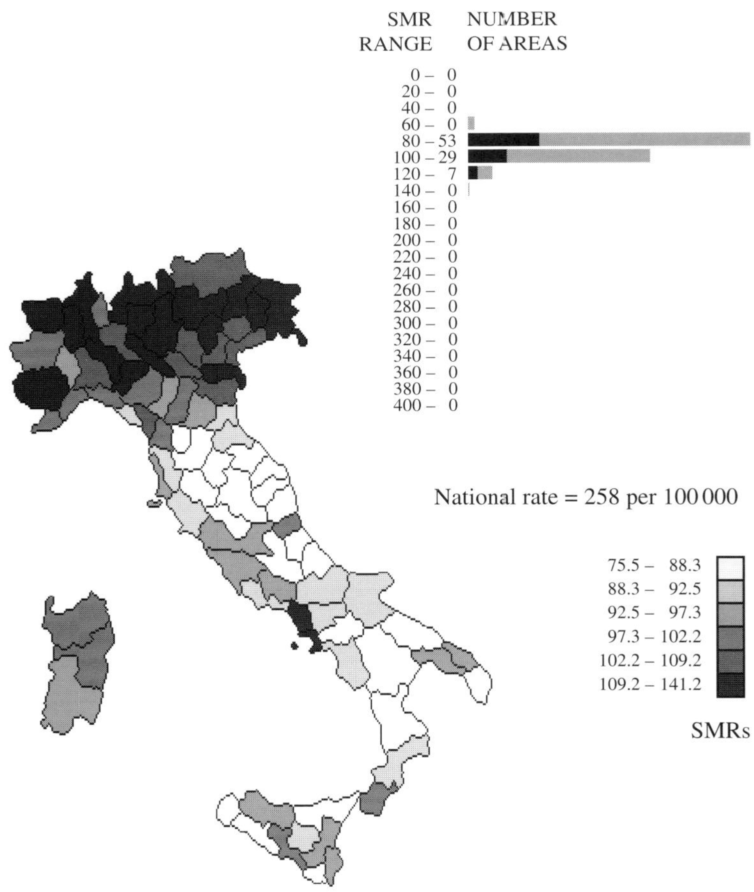

ALL CAUSES MORTALITY ALL AGES: 1985–89

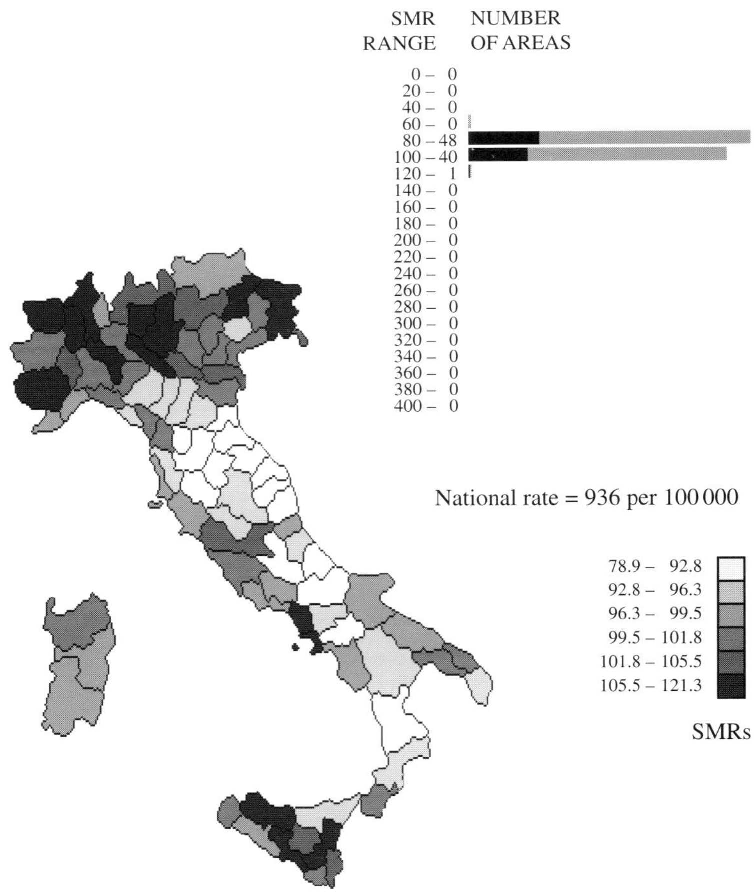

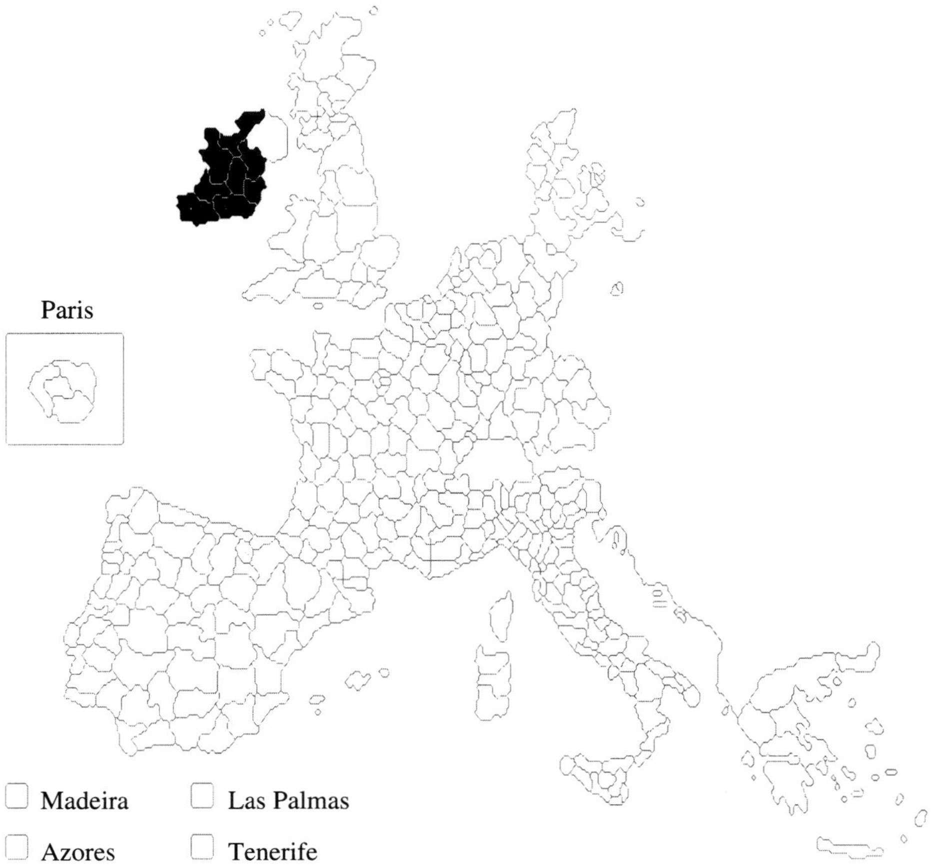

KEY MAP: IRELAND

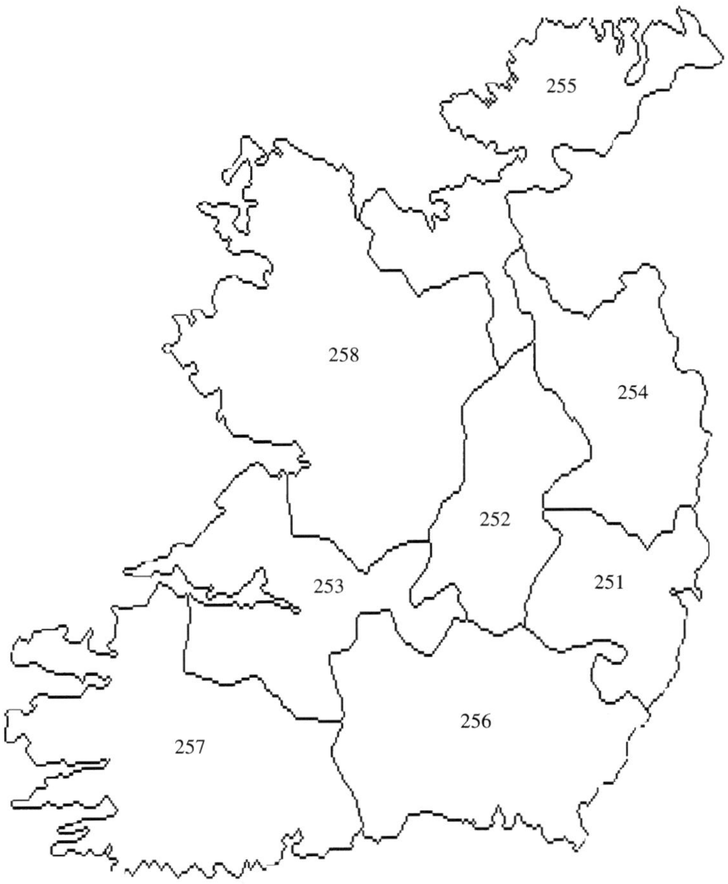

TUBERCULOSIS MORTALITY AGES 5–64: 1985–89

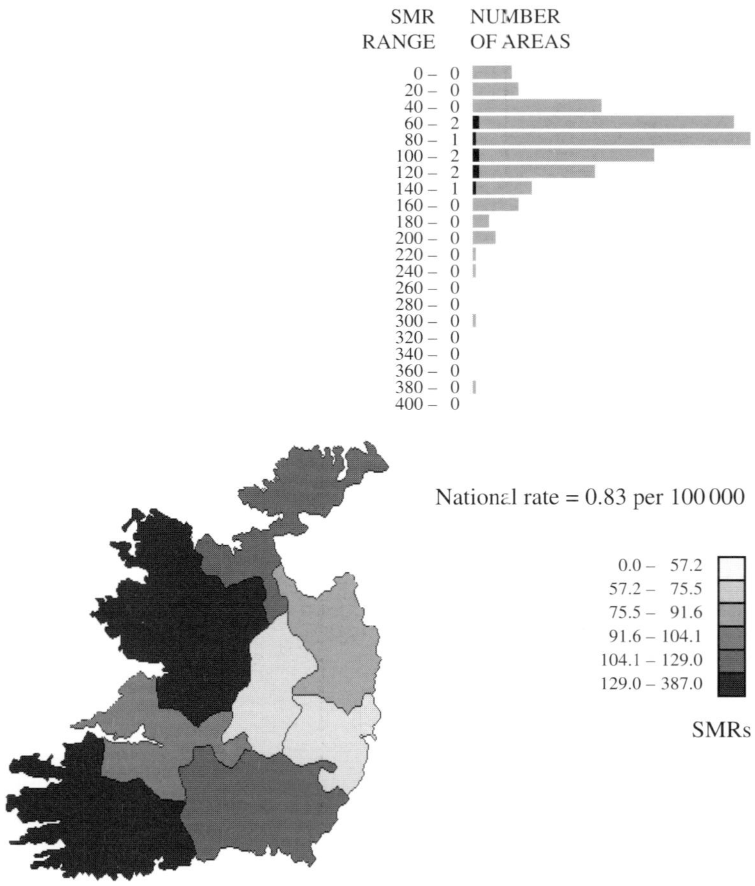

MALIGNANT NEOPLASM OF CERVIX UTERI MORTALITY AGES 15–64: 1985–89

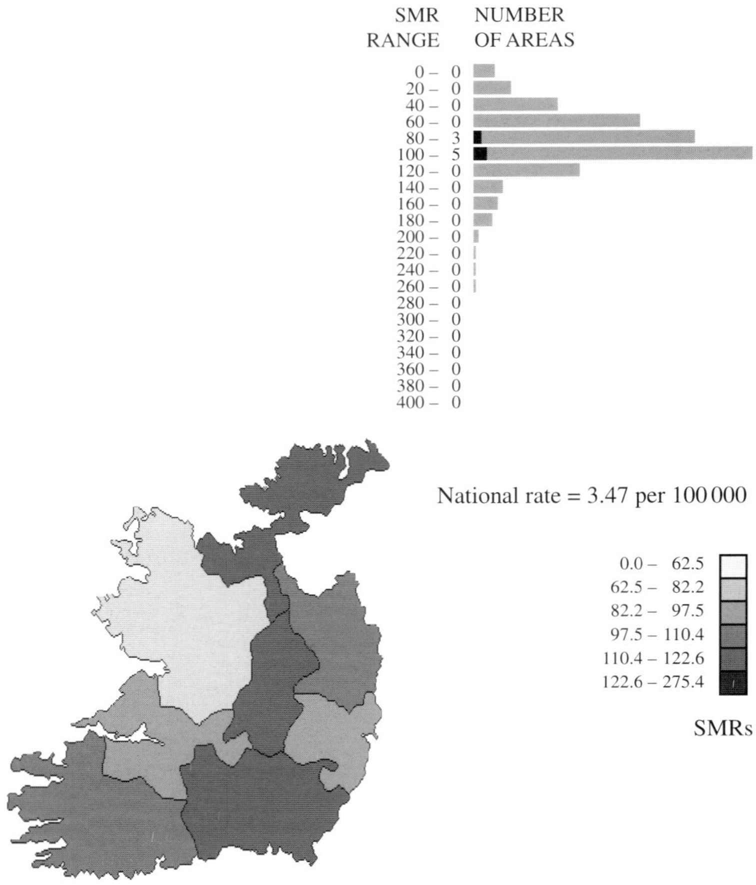

MALIGNANT NEOPLASM OF CERVIX AND BODY OF UTERUS MORTALITY AGES 15–54: 1985–89

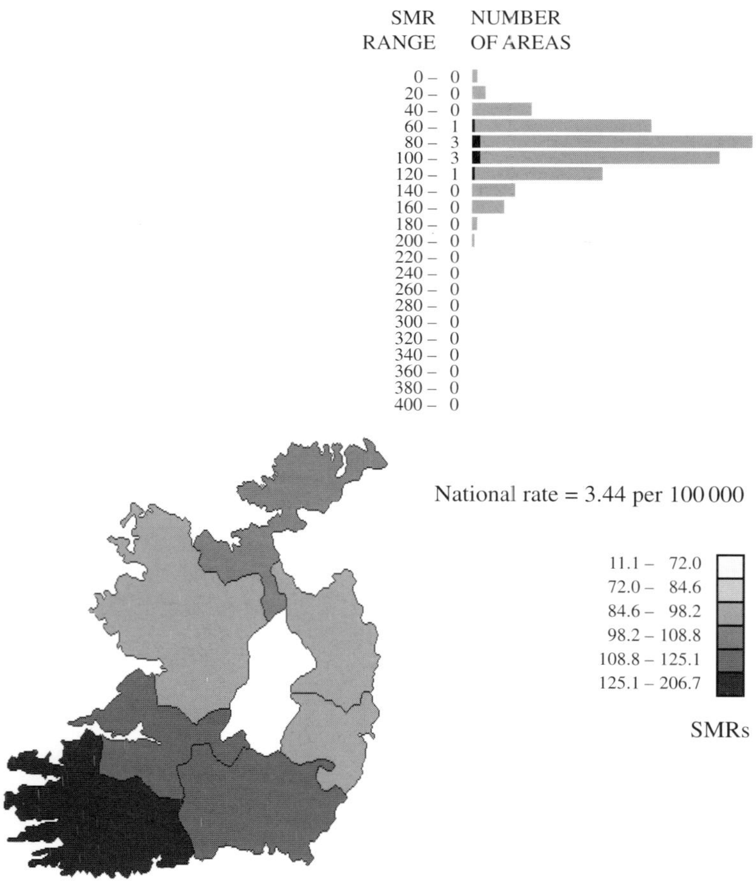

HODGKIN'S DISEASE MORTALITY AGES 5–64: 1985–89

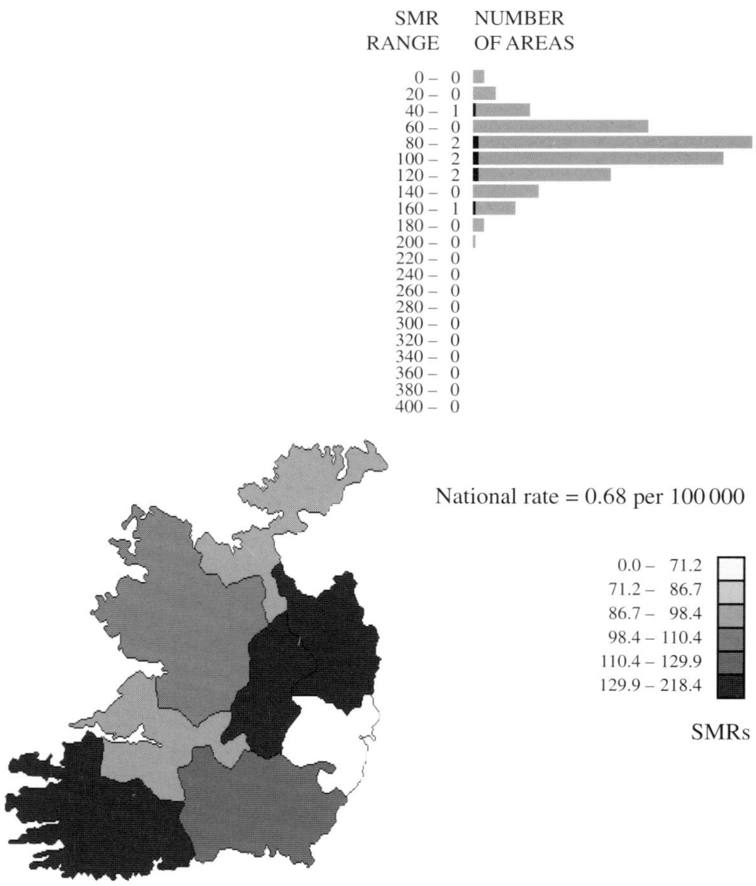

CHRONIC RHEUMATIC HEART DISEASE MORTALITY AGES 5–44: 1985–89

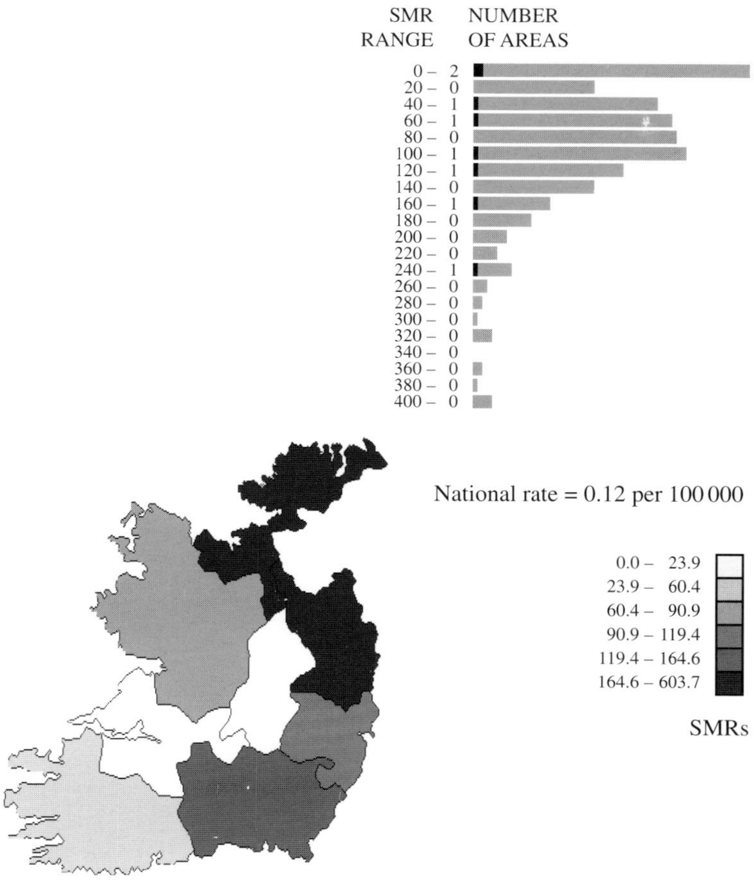

ALL RESPIRATORY DISEASES MORTALITY AGES 1–14: 1985–89

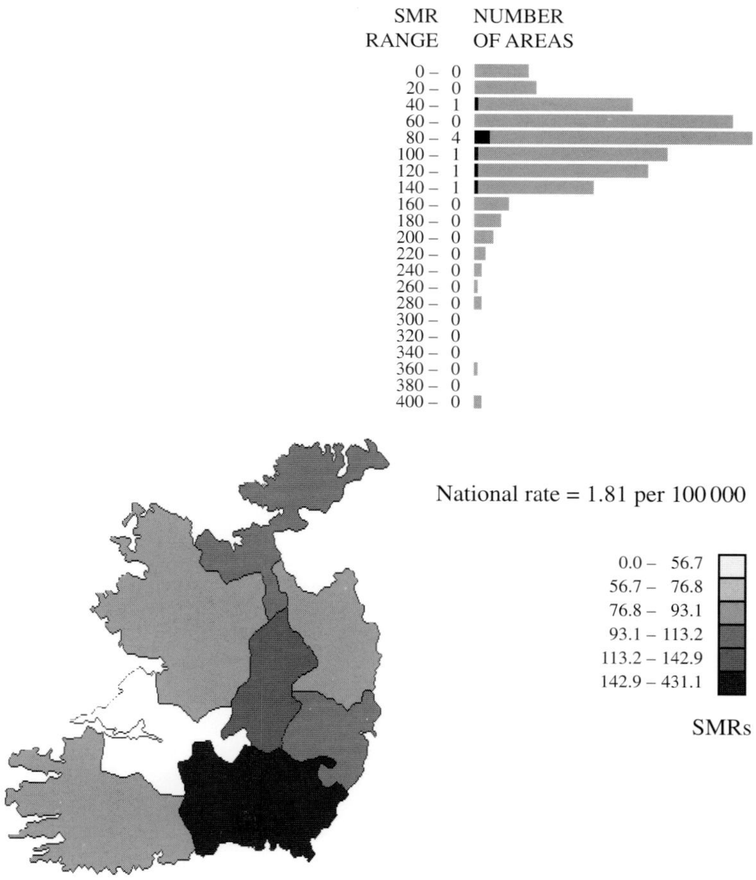

ASTHMA MORTALITY AGES 5–44: 1985–89

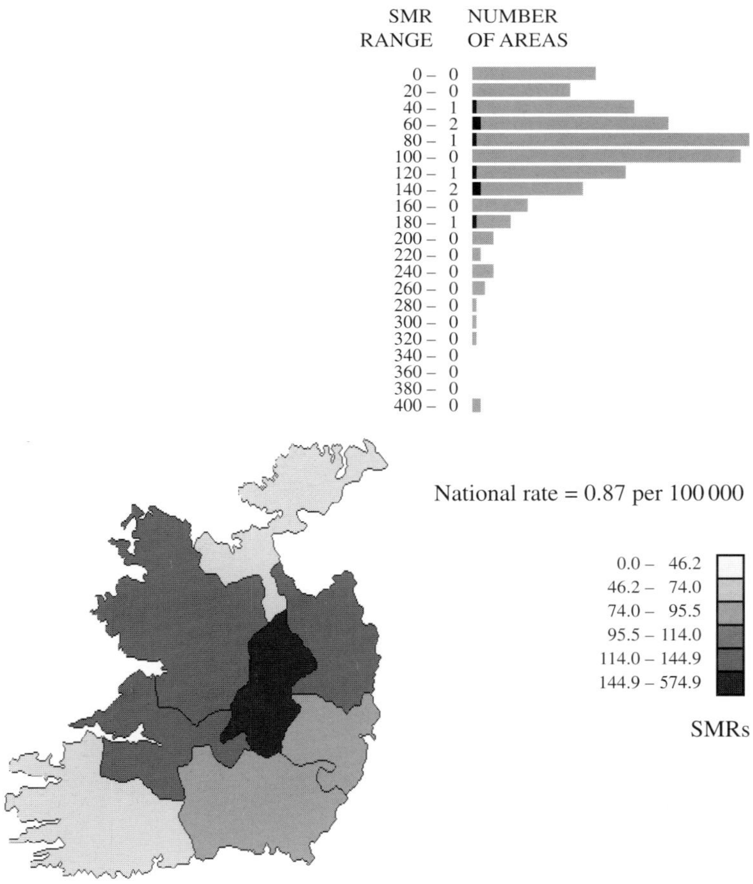

APPENDICITIS MORTALITY AGES 5–64: 1985–89

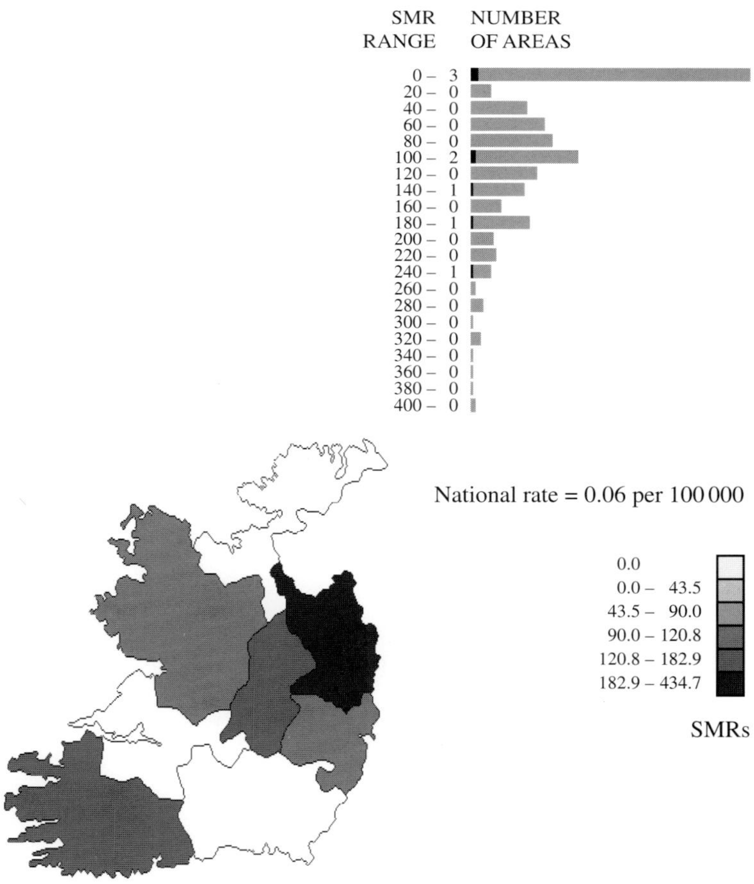

ABDOMINAL HERNIA MORTALITY AGES 5–64: 1985–89

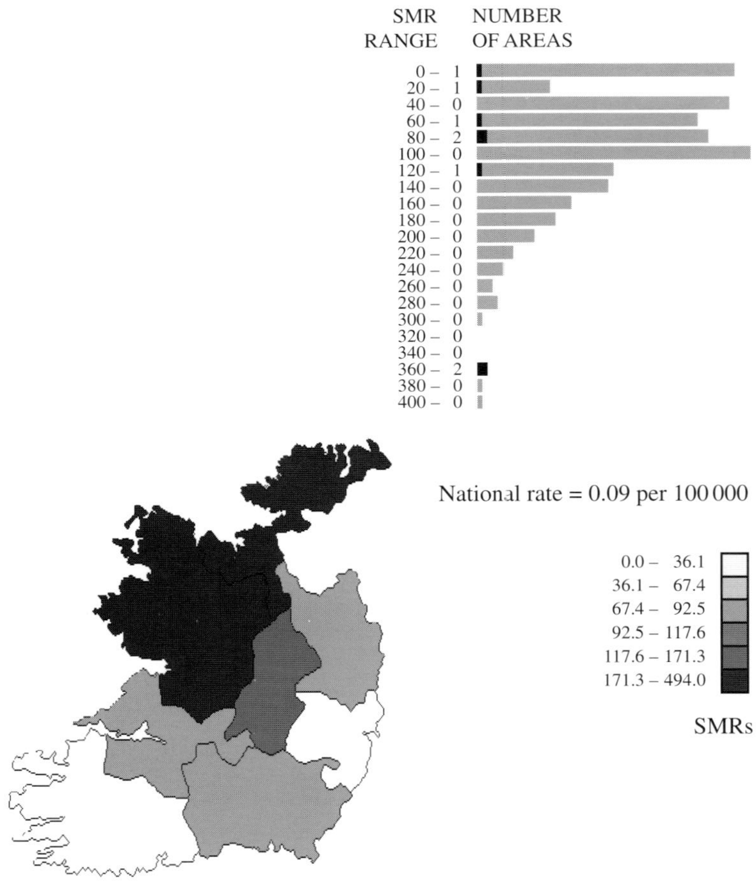

CHOLELITHIASIS AND CHOLECYSTITIS MORTALITY AGES 5–64: 1985–89

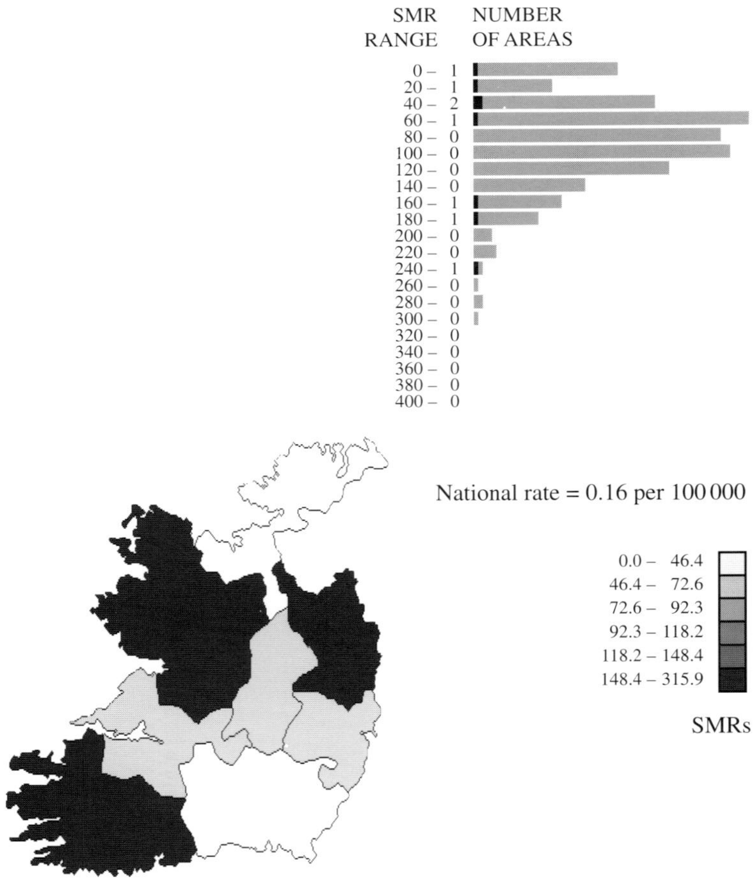

HYPERTENSIVE AND CEREBROVASCULAR DISEASES MORTALITY AGES 35–64: 1985–89

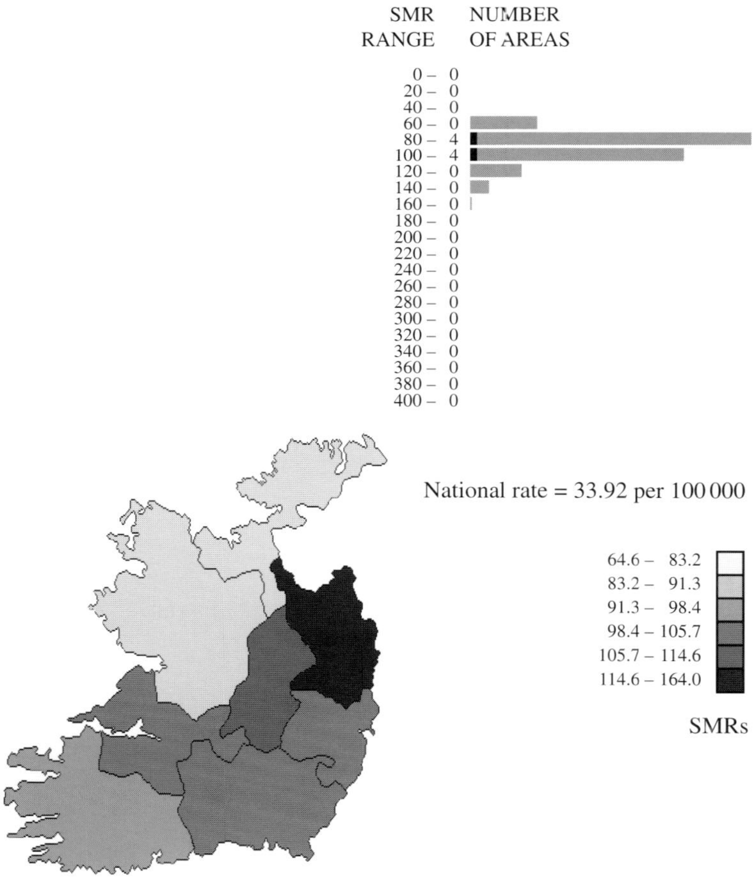

MATERNAL MORTALITY ALL AGES: 1985–89

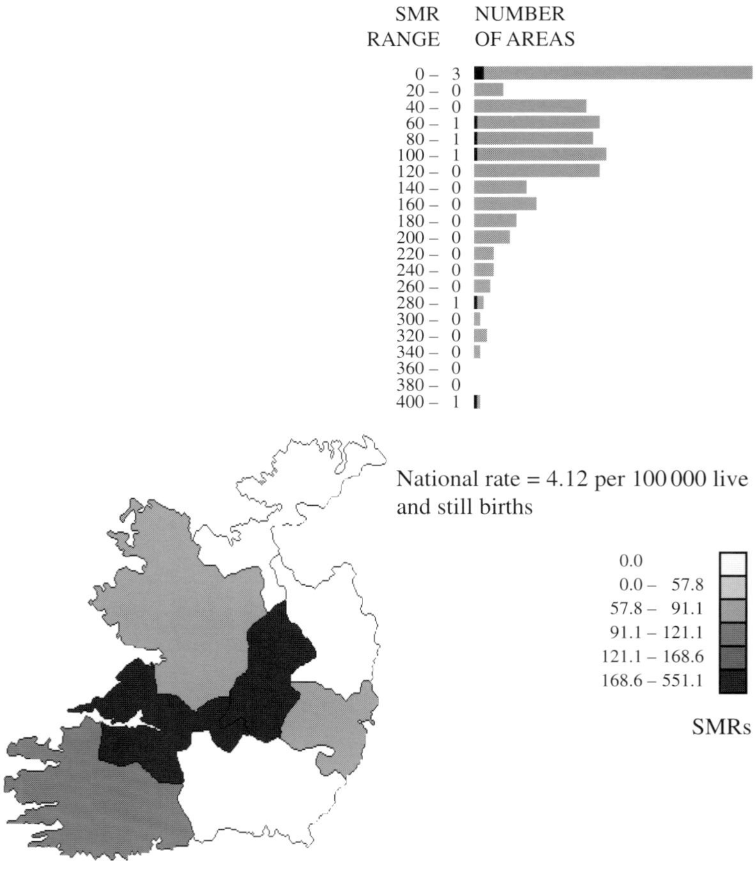

PERINATAL MORTALITY: 1985–89

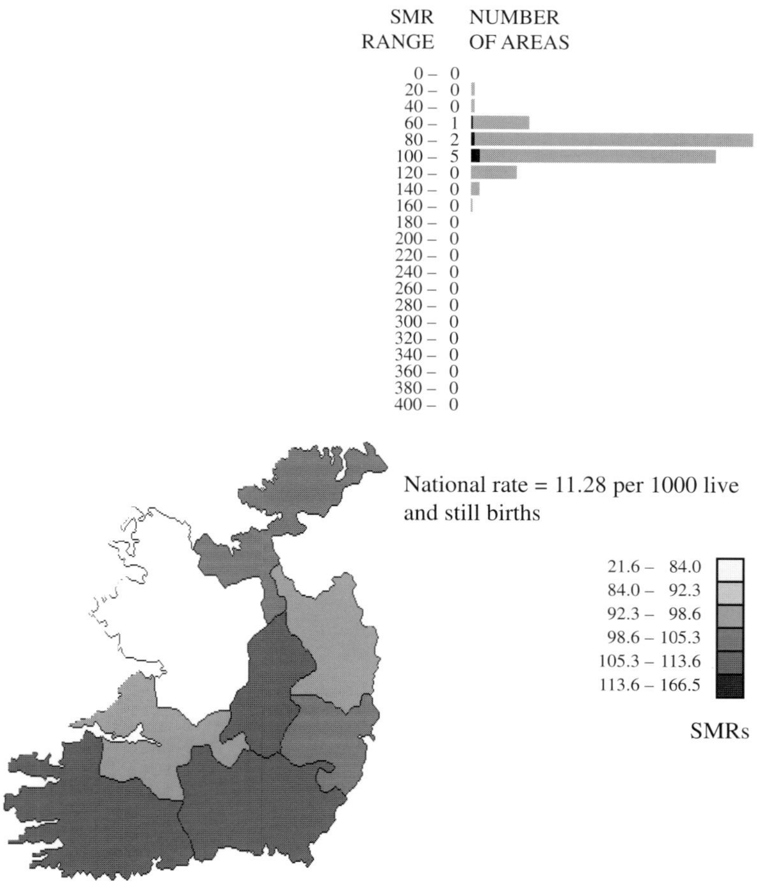

CANCER OF THE BREAST MORTALITY AGES 25–64: 1985–89

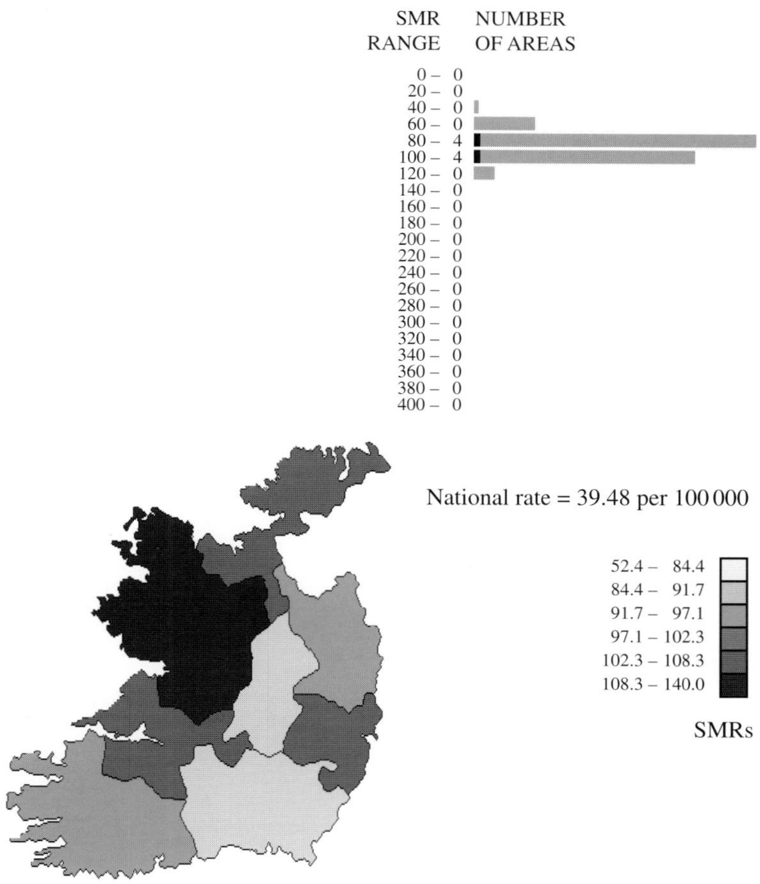

ISCHAEMIC HEART DISEASE MORTALITY AGES 35–64: 1985–89

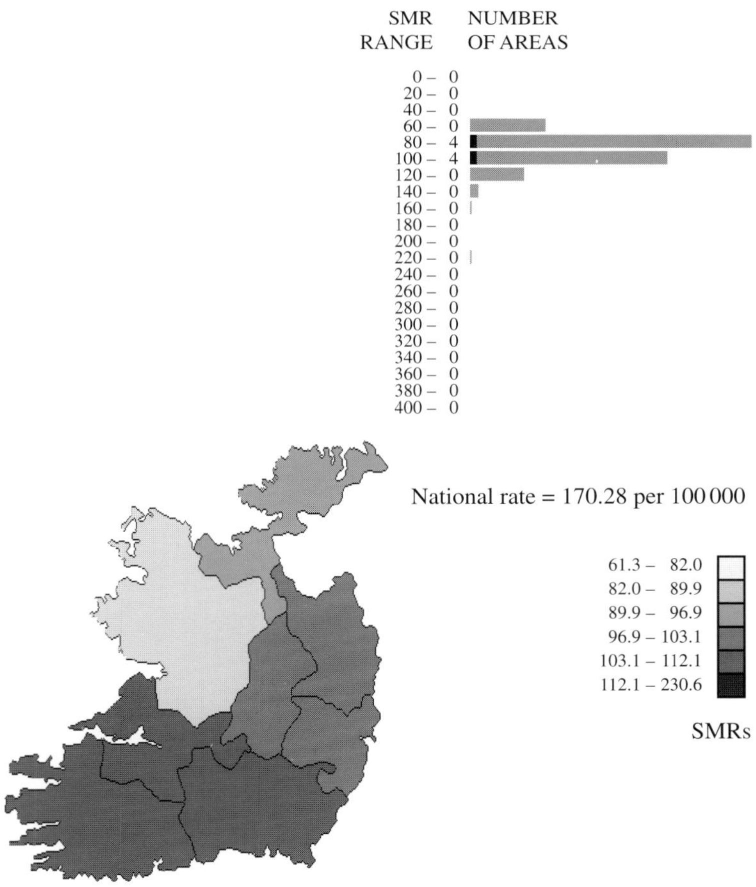

PEPTIC ULCERS MORTALITY AGES 25–64: 1985–89

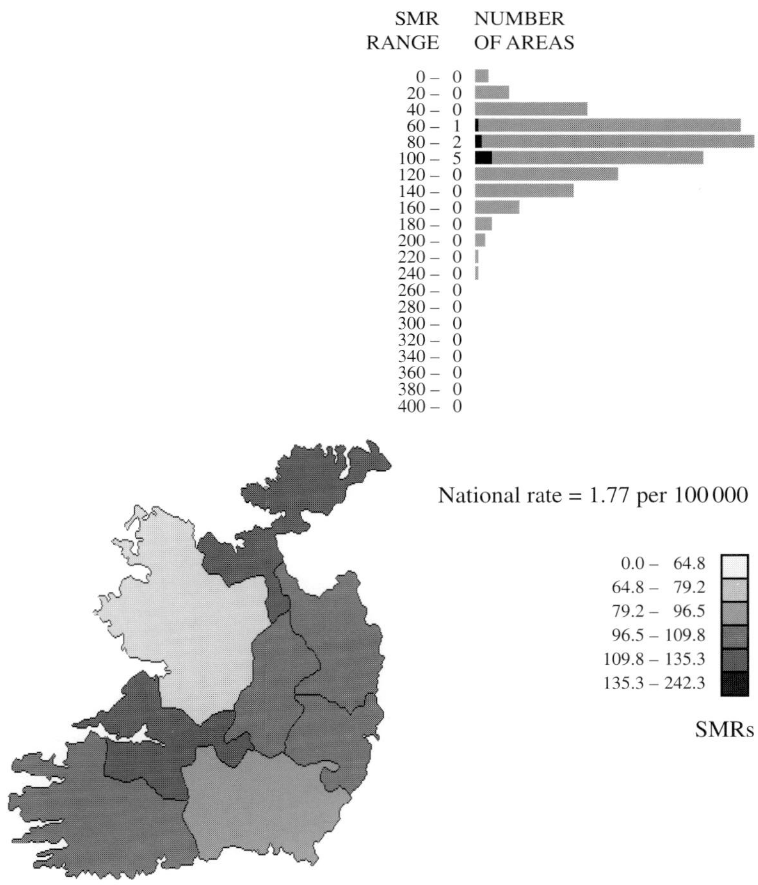

ALL CAUSES MORTALITY AGES 5–64: 1985–89

SMR RANGE	NUMBER OF AREAS
0 –	0
20 –	0
40 –	0
60 –	0
80 –	3
100 –	5
120 –	0
140 –	0
160 –	0
180 –	0
200 –	0
220 –	0
240 –	0
260 –	0
280 –	0
300 –	0
320 –	0
340 –	0
360 –	0
380 –	0
400 –	0

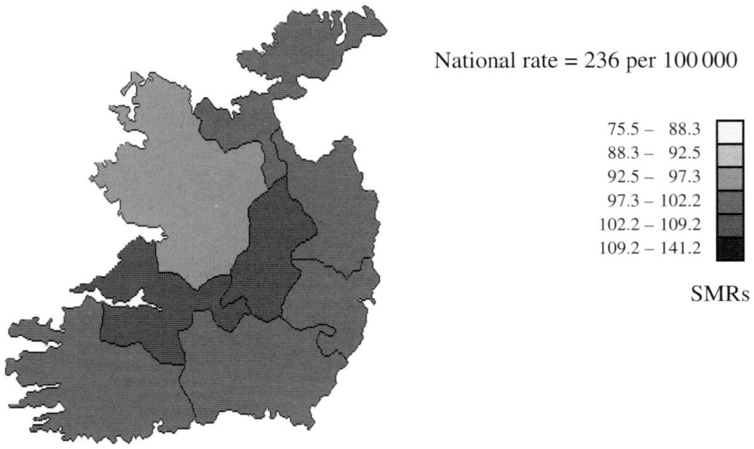

ALL CAUSES MORTALITY ALL AGES: 1985–89

SMR RANGE	NUMBER OF AREAS
0 –	0
20 –	0
40 –	0
60 –	0
80 –	3
100 –	5
120 –	0
140 –	0
160 –	0
180 –	0
200 –	0
220 –	0
240 –	0
260 –	0
280 –	0
300 –	0
320 –	0
340 –	0
360 –	0
380 –	0
400 –	0

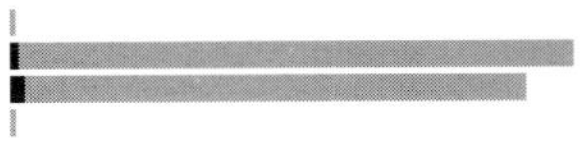

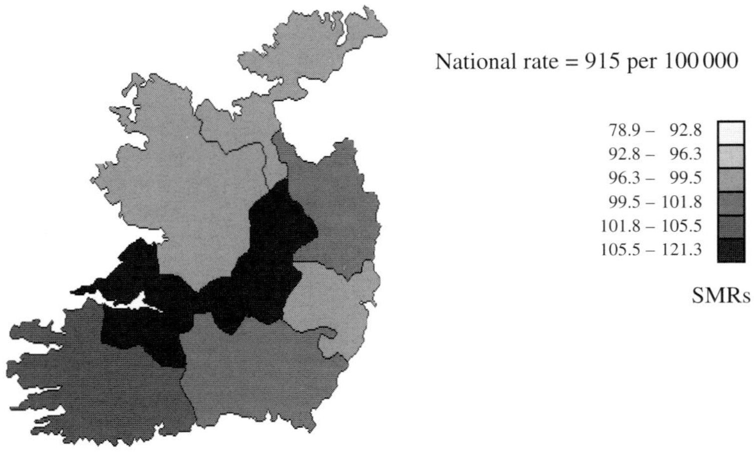

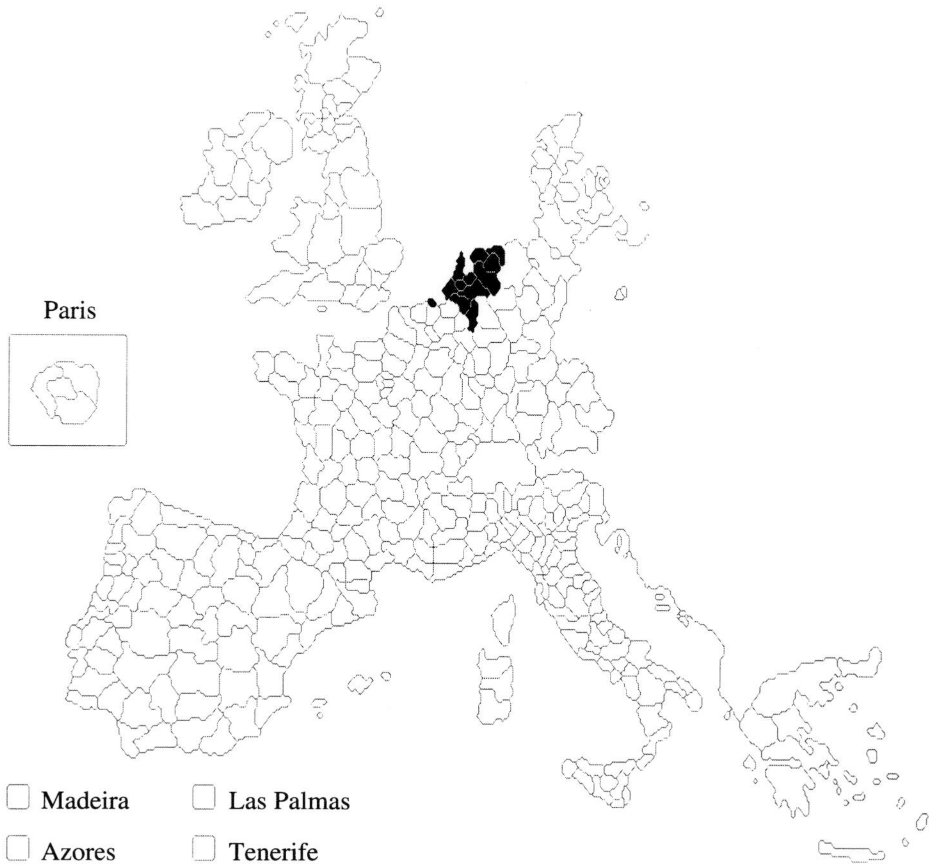

KEY MAP: NETHERLANDS

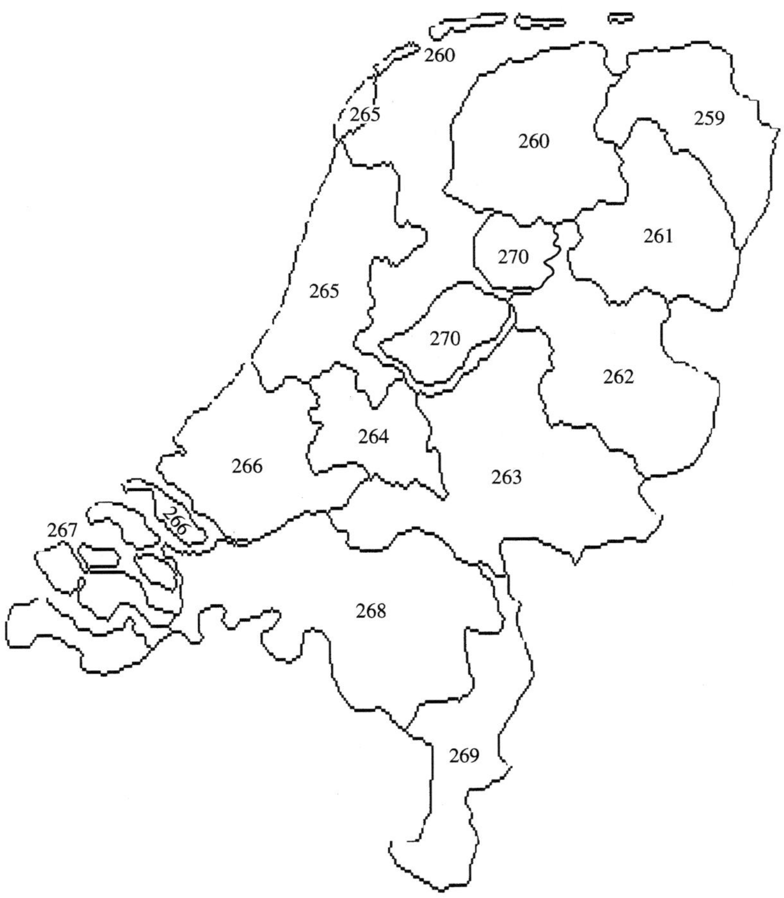

TUBERCULOSIS MORTALITY AGES 5–64: 1985–89

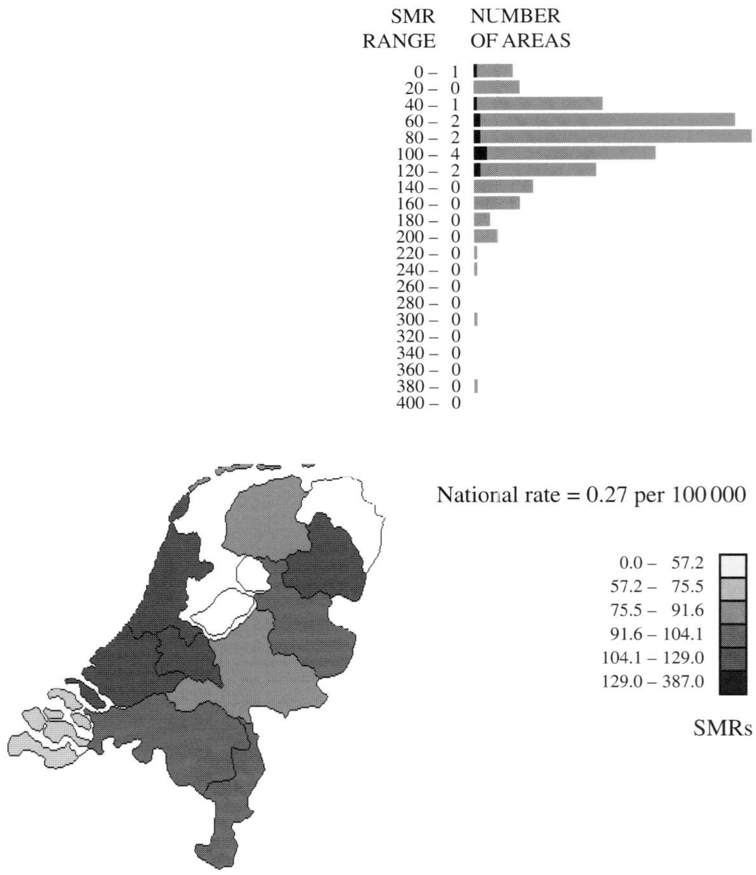

MALIGNANT NEOPLASM OF CERVIX UTERI MORTALITY AGES 15–64: 1985–89

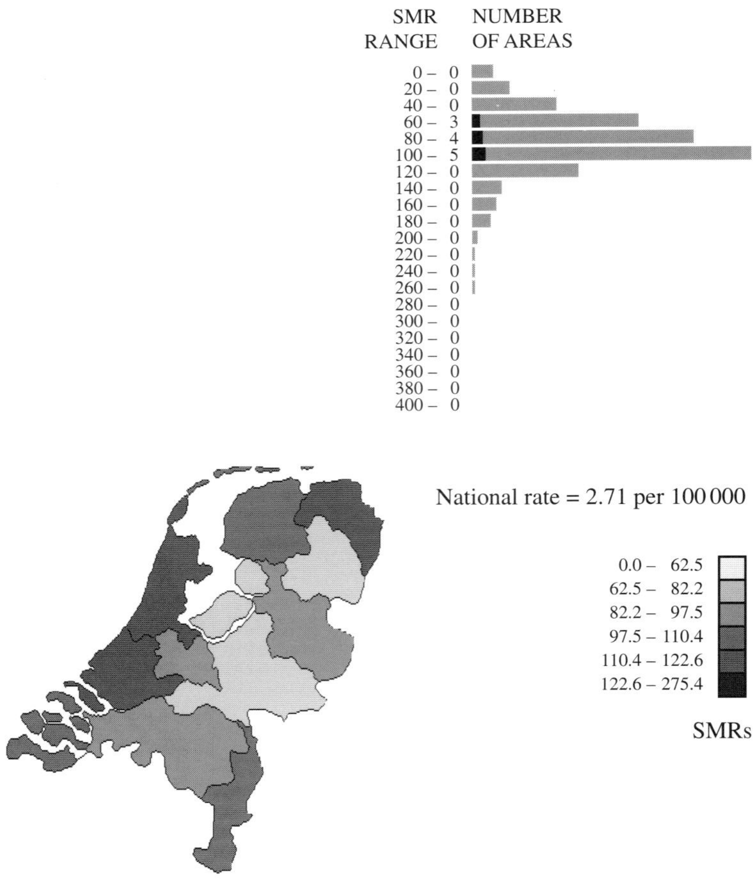

MALIGNANT NEOPLASM OF CERVIX AND BODY OF UTERUS MORTALITY AGES 15–54: 1985–89

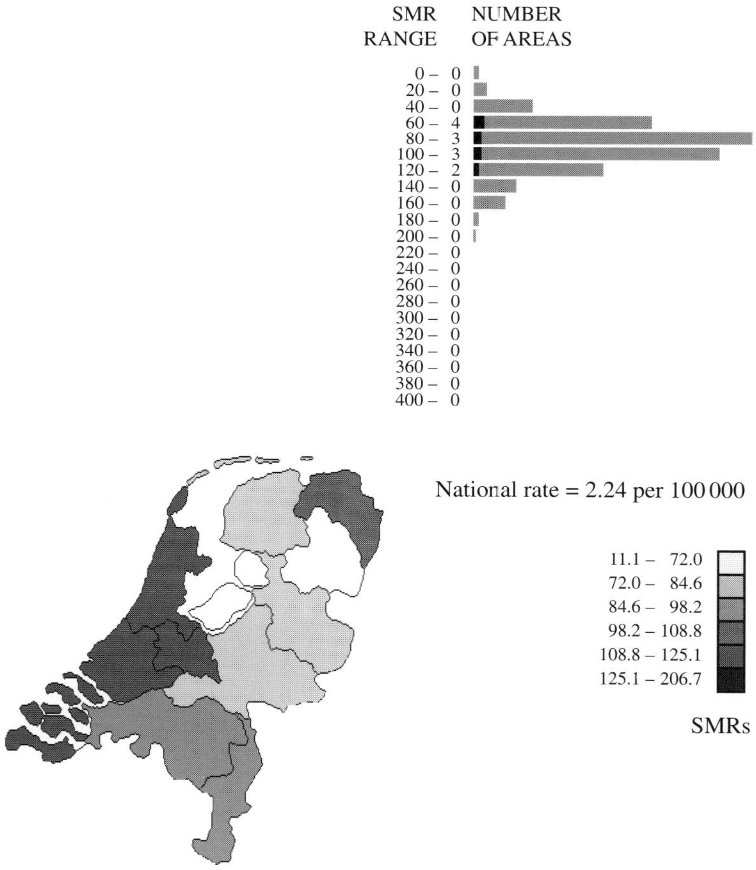

HODGKIN'S DISEASE MORTALITY AGES 5–64: 1985–89

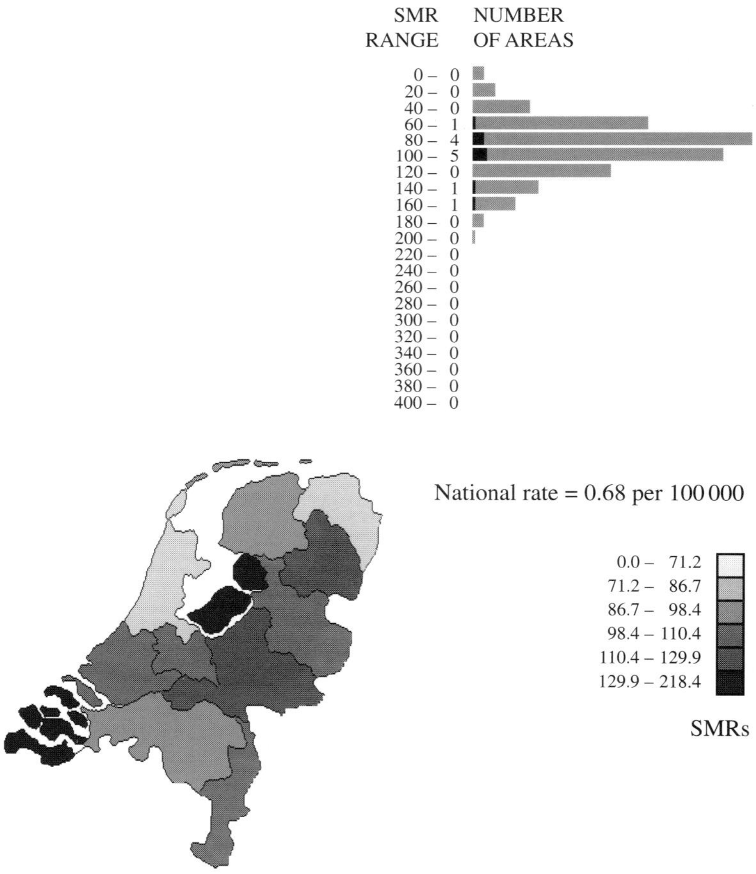

CHRONIC RHEUMATIC HEART DISEASE MORTALITY AGES 5–44: 1985–89

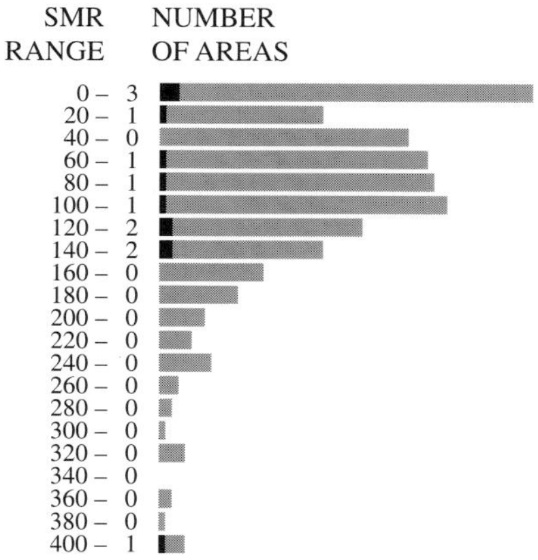

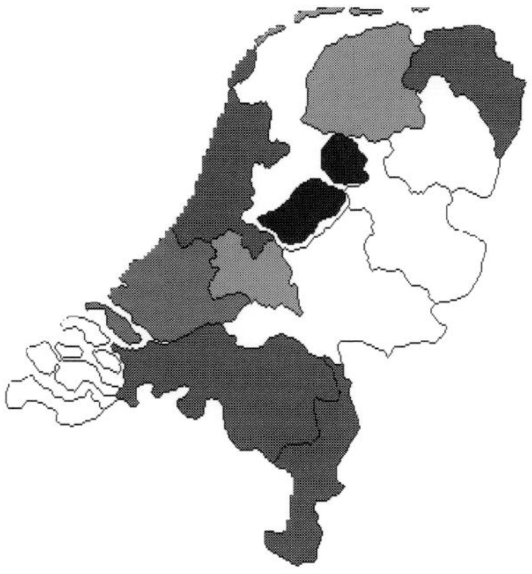

National rate = 0.10 per 100 000

0.0 – 23.9
23.9 – 60.4
60.4 – 90.9
90.9 – 119.4
119.4 – 164.6
164.6 – 603.7

SMRs

ALL RESPIRATORY DISEASES MORTALITY AGES 1–14: 1985–89

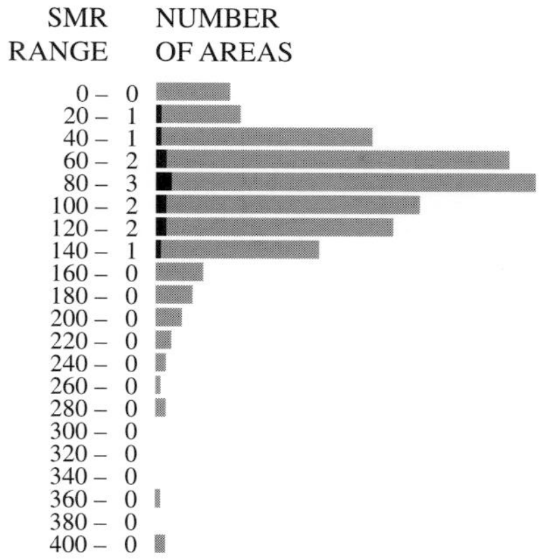

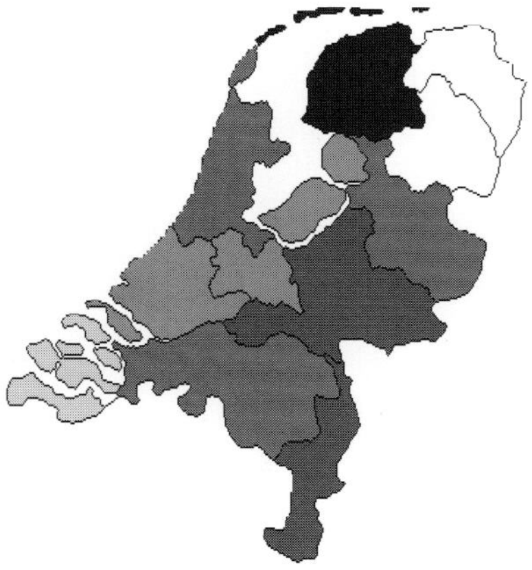

National rate = 1.12 per 100 000

0.0 – 56.7
56.7 – 76.8
76.8 – 93.1
93.1 – 113.2
113.2 – 142.9
142.9 – 431.1

SMRs

ASTHMA MORTALITY AGES 5–44: 1985–89

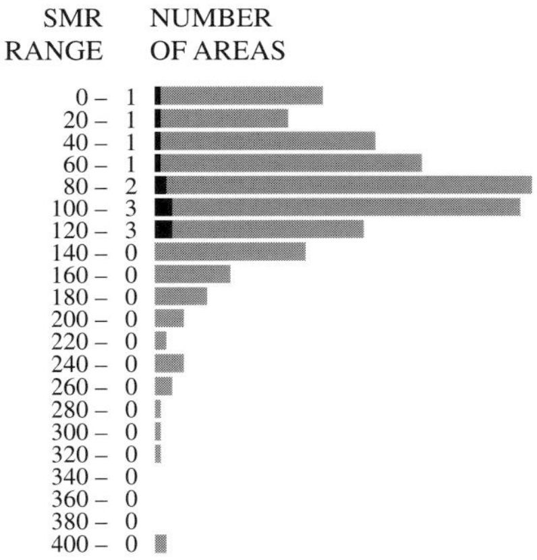

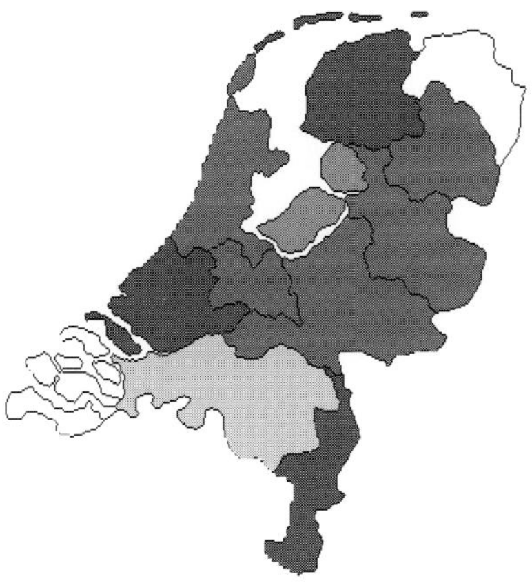

National rate = 0.27 per 100 000

0.0 – 46.2
46.2 – 74.0
74.0 – 95.5
95.5 – 114.0
114.0 – 144.9
144.9 – 574.9

SMRs

APPENDICITIS MORTALITY AGES 5–64: 1985–89

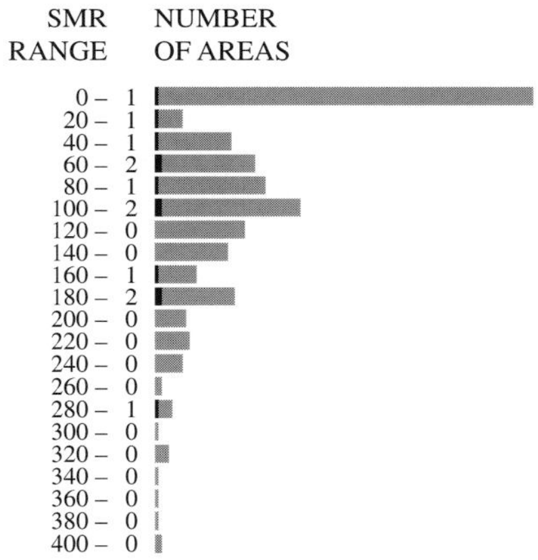

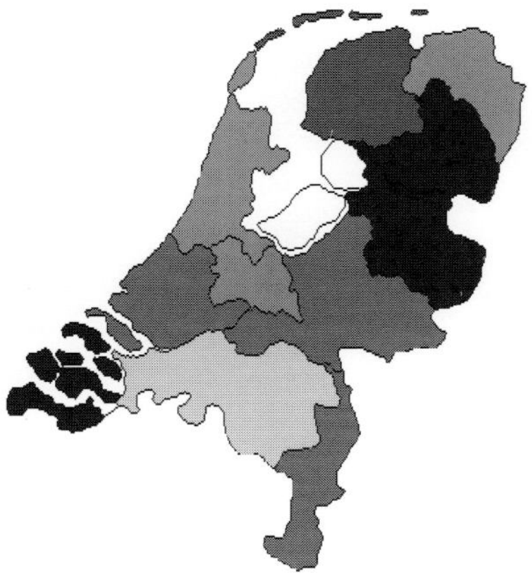

National rate = 0.09 per 100 000

0.0
0.0 – 43.5
43.5 – 90.0
90.0 – 120.8
120.8 – 182.9
182.9 – 434.7

SMRs

ABDOMINAL HERNIA MORTALITY AGES 5–64: 1985–89

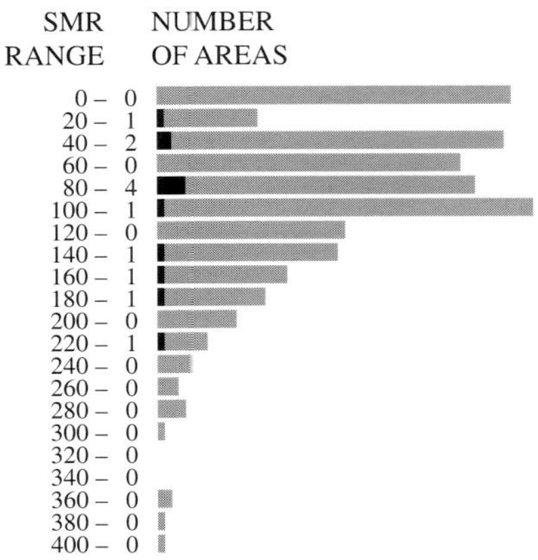

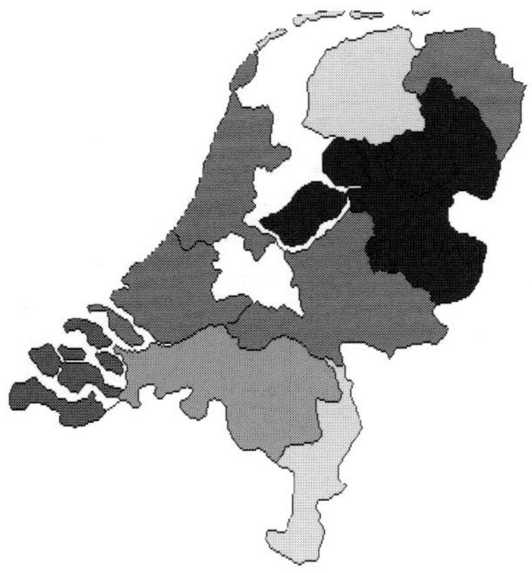

National rate = 0.11 per 100 000

0.0 – 36.1
36.1 – 67.4
67.4 – 92.5
92.5 – 117.6
117.6 – 171.3
171.3 – 494.0

SMRs

CHOLELITHIASIS AND CHOLECYSTITIS MORTALITY AGES 5–64: 1985–89

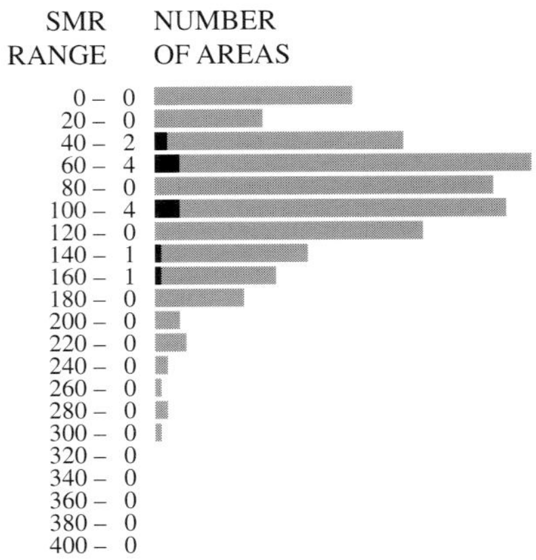

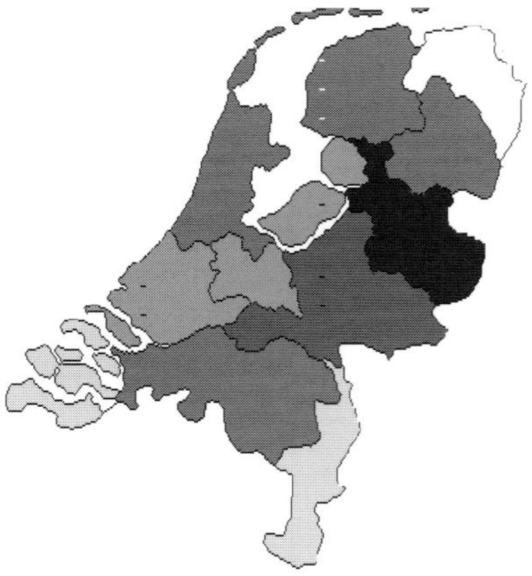

National rate = 0.26 per 100 000

0.0 – 46.4
46.4 – 72.6
72.6 – 92.3
92.3 – 118.2
118.2 – 148.4
148.4 – 315.9

SMRs

HYPERTENSIVE AND CEREBROVASCULAR DISEASES MORTALITY AGES 35–64: 1985–89

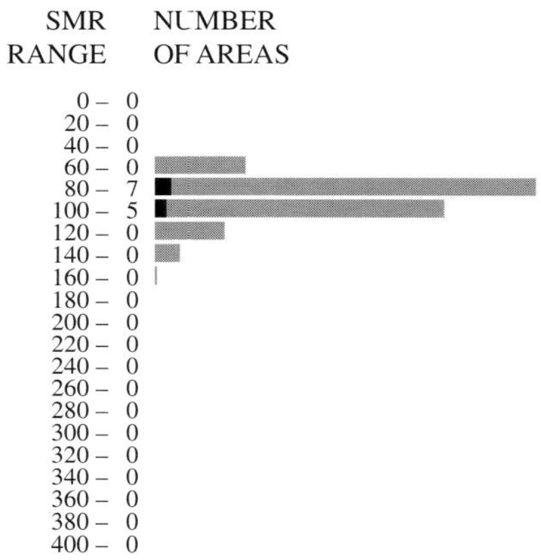

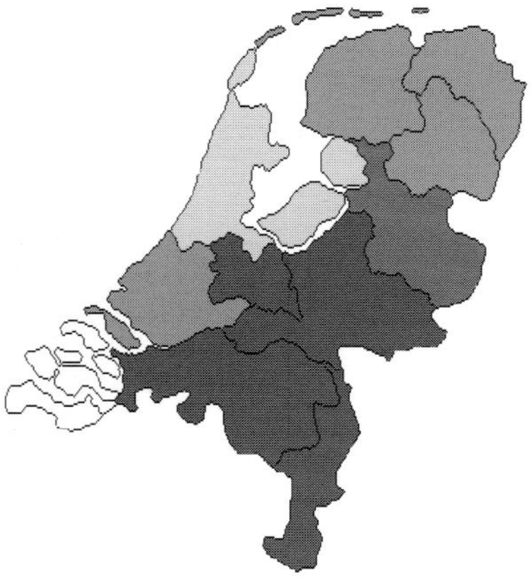

National rate = 22.77 per 100 000

64.6 – 83.2
83.2 – 91.3
91.3 – 98.4
98.4 – 105.7
105.7 – 114.6
114.6 – 164.0

SMRs

MATERNAL MORTALITY ALL AGES: 1985–89

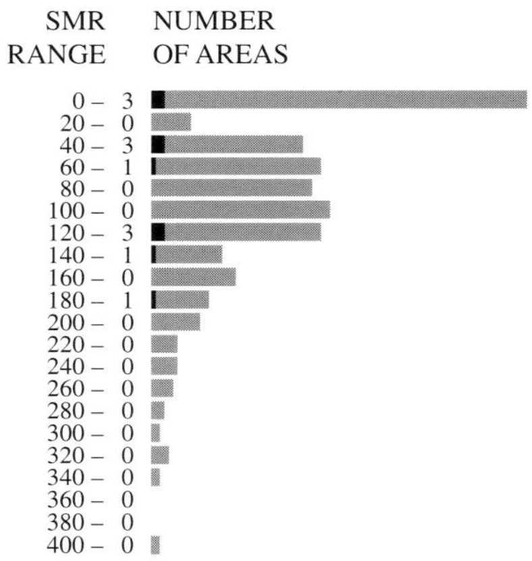

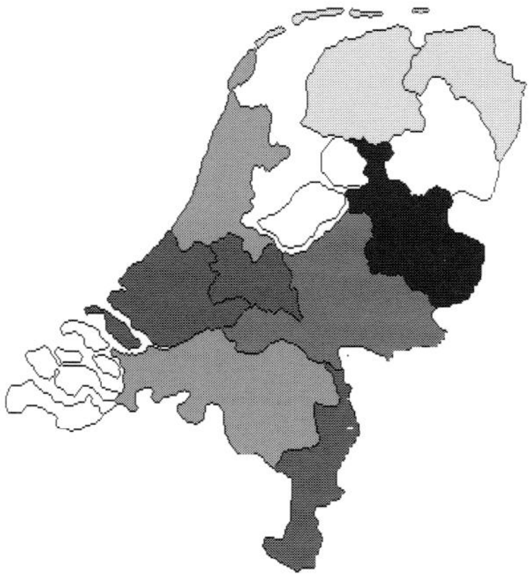

National rate = 7.43 per 100 000 live and still births

0.0
0.0 – 57.8
57.8 – 91.1
91.1 – 121.1
121.1 – 168.6
168.6 – 551.1

SMRs

PERINATAL MORTALITY: 1985–89

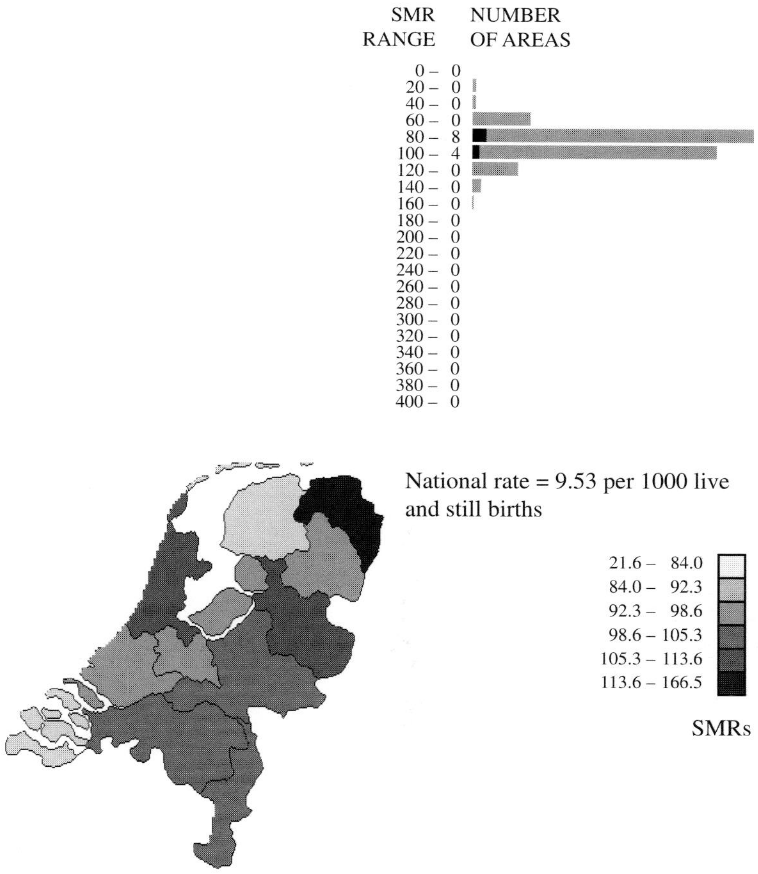

CANCER OF THE BREAST MORTALITY AGES 25–64: 1985–89

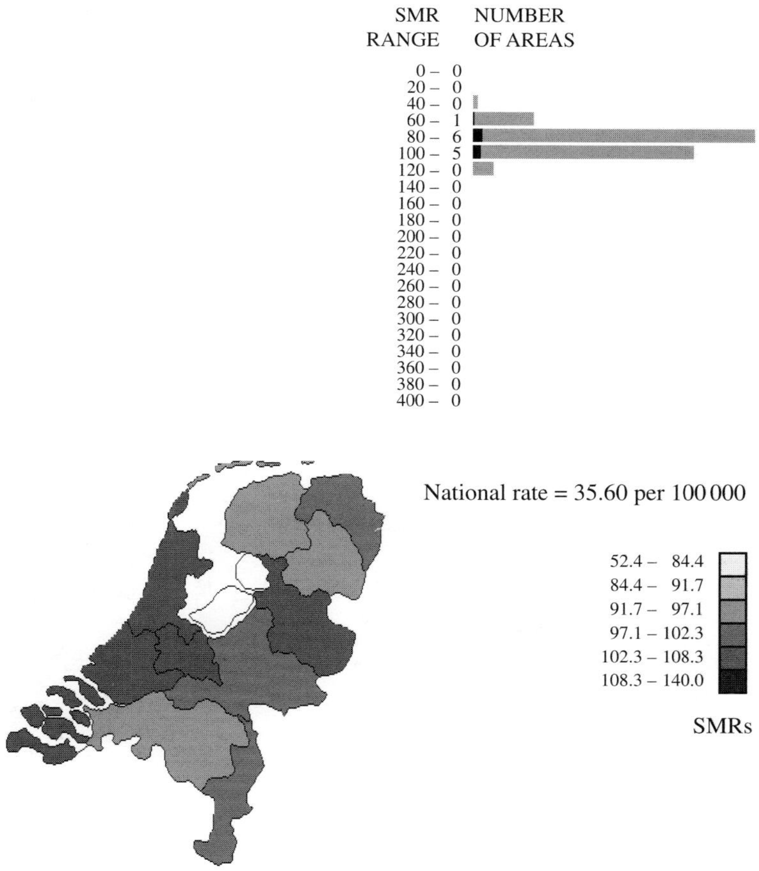

ISCHAEMIC HEART DISEASE MORTALITY AGES 35–64: 1985–89

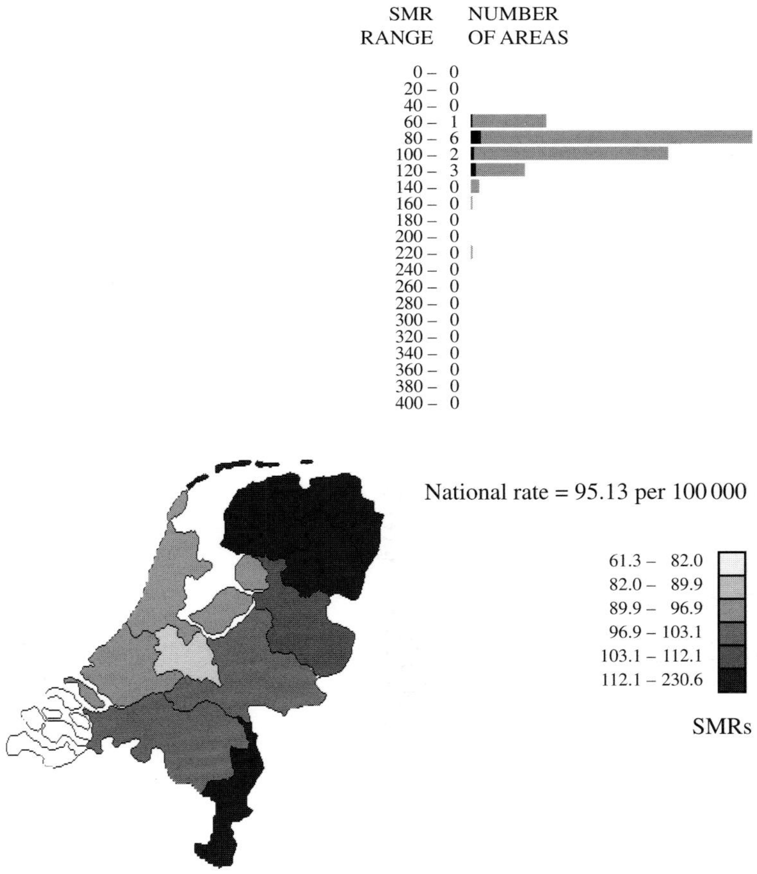

PEPTIC ULCERS MORTALITY AGES 25–64: 1985–89

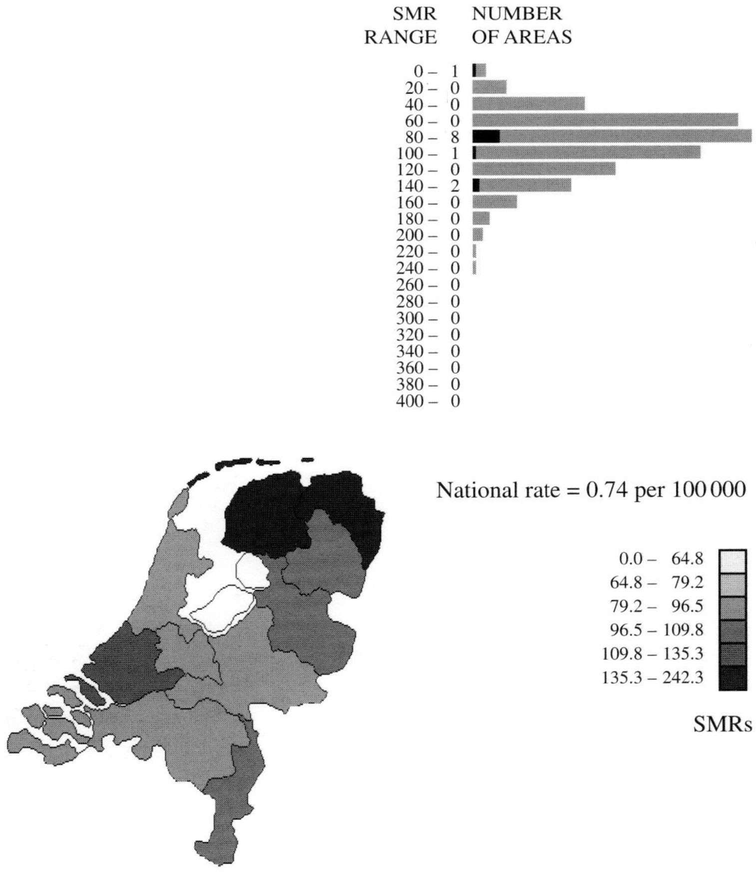

ALL CAUSES MORTALITY AGES 5–64: 1985–89

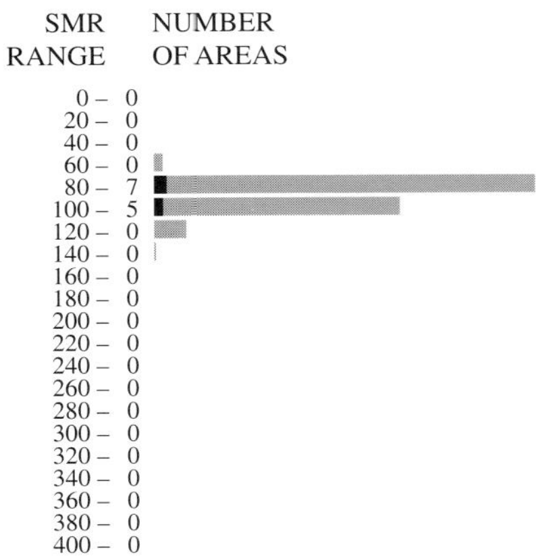

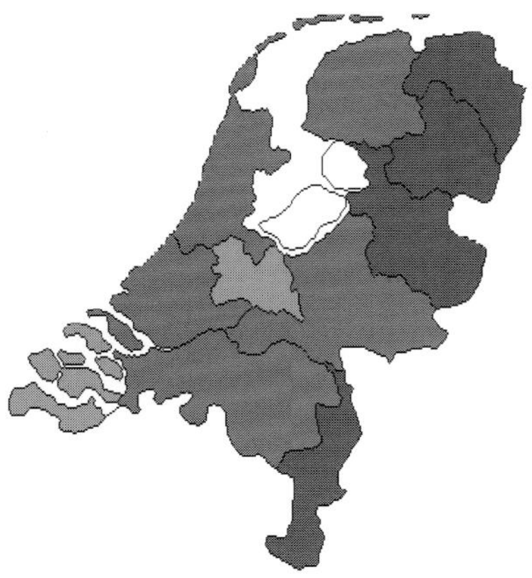

National rate = 219 per 100 000

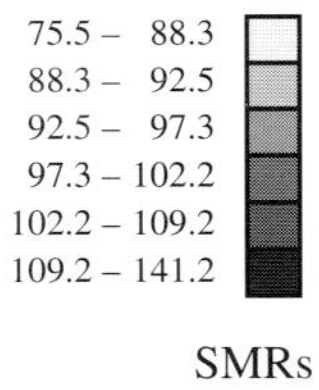

ALL CAUSES MORTALITY ALL AGES: 1985–89

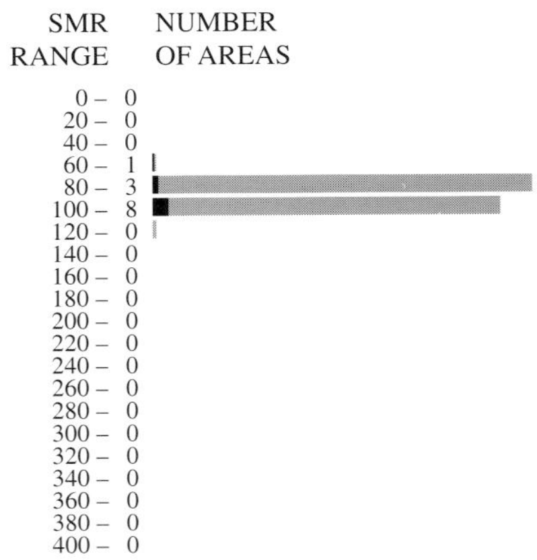

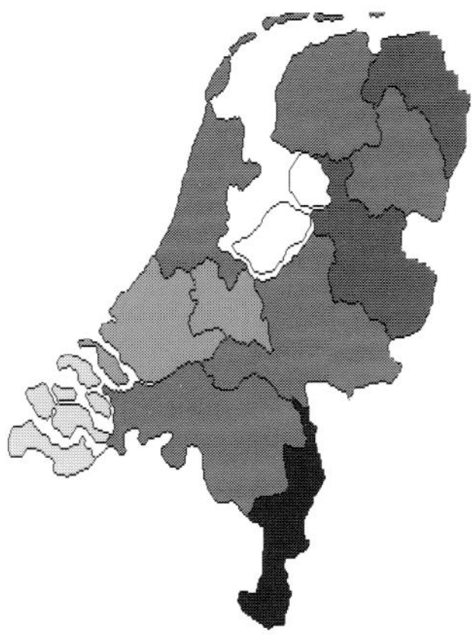

National rate = 843 per 100 000

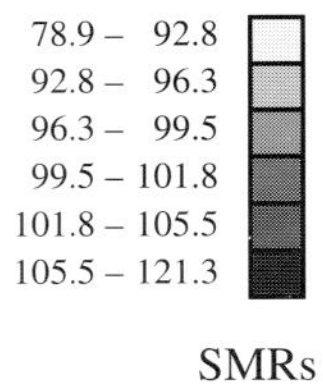

ENGLAND AND WALES

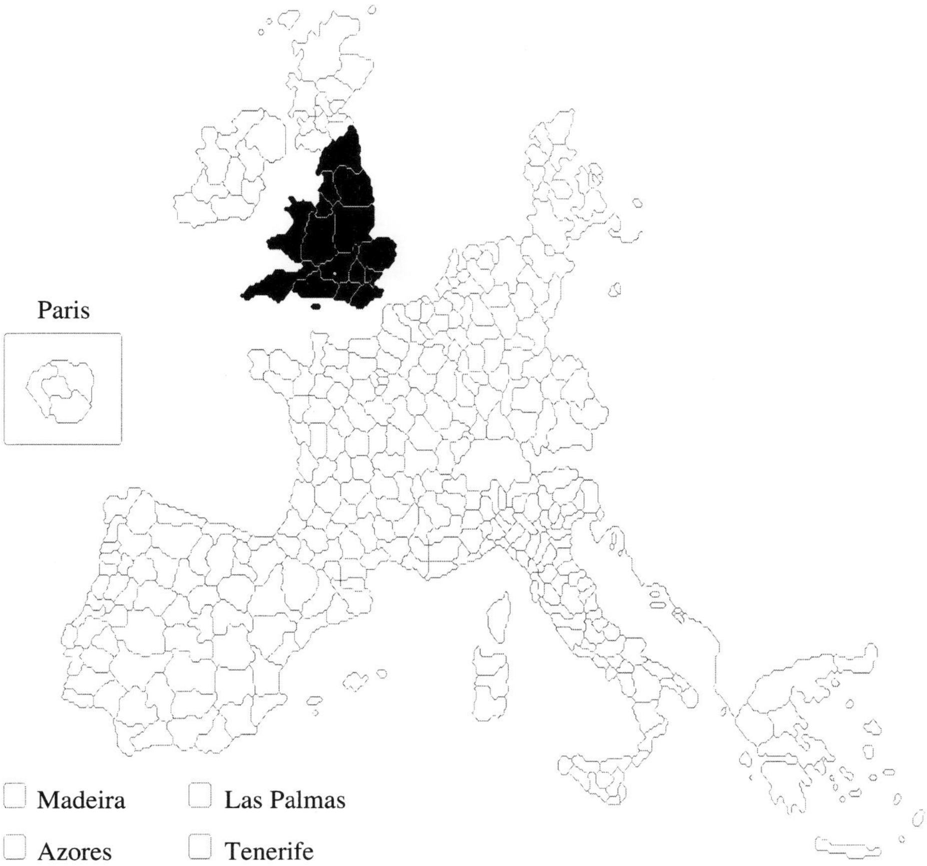

KEY MAP: ENGLAND AND WALES

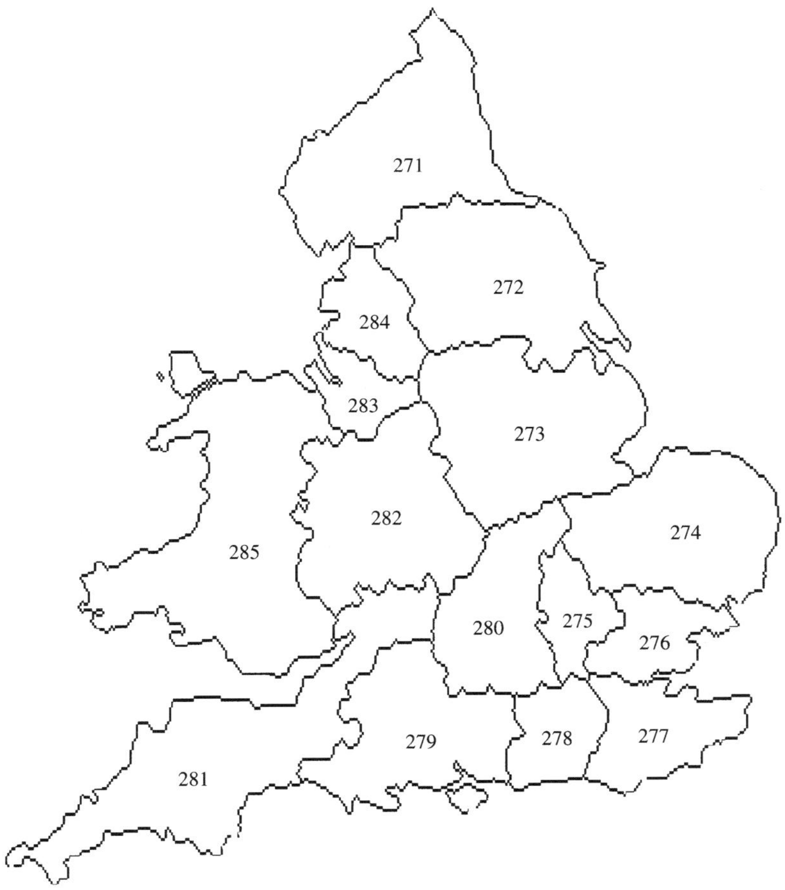

TUBERCULOSIS MORTALITY AGES 5–64: 1985–89

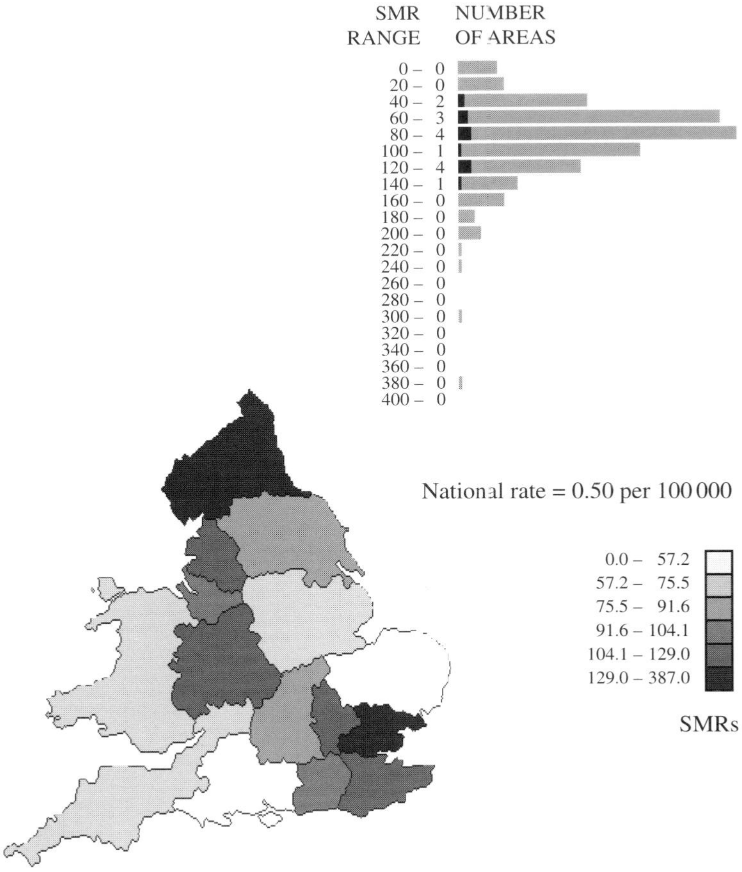

MALIGNANT NEOPLASM OF CERVIX UTERI MORTALITY AGES 15–64: 1985–89

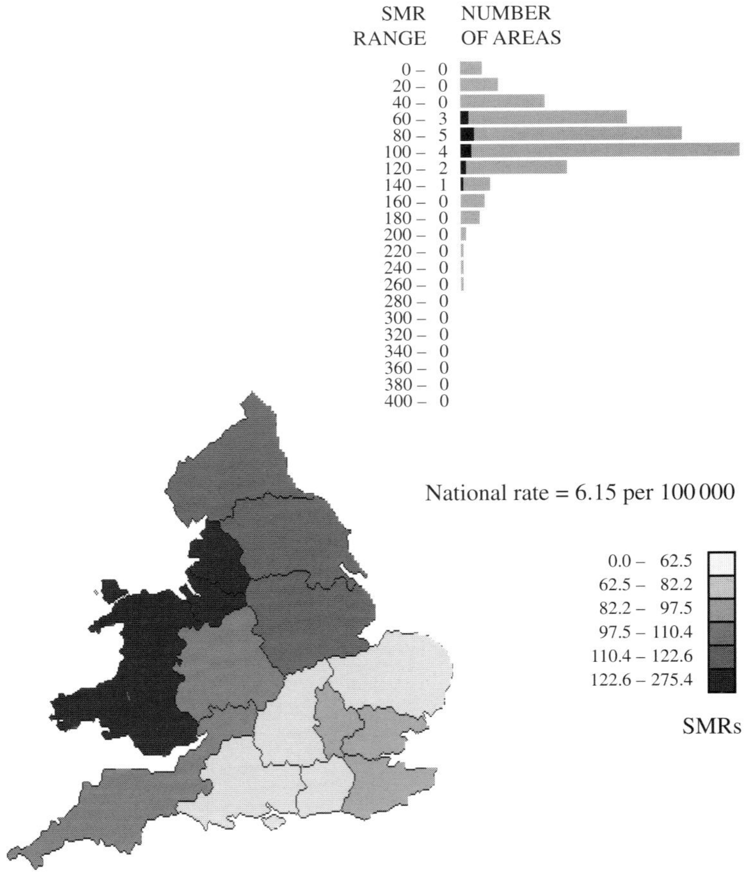

MALIGNANT NEOPLASM OF CERVIX AND BODY OF UTERUS MORTALITY AGES 15–54: 1985–89

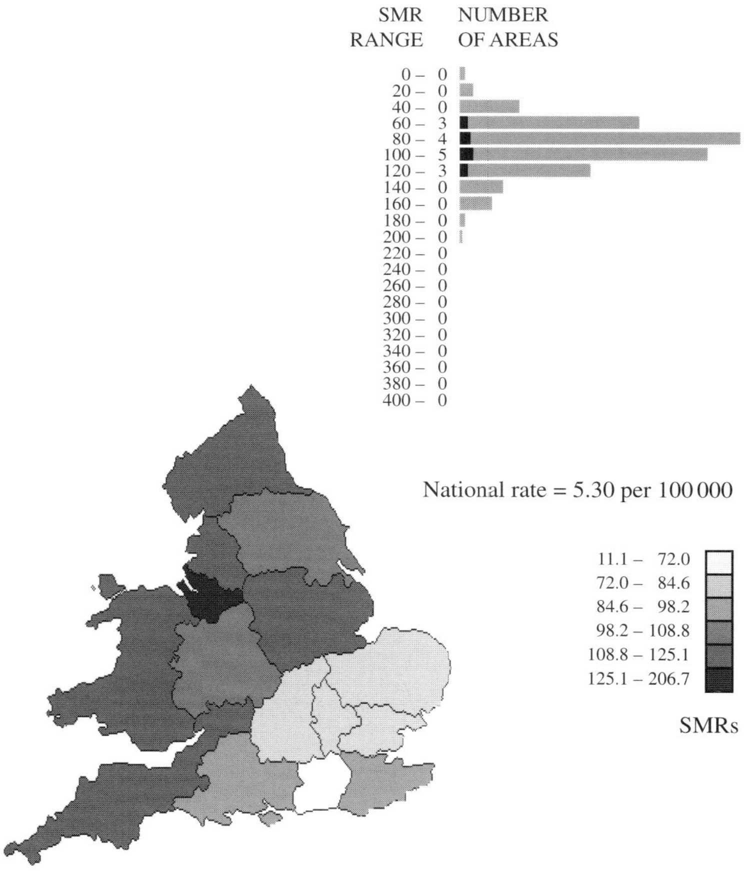

HODGKIN'S DISEASE MORTALITY AGES 5–64: 1985–89

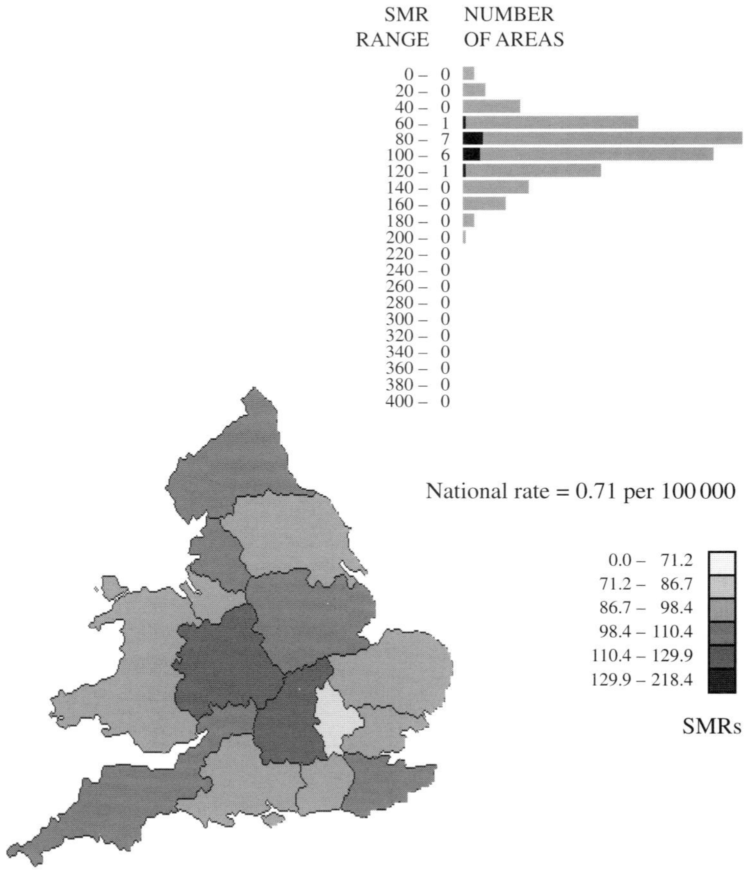

CHRONIC RHEUMATIC HEART DISEASE MORTALITY AGES 5–44: 1985–89

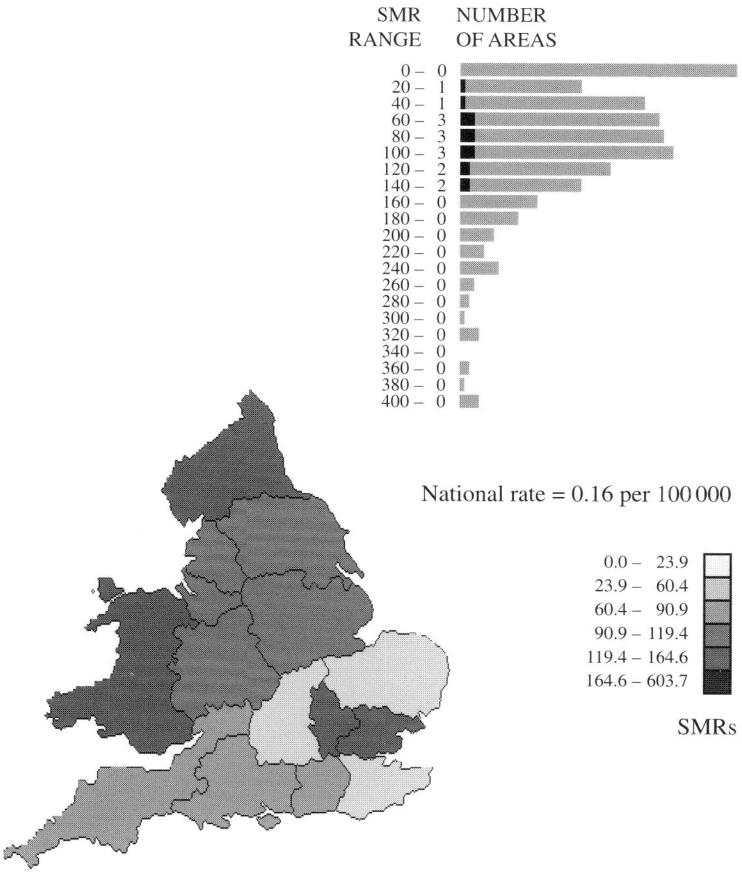

ALL RESPIRATORY DISEASES MORTALITY AGES 1–14: 1985–89

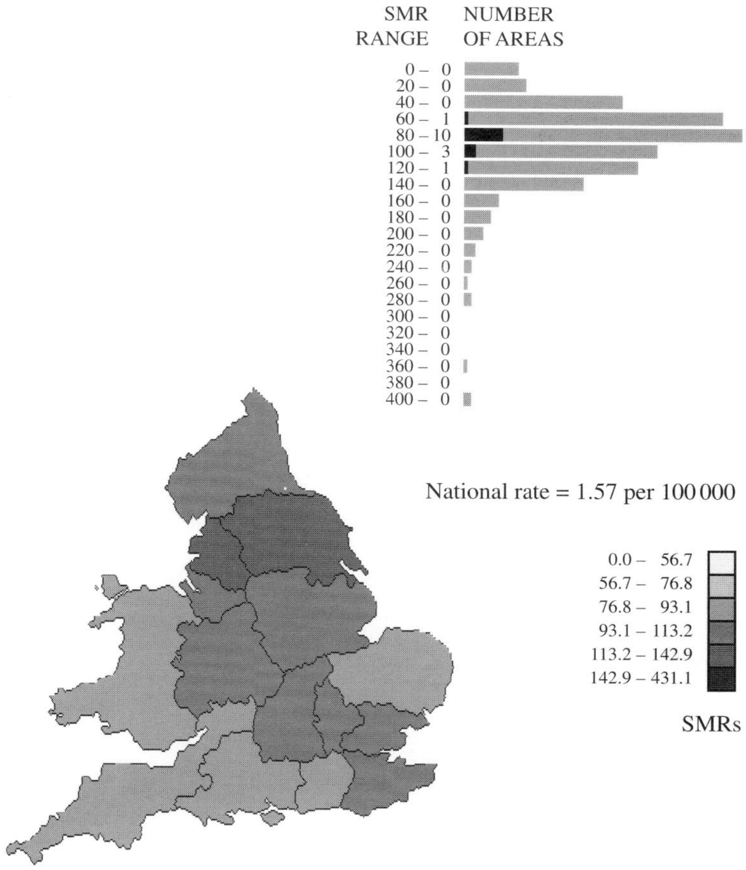

ASTHMA MORTALITY AGES 5–44: 1985–89

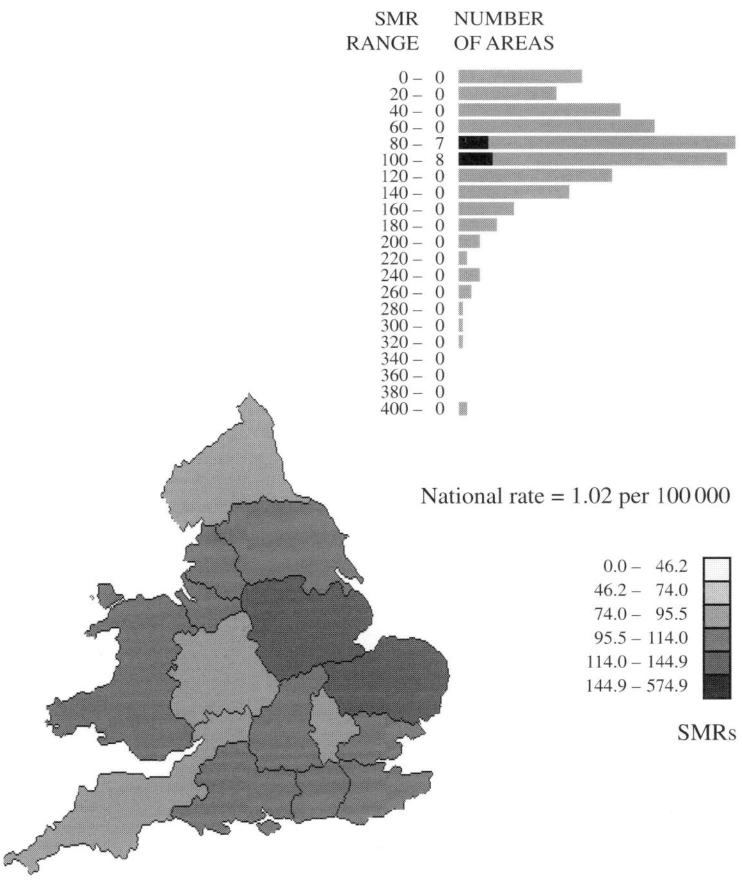

APPENDICITIS MORTALITY AGES 5–64: 1985–89

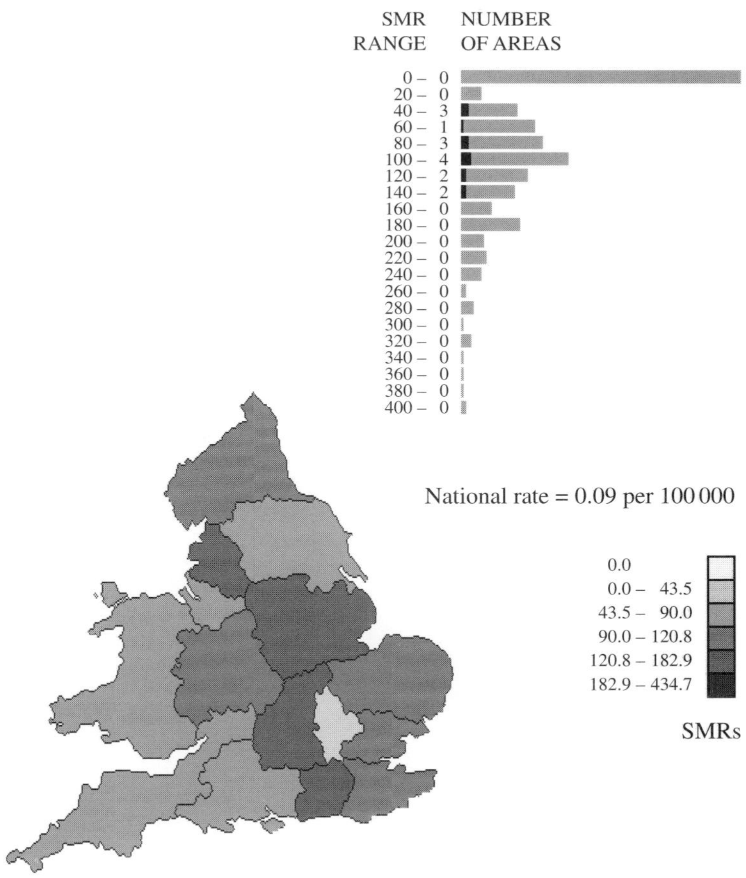

ABDOMINAL HERNIA MORTALITY AGES 5–64: 1985–89

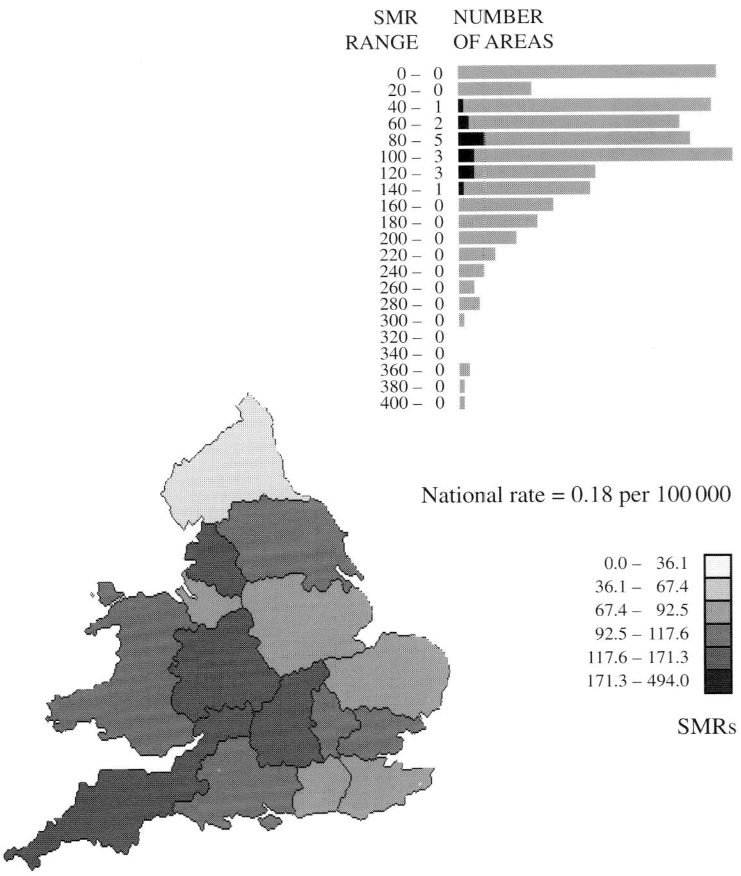

CHOLELITHIASIS AND CHOLECYSTITIS MORTALITY AGES 5–64: 1985–89

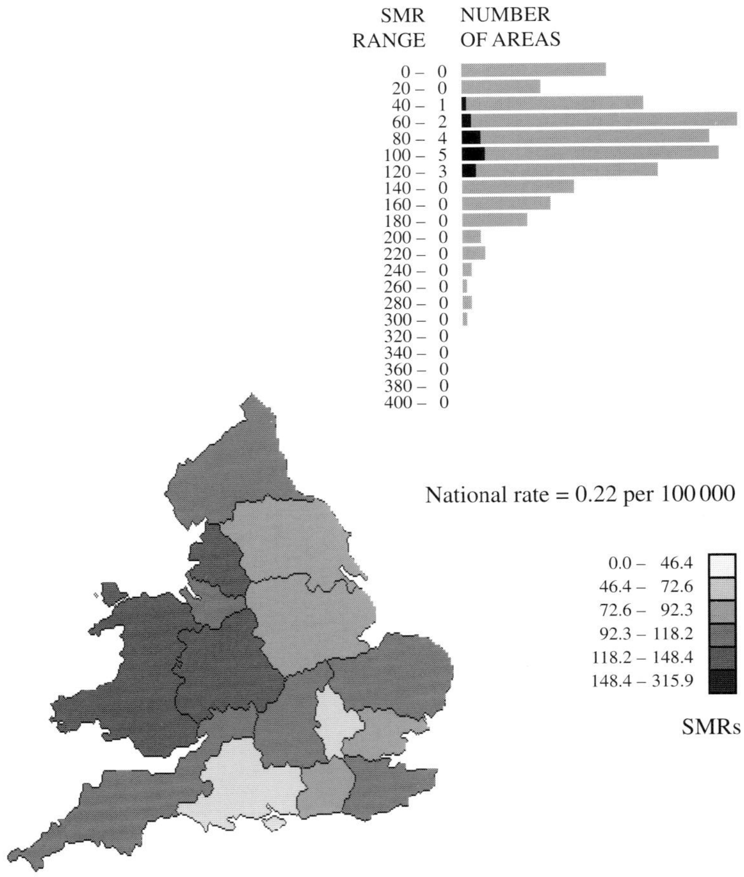

HYPERTENSIVE AND CEREBROVASCULAR DISEASES MORTALITY AGES 35–64: 1985–89

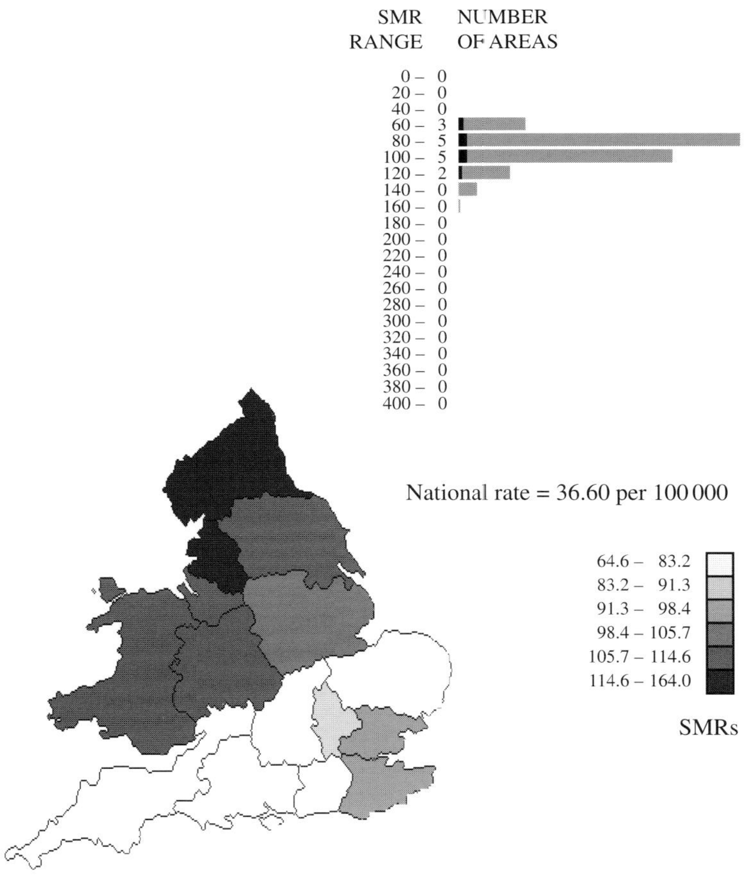

MATERNAL MORTALITY ALL AGES: 1985–89

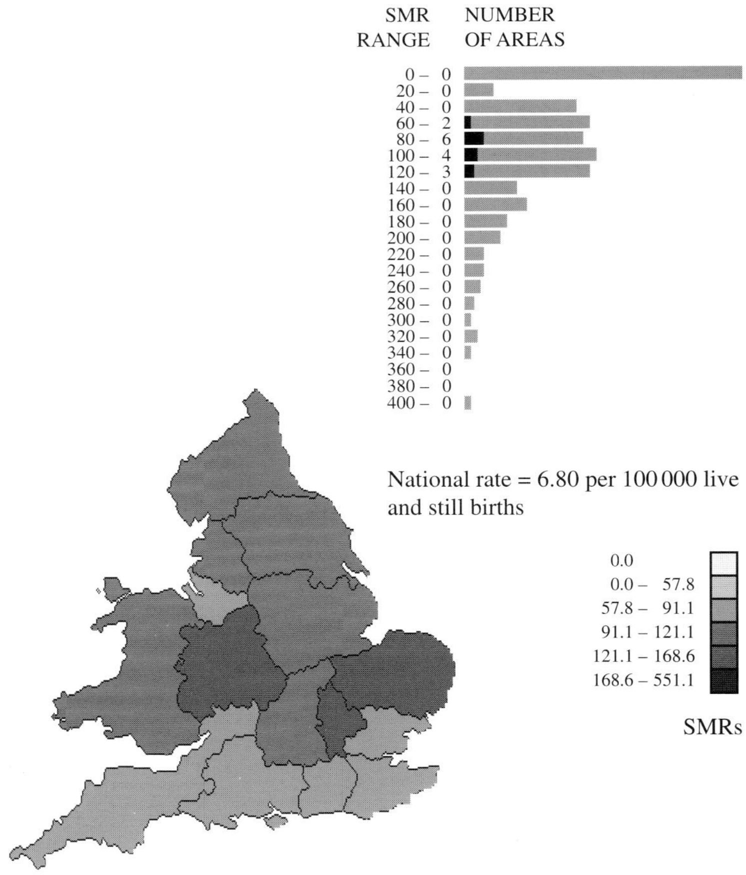

PERINATAL MORTALITY: 1985–89

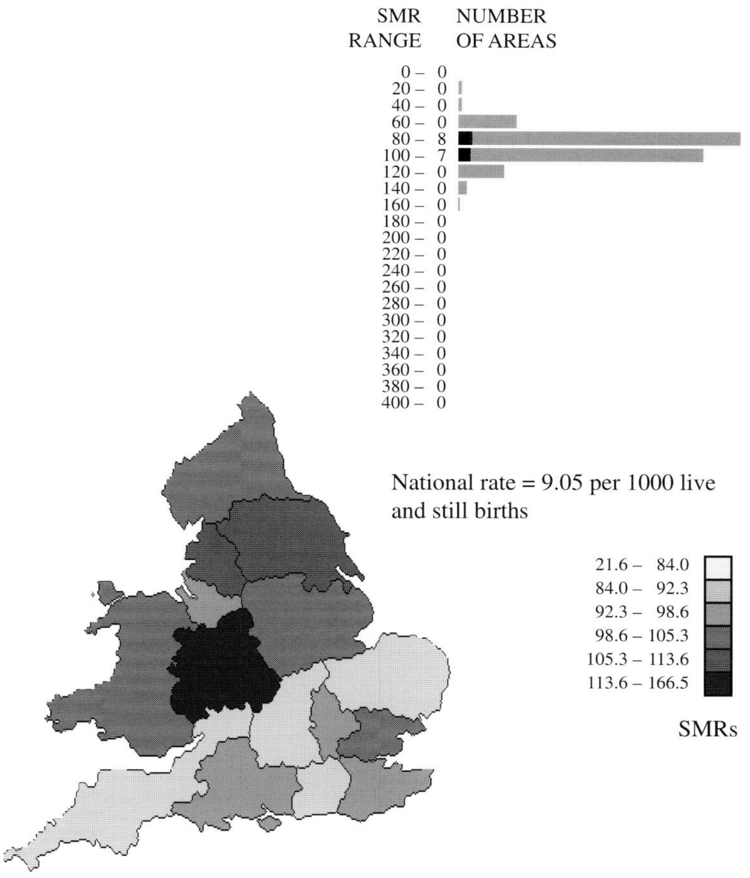

CANCER OF THE BREAST MORTALITY AGES 25–64: 1985–89

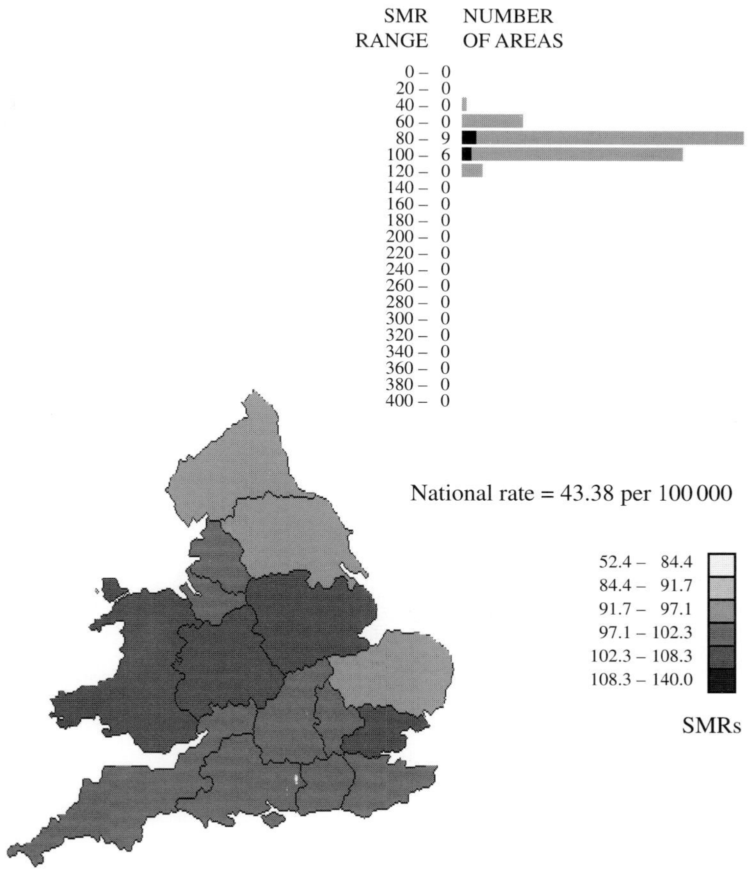

ISCHAEMIC HEART DISEASE MORTALITY AGES 35–64: 1985–89

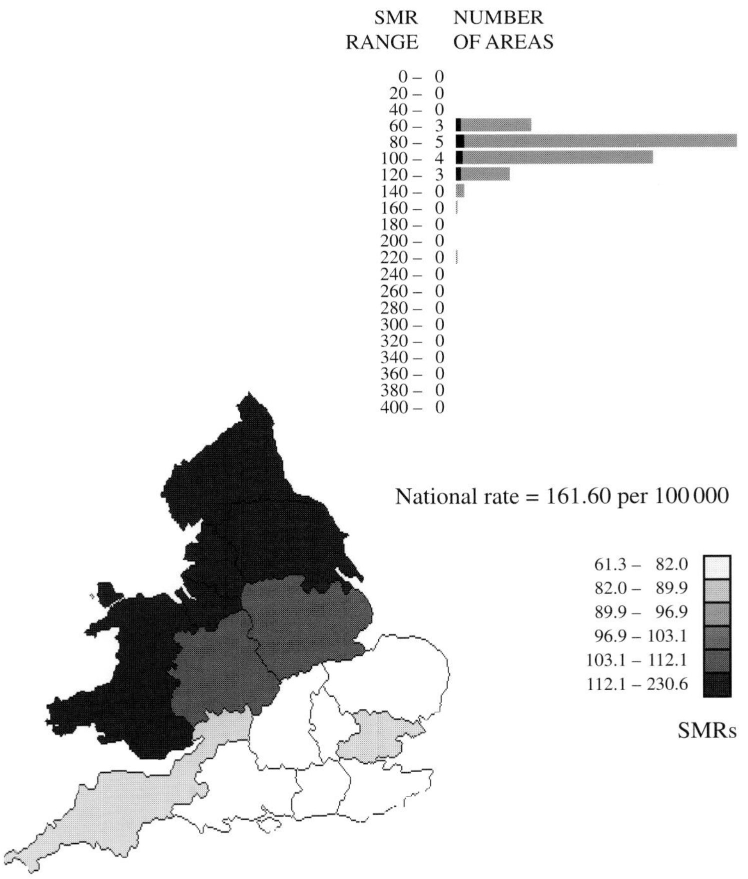

PEPTIC ULCERS MORTALITY AGES 25–64: 1985–89

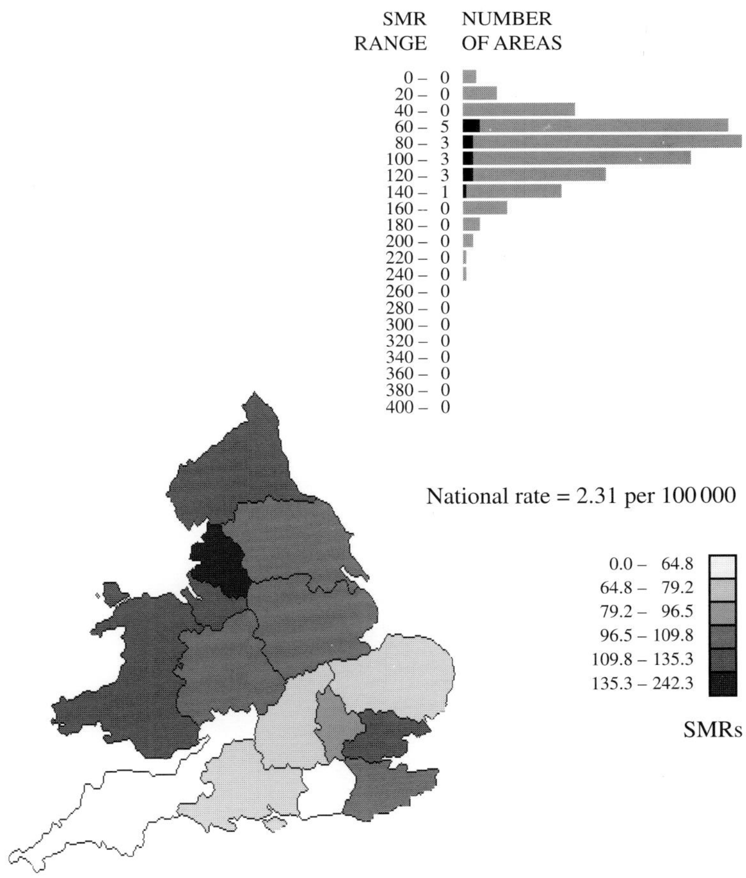

ALL CAUSES MORTALITY AGES 5–64: 1985–89

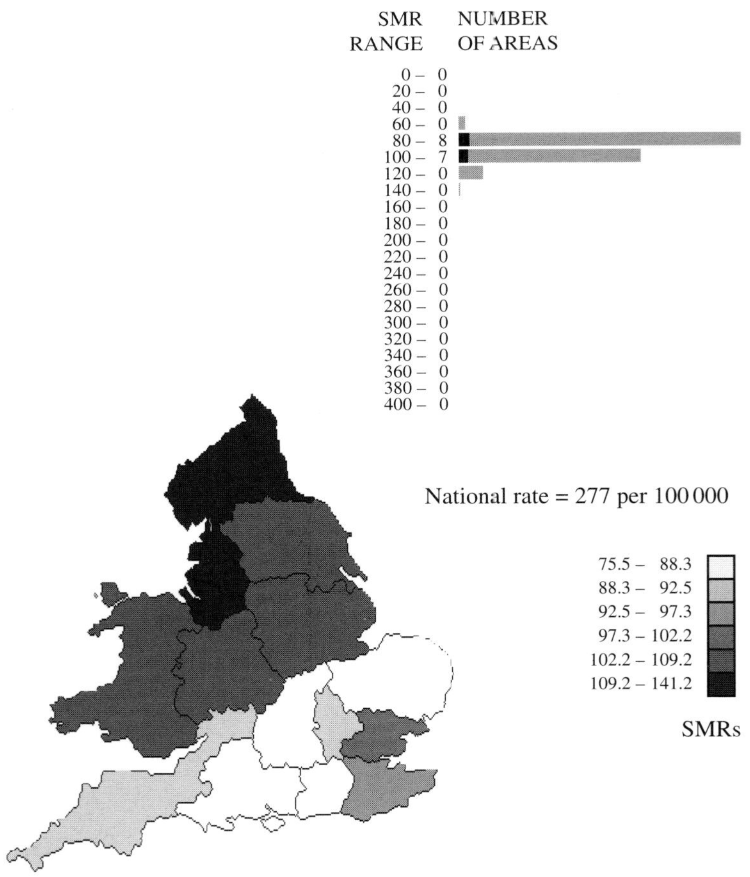

ALL CAUSES MORTALITY ALL AGES: 1985–89

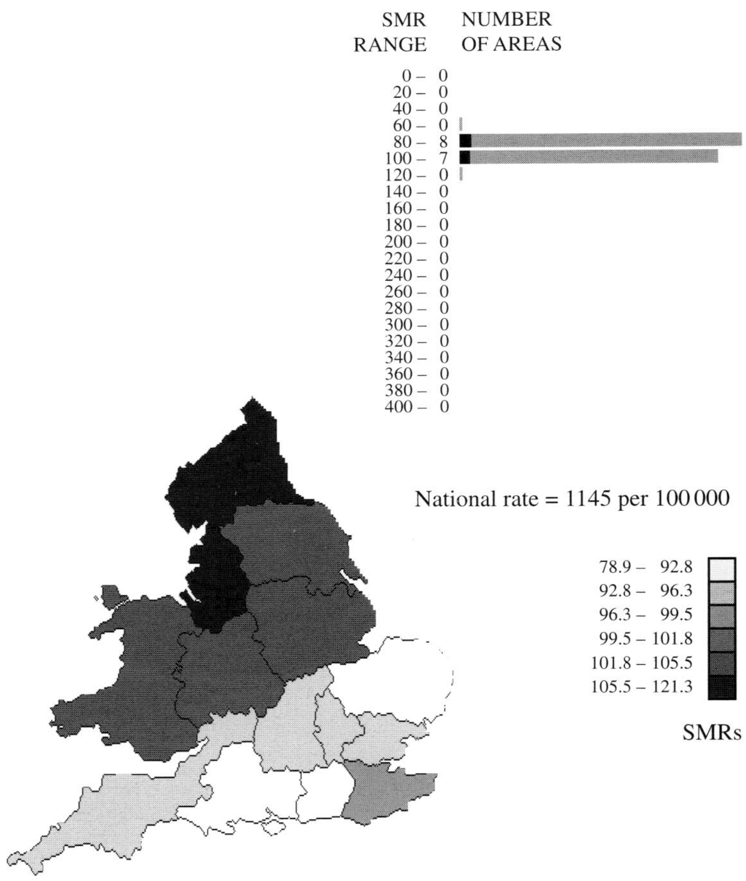

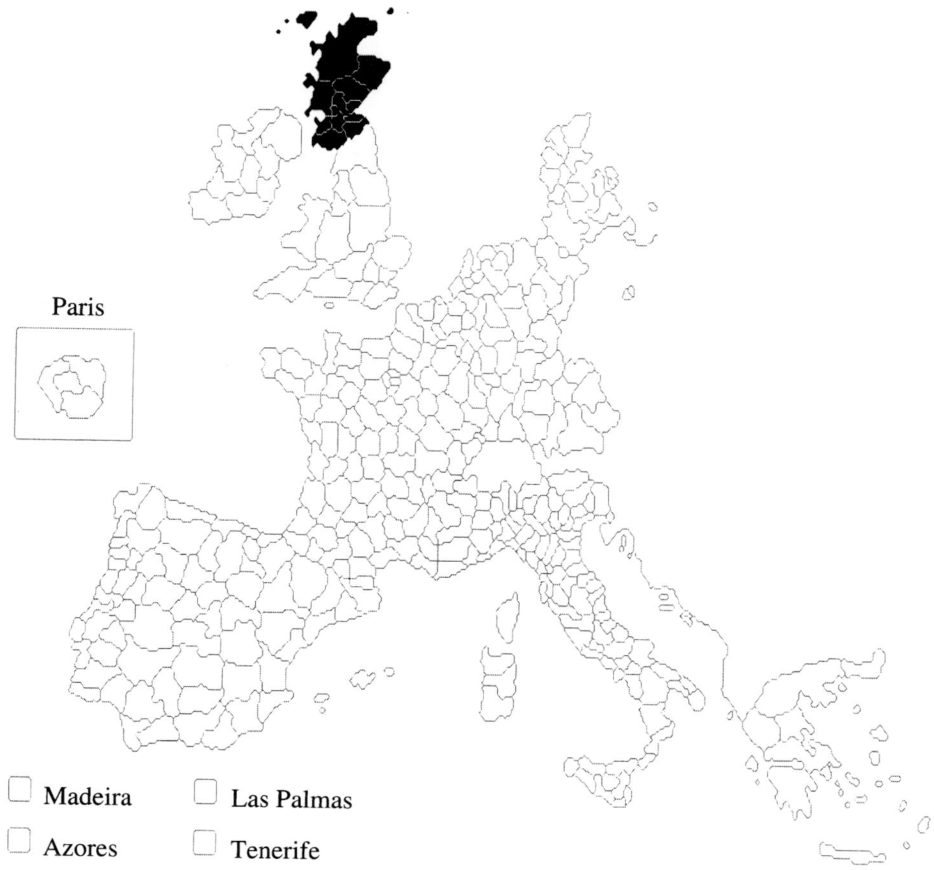

KEY MAP: SCOTLAND

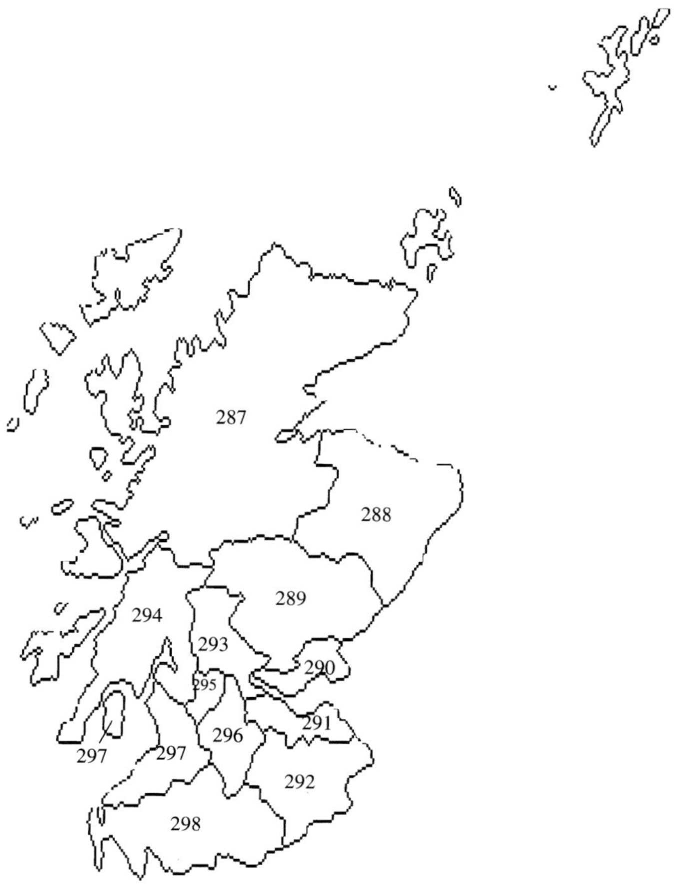

TUBERCULOSIS MORTALITY AGES 5–64: 1985–89

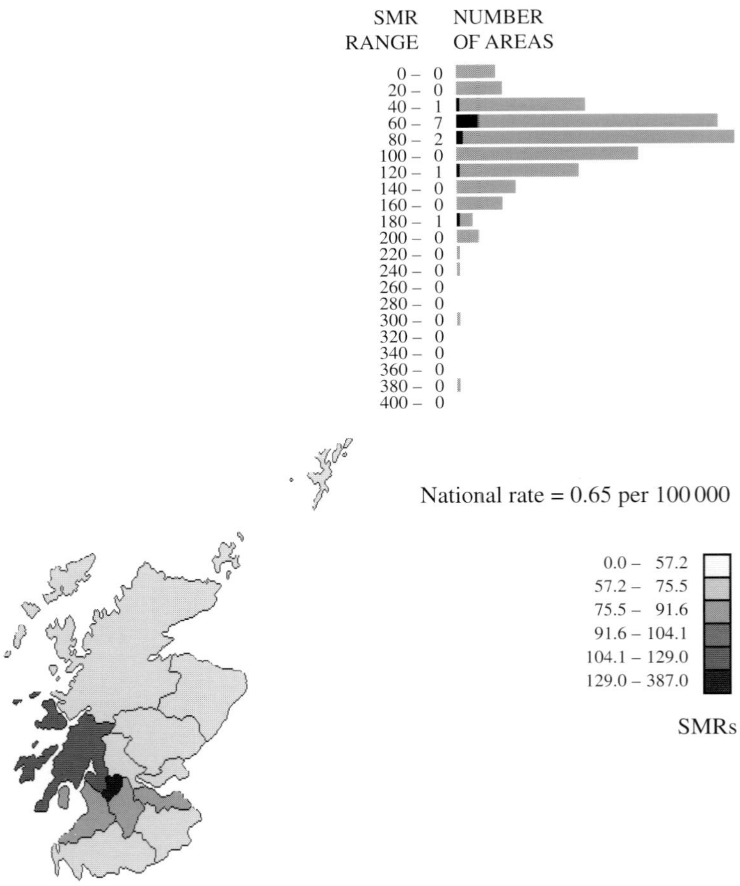

MALIGNANT NEOPLASM OF CERVIX UTERI MORTALITY AGES 15–64: 1985–89

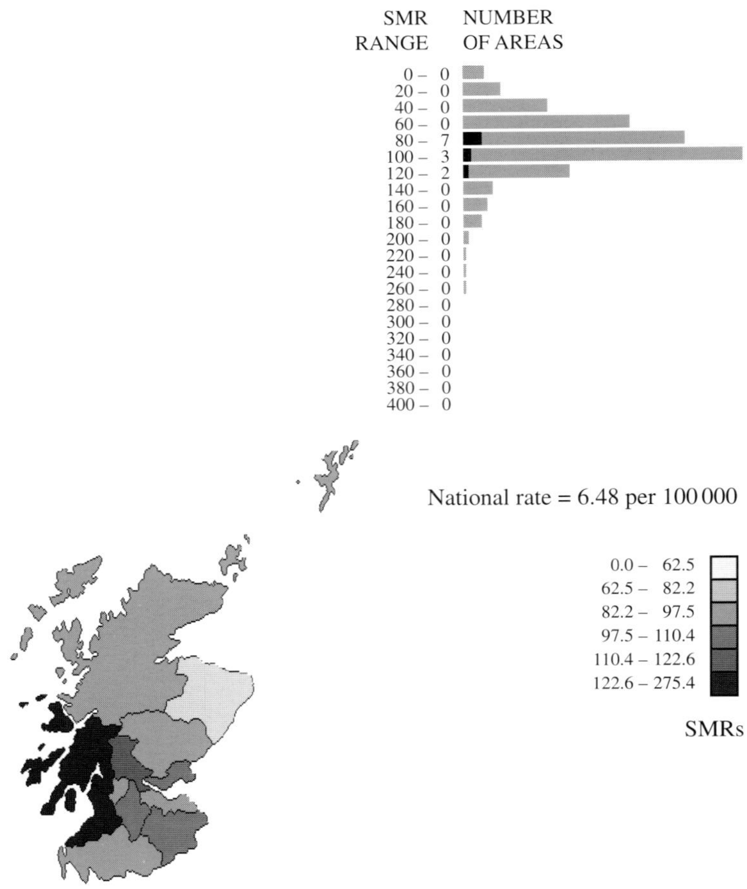

MALIGNANT NEOPLASM OF CERVIX AND BODY OF UTERUS MORTALITY AGES 15–54: 1985–89

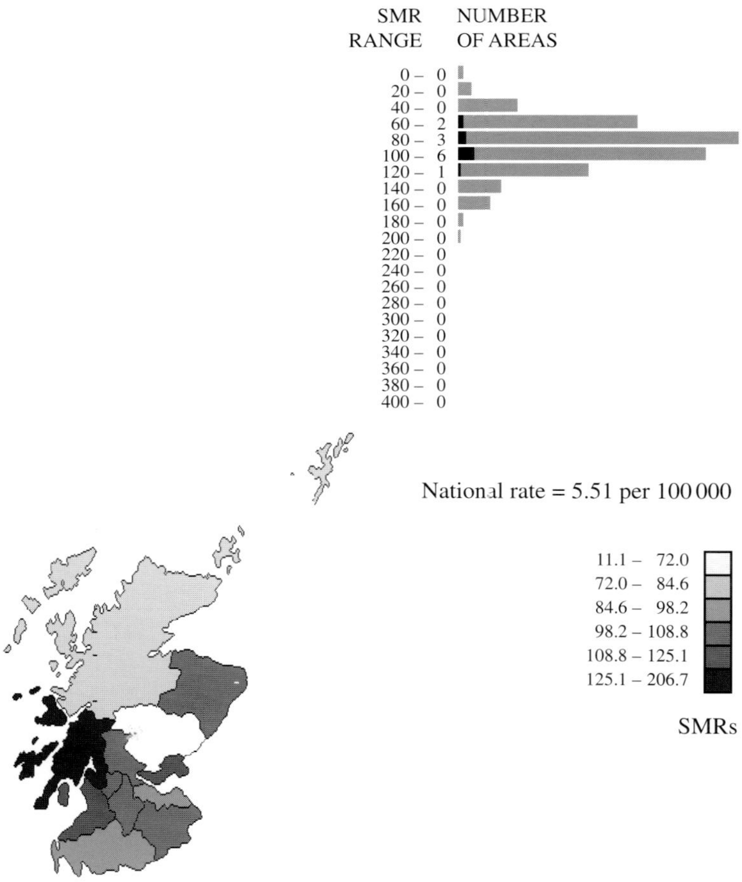

HODGKIN'S DISEASE MORTALITY AGES 5–64: 1985–89

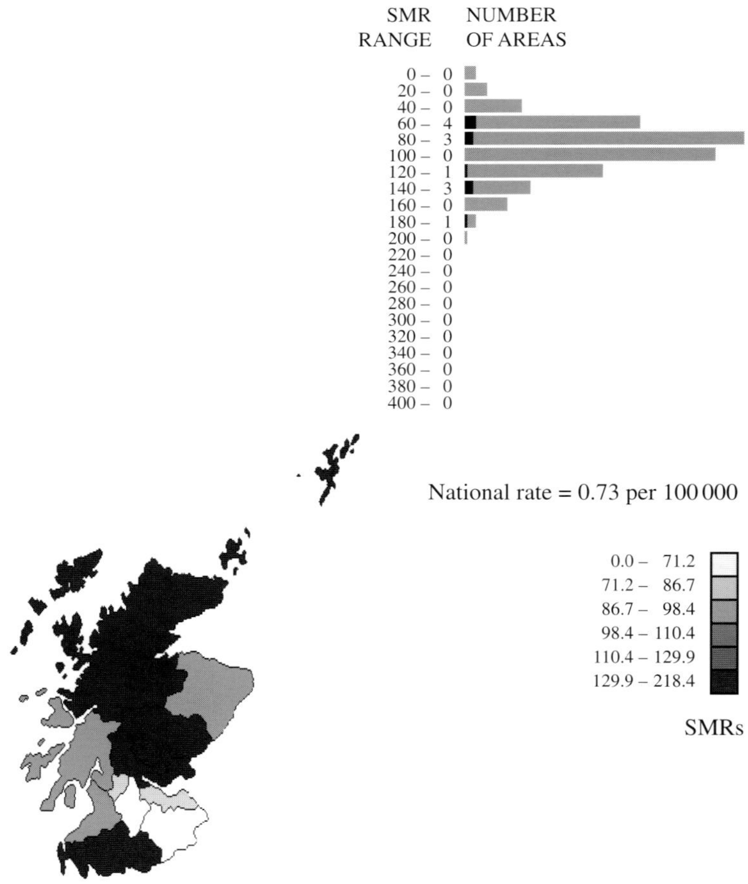

CHRONIC RHEUMATIC HEART DISEASE MORTALITY AGES 5–44: 1985–89

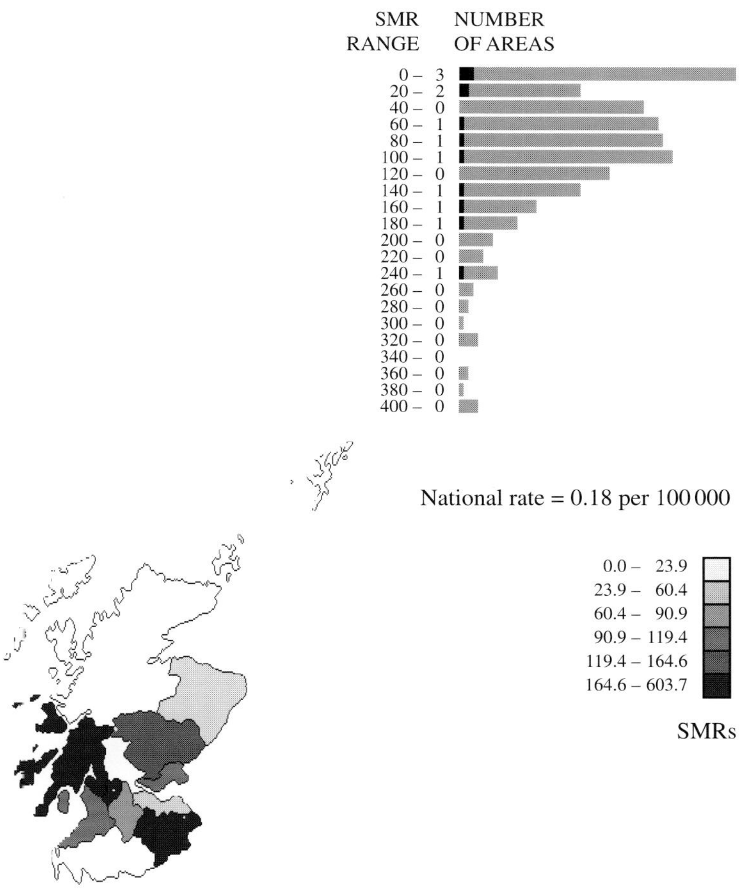

ALL RESPIRATORY DISEASES MORTALITY AGES 1–14: 1985–89

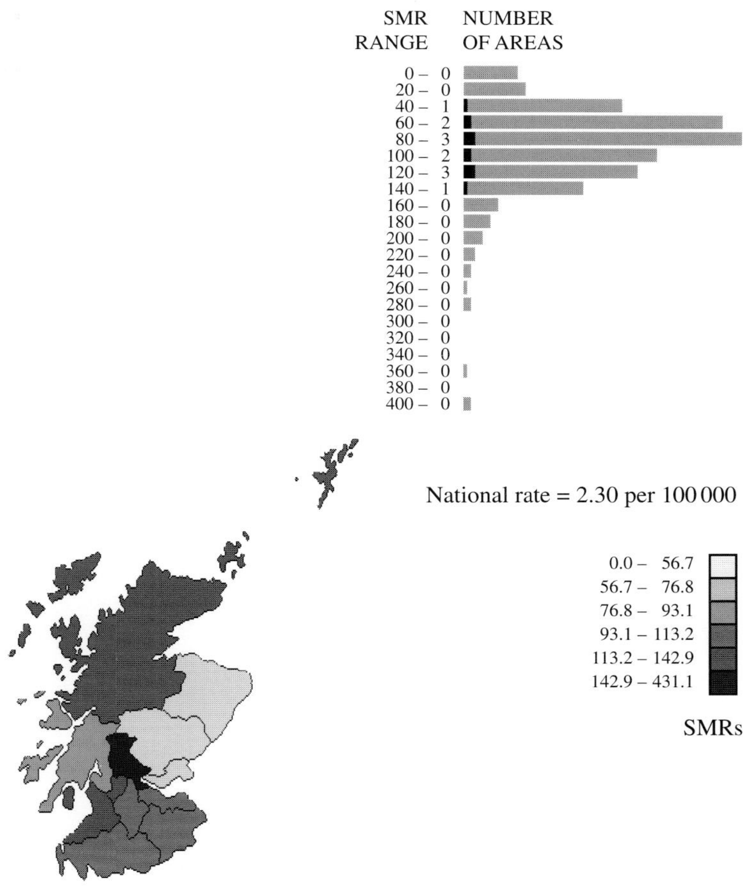

ASTHMA MORTALITY AGES 5–44: 1985–89

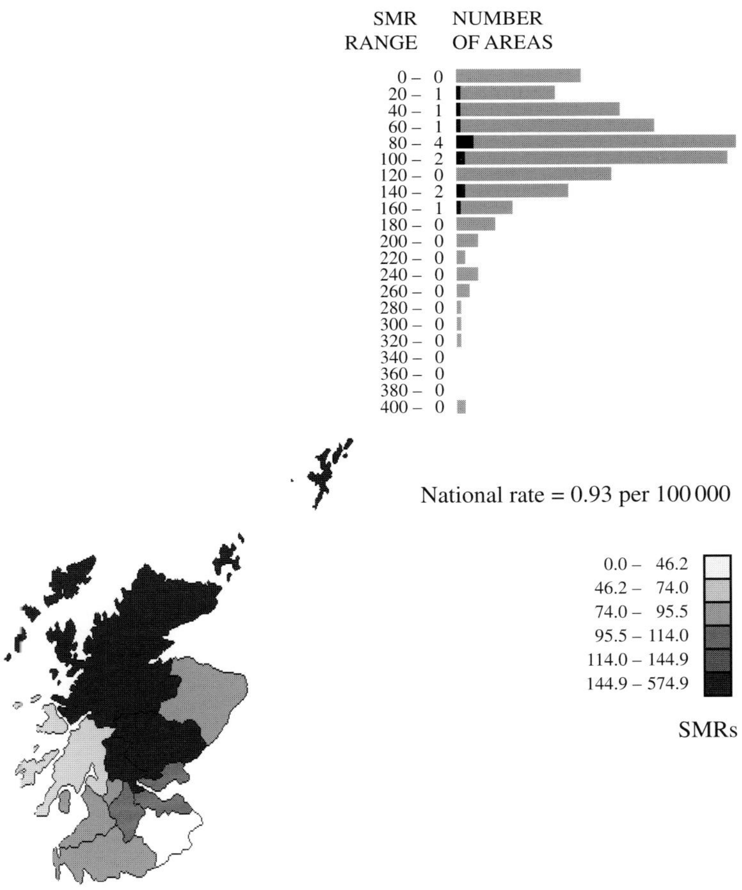

APPENDICITIS MORTALITY AGES 5–64: 1985–89

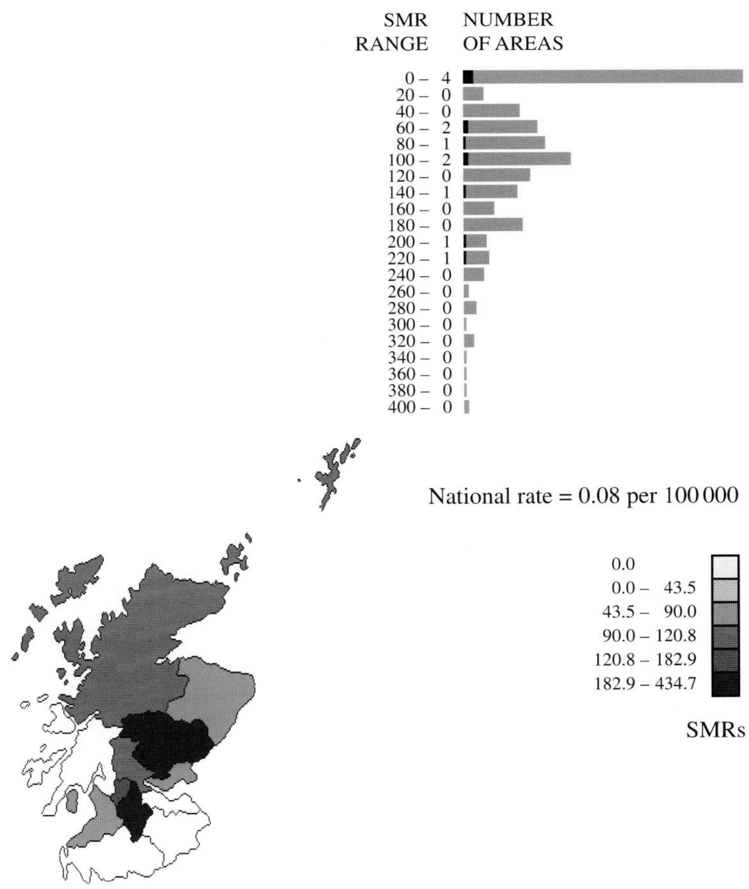

ABDOMINAL HERNIA MORTALITY AGES 5–64: 1985–89

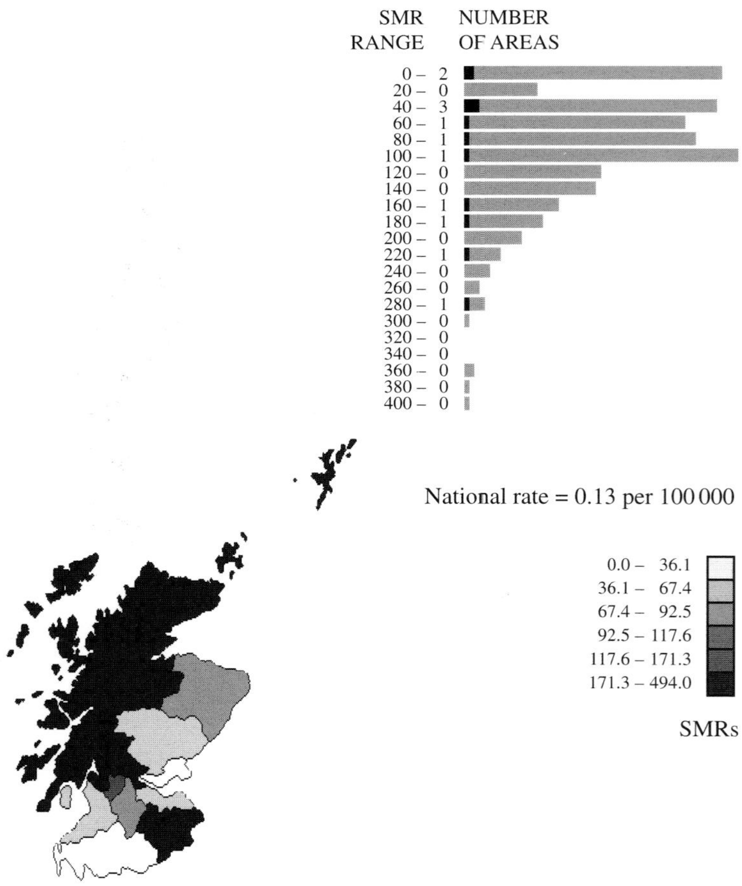

CHOLELITHIASIS AND CHOLECYSTITIS MORTALITY AGES 5–64: 1985–89

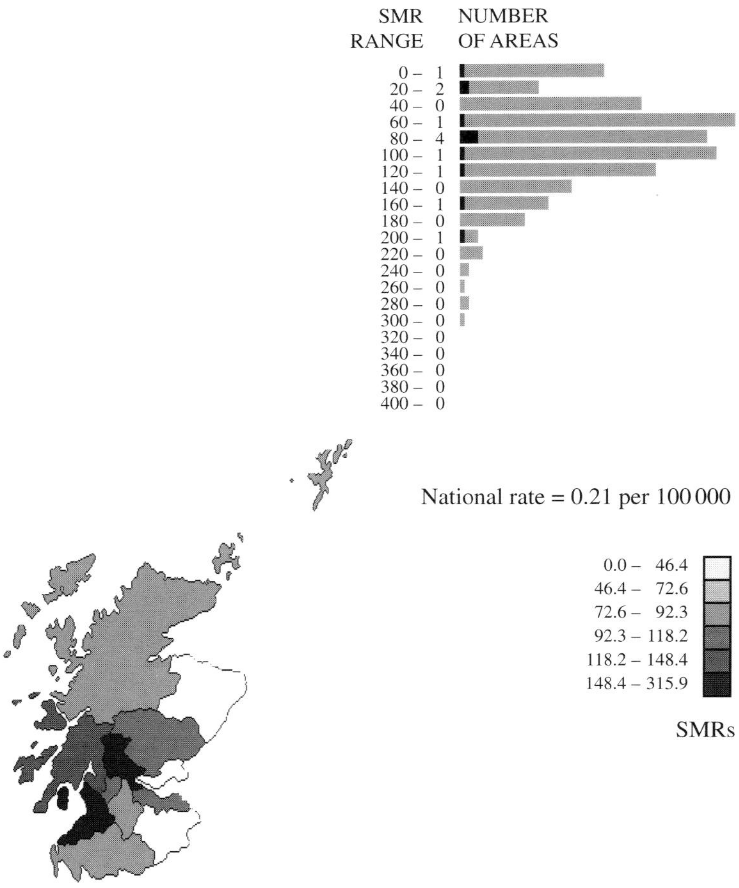

HYPERTENSIVE AND CEREBROVASCULAR DISEASES MORTALITY AGES 35–64: 1985–89

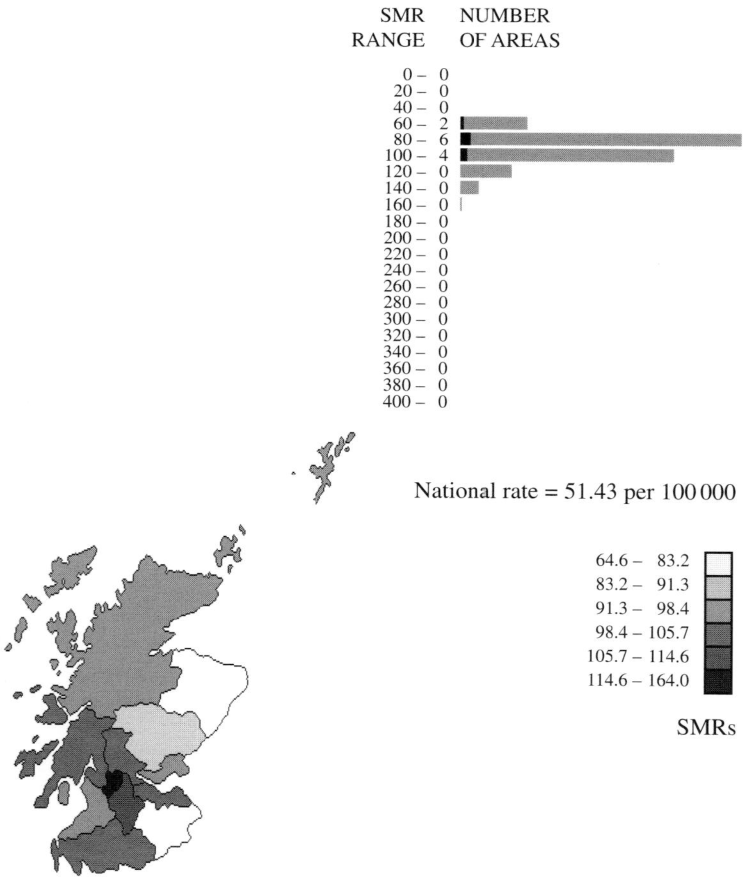

MATERNAL MORTALITY ALL AGES: 1985–89

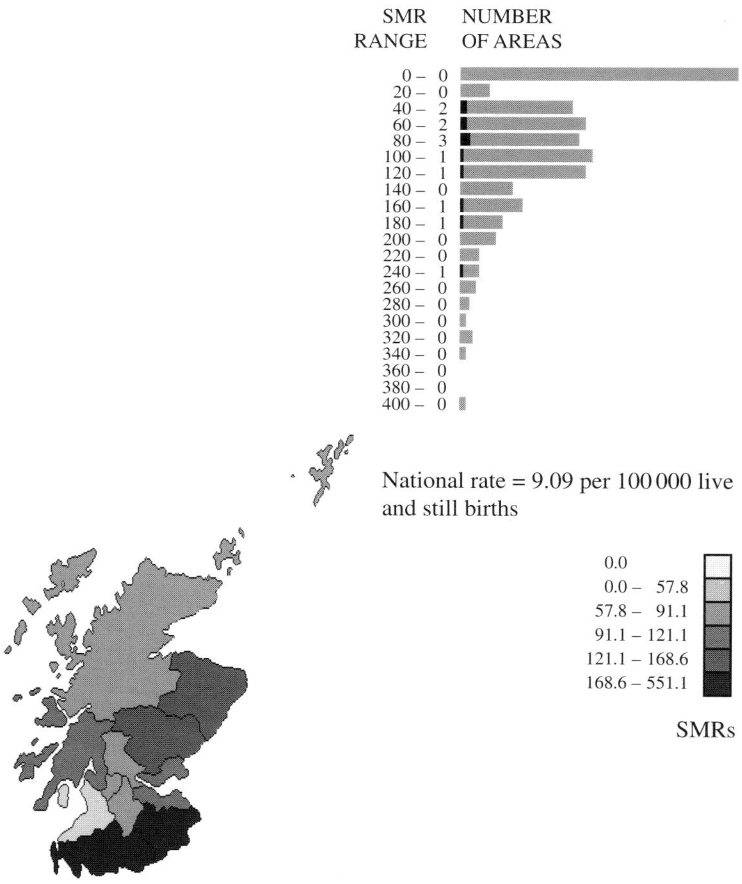

PERINATAL MORTALITY: 1985–89

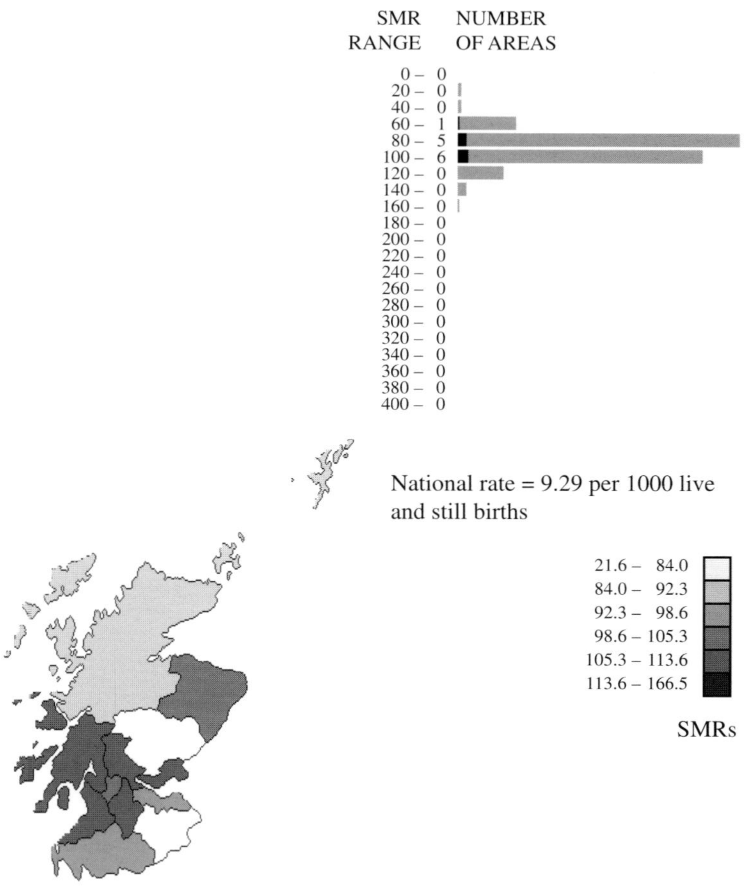

CANCER OF THE BREAST MORTALITY AGES 25–64: 1985–89

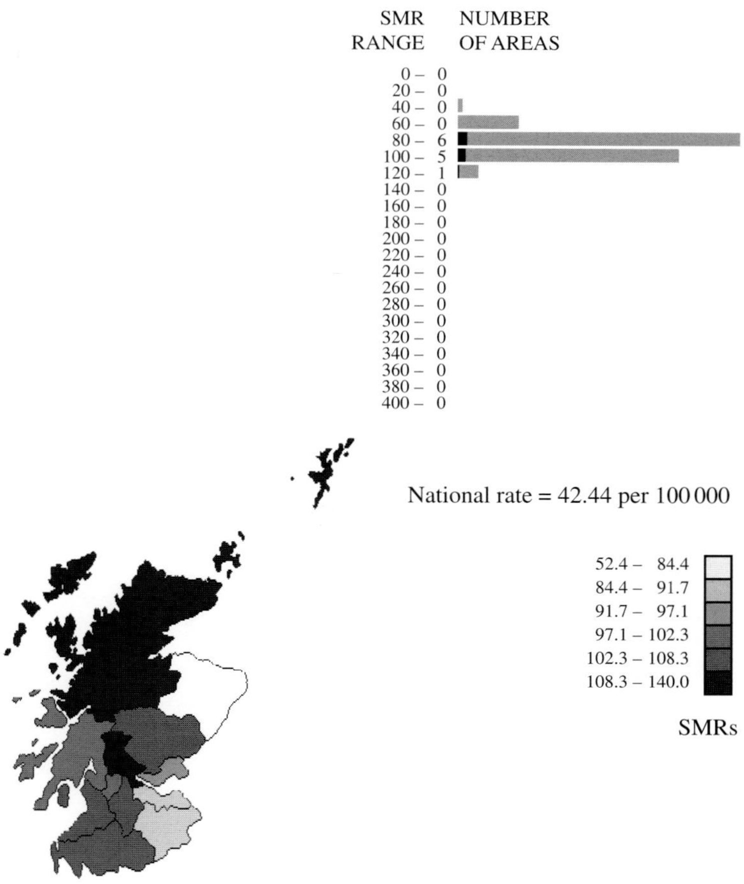

ISCHAEMIC HEART DISEASE MORTALITY AGES 35–64: 1985–89

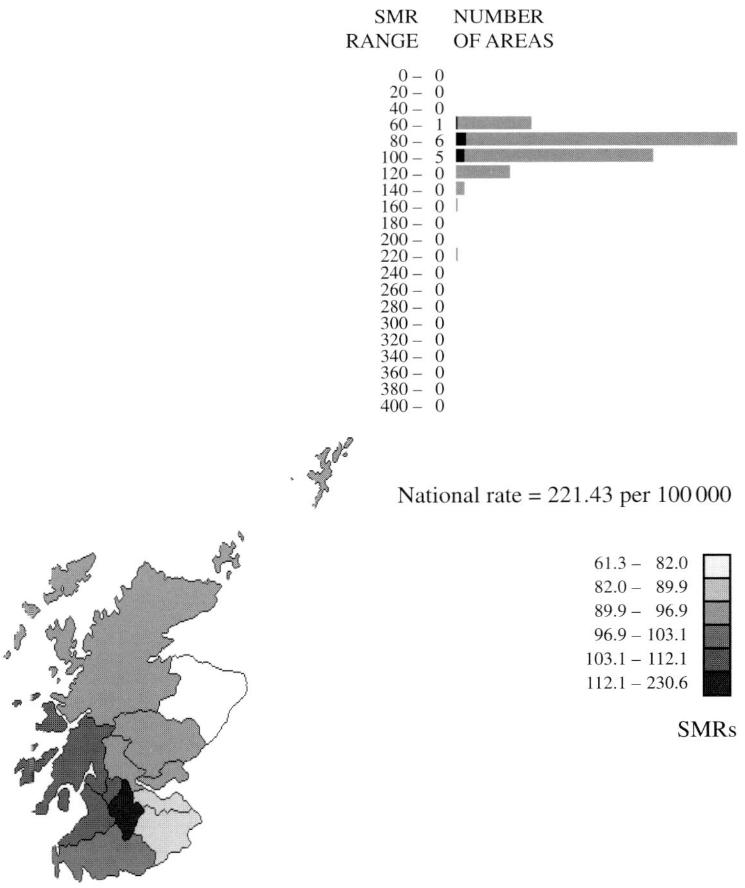

PEPTIC ULCERS MORTALITY AGES 25–64: 1985–89

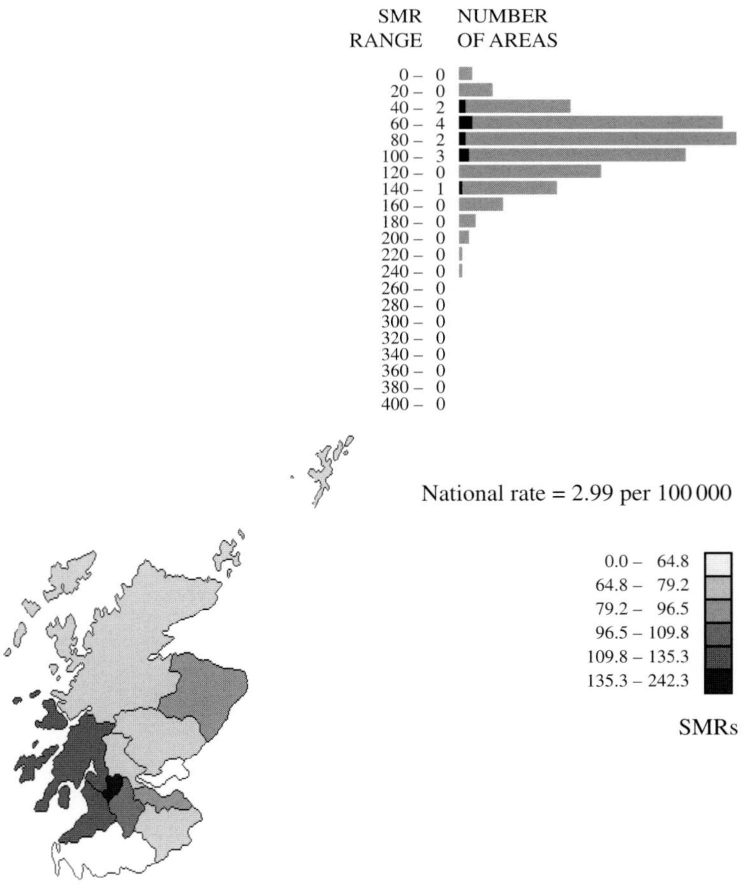

ALL CAUSES MORTALITY AGES 5–64: 1985–89

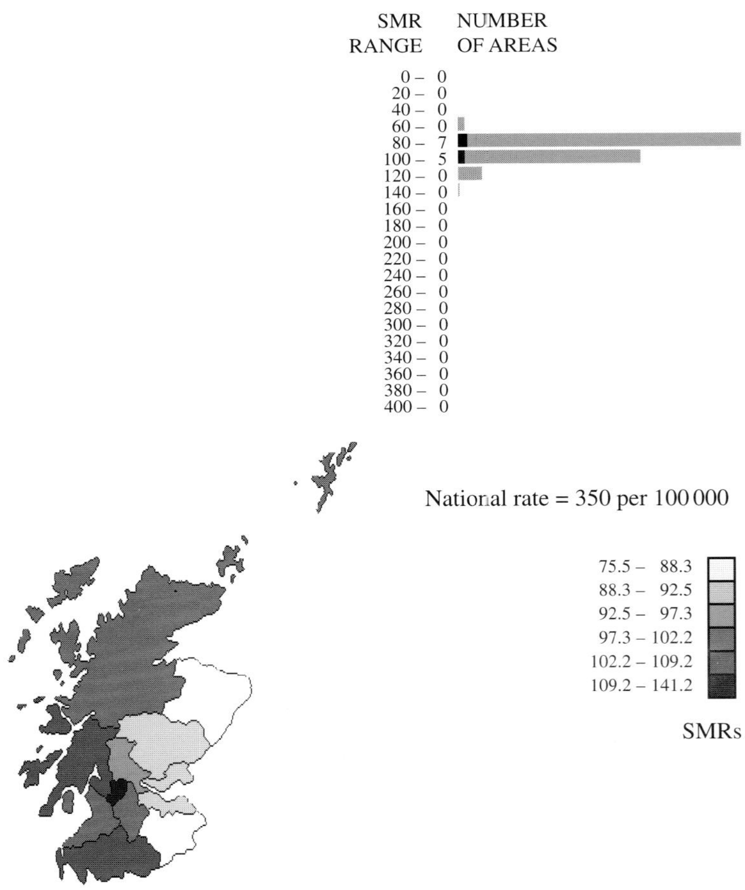

ALL CAUSES MORTALITY ALL AGES: 1985–89

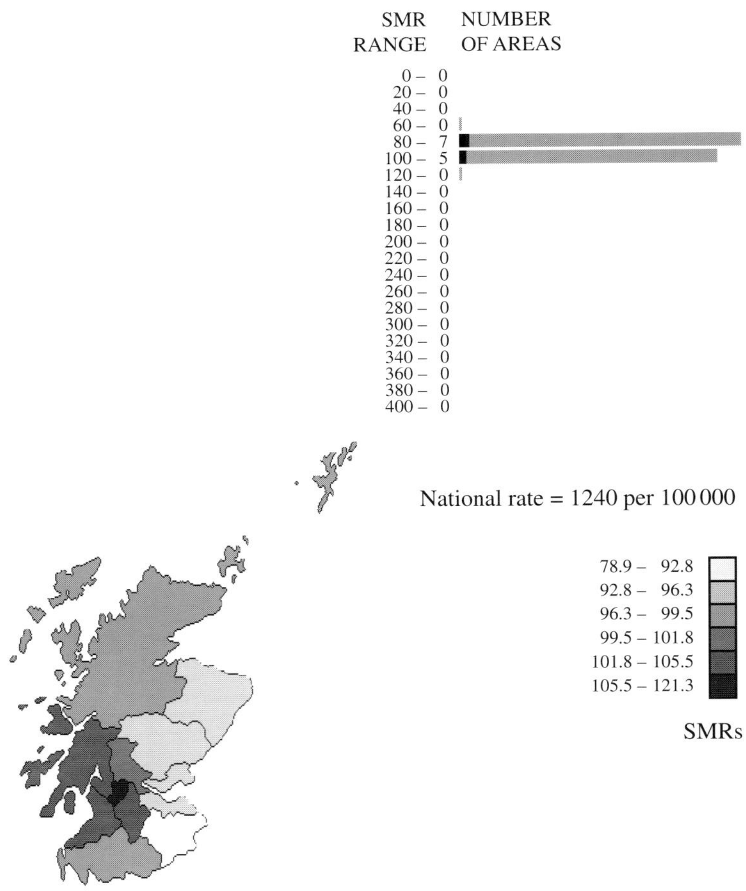

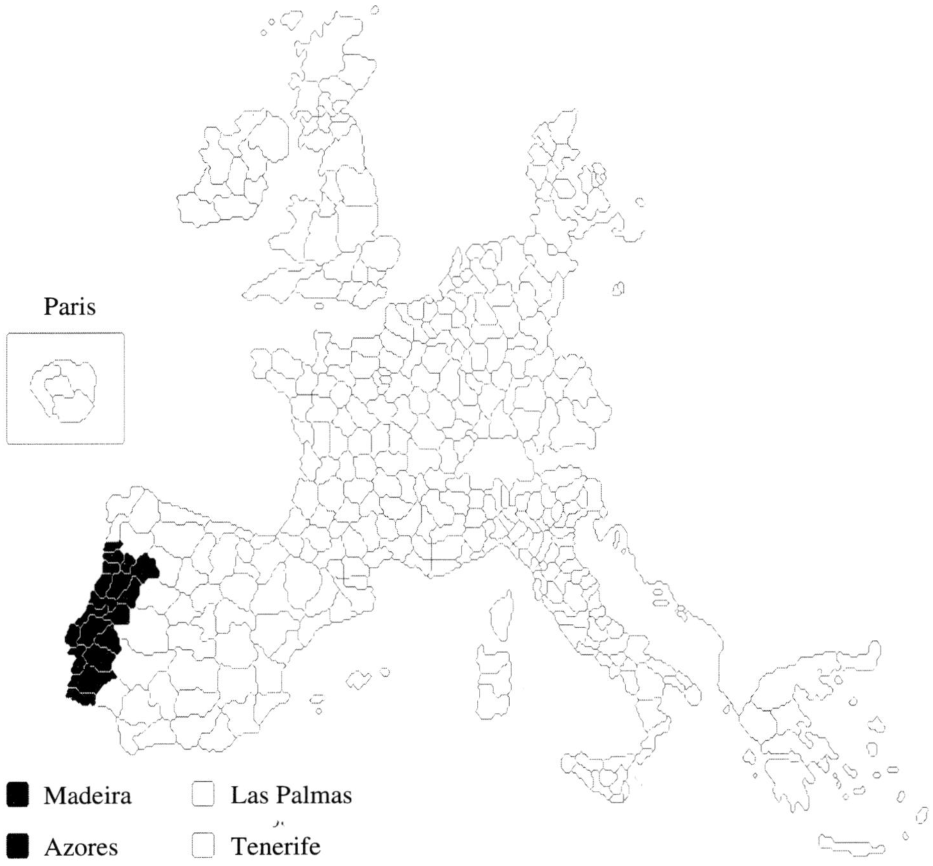

KEY MAP: PORTUGAL

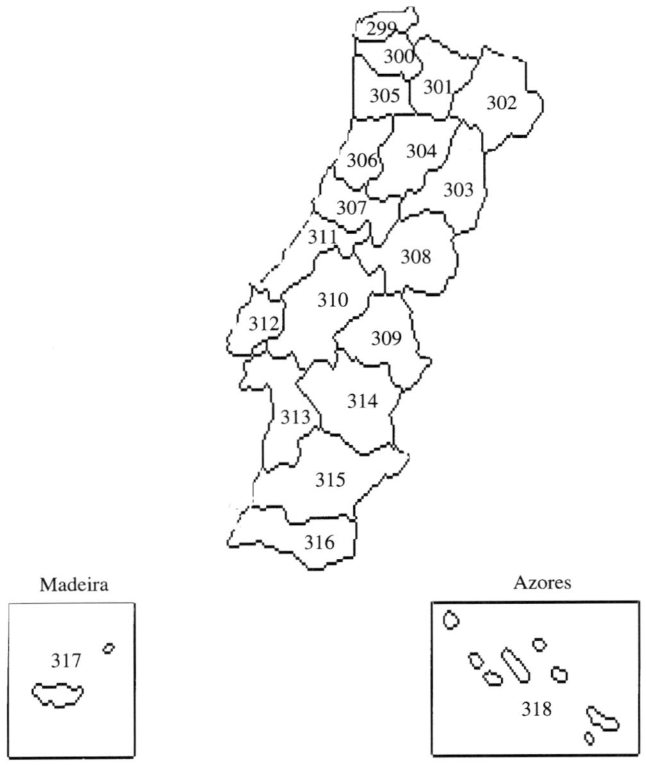

TUBERCULOSIS MORTALITY AGES 5–64: 1985–89

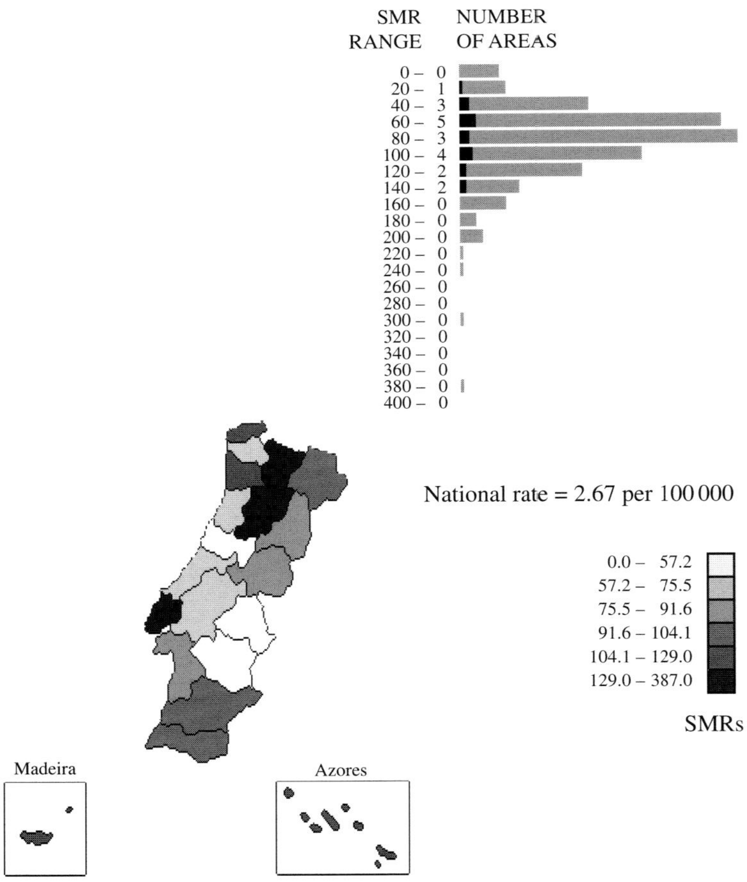

MALIGNANT NEOPLASM OF CERVIX UTERI MORTALITY AGES 15–64: 1985–89

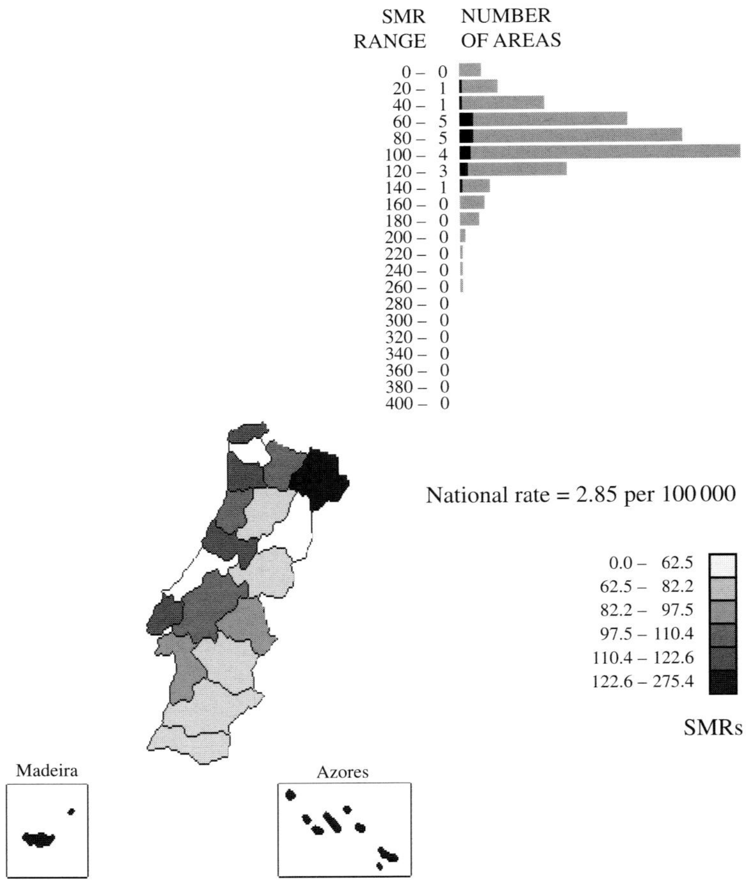

MALIGNANT NEOPLASM OF CERVIX AND BODY OF UTERUS MORTALITY AGES 15–54: 1985–89

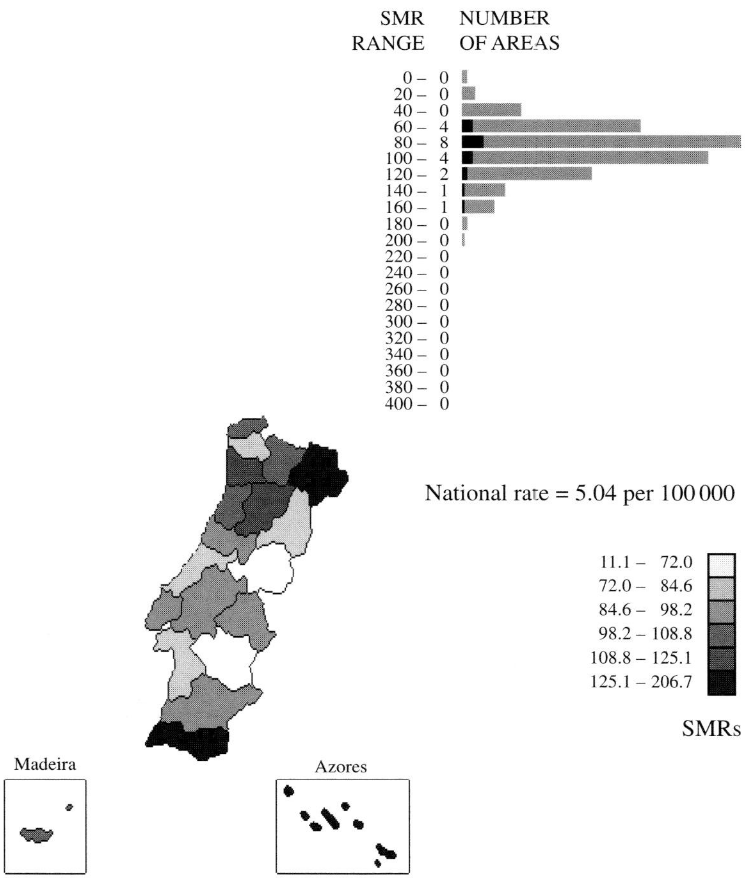

HODGKIN'S DISEASE MORTALITY AGES 5–64: 1985–89

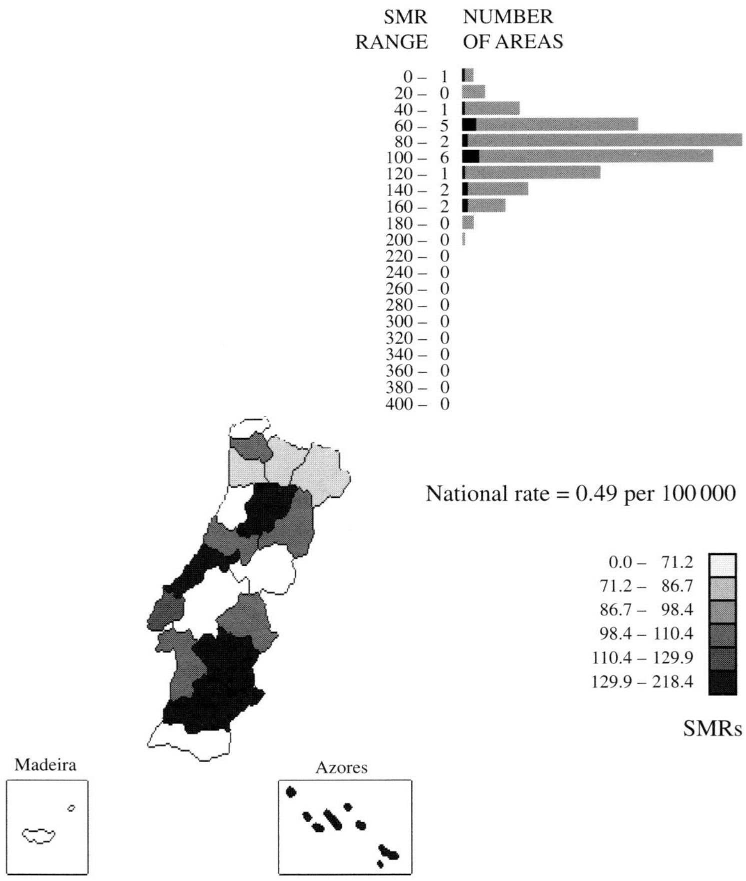

CHRONIC RHEUMATIC HEART DISEASE MORTALITY AGES 5–44: 1985–89

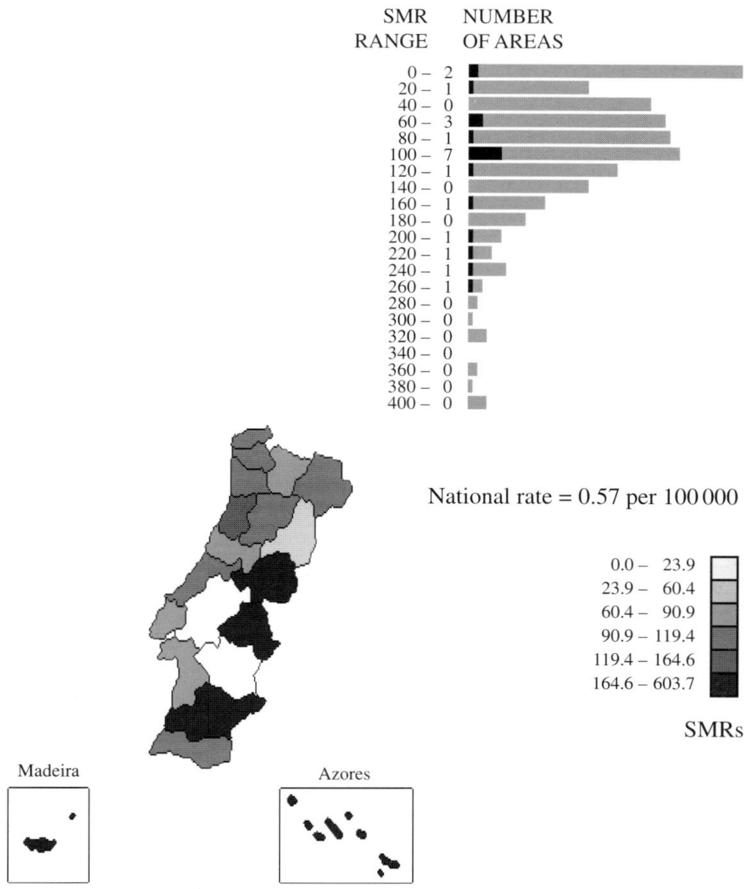

ALL RESPIRATORY DISEASES MORTALITY AGES 1–14: 1985–89

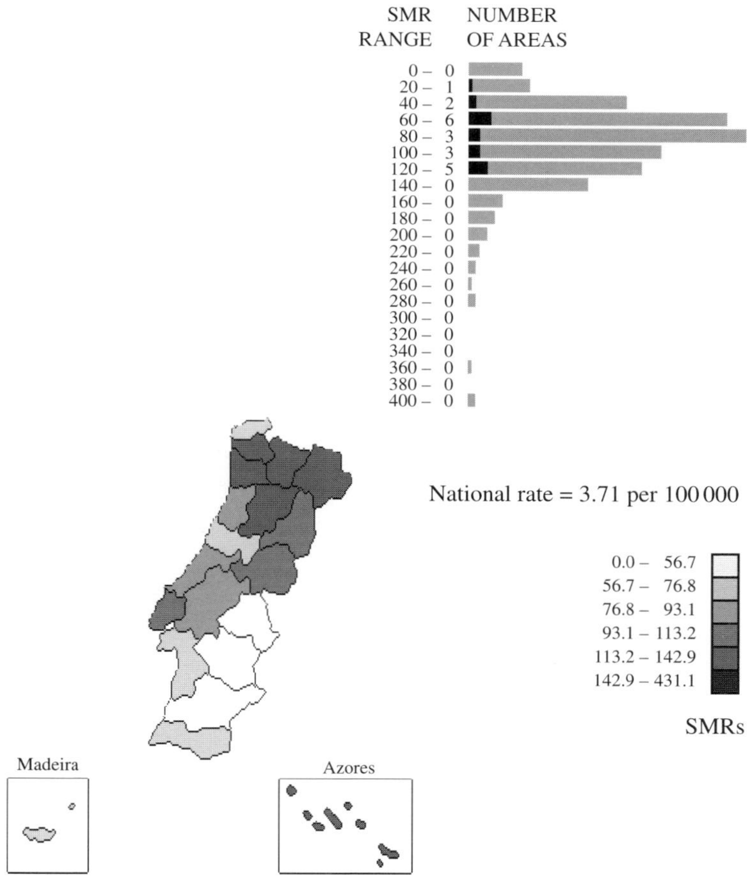

ASTHMA MORTALITY AGES 5–44: 1985–89

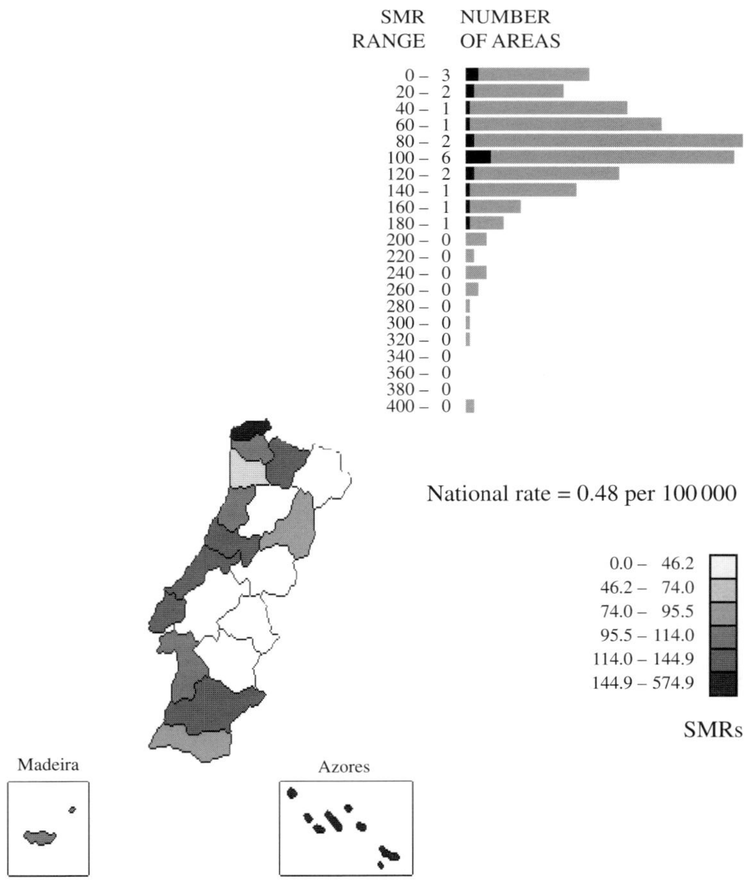

APPENDICITIS MORTALITY AGES 5–64: 1985–89

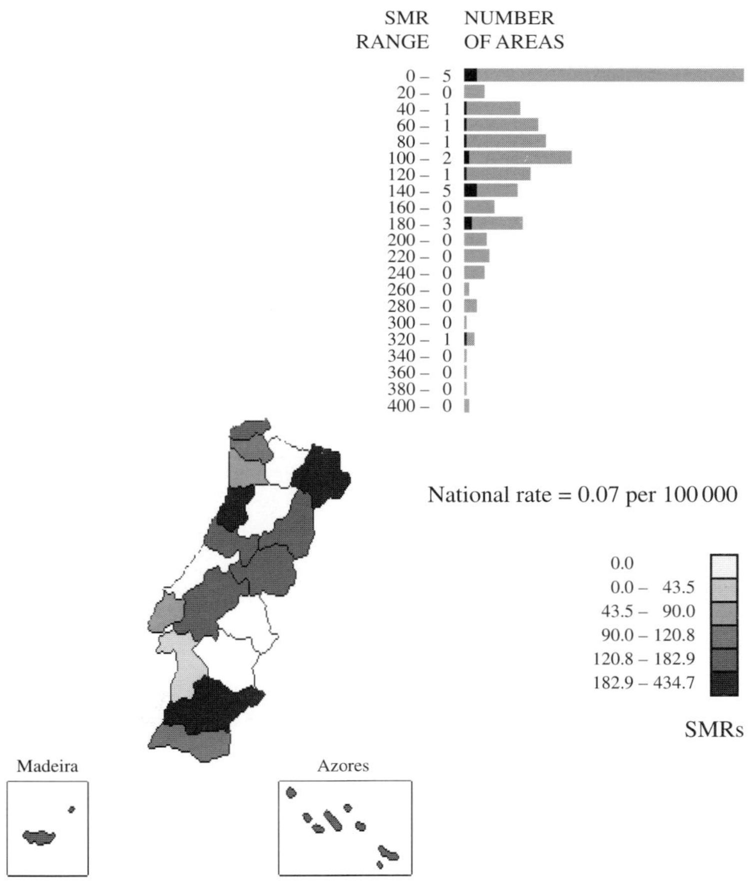

ABDOMINAL HERNIA MORTALITY AGES 5–64: 1985–89

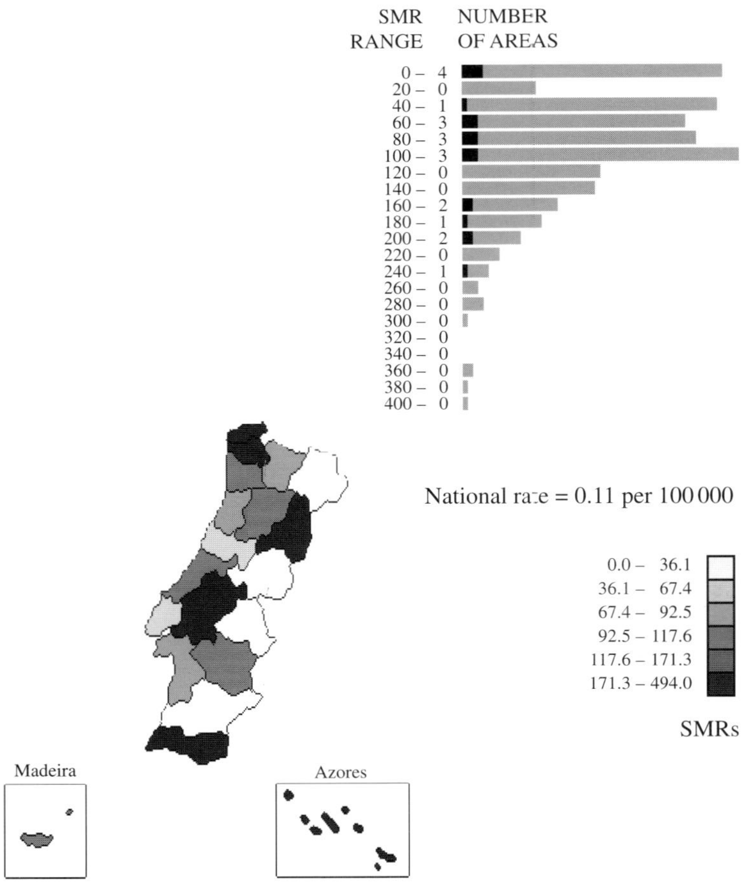

CHOLELITHIASIS AND CHOLECYSTITIS MORTALITY AGES 5–64: 1985–89

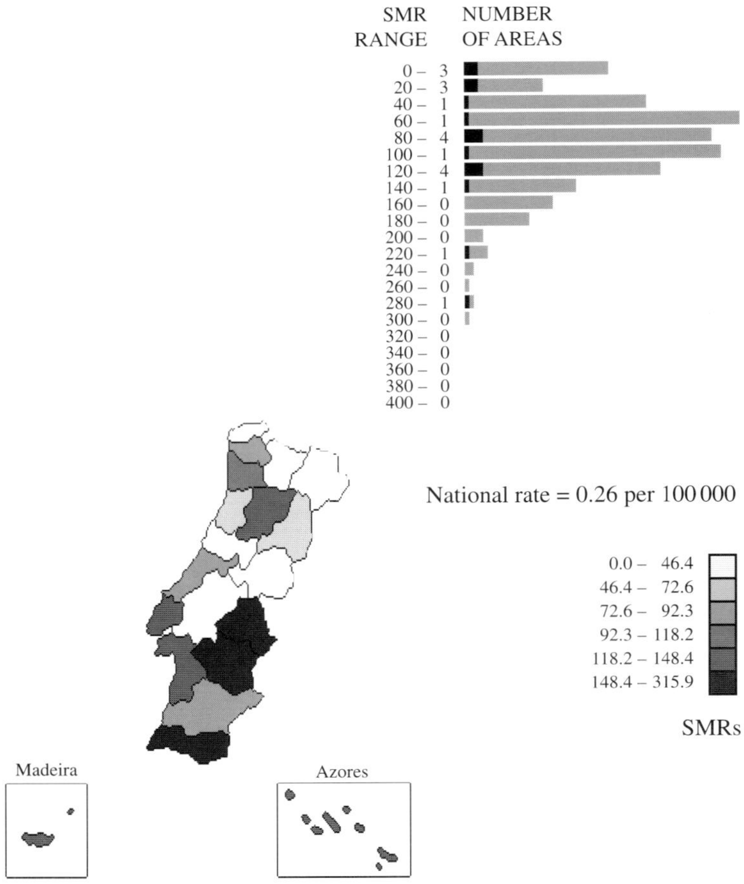

HYPERTENSIVE AND CEREBROVASCULAR DISEASES MORTALITY AGES 35–64: 1985–89

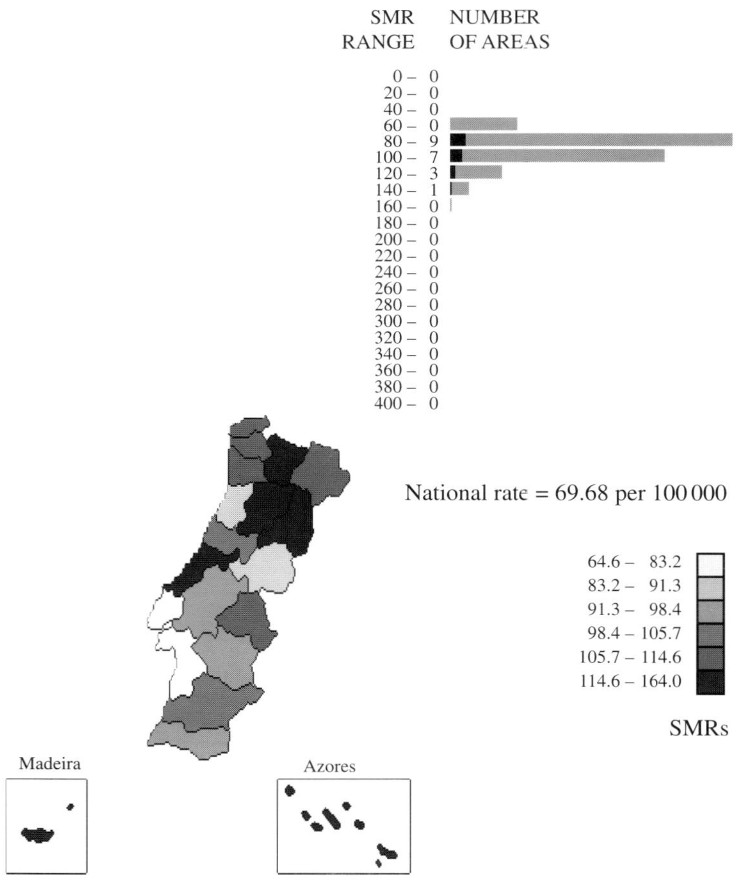

MATERNAL MORTALITY ALL AGES: 1985–89

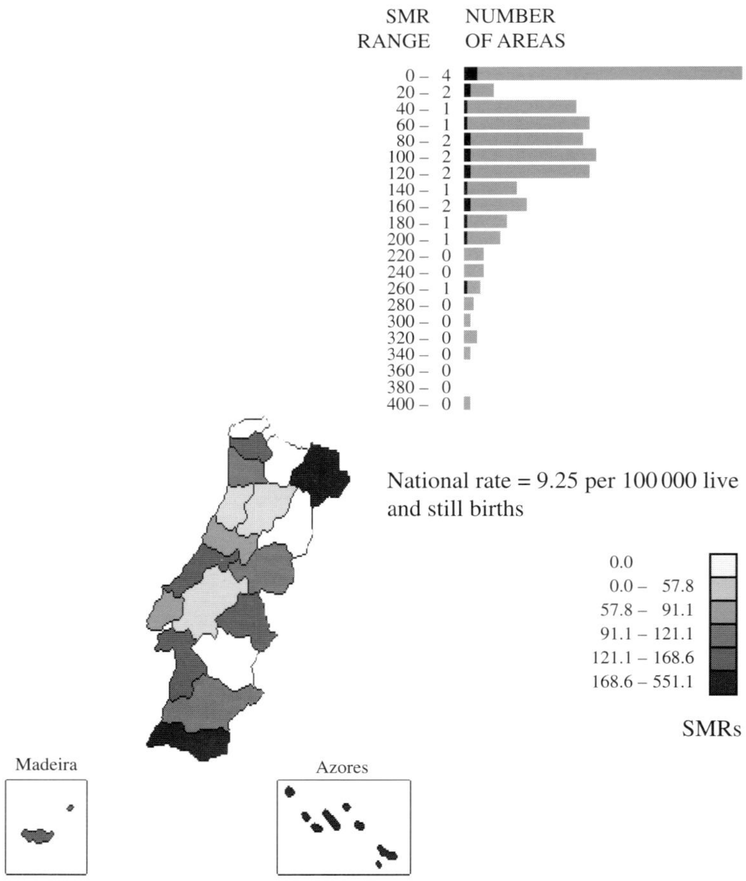

PERINATAL MORTALITY: 1985–89

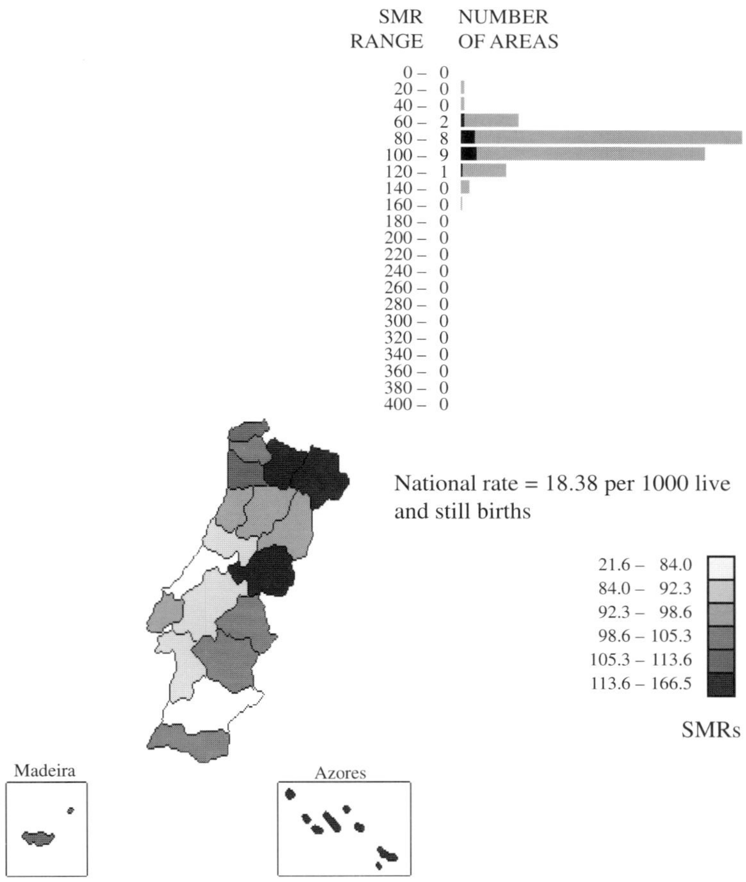

CANCER OF THE BREAST MORTALITY AGES 25–64: 1985–89

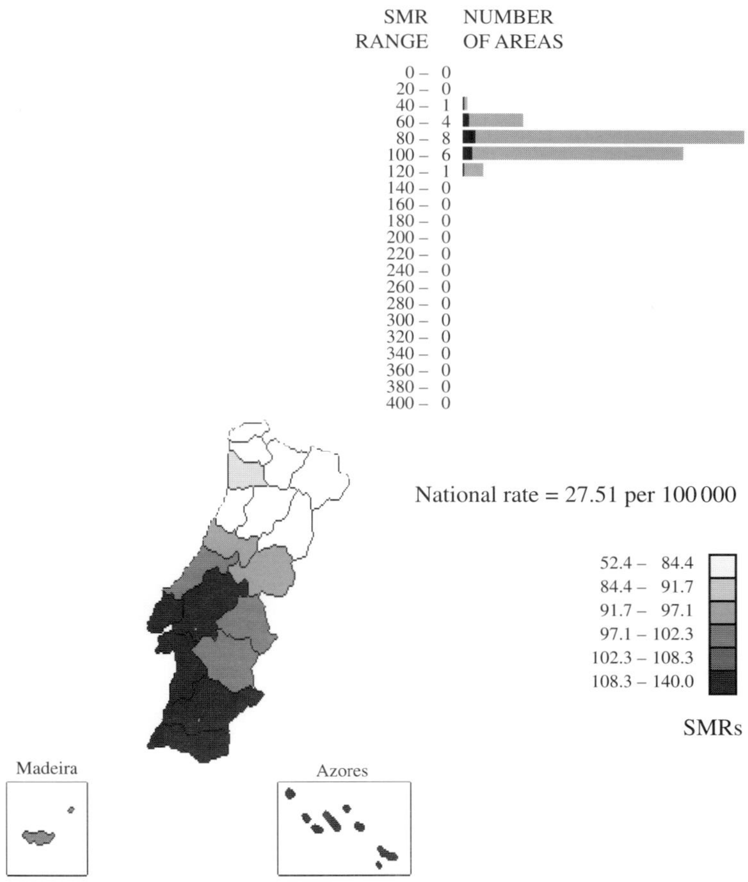

ISCHAEMIC HEART DISEASE MORTALITY AGES 35–64: 1985–89

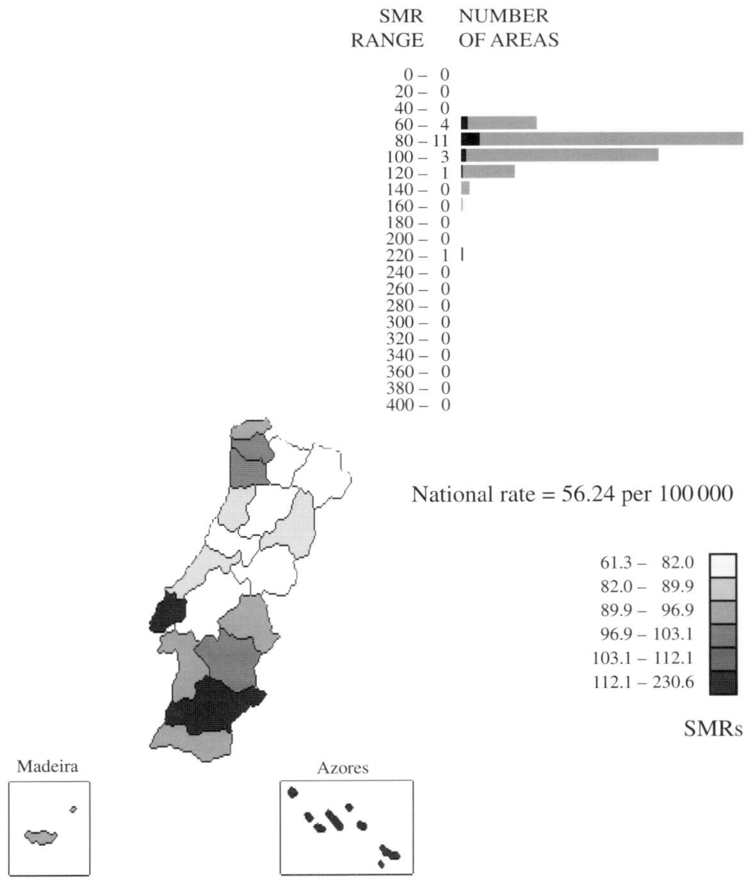

PEPTIC ULCERS MORTALITY AGES 25–64: 1985–89

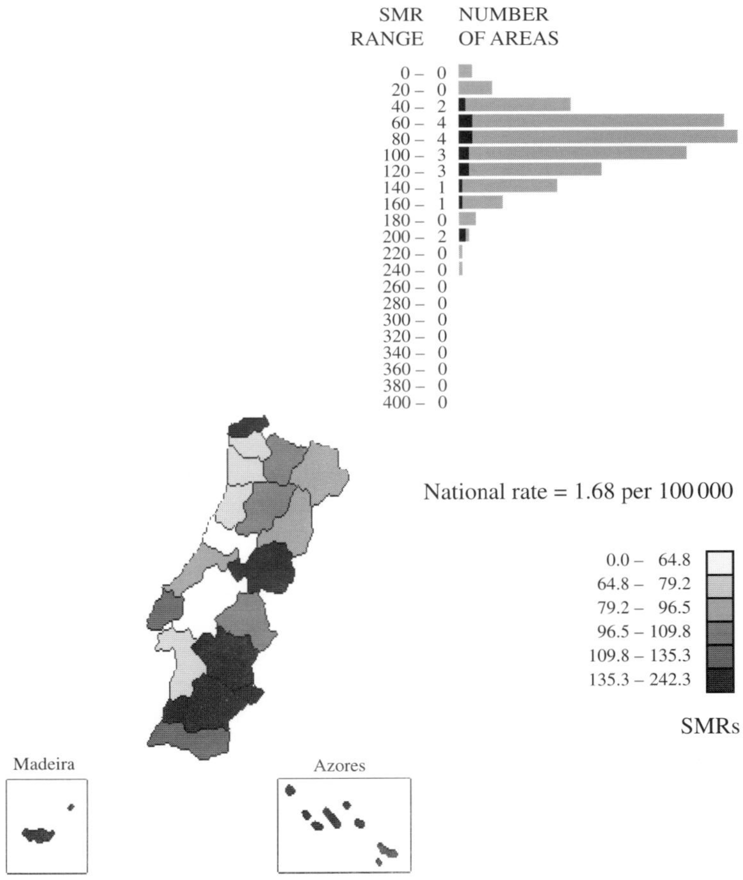

ALL CAUSES MORTALITY AGES 5–64: 1985–89

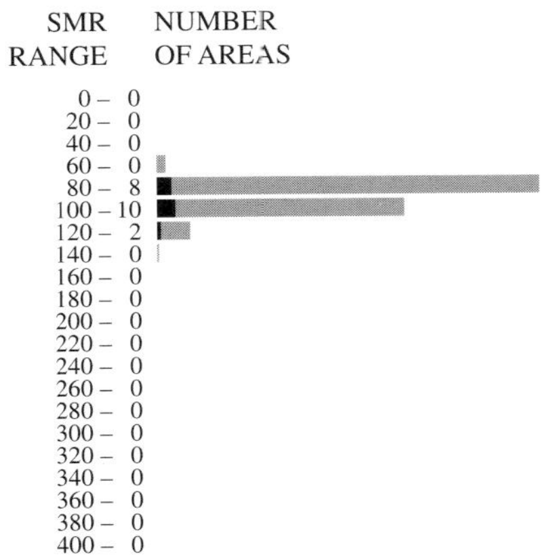

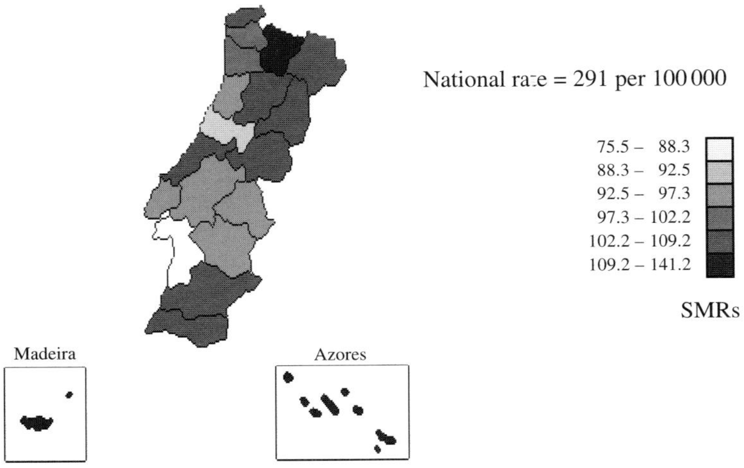

ALL CAUSES MORTALITY ALL AGES: 1985–89

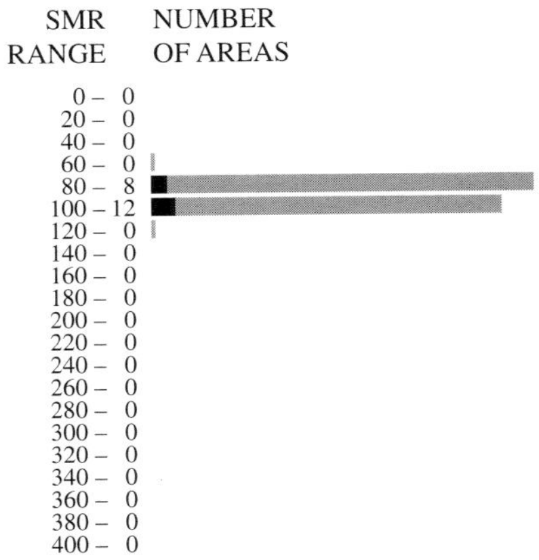

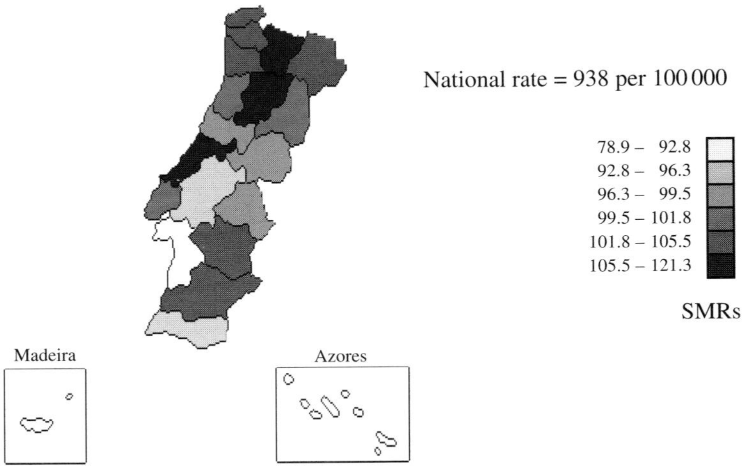

SPAIN

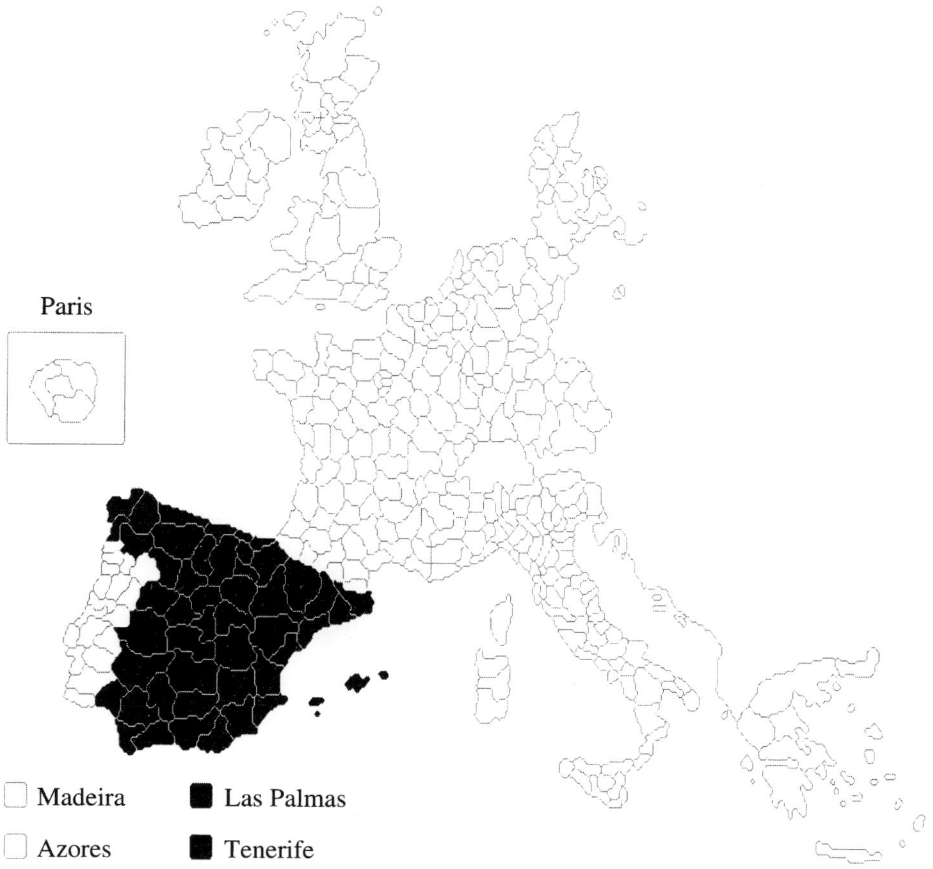

KEY MAP: SPAIN

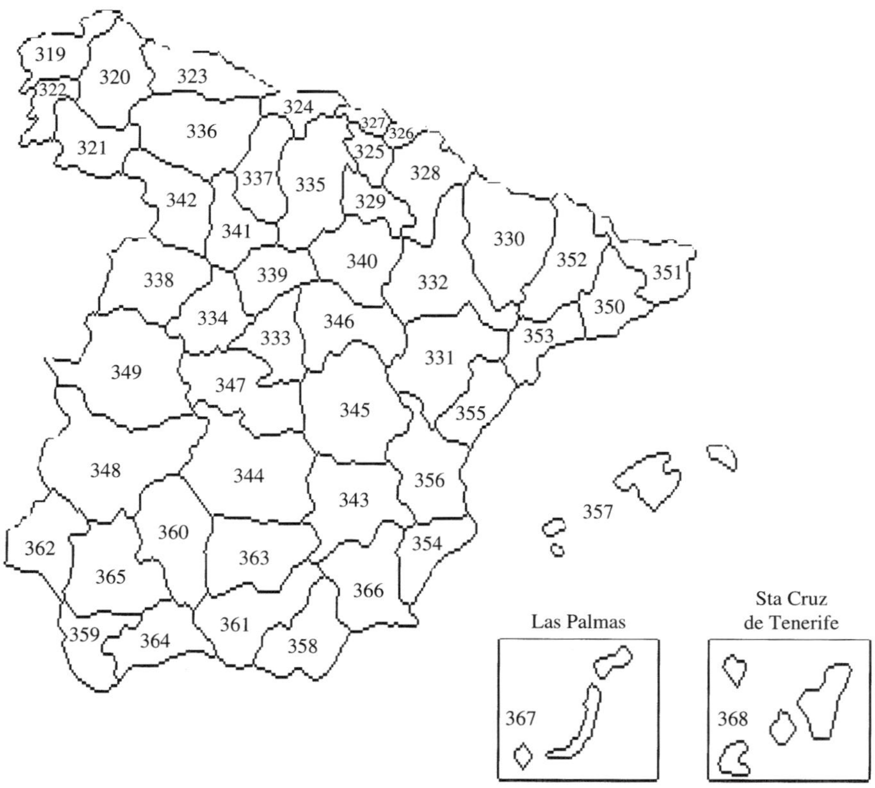

TUBERCULOSIS MORTALITY AGES 5–64: 1985–89

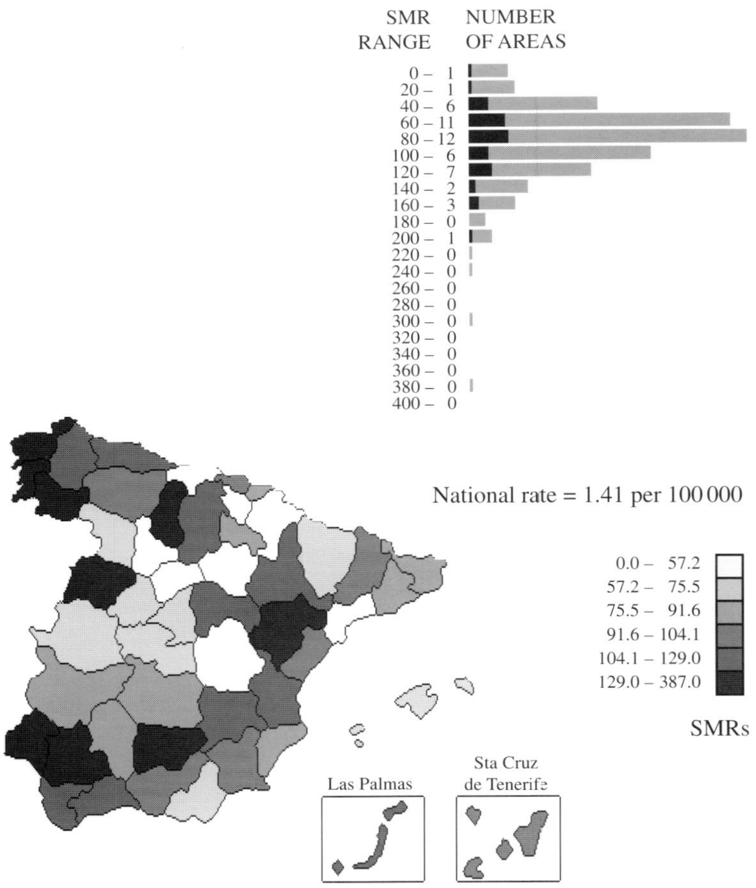

MALIGNANT NEOPLASM OF CERVIX UTERI MORTALITY AGES 15–64: 1985–89

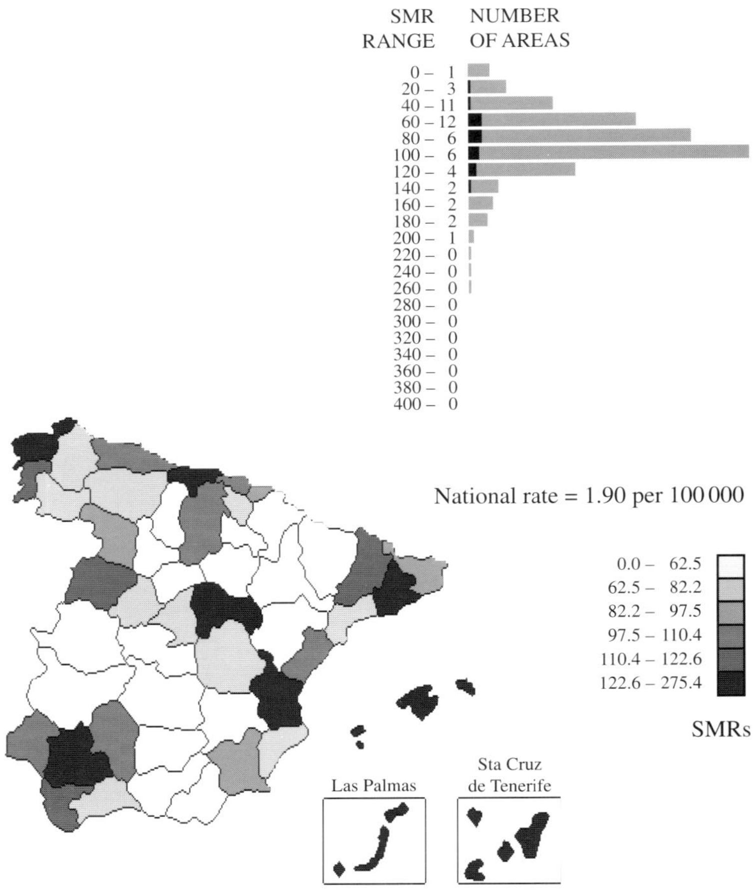

MALIGNANT NEOPLASM OF CERVIX AND BODY OF UTERUS MORTALITY AGES 15–54: 1985–89

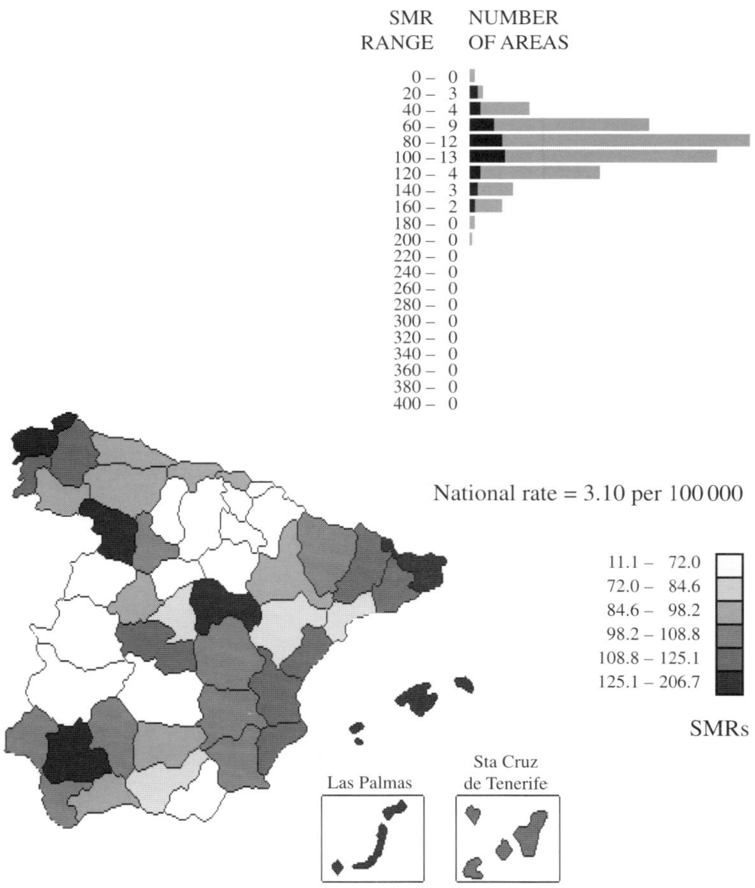

HODGKIN'S DISEASE MORTALITY AGES 5–64: 1985–89

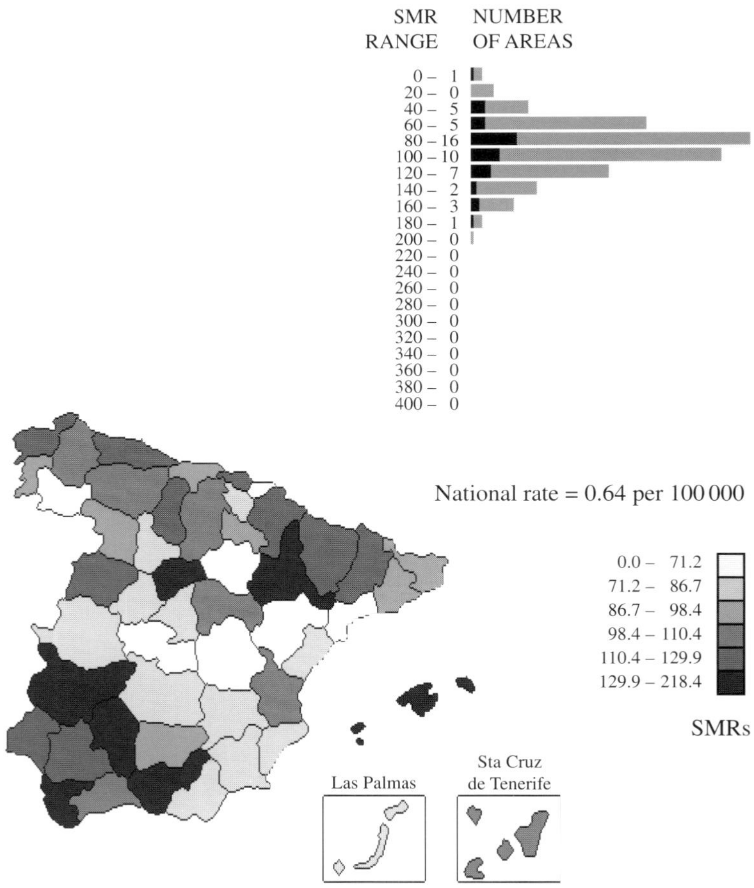

CHRONIC RHEUMATIC HEART DISEASE MORTALITY AGES 5–44: 1985–89

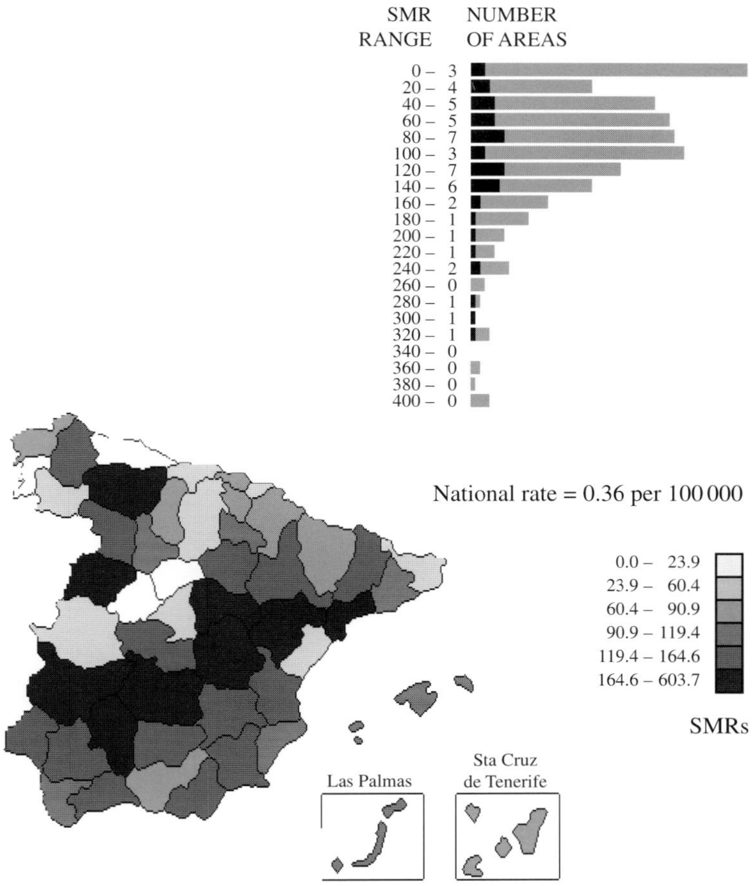

ALL RESPIRATORY DISEASES MORTALITY AGES 1–14: 1985–89

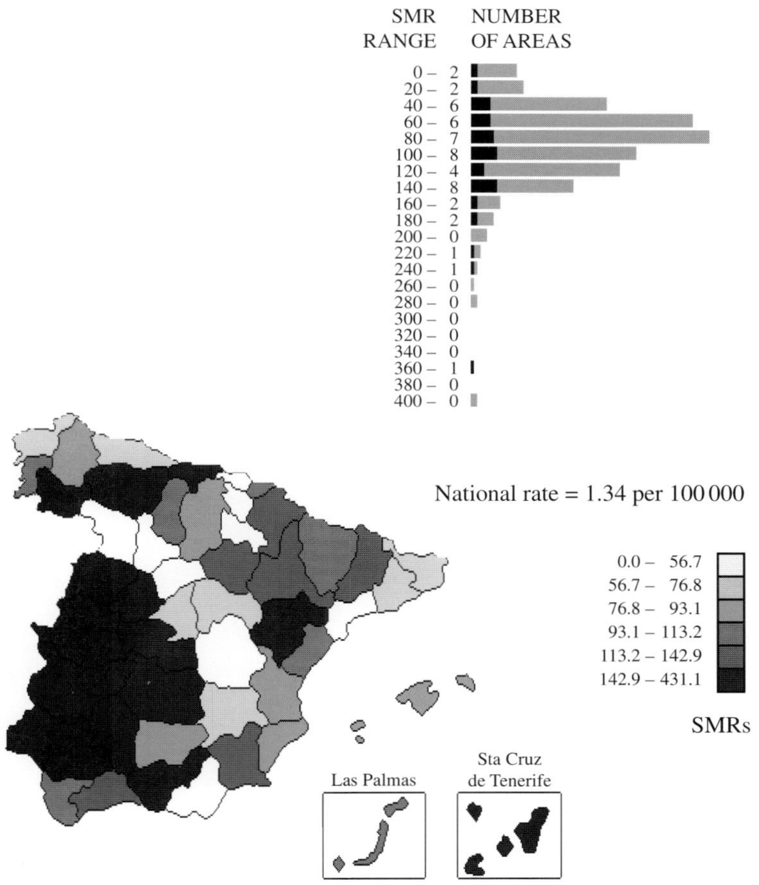

ASTHMA MORTALITY AGES 5–44: 1985–89

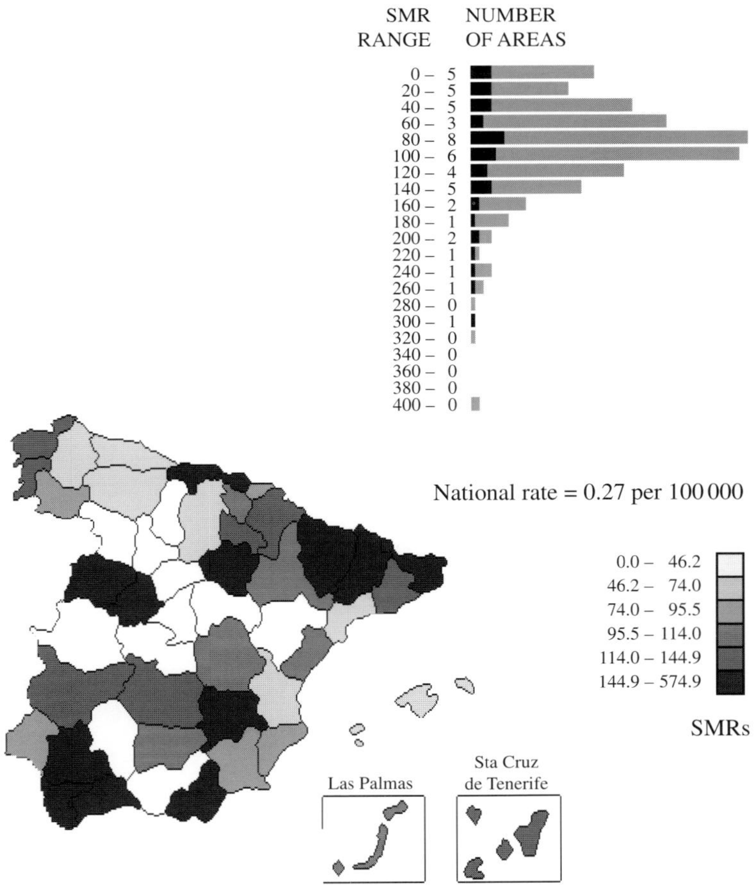

APPENDICITIS MORTALITY AGES 5–64: 1985–89

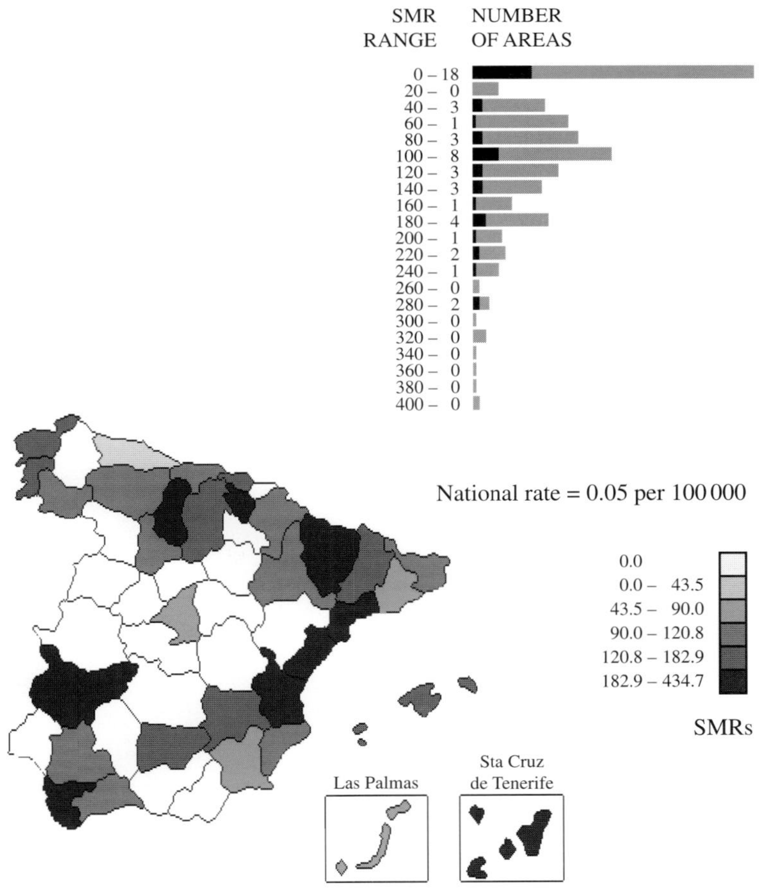

ABDOMINAL HERNIA MORTALITY AGES 5–64: 1985–89

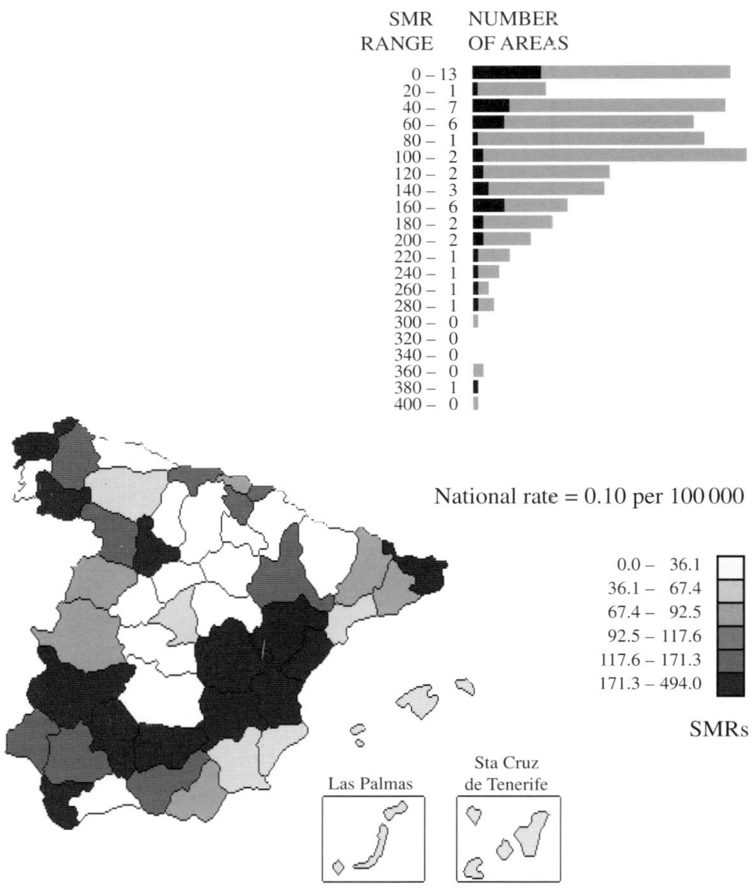

CHOLELITHIASIS AND CHOLECYSTITIS MORTALITY AGES 5–64: 1985–89

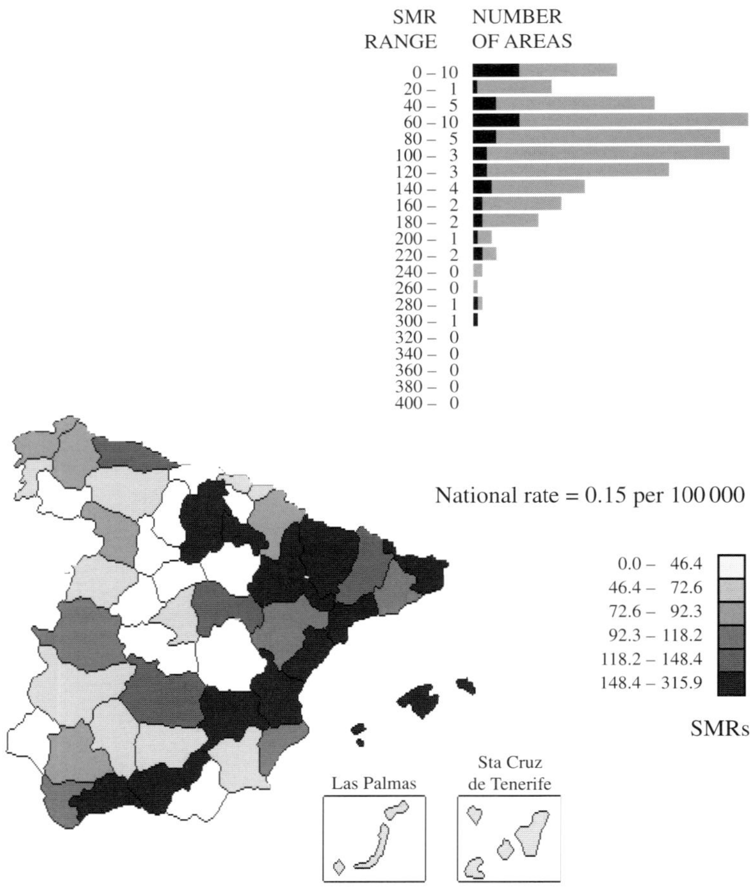

HYPERTENSIVE AND CEREBROVASCULAR DISEASES MORTALITY AGES 35–64: 1985–89

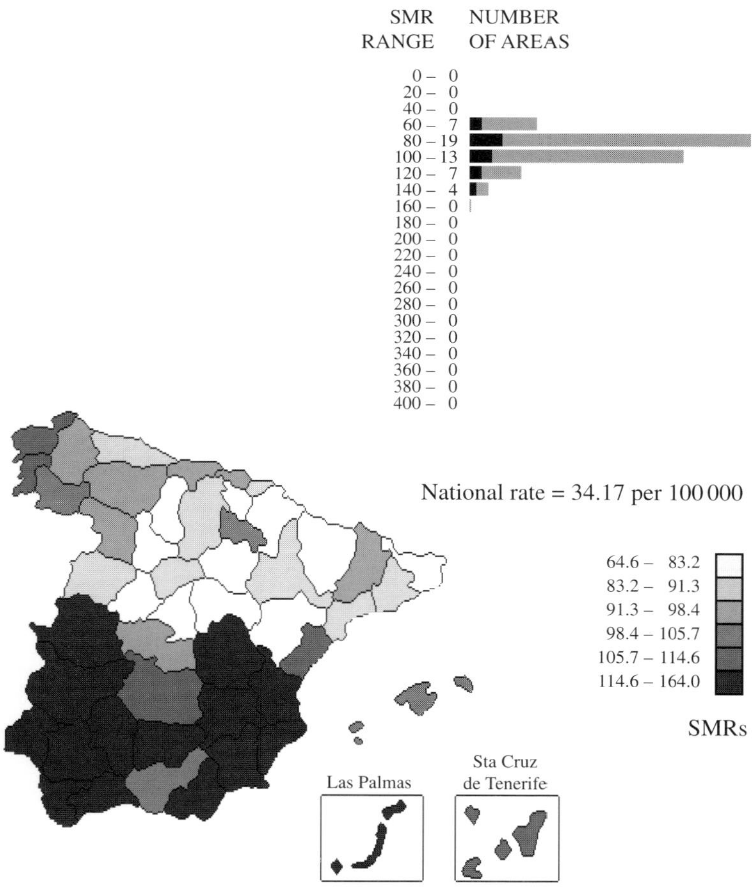

MATERNAL MORTALITY ALL AGES: 1985–89

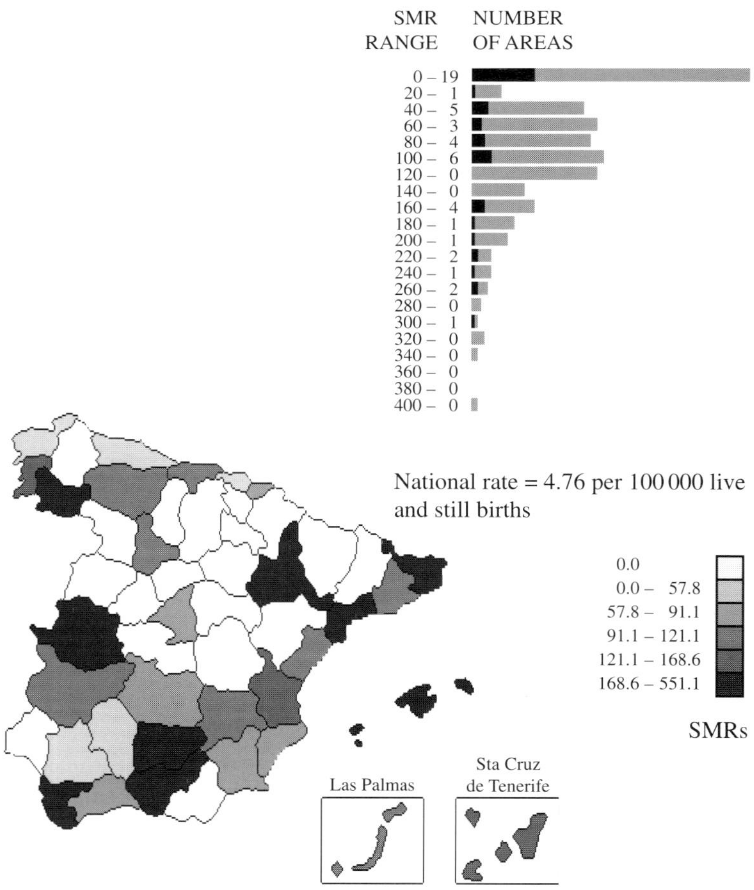

PERINATAL MORTALITY: 1985–89

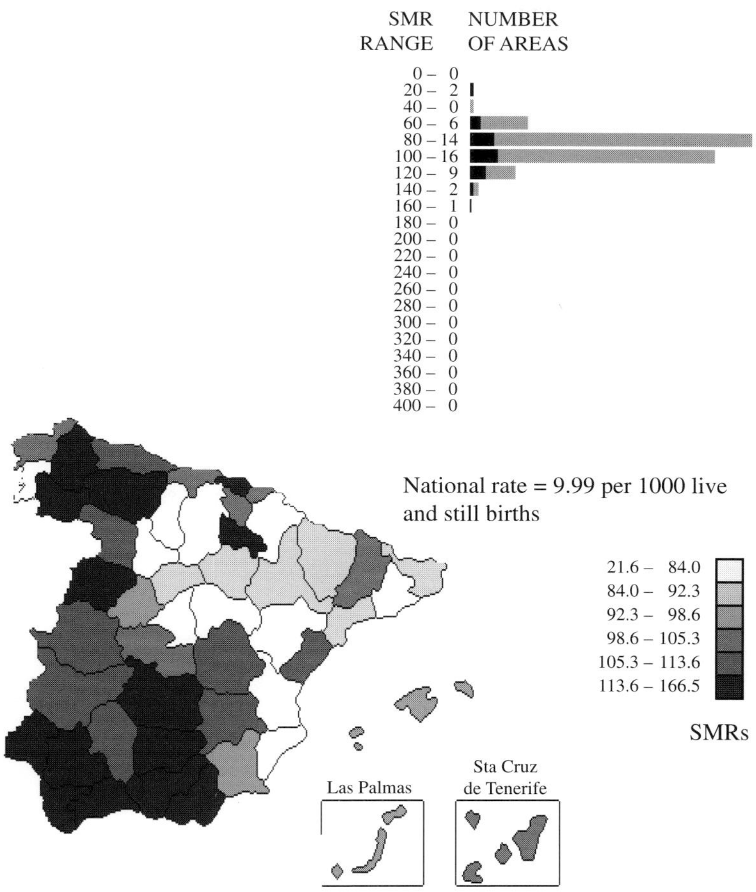

CANCER OF THE BREAST MORTALITY AGES 25–64: 1985–89

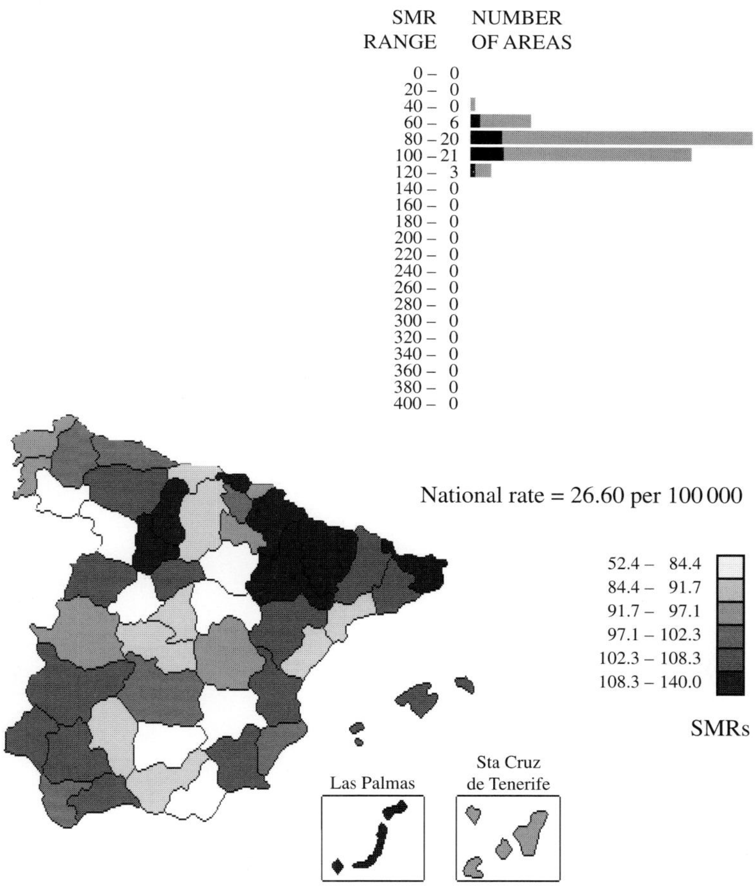

ISCHAEMIC HEART DISEASE MORTALITY AGES 35–64: 1985–89

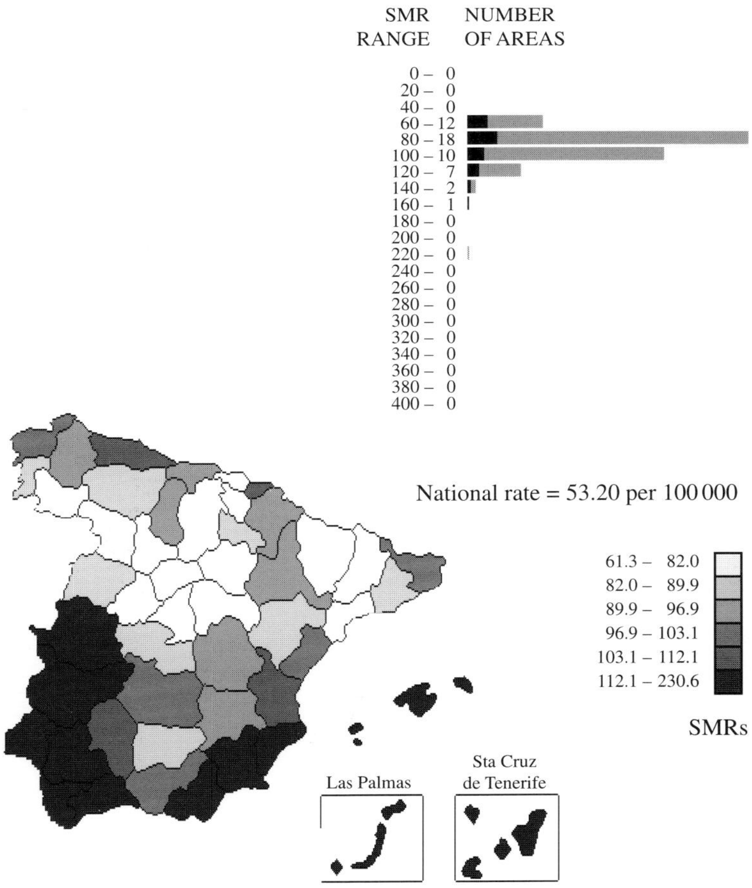

PEPTIC ULCERS MORTALITY AGES 25–64: 1985–89

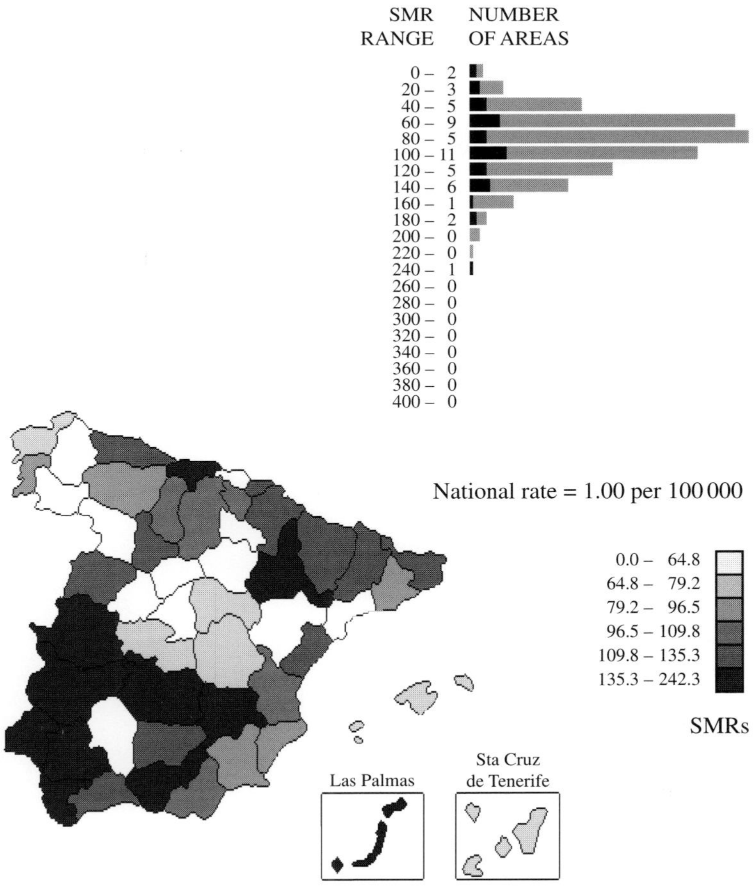

ALL CAUSES MORTALITY AGES 5–64: 1985–89

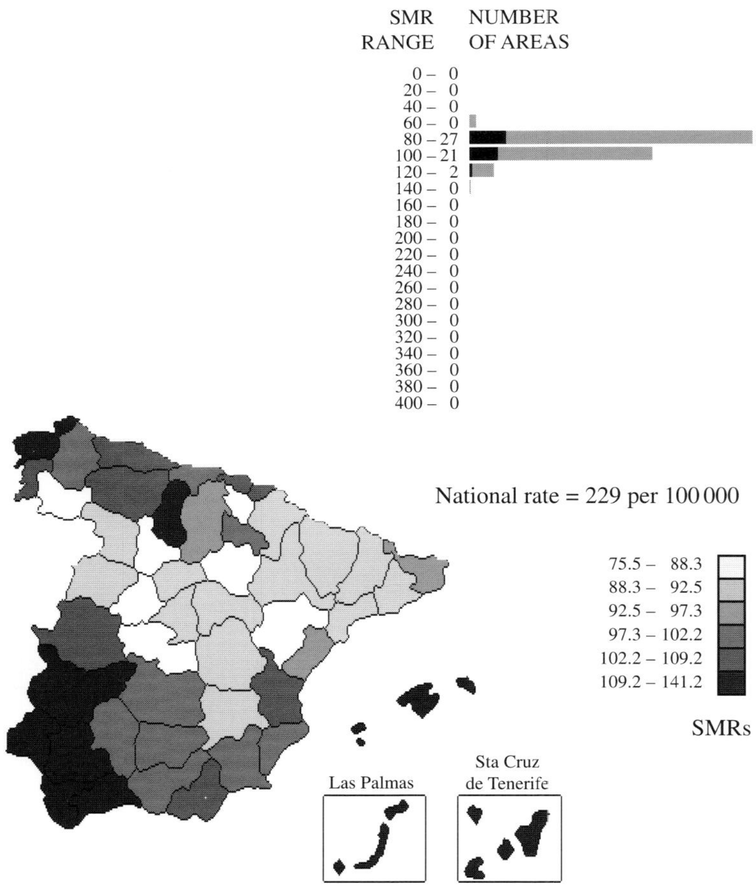

ALL CAUSES MORTALITY ALL AGES: 1985–89

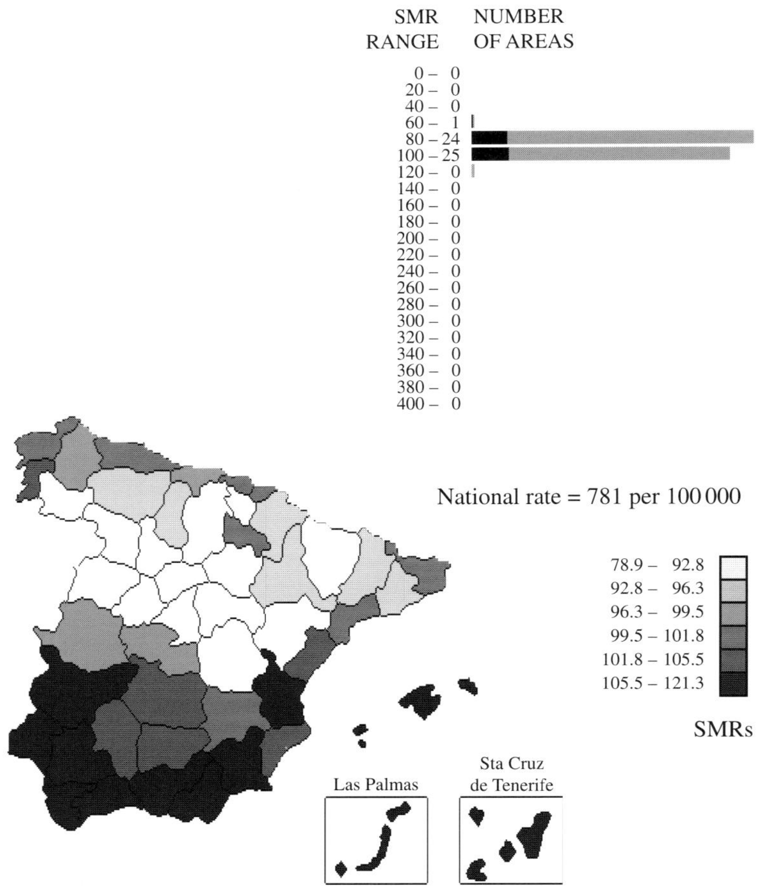

8. TABLES FOR THE PERIOD 1985–89

Table 8.1. Population, total deaths and total 'avoidable deaths' by small area and country.

Table 8.2. Observed numbers of 'avoidable deaths' and 'avoidable death' indicators by disease, small area and country.

Table 8.3. Observed numbers of 'avoidable deaths', age-standardized mortality rates, range and heterogeneity of SMRs (chi-square) by disease and country.

Table 8.1. Population, total deaths and total 'avoidable deaths' by small area and country.

Notes on the use of this table

1. This table shows average populations in thousands, total numbers of all 'avoidable deaths', total numbers of deaths from all causes (age group 5–64) and the percentage of all deaths which are 'avoidable' in the 5–64 age group.

2. The mortality data are for 1985–89 and cover five years, except for The Netherlands (four years, 1985–88) and Spain (four years, 1985–88). The population data are for 1985–89, except for France (1987), Greece (1987), Ireland (1986), and Spain (1986).

3. All countries supplied data according to the 9th revision of the International Classification of Diseases except for Denmark where 8th revision coding rules applied. For key to abbreviations used, please see page xv.

4. The small area numbers are as in the key maps.

Table 8.1

Area		Total population (thousands)			Total avoidable deaths	Total deaths (ages 5-64)	'Avoidable deaths' as a percentage of total deaths (ages 5–64)
		Total	Males	Females			
BELGIUM		9985.4	4875.2	5110.1	33058	122462	27.0
1	Antwerpen	1599.1	787.8	811.2	4980	17560	28.4
2	Brabant	2250.4	1084.1	1166.3	7327	26794	27.3
3	West-Vlaanderen	1107.9	546.1	561.7	3182	12288	25.9
4	Oost-Vlaanderen	1341.0	659.9	681.1	4359	15718	27.7
5	Hainaut	1291.0	622.3	668.7	4795	19336	24.8
6	Liege	1004.6	485.3	519.3	3869	14260	27.1
7	Limburg	741.8	373.0	368.8	2231	7498	29.8
8	Luxembourg (province)	230.2	113.1	117.1	765	3023	25.3
9	Namur	419.4	203.6	215.8	1550	5985	25.9
LUXEMBOURG		371.3	180.7	190.6	1465	5007	29.3
10	Luxembourg	371.3	180.7	190.6	1465	5007	29.3
FEDERAL REPUBLIC OF GERMANY		61401.4	29466.5	31934.9	216885	755733	28.7
11	Schleswig-Holstein	2583.1	1246.8	1336.4	9222	30890	29.9
12	Hamburg	1592.4	746.2	846.2	5212	21922	23.8
13	Braunschweig	1595.2	765.9	829.3	5820	19645	29.6
14	Hannover	2011.6	956.0	1055.6	7251	25593	28.3
15	Lüneburg	1460.5	712.1	748.4	4882	17573	27.8
16	Weser-Ems	2131.1	1033.4	1097.7	7397	24873	29.7
17	Bremen	661.3	312.1	349.2	2350	9327	25.2
18	Düsseldorf	5078.4	2412.1	2666.3	20354	69586	29.3
19	Köln	3890.9	1876.7	2014.2	13839	46984	29.5
20	Munster	2404.2	1160.2	1244.0	9149	31000	29.5
21	Detmold	1802.1	859.8	942.3	6279	21488	29.2
22	Arnsberg	3605.7	1727.1	1878.6	15150	49906	30.4
23	Darmstadt	3413.5	1642.9	1770.5	11500	40915	28.1
24	Giessen	961.8	467.0	494.8	3332	11199	29.8
25	Kassel	1168.6	561.7	606.9	3985	13748	29.0
26	Koblenz	1353.9	651.0	702.9	5208	16962	30.7
27	Trier	471.7	226.6	245.0	1707	6051	28.2
28	Rheinhessen-Pfalz	1812.2	871.4	940.8	6851	23147	29.6
29	Stuttgart	3511.0	1706.3	1804.7	10647	37030	28.8
30	Karlsruhe	2418.1	1162.3	1255.8	8290	28378	29.2
31	Freiburg	1888.2	905.5	982.7	5615	20111	27.9
32	Tübingen	1541.4	747.7	793.7	4356	15335	28.4
33	Oberbayern	3689.2	1777.6	1911.6	10768	39986	26.9
34	Niederbayern	1026.6	492.8	533.8	3553	12783	27.8
35	Oberpfalz	969.6	467.4	502.2	3731	12801	29.1
36	Oberfranken	1039.6	493.9	545.7	4235	14125	30.0
37	Mittelfranken	1529.4	730.5	798.9	5637	19095	29.5
38	Unterfranken	1208.4	584.1	624.2	3852	13682	28.2
39	Schwaben	1555.1	747.4	807.8	4989	17747	28.1
40	Saarland	1051.6	502.8	548.8	4664	15023	31.0
41	Berlin (West)	1974.9	919.1	1055.8	7060	28828	24.5

Table 8.1—*cont.*

Area		Total population (thousands)			Total avoidable deaths	Total deaths (ages 5-64)	'Avoidable deaths' as a percentage of total deaths (ages 5–64)
		Total	Males	Females			
DENMARK		5126.3	2527.0	2599.3	20279	66033	30.7
42	Kobenhavn and Frederiksberg (M)	556.7	259.7	297.0	2383	9565	24.9
43	Kobenhavns County	605.9	294.6	311.3	2381	8240	28.9
44	Frederiksborg County	339.1	168.5	170.5	1220	4059	30.1
45	Roskilde County	213.8	106.7	107.1	807	2557	31.6
46	Vestsjællands County	282.0	140.6	141.4	1200	3676	32.6
47	Storstroms County	257.3	127.6	129.6	1164	3759	31.0
48	Bornholms County	46.7	23.3	23.4	217	524	41.4
49	Fyns County	456.8	225.6	231.2	1670	5575	30.0
50	Sonderjyllands County	249.9	124.4	125.5	1036	3056	33.9
51	Ribe County	219.3	111.3	108.0	855	2463	34.7
52	Vejle County	328.9	163.1	165.8	1222	3995	30.6
53	Ringkobing County	266.1	133.8	132.3	1053	3077	34.2
54	Århus County	590.0	290.8	299.3	2115	6717	31.5
55	Viborg County	230.6	115.9	114.8	920	2690	34.2
56	Nordjyllands County	483.3	241.1	242.2	2036	6080	33.5
FRANCE		55693.9	27139.1	28554.6	138746	647667	21.4
57	Ain	452.4	225.3	227.0	999	4585	21.8
58	Aisne	536.3	264.1	272.2	1519	7363	20.6
59	Allier	363.9	176.0	187.9	984	4700	20.9
60	Alpes-de-Haute-Provence	126.9	62.7	64.2	272	1389	19.6
61	Hautes-Alpes	110.3	54.9	55.4	258	1200	21.5
62	Alpes-Maritimes	934.7	438.7	496.0	2143	10470	20.5
63	Ardèche	273.6	134.2	139.4	649	3009	21.6
64	Ardennes	299.5	147.8	151.7	830	4090	20.3
65	Ariège	136.4	67.1	69.3	321	1454	22.1
66	Aube	290.6	142.6	148.0	734	3446	21.3
67	Aude	288.9	141.7	147.3	715	3039	23.5
68	Aveyron	273.6	134.2	139.5	636	2642	24.1
69	Bouches-du-Rhône	1740.4	845.0	895.5	4098	19523	21.0
70	Calvados	607.4	293.7	313.6	1394	6956	20.0
71	Cantal	160.3	79.1	81.2	490	2004	24.5
72	Charente	340.9	166.0	174.8	814	3958	20.6
73	Charente-Maritime	520.8	253.3	267.5	1224	5867	20.9
74	Cher	320.8	157.1	163.7	811	3918	20.7
75	Corrèze	239.8	116.4	123.4	647	2813	23.0
76	Corse	245.8	122.7	123.0	669	2938	22.8
77	Côte-d'Or	486.5	236.9	249.6	1121	5257	21.3
78	Côtes-du-Nord	539.7	261.5	278.2	1376	7653	18.0
79	Creuse	134.9	66.0	68.9	330	1810	18.2
80	Dordogne	383.4	186.1	197.3	1045	4616	22.6
81	Doubs	482.2	238.0	244.2	1216	4988	24.4
82	Drôme	413.2	202.3	210.9	937	4209	22.3
83	Eure	490.9	243.3	247.6	1244	6058	20.5
84	Eure-et-Loir	382.6	189.6	193.0	852	4182	20.4
85	Finistère	836.1	405.7	430.5	2026	11864	17.1
86	Gard	562.9	274.4	288.5	1448	6327	22.9
87	Haute-Garonne	884.3	429.4	454.9	1863	7946	23.4
88	Gers	174.5	86.6	87.9	416	1817	22.9
89	Gironde	1179.4	566.7	612.7	2670	12729	21.0
90	Hérault	761.5	365.9	395.6	1871	7716	24.2
91	Ille-et-Vilaine	778.1	377.3	400.9	1758	8589	20.5
92	Indre	239.6	117.1	122.5	575	2835	20.3
93	Indre-et-Loire	522.0	253.0	269.0	1048	5234	20.0
94	Isère	984.4	485.4	499.0	2149	9913	21.7
95	Jura	247.6	121.7	125.9	615	2732	22.5
96	Landes	306.6	149.7	156.9	749	3531	21.2
97	Loir-et-Cher	302.0	148.1	153.9	666	3297	20.2
98	Loire	745.3	360.9	384.4	1814	8285	21.9

Table 8.1—*cont.*

	Area	Total population (thousands)			Total avoidable deaths	Total deaths (ages 5-64)	'Avoidable deaths' as a percentage of total deaths (ages 5–64)
		Total	Males	Females			
99	Haute-Loire	206.6	101.5	105.1	537	2581	20.8
100	Loire-Atlantique	1032.6	500.0	532.6	2319	12436	18.6
101	Loiret	561.6	276.2	285.3	1311	6000	21.9
102	Lot	154.7	75.3	79.4	394	1659	23.7
103	Lot-et-Garonne	302.3	147.0	155.3	686	3137	21.9
104	Lozère	73.4	36.7	36.6	191	823	23.2
105	Maine-et-Loire	696.9	339.7	357.2	1447	6796	21.3
106	Manche	473.7	231.7	242.0	1155	5599	20.6
107	Marne	551.3	270.4	280.9	1435	6638	21.6
108	Haute-Marne	206.6	102.5	104.1	507	2519	20.1
109	Mayenne	275.4	134.6	140.7	575	2896	19.9
110	Meurthe-et-Moselle	716.1	349.2	366.8	1893	8757	21.6
111	Meuse	198.6	98.1	100.5	571	2572	22.2
112	Morbihan	607.6	296.9	310.7	1663	8854	18.8
113	Moselle	1015.5	503.2	512.3	3107	12969	24.0
114	Nièvre	235.8	114.6	121.2	702	3359	20.9
115	Nord	2530.1	1230.9	1299.2	8246	36622	22.5
116	Oise	699.3	348.7	350.6	1763	8133	21.7
117	Orne	295.1	144.3	150.8	703	3506	20.1
118	Pas-de-Calais	1429.9	694.4	735.6	4904	21703	22.6
119	Puy-de-dôme	595.7	290.7	304.9	1595	7536	21.2
120	Pyrénées-Atlantiques	568.4	273.7	294.7	1389	6270	22.2
121	Hautes-Pyrénées	226.8	110.1	116.7	563	2555	22.0
122	Pyrénées-Orientales	350.1	167.8	182.3	879	3801	23.1
123	Bas-Rhin	938.1	456.2	481.9	2470	11036	22.4
124	Haut-Rhin	661.4	323.9	337.5	1928	8191	23.5
125	Rhône	1468.4	710.8	757.6	3404	15290	22.3
126	Haute-Saône	231.2	114.5	116.7	576	2714	21.2
127	Saône-et-Loire	563.3	275.5	287.8	1400	6538	21.4
128	Sarthe	512.5	250.9	261.7	1085	5373	20.2
129	Savoie	339.3	167.5	171.8	735	3830	19.2
130	Haute-Savoie	541.9	268.5	273.4	1297	5824	22.3
131	Paris	2161.6	1004.0	1157.6	5263	26292	20.0
132	Seine-Maritime	1213.9	590.6	623.3	3225	15446	20.9
133	Seine-et-Marne	992.5	491.7	500.8	2294	10588	21.7
134	Yvelines	1260.3	623.0	637.3	2688	12187	22.1
135	Deux-Sèvres	344.1	170.3	173.8	690	3206	21.5
136	Somme	546.6	267.2	279.4	1573	7239	21.7
137	Tarn	341.7	166.4	175.3	799	3311	24.1
138	Tarn-et-Garonne	196.0	96.1	99.9	430	1980	21.7
139	Var	770.6	374.4	396.3	1881	8830	21.3
140	Vaucluse	451.1	220.8	230.4	1066	4946	21.6
141	Vendée	501.0	246.9	254.1	1089	5383	20.2
142	Vienne	376.5	184.6	191.9	778	3631	21.4
143	Haute-Vienne	355.7	171.4	184.3	811	3931	20.6
144	Vosges	389.3	189.8	199.5	964	5009	19.2
145	Yonne	318.6	157.1	161.5	845	4181	20.2
146	Territoire-de-Belfort	132.8	66.0	66.9	324	1540	21.0
147	Essonne	1037.6	514.8	522.8	2307	10281	22.4
148	Hauts-de-Seine	1387.7	666.5	721.2	3417	16024	21.3
149	Seine-Saint-Denis	1359.0	670.5	688.5	3765	16699	22.5
150	Val-de-Marne	1203.1	583.5	619.6	2872	13225	21.7
151	Val-d'Oise	992.6	489.2	503.4	2239	10269	21.8
GREECE		10050.1	4927.1	5123.0	33750	100583	33.6
152	Greater Athens	3069.0	1463.8	1605.2	12227	33204	36.8
153	Rest of Central Greece and Eubea	1179.3	590.4	588.9	3386	10655	31.8
154	Peloponnisos	1050.9	526.2	524.7	2970	9666	30.7
155	Ionian Islands	187.5	91.3	96.2	543	1792	30.3
156	Epirus	333.4	163.0	170.4	908	2947	30.8

Table 8.1—*cont.*

Area		Total population (thousands) Total	Males	Females	Total avoidable deaths	Total deaths (ages 5-64)	'Avoidable deaths' as a percentage of total deaths (ages 5–64)
157	Thessaly	716.7	353.0	363.7	2280	7124	32.0
158	Macedonia	2205.6	1084.6	1121.0	7477	22593	33.1
159	Thrace	340.5	172.0	168.5	1347	4195	32.1
160	Aegean Islands	444.4	224.5	219.9	1322	4017	32.9
161	Crete	522.8	258.3	264.5	1290	4390	29.4
ITALY		57345.1	27861.7	29483.4	185623	630702	29.4
162	Torino	2286.8	1110.0	1176.8	7617	26747	28.5
163	Vercelli	384.5	182.9	201.6	1579	5358	29.5
164	Novara	501.9	240.9	261.0	1790	6660	26.9
165	Cuneo	547.0	269.3	277.7	1926	6914	27.9
166	Asti	210.8	101.6	109.2	692	2403	28.8
167	Alessandria	451.2	215.7	235.6	1592	5759	27.6
168	Aosta	114.2	56.6	57.6	397	1700	23.4
169	Imperia	221.8	105.2	116.6	695	2632	26.4
170	Savona	293.1	139.4	153.7	985	3507	28.1
171	Genova	1003.5	474.9	528.6	3304	12516	26.4
172	La Spezia	235.7	112.7	123.1	746	2637	28.3
173	Varese	793.7	382.1	411.6	2519	8749	28.8
174	Como/Sondrio	961.5	464.9	496.6	3230	11614	27.8
175	Milano	3983.8	1916.5	2067.3	12977	47697	27.2
176	Bergamo	914.9	446.5	468.4	2958	11659	25.4
177	Brescia	1032.4	502.0	530.4	3420	13703	25.0
178	Pavia	501.0	239.2	261.8	1998	7373	27.1
179	Cremona	328.7	158.0	170.7	1312	4930	26.6
180	Mantova	372.4	178.8	193.6	1337	4624	28.9
181	Bolzano	436.2	214.1	222.1	1181	4742	24.9
182	Trento	445.2	216.1	229.0	1422	5670	25.1
183	Verona	783.7	380.0	403.7	2480	9351	26.5
184	Vicenza	738.3	358.9	379.4	2257	8588	26.3
185	Belluno	216.3	103.1	113.2	761	3207	23.7
186	Treviso	733.3	355.4	377.9	1960	8057	24.3
187	Venezia	835.9	405.2	430.7	2315	10054	23.0
188	Padova	817.0	396.8	420.2	2376	9337	25.4
189	Rovigo	250.4	121.5	128.8	831	3220	25.8
190	Udine/Gorizia	667.8	320.4	347.3	2188	9133	24.0
191	Trieste	269.1	124.8	144.3	815	3663	22.2
192	Pordenone	276.0	133.4	142.6	755	3364	22.4
193	Piacenza	273.0	131.9	141.0	1053	3710	28.4
194	Parma	396.3	190.9	205.4	1390	4810	28.9
195	Reggio Emilia	415.0	201.4	213.5	1244	4716	26.4
196	Modena	596.8	289.3	307.5	1993	6892	28.9
197	Bologna	916.1	439.5	476.7	3026	10723	28.2
198	Ferrara	371.3	178.1	193.2	1320	4812	27.4
199	Ravenna	353.3	171.1	182.2	968	3777	25.6
200	Forli	608.2	296.3	312.0	1595	6283	25.4
201	Pesaro	335.6	164.7	170.9	890	3352	26.6
202	Ancona	437.9	211.0	226.8	1228	4324	28.4
203	Macerata	294.9	142.9	152.0	843	2871	29.4
204	Ascoli Piceno	359.3	174.9	184.3	1004	3400	29.5
205	Massa-Carrara	205.1	98.7	106.4	643	2516	25.6
206	Lucca	382.8	182.7	200.1	1170	4525	25.9
207	Pistoia	265.6	127.6	138.1	760	2696	28.2
208	Firenze	1196.8	574.4	622.3	3321	12110	27.4
209	Livorno	344.7	166.1	178.6	1034	3756	27.5
210	Pisa	388.4	187.5	200.9	1181	4124	28.6
211	Arezzo	313.7	152.9	160.8	876	3292	26.6
212	Siena	253.1	122.6	130.5	732	2705	27.1
213	Grosseto	220.2	106.9	113.3	657	2423	27.1
214	Perugia	591.8	288.9	302.9	1877	6263	30.0

Table 8.1—*cont.*

Area		Total population (thousands) Total	Males	Females	Total avoidable deaths	Total deaths (ages 5-64)	'Avoidable deaths' as a percentage of total deaths (ages 5–64)
215	Terni	226.3	109.8	116.5	704	2301	30.6
216	Viterbo/Rieti	422.2	206.9	215.3	1410	4712	29.9
217	Roma	3760.7	1811.9	1948.7	12013	40180	29.9
218	Latina	464.7	229.3	235.4	1325	4430	29.9
219	Frosinone	479.8	235.9	243.9	1526	4858	31.4
220	Caserta	807.5	400.3	407.2	3112	9063	34.3
221	Benevento	298.2	145.7	152.5	1092	3007	36.3
222	Napoli	3100.5	1530.9	1569.6	12136	34276	35.4
223	Avellino	448.4	221.1	227.2	1502	4159	36.1
224	Salerno	1056.3	522.3	534.0	3826	10367	36.9
225	L'Aquila	298.4	144.8	153.7	999	3360	29.7
226	Teramo	279.8	137.9	141.8	764	2561	29.8
227	Pescara	294.1	142.8	151.3	963	2926	32.9
228	Chieti	383.8	187.0	196.7	1045	3498	29.9
229	Isernia/Campobasso	334.3	163.4	170.9	1101	3371	32.7
230	Foggia	700.3	344.0	356.3	2212	6540	33.8
231	Bari	1519.0	740.8	778.2	4245	13244	32.1
232	Taranto	596.6	294.0	302.7	1773	5579	31.8
233	Brindisi	407.0	197.5	209.5	1284	3895	33.0
234	Lecce	808.6	388.7	419.9	2363	7387	32.0
235	Potenza/Matera	620.7	307.4	313.3	1996	5906	33.8
236	Cosenza	777.7	384.0	393.7	2413	6714	35.9
237	Catanzaro	772.3	382.6	389.7	2355	7060	33.4
238	Reggio Calabria	590.7	290.8	299.9	1932	6189	31.2
239	Trapani	437.1	213.5	223.5	1362	3846	35.4
240	Palermo	1252.7	609.7	643.0	4025	12379	32.5
241	Messina	689.3	334.6	354.6	2399	6624	36.2
242	Agrigento	489.6	240.7	249.0	1539	4400	35.0
243	Caltanisetta	294.1	143.6	150.5	1053	3040	34.6
244	Enna	197.4	95.8	101.6	741	1950	38.0
245	Catania	1064.0	520.9	543.1	4027	10843	37.1
246	Ragusa	288.9	141.3	147.6	971	2634	36.9
247	Siracusa	409.6	201.8	207.8	1435	3970	36.1
248	Sassari	448.9	221.2	227.7	1374	4396	31.3
249	Nuoro	277.1	137.0	140.2	837	2790	30.0
250	Cagliari/Oristano	920.4	454.2	466.2	2549	8599	29.6
IRELAND		3540.7	1769.7	1771.0	15932	36457	43.7
251	Eastern	1232.2	598.8	633.4	5337	12206	43.7
252	Midland	208.0	106.6	101.4	1015	2289	44.3
253	Mid-Western	315.4	159.9	155.5	1469	3420	43.0
254	North-Eastern	302.0	153.7	148.3	1342	3100	43.3
255	North-Western	212.7	108.3	104.5	949	2232	42.5
256	South-Eastern	385.0	194.9	190.1	1855	4002	46.4
257	Southern	536.9	269.8	267.1	2564	5733	44.7
258	Western	348.3	177.7	170.6	1401	3475	40.3
THE NETHERLANDS		14664.5	7248.6	7415.9	38796	111281	34.9
259	Groningen	557.5	275.9	281.7	1672	4330	38.6
260	Friesland	598.8	297.7	301.1	1597	4288	37.2
261	Drenthe	435.5	217.2	218.3	1299	3581	36.3
262	Overijssel	1006.8	501.4	505.5	2881	7741	37.2
263	Gelderland	1777.9	878.7	899.3	4748	13381	35.5
264	Utrecht	967.0	471.3	495.8	2337	6869	34.0
265	Noord Holland	2343.9	1149.3	1194.6	5936	18184	32.6
266	Zuid Holland	3189.8	1565.7	1624.1	8103	23817	34.0
267	Zeeland	355.5	176.4	179.2	809	2517	32.1
268	Noord Brabant	2148.3	1075.5	1072.8	5586	16080	34.7
269	Limburg	1093.6	544.2	549.4	3425	9438	36.3
270	Flevoland	189.8	95.5	94.3	403	1055	38.2

Table 8.1—*cont.*

Area		Total population (thousands)			Total avoidable deaths	Total deaths (ages 5-64)	'Avoidable deaths' as a percentage of total deaths (ages 5–64)
		Total	Males	Females			
UK: ENGLAND AND WALES		50239.6	24494.3	25745.3	248172	579155	42.9
271	Northern	3077.4	1499.0	1578.4	19068	42759	44.6
	Hartlepool	89.8	43.6	46.2	614	1410	43.5
	North Tees	176.2	86.5	89.7	1002	2295	43.7
	South Tees	289.5	142.3	147.3	1813	4156	43.6
	East Cumbria	178.4	86.3	92.1	961	2250	42.7
	South Cumbria	172.4	83.4	89.1	828	1991	41.6
	West Cumbria	136.9	67.6	69.3	881	1931	45.6
	Darlington	124.3	60.7	63.5	745	1633	45.6
	Durham	235.2	115.0	120.1	1535	3266	47.0
	North-West Durham	86.0	41.6	44.3	595	1233	48.3
	South-West Durham	153.2	75.2	78.0	1026	2243	45.7
	Northumberland	301.5	147.4	154.1	1724	3933	43.8
	Gateshead	206.9	100.8	106.1	1468	3149	46.6
	Newcastle	280.7	136.0	144.8	1670	3911	42.7
	North Tyneside	192.8	92.2	100.5	1154	2741	42.1
	South Tyneside	156.4	76.2	80.2	1142	2505	45.6
	Sunderland	297.2	144.0	153.2	1910	4112	46.4
272	Yorkshire	3614.1	1759.4	1854.7	19912	44592	44.7
	Hull	302.6	146.8	155.8	1746	4004	43.6
	East Yorkshire	193.9	93.4	100.5	923	2044	45.2
	Grimsby	158.6	77.9	80.7	866	1990	43.5
	Scunthorpe	195.2	95.6	99.6	1204	2516	47.9
	Northallerton	115.2	58.3	56.9	492	1162	42.3
	York	263.3	129.2	134.1	1234	2850	43.3
	Scarborough	144.7	69.0	75.7	764	1692	45.2
	Harrogate	135.3	64.7	70.6	581	1327	43.8
	Bradford	338.1	165.7	172.4	2287	4822	47.4
	Airedale	175.1	84.4	90.7	868	1995	43.5
	Calderdale	194.6	94.2	100.4	1147	2562	44.8
	Huddersfield	212.0	103.0	109.0	1187	2665	44.5
	Dewsbury	164.0	80.0	84.0	1030	2065	49.9
	Leeds Western	363.8	176.7	187.1	1951	4541	43.0
	Leeds Eastern	346.6	168.3	178.3	1882	4390	42.9
	Wakefield	144.0	70.4	73.6	757	1720	44.0
	Pontefract	167.1	81.8	85.4	993	2247	44.2
273	Trent	4651.1	2287.6	2363.4	24574	55278	44.5
	North Derbyshire	362.5	178.4	184.1	1912	4359	43.9
	Southern Derbyshire	528.0	260.4	267.5	2849	6426	44.3
	Leicestershire	880.8	435.3	445.5	4177	9332	44.8
	North Lincolnshire	270.6	133.0	137.6	1376	3079	44.7
	South Lincolnshire	303.8	149.1	154.7	1551	3449	45.0
	Bassetlaw	104.9	52.5	52.4	542	1259	43.1
	Central Nottinghamshire	288.5	142.5	146.0	1535	3458	44.4
	Nottingham	615.2	301.4	313.8	3149	7313	43.1
	Barnsley	221.9	109.3	112.6	1424	3014	47.2
	Doncaster	290.6	143.1	147.4	1589	3865	41.1
	Rotherham	252.4	124.2	128.2	1494	3198	46.7
	Sheffield	532.0	258.5	273.6	2976	6526	45.6
274	East Anglian	2009.8	985.0	1024.8	7661	19277	39.7
	Cambridge	273.2	136.1	137.1	887	2375	37.3
	Peterborough	204.3	99.0	105.3	984	2299	42.8
	West Suffolk	226.7	112.0	114.7	821	2121	38.7
	East Suffolk	320.1	156.8	163.3	1178	2915	40.4
	Norwich	468.6	227.4	241.2	1767	4462	39.6
	Great Yarmouth and Waveney	197.3	95.4	101.9	799	2079	38.4
	West Norfolk and Wisbech	187.3	92.2	95.1	827	1945	42.5
	Huntingdon	132.3	66.2	66.1	398	1081	36.8
275	North-West Thames	3483.0	1701.5	1781.5	14607	36435	40.1
	North Bedfordshire	248.1	123.9	124.3	977	2425	40.3

Table 8.1—*cont.*

	Area	Total population (thousands)			Total avoidable deaths	Total deaths (ages 5-64)	'Avoidable deaths' as a percentage of total deaths (ages 5–64)
		Total	Males	Females			
	South Bedfordshire	277.0	137.9	139.0	1194	2901	41.2
	North Hertfordshire	186.4	91.6	94.7	842	1975	42.6
	East Hartfordshire	294.1	146.0	148.1	1169	2773	42.2
	North-West Hertfordshire	261.3	128.1	133.2	1031	2555	40.4
	South-West Hertfordshire	244.6	119.4	125.3	961	2406	39.9
	Barnet	304.7	146.2	158.5	1097	2714	40.4
	Harrow	198.9	96.2	102.7	792	1754	45.2
	Hillingdon	232.3	113.2	119.1	1020	2395	42.6
	Hounslow and Spelthorne	281.7	138.8	142.9	1320	3269	40.4
	Ealing	295.2	144.7	150.5	1318	3232	40.8
	Riverside	282.9	133.0	149.9	1158	3563	32.5
	Parkside	375.8	182.4	193.4	1728	4473	38.6
276	North-East Thames	3768.3	1829.7	1938.6	17287	41958	41.2
	Basildon and Thurrock	281.6	139.0	142.6	1422	3225	44.1
	Mid Essex	288.4	141.6	146.9	1105	2604	42.4
	North-East Essex	305.1	147.9	157.2	1216	3018	40.3
	West Essex	251.9	124.2	127.7	1105	2637	41.9
	Southend	322.6	154.9	167.7	1342	3169	42.3
	Barking, Havering, and Brentwood	454.6	221.3	233.3	2264	5268	43.0
	Hampstead	108.8	50.9	57.9	426	1207	35.3
	Bloomsbury	128.6	60.4	68.2	590	1770	33.3
	Islington	168.6	81.1	87.5	807	2327	34.7
	City and Hackney	193.2	93.8	99.4	979	2498	39.2
	Newham	206.9	100.5	106.4	1165	2612	44.6
	Tower Hamlets	156.9	78.5	78.4	951	2406	39.5
	Enfield	263.0	126.8	136.2	1064	2537	41.9
	Haringey	193.9	94.6	99.3	855	2202	38.8
	Redbridge	229.8	111.2	118.7	994	2276	43.7
	Waltham Forest	214.3	103.1	111.2	1002	2202	45.5
277	South-East Thames	3632.3	1748.9	1883.3	15781	39741	39.7
	Brighton	300.8	141.9	158.9	1152	3266	35.3
	Eastbourne	231.8	106.4	125.4	830	2078	39.9
	Hastings	166.3	76.7	89.6	690	1696	40.7
	South-East Kent	266.6	129.1	137.5	1158	2851	40.6
	Canterbury and Thanet	303.8	144.5	159.3	1338	3295	40.6
	Dartford and Gravesham	218.7	108.1	110.6	1037	2449	42.3
	Maidstone	197.3	97.7	99.6	814	2034	40.0
	Medway	328.2	161.8	166.4	1501	3442	43.6
	Tunbridge Wells	195.6	94.3	101.3	725	1860	39.0
	Bexley	220.0	107.4	112.6	868	2101	41.3
	Greenwich	215.7	103.5	112.2	1035	2549	40.6
	Bromley	298.1	145.3	152.8	1139	2793	40.8
	West Lambeth	160.8	78.7	82.0	786	2199	35.7
	Camberwell	211.6	101.7	109.9	1124	2983	37.7
	Lewisham and North Southwark	316.9	151.8	165.2	1584	4145	38.2
278	South-West Thames	2962.9	1430.5	1532.4	11499	29315	39.2
	North-West Surrey	207.1	101.6	105.5	704	1957	36.0
	West Surrey and North-East Hampshire	276.4	138.0	138.4	910	2312	39.4
	South-West Surrey	182.1	88.0	94.1	645	1683	38.3
	Mid Surrey	166.1	79.5	86.7	622	1652	37.7
	East Surrey	184.0	88.9	95.1	777	1976	39.3
	Chichester	180.0	84.6	95.4	656	1734	37.8
	Mid Downs	275.3	135.5	139.8	1070	2656	40.3
	Worthing	242.8	110.7	132.1	978	2380	41.1
	Croydon	318.4	156.3	162.1	1374	3275	42.0
	Kingston and Esher	177.9	86.0	91.9	653	1680	38.9
	Richmond, Twickenham, and Roehampton	230.8	109.6	121.2	919	2478	37.1
	Wandsworth	188.9	92.2	96.7	843	2172	38.8
	Merton and Sutton	333.1	159.7	173.4	1348	3360	40.1
279	Wessex	2899.8	1413.6	1486.2	12038	28941	41.6

Table 8.1—*cont.*

Area		Total population (thousands)			Total avoidable deaths	Total deaths (ages 5-64)	'Avoidable deaths' as a percentage of total deaths (ages 5–64)
		Total	Males	Females			
	East Dorset	445.7	210.3	235.4	1805	4371	41.3
	West Dorset	199.8	96.7	103.0	808	1970	41.0
	Portsmouth and South-East Hampshire	527.1	260.2	266.9	2352	5454	43.1
	Southampton and South-West Hampshire	418.4	205.1	213.3	1764	4279	41.2
	Winchester	210.3	104.4	105.8	807	2011	40.1
	Basingstoke and North Hampshire	217.9	107.7	110.2	846	2092	40.4
	Salisbury	121.6	59.6	62.0	500	1209	41.4
	Swindon	230.5	112.8	117.6	1003	2409	41.6
	Bath	401.7	196.4	205.3	1564	3778	41.4
	Isle of Wight	126.9	60.4	66.5	589	1368	43.1
280	Oxford	2495.2	1239.4	1255.7	9425	23555	40.0
	East Berkshire	362.0	180.0	182.0	1538	3706	41.5
	West Berkshire	447.4	224.5	222.9	1609	3996	40.3
	Aylesbury Vale	143.8	71.2	72.7	492	1308	37.6
	Wycombe	270.0	133.0	137.0	1010	2532	39.9
	Milton Keynes	169.1	84.5	84.6	562	1436	39.1
	Kettering	255.5	124.8	130.7	1248	2983	41.8
	Northampton	306.3	151.2	155.1	1241	3073	40.4
	Oxfordshire	541.0	270.3	270.7	1725	4521	38.2
281	South-Western	3204.3	1547.4	1657.0	14093	33439	42.1
	Bristol and Weston	365.6	175.6	190.0	1669	3926	42.5
	Frenchay	220.4	107.5	112.9	998	2187	45.6
	Southmead	232.2	114.2	118.0	991	2463	40.2
	Cornwall and Isles of Scilly	454.0	217.1	236.9	2138	4911	43.5
	Exeter	306.3	146.8	159.5	1258	3094	40.7
	North Devon	133.6	65.3	68.3	553	1384	40.0
	Plymouth	330.0	162.6	167.5	1551	3537	43.9
	Torbay	239.7	112.2	127.5	1097	2550	43.0
	Cheltenham and District	210.5	101.1	109.5	875	2161	40.5
	Gloucester	311.0	151.3	159.7	1322	3202	41.3
	Somerset	400.9	193.6	207.3	1641	4024	40.8
282	West Midlands	5196.9	2564.3	2632.6	28225	63268	44.6
	Bromsgrove and Redditch	165.6	82.3	83.3	718	1618	44.4
	Herefordshire	155.6	76.8	78.8	713	1682	42.4
	Kidderminster and District	102.1	49.8	52.3	473	1116	42.4
	Worcester and District	240.1	117.0	123.1	1073	2501	42.9
	Shropshire	396.7	195.9	200.8	1935	4346	44.5
	Mid Staffordshire	311.2	154.5	156.7	1411	3360	42.0
	North Staffordshire	461.9	226.7	235.2	3004	6399	46.9
	South-East Staffordshire	255.0	126.7	128.3	1305	2866	45.5
	Rugby	85.6	42.8	42.8	403	936	43.1
	North Warwickshire	174.1	86.2	87.9	932	2133	43.7
	South Warwickshire	222.7	108.9	113.9	911	2335	39.0
	Central Birmingham	180.2	89.6	90.6	1040	2282	45.6
	East Birmingham	198.7	99.3	99.4	1300	2730	47.6
	North Birmingham	163.7	80.5	83.2	863	1905	45.3
	South Birmingham	247.2	121.1	126.1	1420	3143	45.2
	West Birmingham	209.4	103.6	105.8	1330	2897	45.9
	Coventry	308.4	153.0	155.4	1692	3992	42.4
	Dudley	302.8	149.6	153.2	1631	3673	44.4
	Sandwell	298.9	146.1	152.8	1938	4292	45.2
	Solihull	203.5	99.6	103.9	934	2074	45.0
	Walsall	262.5	130.2	132.3	1667	3622	46.0
	Wolverhampton	251.0	124.2	126.8	1532	3366	45.5
283	Mersey	2411.4	1168.3	1243.0	14232	32008	44.5
	Chester	176.5	85.7	90.8	986	2209	44.6
	Crewe	248.3	122.1	126.3	1345	2901	46.4
	Halton	143.1	70.5	72.6	831	1767	47.0
	Macclesfield	179.2	87.1	92.1	816	1967	41.5
	Warrington	184.7	91.2	93.5	1086	2293	47.4

Table 8.1—*cont.*

Area		Total population (thousands)			Total avoidable deaths	Total deaths (ages 5-64)	'Avoidable deaths' as a percentage of total deaths (ages 5–64)
		Total	Males	Females			
	Liverpool	477.2	230.0	247.2	3165	7541	42.0
	St Helens and Knowsley	349.5	170.2	179.3	2346	5060	46.4
	North Sefton	119.4	56.0	63.4	640	1406	45.5
	South Sefton	178.8	86.0	92.8	1097	2466	44.5
	Wirral	354.7	169.5	185.1	1920	4398	43.7
284	North-Western	3993.4	1941.8	2051.6	23841	53108	44.9
	Lancaster	130.2	62.7	67.5	680	1617	42.1
	Blackpool Wyre and Fylde	318.9	150.2	168.7	1942	4444	43.7
	Preston	126.5	61.3	65.2	809	1774	45.6
	Blackburn, Hyndburn, and Ribble Valley	268.5	131.2	137.3	1635	3666	44.6
	Burnley, Pendle, and Rossendale	230.2	112.4	117.8	1457	3080	47.3
	West Lancashire	106.2	51.8	54.4	580	1287	45.1
	Chorley and South Ribble	195.0	96.1	98.9	1066	2281	46.7
	Bolton	262.7	128.2	134.6	1661	3519	47.2
	Bury	174.2	84.7	89.5	997	2110	47.3
	North Manchester	142.4	69.8	72.6	1094	2427	45.1
	Central Manchester	124.1	63.5	60.6	783	1900	41.2
	South Manchester	181.9	87.0	94.9	986	2380	41.4
	Oldham	219.9	107.3	112.6	1368	2988	45.8
	Rochdale	214.2	104.8	109.4	1330	2834	46.9
	Salford	237.5	115.6	121.9	1562	3611	43.3
	Stockport	290.9	140.5	150.4	1464	3315	44.2
	Tameside and Glossop	246.2	119.6	126.6	1488	3296	45.1
	Trafford	216.3	104.3	112.0	1095	2560	42.8
	Wigan	307.5	150.6	156.9	1844	4019	45.9
285	Wales	2839.9	1377.9	1461.9	15929	35481	44.9
	Clwyd	403.7	194.9	208.8	2134	4754	44.9
	East Dyfed	232.5	112.5	120.0	1303	2958	44.1
	Pembrokeshire	111.4	53.6	57.8	641	1407	45.6
	Gwent	443.5	216.6	226.8	2633	5766	45.7
	Gwynedd	236.9	113.9	123.0	1210	2791	43.4
	Mid Glamorgan	535.4	261.2	274.2	3322	7243	45.9
	Powys	113.8	56.5	57.2	589	1259	46.8
	South Glamorgan	399.5	193.4	206.1	1954	4598	42.5
	West Glamorgan	363.3	175.3	188.0	2143	4705	45.5
UK: NORTHERN IRELAND		1572.2	771.3	800.8	8378	18862	44.4
286	Northern Ireland	1572.2	771.3	800.8	8378	18862	44.4
UK: SCOTLAND		5110.9	2469.8	2641.1	31850	74015	43.0
287	Highlands and Islands	274.0	134.6	139.4	1615	3901	41.4
288	Grampian	502.2	246.3	255.9	2422	6159	39.3
289	Tayside	393.3	188.3	205.0	2287	5325	42.9
290	Fife	344.4	167.5	176.9	2067	4495	46.0
291	Lothian	743.0	357.2	385.8	4002	9595	41.7
292	Borders	102.2	49.0	53.2	531	1244	42.7
293	Forth Valley	271.8	132.0	139.9	1701	3883	43.8
294	Argyll and Clyde	443.6	214.4	229.2	2998	6809	44.0
295	Greater Glasgow	950.5	454.5	496.0	6758	16459	41.1
296	Lanarkshire	563.9	274.5	289.4	3917	8207	47.7
297	Ayrshire and Arran	374.8	180.2	194.6	2578	5518	46.7
298	Dumfries and Galloway	147.1	71.3	75.8	974	2420	40.2
PORTUGAL		10265.9	4957.9	5308.1	40453	132277	30.6
299	Viana do Castelo	266.0	123.3	142.8	1047	3480	30.1
300	Braga	770.9	376.0	394.9	2850	8916	32.0
301	Vila Real	262.9	130.4	132.4	1068	3929	27.2
302	Bragança	184.6	93.5	91.1	717	2533	28.3
303	Guarda	196.2	95.5	100.7	756	2801	27.0
304	Viseu	423.1	206.8	216.3	1682	5653	29.8

Table 8.1—*cont.*

	Area	Total population (thousands) Total	Males	Females	Total avoidable deaths	Total deaths (ages 5-64)	'Avoidable deaths' as a percentage of total deaths (ages 5–64)
305	Porto	1670.2	806.9	863.3	6571	20417	32.2
306	Aveiro	665.1	323.2	341.9	2210	7875	28.1
307	Coimbra	446.3	212.1	234.3	1566	5342	29.3
308	Castelo Branco	223.6	108.8	114.8	837	3198	26.2
309	Portalegre	137.3	67.4	69.9	597	1820	32.8
310	Santarem	460.0	222.8	237.2	1672	6081	27.5
311	Leiria	435.8	213.7	222.1	1623	5956	27.2
312	Lisboa	2125.9	1003.1	1122.8	8853	27704	32.0
313	Setubal	779.9	380.8	399.1	2774	9067	30.6
314	Evora	174.4	85.1	89.2	740	2363	31.3
315	Beja	177.7	89.0	88.7	765	2657	28.8
316	Faro	341.1	167.9	173.2	1413	4893	28.9
317	Madeira	271.4	126.1	145.3	1175	3863	30.4
318	Azores	253.5	125.6	127.9	1537	3729	41.2
SPAIN		39788.6	19566.9	20221.7	79591	311116	25.6
319	La Coruña	1128.2	547.1	581.1	2377	9911	24.0
320	Lugo	396.0	195.2	200.8	908	3682	24.7
321	Orense	424.5	207.3	217.2	807	3281	24.6
322	Pontevedra	942.3	455.4	486.9	1688	7627	22.1
323	Asturias	1172.7	570.0	602.7	2547	10724	23.8
324	Cantabria	537.9	264.4	273.5	1026	4332	23.7
325	Alava	294.6	147.9	146.7	413	1836	22.5
326	Guipuzcoa	733.5	364.4	369.1	1317	5857	22.5
327	Vizcaya	1275.0	631.1	643.9	2282	10429	21.9
328	Navarra	532.8	265.4	267.4	898	3911	23.0
329	Rioja	265.1	133.0	132.1	561	2180	25.7
330	Huesca	211.6	107.0	104.6	431	1754	24.6
331	Teruel	143.7	72.6	71.1	278	1086	25.6
332	Zaragoza	868.8	426.2	442.6	1791	6663	26.9
333	Madrid Centro	5260.6	2549.1	2711.5	7724	36108	21.4
334	Avila	170.6	86.5	84.1	322	1279	25.2
335	Burgos	364.5	183.5	181.0	597	2940	20.3
336	Leon	504.1	249.1	255.0	1235	4883	25.3
337	Palencia	182.1	90.1	92.0	352	1720	20.5
338	Salamanca	356.2	174.1	182.1	752	2656	28.3
339	Segovia	143.3	71.8	71.5	242	1114	21.7
340	Soria	92.9	46.2	46.7	145	681	21.3
341	Valladolid	522.3	258.3	264.0	660	3272	20.2
342	Zamora	213.4	105.3	108.1	414	1752	23.6
343	Albacete	338.3	168.1	170.2	747	2492	30.0
344	Ciudad Real	456.7	223.2	233.5	1112	3920	28.4
345	Cuenca	199.6	99.5	100.1	444	1591	27.9
346	Guadalajara	140.0	71.2	68.8	191	1018	18.8
347	Toledo	473.2	235.2	238.0	966	3485	27.7
348	Badajoz	615.2	303.3	311.9	1709	5638	30.3
349	Caceres	399.3	198.0	201.3	967	3412	28.3
350	Barcelona	5045.1	2475.5	2569.6	8650	36227	23.9
351	Gerona	498.7	247.2	251.5	1003	4015	25.0
352	Lerida	356.5	178.2	178.3	742	2902	25.6
353	Tarragona	560.7	278.5	282.2	970	4013	24.2
354	Alicante	1290.0	635.1	654.9	2825	9711	29.1
355	Castellon de la Plana	458.0	226.3	231.7	979	3439	28.5
356	Valencia	2240.6	1098.6	1142.0	4756	17965	26.5
357	Baleares	731.6	361.4	370.2	1796	6389	28.1
358	Almeria	429.3	212.9	216.4	933	3367	27.7
359	Cadiz	1051.1	523.4	527.7	2890	8894	32.5
360	Cordoba	715.2	349.4	365.8	1669	5755	29.0
361	Granada	767.4	376.1	391.3	1743	6265	27.8
362	Huelva	426.7	211.0	215.7	1103	3529	31.3

Table 8.1—*cont.*

Area		Total population (thousands)			Total avoidable deaths	Total deaths (ages 5-64)	'Avoidable deaths' as a percentage of total deaths (ages 5–64)
		Total	Males	Females			
363	Jaen	625.7	308.3	317.4	1424	5006	28.4
364	Malaga	1129.6	557.3	572.3	2792	9842	28.4
365	Sevilla	1558.9	765.9	793.0	3917	12826	30.5
366	Murcia	1027.5	505.5	522.0	2200	7671	28.7
367	Las Palmas	810.2	408.8	401.4	1809	6347	28.5
368	Sta Cruz de Tenerife	706.8	348.0	358.8	1487	5719	26.0
EC		325155.8	158256.0	166899.8	1092978	3591350	30.4

Table 8.2. Observed numbers of 'avoidable deaths' and 'avoidable death' indicators by disease, small area and country.

Notes on the use of this table

1. This table shows observed numbers of deaths (totals for years in 2, below) and SMRs standardized to the EC standard (the value for the whole EC being 100) and to own country's standard (the value for the whole country being 100).

2. The mortality data are for 1985-89 and cover five years, except for Netherlands (four years, 1985-88) and Spain (four years, 1985-88). The population data are for 1985-89, except for France (1987), Greece (1987), Ireland (1986), and Spain (1986).

3. All countries supplied data according to the 9th revision of the International Classification of Diseases except for Denmark where 8th revision coding rules applied. For key to abbreviations used, please see page xv.

4. The small area numbers are as in the key maps.

5. The indicators have been tested for indicating significantly different mortality relative to EC or national rates, as appropriate. The p-values achieved for two-tail tests are indicated as follows: *p<0.05; **p<0.01; ***p<0.001.

Table 8.2(a)

Area	TUB			CERV			UTER		
	Deaths	SMR to EC std	SMR to own std	Deaths	SMR to EC std	SMR to own std	Deaths	SMR to EC std	SMR to own std
BELGIUM	205	62***	100	507	93	100	440	88**	100
1 Antwerpen	12	23***	36***	104	120	129*	73	90	102
2 Brabant	62	82	132*	106	84	90	107	92	105
3 West-Vlaanderen	15	41***	66	29	49***	52***	51	92	104
4 Oost-Vlaanderen	14	32***	51**	90	124	133*	67	99	112
5 Hainaut	57	131	210***	53	74*	79	51	82	94
6 Liege	31	91	146	61	108	116	33	66*	75
7 Limburg	7	31***	50	33	88	96	35	94	107
8 Luxembourg (province)	1	14*	22	9	76	82	9	87	100
9 Namur	6	44*	72	22	98	106	14	70	80
LUXEMBOURG	8	65	100	26	125	100	21	106	100
10 Luxembourg	8	65	100	26	125	100	21	106	100
FEDERAL REPUBLIC OF GERMANY	1855	89***	100	4297	122***	100	3392	100	100
11 Schleswig-Holstein	48	56***	63***	206	141***	116*	171	118*	118*
12 Hamburg	45	81	91	142	148***	122*	103	111	112
13 Braunschweig	62	113	127	117	127*	105	98	114	114
14 Hannover	57	81	92	193	163***	134***	147	130**	130**
15 Lüneburg	31	63**	71	95	115	95	66	82	83
16 Weser-Ems	60	88	100	147	128**	105	98	89	89
17 Bremen	28	123	138	66	168***	138*	42	112	113
18 Düsseldorf	155	85*	95	431	140***	115**	315	107	107
19 Köln	92	68***	77*	268	118**	97	203	91	91
20 Munster	49	60***	68**	142	105	86	116	91	91
21 Detmold	30	49***	55***	89	87	71***	81	84	84
22 Arnsberg	103	80*	90	263	124***	101	210	105	106
23 Darmstadt	105	89	100	228	114	93	176	89	89
24 Giessen	24	74	84	51	96	79	55	110	110
25 Kassel	33	82	92	74	111	91	54	88	88
26 Koblenz	29	61**	69*	91	116	95	76	105	105
27 Trier	14	86	97	33	123	101	25	105	106
28 Rheinhessen-Pfalz	53	84	95	118	112	92	105	105	106
29 Stuttgart	100	85	96	180	91	75***	165	84*	84*
30 Karlsruhe	105	128*	144***	131	94	78**	109	81*	81*
31 Freiburg	65	105	119	117	112	92	83	82	82
32 Tübingen	40	82	93	76	92	76*	69	85	85
33 Oberbayern	112	91	102	201	94	77***	180	84*	84*
34 Niederbayern	62	185***	209***	70	123	101	59	113	113
35 Oberpfalz	46	142*	161**	76	140**	115	63	125	126
36 Oberfranken	53	146*	165***	82	135**	111	70	126	127

Table 8.2(a)—*cont.*

Area		TUB			CERV			UTER		
		Deaths	SMR to EC std	SMR to own std	Deaths	SMR to EC std	SMR to own std	Deaths	SMR to EC std	SMR to own std
37	Mittelfranken	97	186***	210***	134	152***	125*	109	128*	129*
38	Unterfranken	28	70	79	73	109	90	50	80	80
39	Schwaben	30	59**	66*	77	89	73**	52	63***	64***
40	Saarland	38	100	113	80	126*	103	56	95	95
41	Berlin (West)	61	98	110	246	222***	182***	186	164***	164***
DENMARK		79	50***	100	578	216***	100	334	127***	100
42	Kobenhavn and Frederiksberg (M)	18	110	214**	69	253***	113	44	183***	139*
43	Kobenhavns County	11	53*	106	51	143*	66**	26	74	59**
44	Frederiksborg County	1	9***	20	23	125	60*	20	100	80
45	Roskilde County	1	16*	34	22	193**	94	17	134	108
46	Vestsjællands County	4	46	91	36	246***	113	18	126	100
47	Storstroms County	4	47	92	30	216***	99	14	107	85
48	Bornholms County	0	0	0	5	206	94	4	173	137
49	Fyns County	8	57	113	57	241***	111	29	125	99
50	Sonderjyllands County	7	89	176	35	270***	124	22	172*	135
51	Ribe County	6	93	185	25	232***	107	16	149	117
52	Vejle County	1	10***	20	40	236***	109	23	137	108
53	Ringkobing County	2	26*	51	22	167*	78	14	106	84
54	Århus County	8	47*	95	79	268***	125	46	154**	121
55	Viborg County	3	43	84	28	241***	111	12	107	84
56	Nordjyllands County	5	34**	67	56	226***	104	29	120	95
FRANCE		1661	97	100	2141	75***	100	2514	94**	100
57	Ain	10	75	78	13	59	79	15	71	75
58	Aisne	13	80	82	22	82	110	24	100	106
59	Allier	10	80	82	16	79	105	18	104	110
60	Alpes-de-Haute-Provence	2	47	48	6	88	117	3	49	51
61	Hautes-Alpes	4	114	117	0	0**	0*	2	38	41
62	Alpes-Maritimes	30	95	97	45	84	112	48	103	109
63	Ardèche	5	55	57	10	69	93	7	55	58
64	Ardennes	9	99	102	13	88	117	18	133	141
65	Ariège	5	104	108	5	67	89	6	97	103
66	Aube	8	91	94	16	109	146	19	140	149
67	Aude	8	80	82	11	69	92	10	75	79
68	Aveyron	9	95	97	8	53	71	11	86	91
69	Bouches-du-Rhône	52	95	98	56	61***	81	74	85	90
70	Calvados	22	124	129	34	113	152*	34	120	128
71	Cantal	4	74	77	5	59	79	8	110	117
72	Charente	7	63	65	14	78	104	18	111	118
73	Charente-Maritime	13	75	77	14	50**	66	17	70	74
74	Cher	5	48	50	6	36**	48	12	80	85
75	Corrèze	1	12**	12**	6	45*	59	14	125	132
76	Corse	1	12**	13**	7	54	72	12	103	110
77	Côte-d'Or	14	98	102	32	134	179**	26	115	122
78	Côtes-du-Nord	17	93	96	14	48**	64	19	77	81
79	Creuse	5	101	104	6	80	106	6	102	107
80	Dordogne	7	51	53	13	60	79	23	128	135
81	Doubs	10	72	74	18	77	103	16	70	74
82	Drôme	2	16***	16***	19	89	119	25	125	133
83	Eure	17	121	125	29	123	166*	38	167**	179**
84	Eure-et-Loir	10	90	93	7	38**	51	12	69	74
85	Finistère	42	156**	161**	35	79	105	35	91	96
86	Gard	22	120	123	20	66	88	33	121	129
87	Haute-Garonne	12	45**	46**	29	63*	85	30	68*	73
88	Gers	3	48	49	8	82	109	13	156	164
89	Gironde	23	63*	65*	44	72*	96	48	85	90
90	Hérault	19	79	81	34	84	112	31	85	91
91	Ille-et-Vilaine	20	87	90	30	77	104	34	94	100
92	Indre	7	87	89	3	23**	31*	8	72	76
93	Indre-et-Loire	14	90	92	18	69	92	28	114	122

Table 8.2(a)—*cont.*

	Area	TUB			CERV			UTER		
		Deaths	SMR to EC std	SMR to own std	Deaths	SMR to EC std	SMR to own std	Deaths	SMR to EC std	SMR to own std
94	Isère	22	76	78	45	92	123	38	80	85
95	Jura	7	90	93	8	63	84	13	114	121
96	Landes	7	66	68	9	53	71	9	61	65
97	Loir-et-Cher	5	52	54	21	135	181*	27	195**	207***
98	Loire	18	76	79	36	92	122	38	106	112
99	Haute-Loire	5	72	75	5	46	61	6	64	67
100	Loire-Atlantique	40	131	135	20	38***	51**	26	53***	56**
101	Loiret	19	114	118	17	61*	82	25	95	101
102	Lot	4	72	74	1	11**	15*	1	14*	15*
103	Lot-et-Garonne	2	19**	20**	8	48*	64	11	76	80
104	Lozère	1	41	43	2	54	72	4	124	132
105	Maine-et-Loire	18	91	94	10	30***	40**	19	61*	65
106	Manche	9	59	61	25	102	136	23	107	113
107	Marne	18	115	119	23	87	117	30	118	126
108	Haute-Marne	13	206*	213*	8	79	105	5	54	58
109	Mayenne	8	95	98	9	65	87	6	48	51
110	Meurthe-et-Moselle	16	74	76	29	80	107	31	91	96
111	Meuse	5	80	83	9	89	120	9	102	108
112	Morbihan	24	124	128	24	75	101	21	75	80
113	Moselle	33	106	109	38	74	99	33	67*	72
114	Nièvre	7	88	91	11	87	116	10	94	99
115	Nord	124	171***	177***	110	90	120	130	114	122*
116	Oise	20	104	107	27	83	112	41	126	135
117	Orne	7	74	77	8	53	70	8	59	63
118	Pas-de-Calais	72	169***	175***	69	97	129*	71	110	118
119	Puy-de-dôme	18	94	97	22	70	93	27	93	99
120	Pyrénées-Atlantiques	26	139	143	21	68	91	25	90	95
121	Hautes-Pyrénées	3	38	39	8	62	83	17	150	158
122	Pyrénées-Orientales	17	139	143	9	45*	60	12	72	75
123	Bas-Rhin	27	97	101	46	98	131	44	99	105
124	Haut-Rhin	28	139	143	28	83	111	35	110	117
125	Rhône	43	98	101	56	75*	100	64	88	93
126	Haute-Saône	2	28	29	12	105	140	9	87	92
127	Saône-et-Loire	12	65	67	21	71	94	20	76	80
128	Sarthe	7	45*	47*	24	94	125	22	93	99
129	Savoie	6	57	59	15	86	115	13	79	84
130	Haute-Savoie	18	114	118	20	74	100	28	104	112
131	Paris	101	149***	153***	108	90	121	130	115	122*
132	Seine-Maritime	42	120	124	45	75	101	55	97	103
133	Seine-et-Marne	24	91	94	23	50***	67	43	88	95
134	Yvelines	23	64*	66*	34	54***	73	48	72*	76
135	Deux-Sèvres	11	101	104	11	63	84	9	57	61
136	Somme	17	105	109	33	124	166**	39	159**	170**
137	Tarn	2	17**	17**	6	31***	42*	7	42*	45*
138	Tarn-et-Garonne	6	91	94	3	28*	38	4	44	46
139	Var	29	111	114	28	65*	87	35	93	98
140	Vaucluse	10	70	72	23	97	129	24	108	115
141	Vendée	10	64	66	8	31***	42**	13	58*	62
142	Vienne	11	95	98	19	101	135	18	106	112
143	Haute-Vienne	8	67	69	6	31***	41*	11	65	68
144	Vosges	9	75	78	10	51*	68	20	112	119
145	Yonne	14	140	145	18	112	150	12	87	92
146	Territoire-de-Belfort	2	50	52	5	75	100	6	95	101
147	Essonne	27	92	95	37	72*	97	52	94	100
148	Hauts-de-Seine	36	81	84	63	83	112	74	102	108
149	Seine-Saint-Denis	44	112	116	59	88	119	72	106	113
150	Val-de-Marne	36	98	101	51	81	108	61	97	103
151	Val-d'Oise	26	95	98	31	65*	87	35	70*	74
GREECE		298	99	100	289	55***	100	439	79***	100
152	Greater Athens	84	90	90	125	74***	133**	153	86	108

Table 8.2(a)—*cont.*

Area		TUB			CERV			UTER		
		Deaths	SMR to EC std	SMR to own std	Deaths	SMR to EC std	SMR to own std	Deaths	SMR to EC std	SMR to own std
153	Rest of Central Greece and Eubea	20	57**	57**	20	34***	61*	42	68**	86
154	Peloponnisos	32	100	100	25	48***	86	36	68*	85
155	Ionian Islands	5	80	80	7	68	123	5	50	63
156	Epirus	11	110	111	2	12***	21**	16	89	112
157	Thessaly	22	100	101	11	29***	53*	27	68*	87
158	Macedonia	74	117	120	75	67***	121	110	87	109
159	Thrace	29	306***	313***	5	30**	54	21	115	145
160	Aegean Islands	9	67	67	10	46**	84	13	62	77
161	Crete	12	78	77	9	35***	63	16	61*	77
ITALY		1580	82***	100	1010	31***	100	2193	72***	100
162	Torino	67	81	99	59	43***	136*	83	62***	85
163	Vercelli	16	110	133	7	29***	93	15	70	96
164	Novara	24	135	164*	10	34***	107	17	61*	84
165	Cuneo	35	177**	215***	15	47**	151	25	88	121
166	Asti	12	153	185	11	87	275**	5	45	62
167	Alessandria	10	58	70	10	36***	114	16	65	89
168	Aosta	13	317***	387***	4	60	191	7	112	155
169	Imperia	6	71	86	11	79	250*	9	73	99
170	Savona	11	97	117	5	27***	85	15	90	121
171	Genova	41	105	127	22	34***	108	49	86	117
172	La Spezia	10	111	134	8	54	173	12	95	129
173	Varese	20	74	90	15	32***	104	27	60**	83
174	Como/Sondrio	15	46**	57*	16	29***	94	28	53***	74
175	Milano	90	63***	78*	72	30***	95	151	63***	87
176	Bergamo	25	84	103	12	24***	76	27	55***	76
177	Brescia	45	129	158**	21	36***	114	40	71*	99
178	Pavia	19	99	120	16	51**	161	26	93	127
179	Cremona	8	65	79	2	10***	32	11	61	83
180	Mantova	8	59	71	6	27***	85	15	74	102
181	Bolzano	15	110	136	15	66	211*	9	41**	57
182	Trento	30	199***	243***	9	36***	115	10	44**	61
183	Verona	15	56*	68	12	27***	86	24	57**	79
184	Vicenza	16	66	81	12	29***	94	14	36***	49**
185	Belluno	12	157	192	2	16***	50	6	53	74
186	Treviso	19	78	96	14	34***	110	21	55**	76
187	Venezia	23	79	97	6	12***	39*	13	28***	39***
188	Padova	20	73	90	19	41***	132	18	41***	57*
189	Rovigo	5	55	67	3	20***	65	5	39*	53
190	Udine/Gorizia	18	75	91	15	38***	120	27	74	102
191	Trieste	15	145	175	10	58	183	9	59	80
192	Pordenone	6	64	79	4	26**	82	12	82	114
193	Piacenza	1	9***	11**	6	35**	112	9	61	83
194	Parma	11	73	89	9	37***	117	16	74	101
195	Reggio Emilia	6	39*	48	8	32***	103	13	58*	80
196	Modena	6	27***	33**	9	25***	80	19	57*	79
197	Bologna	22	62*	75	30	51***	162*	36	67*	92
198	Ferrara	4	28**	34*	17	72	229**	7	33***	45*
199	Ravenna	2	15***	18**	5	23***	73	13	65	89
200	Forli	10	46**	56	12	34***	107	22	66*	91
201	Pesaro	4	33*	41	6	31***	99	6	34**	47
202	Ancona	7	44*	53	3	11***	36	12	50*	69
203	Macerata	2	18**	22*	6	34**	108	7	44*	60
204	Ascoli Piceno	3	23**	28*	1	5***	15*	9	47*	64
205	Massa-Carrara	6	80	97	0	0***	0*	13	121	165
206	Lucca	19	137	166	10	44**	139	9	44**	60
207	Pistoia	3	31*	38	6	38**	121	5	34**	47
208	Firenze	25	57**	69	15	20***	65	35	51***	71*
209	Livorno	8	64	77	2	10***	31	12	63	87
210	Pisa	11	78	94	9	39**	123	15	70	96
211	Arezzo	12	103	125	10	53*	170	11	66	91

Table 8.2(a)—*cont.*

Area		TUB			CERV			UTER		
		Deaths	SMR to EC std	SMR to own std	Deaths	SMR to EC std	SMR to own std	Deaths	SMR to EC std	SMR to own std
212	Siena	5	50	61	3	19***	60	8	58	79
213	Grosseto	4	47	57	1	7***	23	15	123	169
214	Perugia	21	95	116	13	36***	116	15	47**	65
215	Terni	3	35	42	3	21***	68	1	8***	11**
216	Viterbo/Rieti	8	52	64	9	37***	117	12	56*	77
217	Roma	122	94	115	75	34***	107	152	70***	97
218	Latina	8	56	69	10	41**	133	25	105	147
219	Frosinone	19	121	148	9	35***	113	27	116	162*
220	Caserta	23	99	122	10	26***	82	38	101	141
221	Benevento	9	91	111	3	19***	60	12	86	118
222	Napoli	98	114	141**	52	35***	114	158	109	154***
223	Avellino	8	56	68	8	34***	110	13	62	86
224	Salerno	23	70	85	9	17***	53	59	117	162***
225	L'Aquila	19	183*	222**	7	41*	131	10	69	96
226	Teramo	7	75	91	5	33**	106	10	71	98
227	Pescara	11	109	133	6	36**	115	20	130	178*
228	Chieti	9	68	83	7	33***	104	8	42**	58
229	Isernia/Campobasso	9	80	97	3	16***	52	15	93	127
230	Foggia	15	74	90	11	32***	103	31	96	134
231	Bari	54	123	152**	18	24***	77	63	86	120
232	Taranto	20	114	141	7	23***	75	32	108	151*
233	Brindisi	17	139	171	12	57*	184	18	90	126
234	Lecce	23	91	112	16	37***	119	37	90	125
235	Potenza/Matera	17	86	106	15	47**	149	26	88	121
236	Cosenza	14	60*	73	5	13***	41*	29	79	110
237	Catanzaro	30	136	167*	4	11***	35*	31	90	125
238	Reggio Calabria	18	101	124	1	3***	11**	30	112	156*
239	Trapani	10	73	89	1	4***	14*	21	99	137
240	Palermo	20	53**	65	17	26***	85	54	88	123
241	Messina	8	36***	43*	6	16***	51	36	107	149*
242	Agrigento	7	46*	57	5	20***	64	17	73	101
243	Caltanisetta	8	90	110	4	27**	86	14	100	139
244	Enna	2	32	40	1	10***	31	5	53	74
245	Catania	21	65*	79	10	18***	59	55	107	150**
246	Ragusa	3	33*	40	7	46*	147	19	133	185*
247	Siracusa	4	32*	40	1	5***	15*	27	134	188**
248	Sassari	13	97	119	8	35***	112	8	35***	50*
249	Nuoro	13	158	194*	5	36*	116	3	23**	31*
250	Cagliari/Oristano	26	98	121	16	35***	113	24	53***	75
IRELAND		118	136**	100	183	126**	100	157	110	100
251	Eastern	28	95	71	63	120	96	50	94	85
252	Midland	5	96	70	12	145	115	6	77	69
253	Mid-Western	11	141	103	14	110	87	16	129	117
254	North-Eastern	9	123	91	16	134	106	12	103	93
255	North-Western	8	151	109	12	143	114	9	114	103
256	South-Eastern	16	166	122	23	147	117	19	126	114
257	Southern	24	178*	131	29	131	104	32	150*	135
258	Western	17	194*	140	14	101	80	13	101	91
THE NETHERLANDS		131	38***	100	541	92*	100	382	65***	100
259	Groningen	2	16***	41	22	102	111	15	71	109
260	Friesland	4	30**	78	21	92	101	12	54*	82
261	Drenthe	5	47	123	12	67	73	7	40**	61
262	Overijssel	9	38**	101	32	81	88	19	49***	75
263	Gelderland	14	34***	89	50	70*	77	35	50***	76
264	Utrecht	10	45**	121	32	84	92	30	78	119
265	Noord Holland	23	41***	109	104	109	119	68	72**	110
266	Zuid Holland	33	44***	116	136	106	115	100	79*	121
267	Zeeland	2	24*	61	13	92	99	11	81	124
268	Noord Brabant	18	35***	95	79	80	88	54	61***	93

Table 8.2(a)—*cont.*

	Area	TUB			CERV			UTER		
		Deaths	SMR to EC std	SMR to own std	Deaths	SMR to EC std	SMR to own std	Deaths	SMR to EC std	SMR to own std
269	Limburg	11	39***	104	45	96	104	28	61**	93
270	Flevoland	0	0*	0	4	60	67	3	44	69
	UK: ENGLAND AND WALES	973	62***	100	5054	196***	100	3624	148***	100
271	Northern	84	85	136**	358	221***	113*	250	166***	112
	Hartlepool	5	174	278	22	473***	242***	14	321***	218*
	North Tees	6	111	178	21	233***	118	15	172	115
	South Tees	12	134	213*	45	304***	155**	31	222***	150*
	East Cumbria	3	52	83	22	231***	118	18	204**	138
	South Cumbria	0	0**	0	17	185*	95	18	216**	146
	West Cumbria	0	0*	0	13	180	92	8	119	80
	Darlington	6	148	235	15	229**	117	8	133	90
	Durham	11	145	233*	22	177*	90	18	152	103
	North-West Durham	3	106	169	8	174	89	4	94	64
	South-West Durham	3	60	96	15	183*	94	14	185*	125
	Northumberland	4	41	66	36	225***	115	24	159*	108
	Gateshead	8	117	186	24	217***	111	11	109	74
	Newcastle	5	58	92	31	220***	112	18	139	94
	North Tyneside	4	62	98	18	170*	87	19	199**	135
	South Tyneside	8	152	239*	16	190*	98	12	161	110
	Sunderland	6	65	104	33	214***	109	18	123	83
272	Yorkshire	58	52***	83	402	218***	111*	271	156***	105
	Hull	2	22*	34	42	278***	142*	26	187**	126
	East Yorkshire	4	63	100	18	169	86	10	99	67
	Grimsby	2	40	65	37	461***	236***	23	305***	206**
	Scunthorpe	4	64	102	33	322***	164*	20	205**	138
	Northallerton	1	30	48	13	230*	117	7	127	86
	York	1	12**	20	19	140	71	14	107	72
	Scarborough	0	0*	0	6	78	40*	5	72	49
	Harrogate	3	70	113	6	83	43*	1	15*	10***
	Bradford	14	144	229**	39	245***	124	28	187**	125
	Airedale	0	0**	0	17	186*	95	9	106	71
	Calderdale	2	34	54	20	204**	104	16	174	117
	Huddersfield	6	92	148	26	241***	123	19	187*	126
	Dewsbury	3	61	99	18	222**	113	11	139	94
	Leeds Western	5	45	71	22	120	61*	18	104	70
	Leeds Eastern	9	83	133	40	226***	116	27	161*	109
	Wakefield	2	45	72	18	242**	123	15	207*	139
	Pontefract	0	0**	0	28	320***	164*	22	267***	181*
273	Trent	64	44***	70**	524	220***	112*	371	164***	110
	North Derbyshire	5	42*	67	33	171**	87	27	148	100
	Southern Derbyshire	8	48*	77	55	204***	104	39	153*	103
	Leicestershire	14	53*	85	82	188***	95	52	122	82
	North Lincolnshire	3	35	56	35	250***	127	28	212***	143
	South Lincolnshire	5	51	82	38	237***	121	29	193**	131
	Bassetlaw	1	30	48	6	110	56	5	96	65
	Central Nottinghamshire	2	22*	35	21	140	71	18	126	85
	Nottingham	8	42**	67	76	244***	125	49	166**	112
	Barnsley	5	70	112	30	257***	131	22	200**	135
	Doncaster	4	44	69	44	293***	150*	30	211***	143
	Rotherham	0	0***	0*	45	345***	176***	34	273***	185**
	Sheffield	9	54	86	59	217***	111	38	151*	102
274	East Anglian	19	31***	50***	146	143***	73***	106	111	74**
	Cambridge	3	37	60	15	111	56*	11	83	56*
	Peterborough	4	66	106	22	217**	110	15	153	102
	West Suffolk	3	47	75	10	93	47**	9	87	57
	East Suffolk	3	31*	49	13	81	41***	9	60	40**
	Norwich	3	20***	32*	49	197***	101	35	154*	105
	Great Yarmouth and Waveney	2	31	50	20	191*	98	15	159	108
	West Norfolk and Wisbech	0	0**	0*	12	122	63	9	101	68
	Huntingdon	1	28	46	5	80	40*	3	47	31*

Table 8.2(a)—*cont.*

	Area	TUB			CERV			UTER		
		Deaths	SMR to EC std	SMR to own std	Deaths	SMR to EC std	SMR to own std	Deaths	SMR to EC std	SMR to own std
275	North-West Thames	85	80*	129*	290	163***	83**	216	124**	83**
	North Bedfordshire	4	54	87	13	105	53*	12	98	65
	South Bedfordshire	4	49	80	39	292***	148*	27	201**	134
	North Hertfordshire	1	17*	28	13	134	68	10	107	72
	East Hartfordshire	5	53	85	24	154	78	20	130	88
	North-West Hertfordshire	3	35	57	19	136	69	14	103	70
	South-West Hertfordshire	1	13**	20	14	108	55*	12	98	66
	Barnet	9	99	159	20	128	65	19	125	83
	Harrow	5	83	135	10	98	50*	8	78	53
	Hillingdon	2	28	45	18	151	77	13	113	76
	Hounslow and Spelthorne	9	101	162	21	144	74	20	140	95
	Ealing	10	116	187	24	166*	83	15	104	69
	Riverside	13	157	255**	37	259***	130	20	141	93
	Parkside	19	173*	280***	38	206***	104	26	139	92
276	North-East Thames	110	95	153***	311	162***	83***	224	122**	82**
	Basildon and Thurrock	6	69	111	13	89	45**	11	78	52*
	Mid Essex	4	47	76	18	123	62*	17	115	77
	North-East Essex	2	21**	34	24	154	79	17	120	81
	West Essex	5	60	95	21	152	78	16	122	83
	Southend	4	40	63	29	172**	88	20	127	86
	Barking, Havering, and Brentwood	7	46*	72	50	199***	102	34	147*	100
	Hampstead	4	131	212	6	110	55	4	74	49
	Bloomsbury	12	307**	491***	11	170	86	5	79	53
	Islington	6	122	196	20	240***	121	14	172	113
	City and Hackney	14	262**	423***	21	239***	120	16	184*	121
	Newham	9	155	249*	23	240***	121	14	150	99
	Tower Hamlets	18	404***	644***	14	205*	103	6	95	62
	Enfield	3	37	60	14	103	53*	10	75	51*
	Haringey	7	123	200	13	135	68	11	111	74
	Redbridge	4	55	88	12	99	51*	16	140	94
	Waltham Forest	5	81	132	22	213**	108	13	128	85
277	South-East Thames	85	76**	121	334	179***	91	243	139***	94
	Brighton	4	43	68	26	167*	86	19	137	92
	Eastbourne	0	0**	0*	11	89	46**	9	83	57
	Hastings	1	19	30	12	138	71	12	163	111
	South-East Kent	0	0***	0*	38	275***	141	23	182*	122
	Canterbury and Thanet	3	32*	50	26	165*	85	21	151	102
	Dartford and Gravesham	5	72	116	22	192**	98	13	117	79
	Maidstone	7	114	185	26	253***	129	21	205**	139
	Medway	6	63	102	36	225***	114	28	176**	117
	Tunbridge Wells	3	47	76	13	123	63	6	60	41*
	Bexley	6	87	140	20	173*	88	16	142	96
	Greenwich	9	142	227*	22	206**	104	15	149	99
	Bromley	5	50	81	20	121	62*	16	102	70
	West Lambeth	10	220*	356**	12	163	82	8	110	72
	Camberwell	11	181	290**	24	237***	120	15	155	103
	Lewisham and North Southwark	15	158	250**	26	167*	85	21	146	98
278	South-West Thames	55	59***	95	202	130***	66***	155	104	70***
	North-West Surrey	2	30	48	9	81	42**	5	47	32**
	West Surrey and North-East Hampshire	2	25*	40	18	130	66	14	97	65
	South-West Surrey	2	35	56	15	155	79	13	142	96
	Mid Surrey	5	89	142	13	139	71	8	91	62
	East Surrey	3	50	79	8	79	41**	8	84	57
	Chichester	3	51	79	13	132	68	9	106	72
	Mid Downs	7	81	130	19	131	67	16	115	77
	Worthing	2	26*	41	18	139	72	12	109	75
	Croydon	8	83	134	20	123	62*	14	87	58*
	Kingston and Esher	1	18*	28	16	168	86	11	121	82
	Richmond, Twickenham, and Roehampton	5	69	111	19	154	78	13	110	74
	Wandsworth	6	114	186	15	170	85	12	135	89
	Merton and Sutton	9	87	140	19	109	55**	20	119	80

Table 8.2(a)—*cont.*

	Area	TUB			CERV			UTER		
		Deaths	SMR to EC std	SMR to own std	Deaths	SMR to EC std	SMR to own std	Deaths	SMR to EC std	SMR to own std
279	Wessex	29	33***	52***	240	161***	82**	178	128**	86*
	East Dorset	6	42*	66	43	180***	93	34	163*	111
	West Dorset	0	0**	0*	22	213**	109	16	175*	119
	Portsmouth and South-East Hampshire	7	45*	72	57	216***	110	38	151*	102
	Southampton and South-West Hampshire	4	31**	49	39	180***	92	28	139	94
	Winchester	1	15*	25	12	109	56*	9	84	57
	Basingstoke and North Hampshire	2	31	51	8	73	37**	6	54	36**
	Salisbury	1	27	43	10	161	82	8	139	94
	Swindon	3	44	71	20	175*	89	17	152	101
	Bath	2	16***	26*	24	117	60**	19	98	66
	Isle of Wight	3	72	114	5	72	37*	3	50	34*
280	Oxford	39	53***	87	190	155***	78***	133	109	73***
	East Berkshire	7	63	103	31	169**	86	22	122	82
	West Berkshire	2	15***	25*	29	133	67*	20	91	61*
	Aylesbury Vale	4	95	155	6	84	42*	4	55	37*
	Wycombe	5	57	92	18	123	63*	14	95	65
	Milton Keynes	3	73	121	11	152	75	9	116	75
	Kettering	10	130	209*	36	280***	143	24	194**	130
	Northampton	2	22*	36	32	212***	107	19	128	85
	Oxfordshire	6	39*	64	27	105	53***	21	82	55**
281	South-Western	44	44***	69*	332	198***	101	258	167***	113
	Bristol and Weston	4	36*	57	48	257***	131	42	239***	161**
	Frenchay	0	0**	0*	22	195**	99	13	119	80
	Southmead	4	55	88	20	165*	84	12	105	71
	Cornwall and Isles of Scilly	3	20***	32*	47	190***	98	36	160*	109
	Exeter	2	21**	33	28	175**	90	19	133	91
	North Devon	2	47	75	15	216*	111	14	221*	150
	Plymouth	7	72	115	33	201***	103	29	187**	126
	Torbay	1	13**	20	23	178*	92	20	178*	122
	Cheltenham and District	5	76	121	23	209**	107	20	196**	132
	Gloucester	14	143	228**	32	197***	101	26	169*	114
	Somerset	2	16***	25*	41	194***	99	27	140	95
282	West Midlands	121	74***	119	514	193***	99	379	150***	101
	Bromsgrove and Redditch	2	40	66	11	131	66	8	95	63
	Herefordshire	2	41	65	16	198*	101	14	186*	126
	Kidderminster and District	1	31	50	8	148	75	2	38	25*
	Worcester and District	3	39	63	12	95	49**	9	74	50*
	Shropshire	3	25**	40	40	199***	101	33	170**	115
	Mid Staffordshire	5	51	83	26	158*	80	22	134	90
	North Staffordshire	4	27**	42	54	222***	114	33	146*	99
	South-East Staffordshire	5	65	105	22	170*	86	19	145	98
	Rugby	2	73	117	5	113	58	6	141	96
	North Warwickshire	2	36	59	21	233***	118	18	204**	138
	South Warwickshire	3	42	67	17	143	73	9	78	53
	Central Birmingham	6	114	182	16	189*	96	12	150	101
	East Birmingham	3	49	77	24	251***	128	19	225**	152
	North Birmingham	0	0*	0	17	197*	101	10	123	83
	South Birmingham	5	66	106	19	154	78	16	142	95
	West Birmingham	16	272***	434***	22	234***	119	19	214**	143
	Coventry	10	105	167	26	170*	87	17	120	81
	Dudley	10	101	162	30	186**	95	23	149	101
	Sandwell	12	125	197*	30	195**	100	22	158	107
	Solihull	2	30	48	18	161	82	16	147	100
	Walsall	14	163	261**	42	305***	156**	28	214***	146
	Wolverhampton	11	138	219*	38	302***	155*	24	208**	141
283	Mersey	44	58***	93	362	289***	148***	241	204***	138***
	Chester	0	0**	0	37	392***	201***	32	353***	240***
	Crewe	2	25*	41	23	176*	90	14	111	75
	Halton	3	71	114	17	240**	122	9	131	87
	Macclesfield	3	51	82	17	174*	89	13	137	93
	Warrington	2	36	58	30	326***	165*	22	243***	163*

Table 8.2(a)—*cont.*

Area	TUB			CERV			UTER		
	Deaths	SMR to EC std	SMR to own std	Deaths	SMR to EC std	SMR to own std	Deaths	SMR to EC std	SMR to own std
Liverpool	16	109	172	90	373***	191***	60	274***	185***
St Helens and Knowsley	7	65	103	67	374***	191***	41	241***	163**
North Sefton	2	51	81	17	258***	133	9	148	101
South Sefton	1	17*	28	23	242***	124	16	181*	123
Wirral	8	72	115	41	220***	113	25	144	97
284 North-Western	96	78*	125*	490	243***	124***	348	183***	123***
Lancaster	3	74	117	17	255**	131	9	149	102
Blackpool Wyre and Fylde	8	74	116	34	190***	99	24	154	106
Preston	5	130	207	19	307***	157	17	295***	199*
Blackburn, Hyndburn, and Ribble Valley	8	98	157	50	378***	193***	38	305***	206***
Burnley, Pendle, and Rossendale	9	128	205	39	336***	171**	33	304***	205***
West Lancashire	2	61	99	15	273**	139	12	220*	149
Chorley and South Ribble	2	34	55	23	232***	118	18	183*	122
Bolton	10	127	205	27	208***	106	20	162	108
Bury	5	94	152	14	157	80	9	103	70
North Manchester	6	143	225	26	390***	199**	16	268***	180*
Central Manchester	6	180	285*	11	211*	107	9	183	122
South Manchester	8	152	240*	16	183*	93	6	77	51
Oldham	4	61	97	23	210**	107	15	143	96
Rochdale	4	63	101	23	218**	111	21	208**	139
Salford	8	108	172	30	251***	129	21	192**	130
Stockport	1	11**	17*	31	201***	103	21	141	95
Tameside and Glossop	2	26*	42	24	192**	98	22	186*	125
Trafford	2	29	47	32	281***	144	15	138	94
Wigan	3	32*	51	36	229***	117	22	145	97
285 Wales	40	45***	71*	359	244***	125***	251	185***	125***
Clwyd	5	40*	64	41	197***	101	26	134	90
East Dyfed	3	39	62	34	276***	142	26	238***	162*
Pembrokeshire	3	84	133	16	272***	139	14	255**	173
Gwent	9	64	101	48	207***	106	41	190***	129
Gwynedd	2	27*	43	36	294***	151*	28	254***	173**
Mid Glamorgan	6	36**	57	71	258***	132*	43	167**	113
Powys	2	54	85	15	251**	129	8	147	100
South Glamorgan	6	50	79	41	204***	104	26	139	94
West Glamorgan	4	34*	54	57	297***	152**	39	222***	151*
UK: NORTHERN IRELAND	19	45***	100	98	135**	100	75	107	100
286 Northern Ireland	19	45***	100	98	135**	100	75	107	100
UK: SCOTLAND	132	83*	100	552	206***	100	390	155***	100
287 Highlands and Islands	4	48	58	24	173*	83	15	112	72
288 Grampian	9	60	73	43	169**	81	41	167**	107
289 Tayside	7	56	67	38	181**	88	21	109	71
290 Fife	6	57	69	36	202***	98	29	173**	111
291 Lothian	17	75	91	74	192***	93	49	134	86
292 Borders	2	61	73	12	220*	107	8	159	104
293 Forth Valley	5	59	71	35	242***	117	21	152	98
294 Argyll and Clyde	14	102	122	64	275***	133*	43	193***	126
295 Greater Glasgow	46	153**	182***	96	192***	94	72	159***	103
296 Lanarkshire	11	63	77	64	216***	105	45	157**	101
297 Ayrshire and Arran	8	68	82	51	255***	124	35	184**	119
298 Dumfries and Galloway	3	62	73	15	187*	91	11	150	98
PORTUGAL	1110	356***	100	489	91*	100	719	142***	100
299 Viana do Castelo	30	392***	112	14	101	112	18	145	102
300 Braga	45	242***	67**	18	55**	61*	35	109	78
301 Vila Real	38	504***	144*	11	90	100	16	148	105
302 Bragança	19	335***	97	10	112	124	18	233**	165
303 Guarda	17	279***	81	3	30*	34*	10	118	84
304 Viseu	58	480***	137*	12	60	66	28	155*	110
305 Porto	177	388***	107	87	107	117	139	173***	123*

Table 8.2(a)—*cont.*

Area		TUB			CERV			UTER		
		Deaths	SMR to EC std	SMR to own std	Deaths	SMR to EC std	SMR to own std	Deaths	SMR to EC std	SMR to own std
306	Aveiro	48	258***	72*	29	90	98	44	140*	99
307	Coimbra	28	196**	56***	27	110	121	30	134	94
308	Castelo Branco	20	269***	78	8	66	74	9	89	62
309	Portalegre	9	185	54	6	78	86	8	122	86
310	Santarem	37	238***	68*	24	93	102	32	138	97
311	Leiria	28	205***	58**	9	39**	43**	23	108	76
312	Lisboa	361	504***	141***	139	110	119*	165	135***	94
313	Setubal	70	273***	76*	39	89	96	53	120	84
314	Evora	7	112	32***	6	59	65	8	89	63
315	Beja	20	327***	95	7	74	82	10	122	86
316	Faro	41	363***	104	12	66	72	36	218***	153*
317	Madeira	31	453***	127	14	112	124	18	152	108
318	Azores	26	403***	114	14	133	147	19	196*	139
SPAIN		1806	194***	100	956	61***	100	1311	84***	100
319	La Coruña	109	403***	208***	50	107	175***	64	136*	162***
320	Lugo	25	221***	118	8	44*	70	16	100	116
321	Orense	31	266***	140	8	42**	68	14	78	92
322	Pontevedra	66	315***	161***	27	74	121	37	101	120
323	Asturias	71	229***	120	34	68*	110	35	73	86
324	Cantabria	14	108	56*	19	90	147	16	79	93
325	Alava	6	95	47	4	38*	63	3	26**	32*
326	Guipuzcoa	26	152	78	16	56*	92	13	44***	52*
327	Vizcaya	55	178***	92	32	63**	102	43	80	95
328	Navarra	13	102	52*	7	34**	55	11	55*	66
329	Rioja	10	149	78	3	28*	45	6	58	68
330	Huesca	7	116	62	3	33*	52	7	90	105
331	Teruel	11	277**	149	1	17*	27	4	71	82
332	Zaragoza	48	211***	111	14	38***	61	28	80	94
333	Madrid Centro	174	148***	75***	100	48***	80*	130	61***	73***
334	Avila	6	126	68	3	41	65	5	79	91
335	Burgos	22	238***	125	9	61	97	3	22**	26**
336	Leon	25	177*	95	9	40**	63	18	84	97
337	Palencia	12	254**	134	2	27*	43	3	43	49
338	Salamanca	23	256***	136	11	75	120	8	57	67
339	Segovia	1	27	14*	0	0**	0*	3	53	61
340	Soria	2	81	44	1	26	42	1	28	32
341	Valladolid	11	95	48**	6	31***	50	17	87	104
342	Zamora	7	116	63	5	53	83	11	122	140
343	Albacete	18	223**	117	4	31**	49	11	85	99
344	Ciudad Real	19	163	87	6	33**	52	9	50*	59
345	Cuenca	3	57	31*	4	49	77	7	92	107
346	Guadalajara	7	201	106	6	111	178	6	123	144
347	Toledo	15	124	66	6	32**	51	17	95	110
348	Badajoz	23	157	83	3	13***	21***	14	61	71
349	Caceres	12	124	66	6	38*	61	9	58	67
350	Barcelona	214	179***	92	153	76***	124*	203	100	119*
351	Gerona	20	159	83	11	55*	89	21	111	131
352	Lerida	17	174*	92	11	73	117	13	94	110
353	Tarragona	13	96	50**	10	46**	74	14	67	79
354	Alicante	43	147*	76	23	47***	77	47	97	115
355	Castellon de la Plana	21	188*	98	11	60	98	18	103	122
356	Valencia	119	230***	118	75	85	139**	82	95	113
357	Baleares	23	135	69	32	113	185**	38	138	165**
358	Almeria	11	119	61	5	33**	53	7	43*	51
359	Cadiz	52	252***	127	25	72	119	31	86	102
360	Cordoba	26	155*	81	18	66	106	24	89	104
361	Granada	32	181**	95	9	31***	49*	20	68	80
362	Huelva	31	333***	172**	10	65	106	14	90	106
363	Jaen	37	251***	132	4	17***	27**	19	77	90
364	Malaga	61	248***	127	19	45***	75	31	74	88

Table 8.2(a)—*cont.*

Area		TUB			CERV			UTER		
		Deaths	SMR to EC std	SMR to own std	Deaths	SMR to EC std	SMR to own std	Deaths	SMR to EC std	SMR to own std
365	Sevilla	113	338***	173***	51	90	147*	64	113	134*
366	Murcia	43	190***	98	21	55**	90	33	84	98
367	Las Palmas	32	218***	107	34	131	220***	37	127	153*
368	Sta Cruz de Tenerife	26	187**	94	27	109	181**	26	98	117
EC		9975	100	-	16721	100	-	15991	100	-

Table 8.2(b)

Area	HODG			CRHD			RESP		
	Deaths	SMR to EC std	SMR to own std	Deaths	SMR to EC std	SMR to own std	Deaths	SMR to EC std	SMR to own std
BELGIUM	276	96	100	8	13***	100	127	103	100
1 Antwerpen	45	97	101	0	0***	0	19	98	95
2 Brabant	45	69**	72*	1	7***	54	19	71	69
3 West-Vlaanderen	48	151**	158**	0	0**	0	14	101	98
4 Oost-Vlaanderen	37	96	100	1	12**	92	24	149	145
5 Hainaut	30	81	84	1	13**	98	16	100	98
6 Liege	25	86	89	2	34	255	19	156	151
7 Limburg	36	168**	177**	2	43	329	9	88	86
8 Luxembourg (province)	6	94	99	1	78	604	1	31	30
9 Namur	4	34*	35*	0	0	0	6	108	105
LUXEMBOURG	14	126	100	1	42	100	4	93	100
10 Luxembourg	14	126	100	1	42	100	4	93	100
FEDERAL REPUBLIC OF GERMANY	1908	104	100	156	43***	100	512	83***	100
11 Schleswig-Holstein	67	88	85	5	32**	75	15	60*	72
12 Hamburg	62	129	123	6	61	145	4	31**	38*
13 Braunschweig	73	154***	148**	3	33*	77	9	60	72
14 Hannover	96	160***	153***	4	34*	80	24	130	157*
15 Lüneburg	51	119	114	6	69	161	9	60	72
16 Weser-Ems	62	101	98	7	57	133	32	132	159*
17 Bremen	16	81	78	2	50	119	7	124	149
18 Düsseldorf	130	83*	80**	9	30***	70	37	77	93
19 Köln	80	67***	65***	7	29***	69	32	84	101
20 Munster	73	102	98	7	50	117	17	64	77
21 Detmold	55	104	100	2	20**	46	19	102	123
22 Arnsberg	124	114	109	10	48*	113	37	103	124
23 Darmstadt	126	121*	116	13	59	141	21	65*	78
24 Giessen	32	112	108	3	54	125	10	101	122
25 Kassel	42	123	118	3	46	107	9	78	94
26 Koblenz	43	107	103	7	92	215	9	65	79
27 Trier	13	94	90	2	79	183	0	0*	0*
28 Rheinhessen-Pfalz	53	97	93	12	113	265**	20	109	132
29 Stuttgart	102	98	94	14	65	154	36	96	116
30 Karlsruhe	79	108	104	5	34**	80	24	100	121
31 Freiburg	41	74	71*	3	27**	63	25	123	148
32 Tübingen	35	79	76	2	22*	51	12	68	82
33 Oberbayern	117	105	100	8	33***	78	25	71	85
34 Niederbayern	32	108	104	0	0**	0	6	50	61
35 Oberpfalz	34	120	115	0	0**	0	11	100	120
36 Oberfranken	31	101	97	1	17*	41	9	83	100
37 Mittelfranken	46	101	97	4	44	102	7	46*	55
38 Unterfranken	32	91	87	1	15*	34	6	44*	53
39 Schwaben	46	103	99	0	0***	0*	20	115	139
40 Saarland	30	93	89	3	50	116	5	49	60
41 Berlin (West)	85	148***	142**	7	55	130	15	84	102
DENMARK	118	82*	100	16	47***	100	46	77	100
42 Kobenhavn and Frederiksberg (M)	18	116	141	3	86	191	1	24	31
43 Kobenhavns County	17	94	114	2	47	99	6	89	115
44 Frederiksborg County	6	61	75	1	39	80	2	48	62
45 Roskilde County	4	64	80	0	0	0	4	153	196
46 Vestsjællands County	8	102	124	1	53	114	3	89	115
47 Storstroms County	7	97	117	0	0	0	3	104	134
48 Bornholms County	0	0	0	0	0	0	1	174	225
49 Fyns County	14	110	134	1	34	72	3	57	74
50 Sonderjyllands County	5	72	88	1	63	136	1	31	41
51 Ribe County	1	17*	20	0	0	0	2	70	90
52 Vejle County	8	88	107	0	0	0	1	25	32
53 Ringkobing County	3	41	51	0	0	0	2	56	72
54 Århus County	12	73	90	2	49	107	7	99	127

Table 8.2(b)

Area		HODG			CRHD			RESP		
		Deaths	SMR to EC std	SMR to own std	Deaths	SMR to EC std	SMR to own std	Deaths	SMR to EC std	SMR to own std
55	Viborg County	4	64	78	3	208	458	2	68	87
56	Nordjyllands County	11	82	100	2	64	138	8	136	176
FRANCE		1189	77***	100	207	61***	100	574	74***	100
57	Ain	12	97	125	3	104	169	12	173	236*
58	Aisne	11	75	98	3	97	158	9	108	147
59	Allier	8	78	103	0	0	0	2	47	63
60	Alpes-de-Haute-Provence	4	111	146	0	0	0	2	128	174
61	Hautes-Alpes	1	32	42	0	0	0	1	68	92
62	Alpes-Maritimes	27	103	135	1	18	30	8	79	108
63	Ardèche	4	53	69	0	0	0	3	84	113
64	Ardennes	8	98	128	1	59	96	3	65	88
65	Ariège	3	79	104	2	275	448	0	0	0
66	Aube	6	76	98	2	115	187	3	73	99
67	Aude	4	50	65	0	0	0	7	212	287*
68	Aveyron	4	52	69	0	0	0	2	63	85
69	Bouches-du-Rhône	45	92	119	14	128	208*	10	43**	59
70	Calvados	8	49*	63	3	83	136	4	43	59
71	Cantal	0	0*	0	2	229	373	2	101	136
72	Charente	5	53	69	1	52	85	2	45	61
73	Charente-Maritime	12	83	109	1	34	56	6	90	121
74	Cher	12	135	177	2	108	176	4	96	131
75	Corrèze	6	89	117	0	0	0	3	111	151
76	Corse	2	28	37	3	201	327	1	33	45
77	Côte-d'Or	10	76	98	2	67	110	6	87	119
78	Côtes-du-Nord	8	54	71	2	68	111	2	28	38
79	Creuse	3	79	106	1	151	247	4	299	403*
80	Dordogne	9	83	110	2	97	159	5	115	155
81	Doubs	11	84	108	1	34	55	8	108	146
82	Drôme	5	44	57	0	0	0	6	101	138
83	Eure	11	83	107	0	0	0	8	101	138
84	Eure-et-Loir	8	78	101	1	43	71	6	99	135
85	Finistère	8	35***	46*	3	65	105	8	71	96
86	Gard	11	70	91	6	178	291*	5	68	93
87	Haute-Garonne	20	80	104	0	0**	0	5	46	63
88	Gers	5	100	132	1	106	173	6	319*	431**
89	Gironde	24	73	95	3	41	67	15	98	132
90	Hérault	12	57*	74	2	44	71	8	84	115
91	Ille-et-Vilaine	16	76	99	1	22	35	5	43	59
92	Indre	7	106	139	1	76	125	4	144	194
93	Indre-et-Loire	14	99	129	0	0	0	3	42	57
94	Isère	15	55*	71	5	79	129	7	48*	65
95	Jura	5	74	97	1	70	114	3	86	117
96	Landes	2	23*	30	0	0	0	4	107	145
97	Loir-et-Cher	5	61	80	1	59	96	4	100	136
98	Loire	15	73	95	2	46	75	8	75	102
99	Haute-Loire	2	35	46	0	0	0	5	188	254
100	Loire-Atlantique	18	64	83	2	32	52	9	57	77
101	Loiret	14	92	119	8	232*	379**	7	85	116
102	Lot	3	68	90	1	121	197	0	0	0
103	Lot-et-Garonne	9	106	139	0	0	0	2	53	72
104	Lozère	2	99	130	0	0	0	1	109	148
105	Maine-et-Loire	18	99	129	1	25	41	9	80	108
106	Manche	6	46	61	0	0	0	4	57	78
107	Marne	21	141	182*	1	29	48	5	60	82
108	Haute-Marne	6	107	140	0	0	0	2	65	88
109	Mayenne	4	54	71	2	132	215	3	71	96
110	Meurthe-et-Moselle	8	40**	52	6	140	228	9	87	119
111	Meuse	5	92	120	1	91	149	0	0	0
112	Morbihan	5	30**	39*	0	0	0	9	102	138
113	Moselle	19	66	86	2	33	54	8	53	72

Table 8.2(b)

	Area	HODG			CRHD			RESP		
		Deaths	SMR to EC std	SMR to own std	Deaths	SMR to EC std	SMR to own std	Deaths	SMR to EC std	SMR to own std
114	Nièvre	7	108	142	1	79	129	2	70	95
115	Nord	70	104	135*	6	41*	66	39	93	127
116	Oise	8	43**	55	1	22	36	18	157	214**
117	Orne	9	112	146	1	61	100	4	92	125
118	Pas-de-Calais	45	118	153**	7	87	142	20	84	115
119	Puy-de-dôme	16	95	123	2	54	88	3	39	53
120	Pyrénées-Atlantiques	8	50*	66	1	31	50	4	58	78
121	Hautes-Pyrénées	4	61	81	0	0	0	4	156	210
122	Pyrénées-Orientales	9	92	122	3	159	258	5	122	166
123	Bas-Rhin	20	76	99	3	52	85	14	109	148
124	Haut-Rhin	14	75	97	2	49	80	13	137	186
125	Rhône	20	49***	63*	9	97	158	14	67	92
126	Haute-Saône	3	48	63	1	75	122	5	145	197
127	Saône-et-Loire	11	71	93	2	63	102	4	53	72
128	Sarthe	17	123	161	1	34	56	3	41	55
129	Savoie	5	53	68	2	94	153	6	128	174
130	Haute-Savoie	11	73	93	2	55	89	4	49	67
131	Paris	56	87	112	8	55	89	14	67	92
132	Seine-Maritime	22	67	87	4	55	89	14	74	101
133	Seine-et-Marne	26	98	125	4	59	97	13	79	107
134	Yvelines	23	65*	83	5	57	93	13	65	88
135	Deux-Sèvres	2	21**	28	0	0	0	2	41	56
136	Somme	19	130	169*	2	63	102	4	49	66
137	Tarn	16	166	218**	0	0	0	1	24	32
138	Tarn-et-Garonne	7	128	168	0	0	0	1	41	56
139	Var	18	83	108	5	110	179	4	41	56
140	Vaucluse	13	103	134	3	108	176	2	32	44
141	Vendée	12	89	116	1	36	59	4	53	72
142	Vienne	7	68	89	0	0	0	2	41	55
143	Haute-Vienne	6	60	79	0	0	0	3	76	102
144	Vosges	7	66	86	0	0	0	2	35	48
145	Yonne	6	70	92	0	0	0	3	68	92
146	Territoire-de-Belfort	3	81	105	2	245	399	0	0	0
147	Essonne	27	93	119	4	56	91	8	50*	69
148	Hauts-de-Seine	25	61*	79	5	55	89	8	46*	63
149	Seine-Saint-Denis	23	60*	77	7	79	129	15	71	98
150	Val-de-Marne	26	75	96	7	88	144	8	49*	67
151	Val-d'Oise	22	80	103	9	134	218	4	24***	33*
GREECE		333	124***	100	24	41***	100	125	79**	100
152	Greater Athens	110	127*	104	9	48*	114	26	57**	72
153	Rest of Central Greece and Eubea	35	113	91	2	31	75	12	61	77
154	Peloponnisos	32	118	92	1	19	45	12	73	92
155	Ionian Islands	5	100	76	1	108	263	3	109	137
156	Epirus	8	92	73	0	0	0	3	55	70
157	Thessaly	17	88	71	1	24	58	16	137	173
158	Macedonia	69	118	98	8	61	148	34	97	122
159	Thrace	13	146	122	1	50	119	7	125	158
160	Aegean Islands	20	175*	137	0	0	0	4	59	74
161	Crete	24	179*	142	1	36	87	8	91	114
ITALY		1972	119***	100	646	190***	100	723	107	100
162	Torino	80	114	96	26	180**	95	13	58*	54*
163	Vercelli	11	94	79	8	366**	193	4	121	113
164	Novara	10	67	56	3	101	53	4	82	77
165	Cuneo	24	148	125	7	222	117	4	74	69
166	Asti	6	96	81	1	86	45	0	0	0
167	Alessandria	21	156	131	0	0	0*	4	115	108
168	Aosta	3	86	73	1	140	74	1	91	85
169	Imperia	13	195*	163	3	243	128	2	112	105
170	Savona	16	180*	151	1	61	32	1	45	42

Table 8.2(b)

	Area	HODG			CRHD			RESP		
		Deaths	SMR to EC std	SMR to own std	Deaths	SMR to EC std	SMR to own std	Deaths	SMR to EC std	SMR to own std
171	Genova	41	133	112	11	191	101	8	103	97
172	La Spezia	9	127	107	3	227	120	1	53	49
173	Varese	20	85	71	7	140	74	7	82	77
174	Como/Sondrio	38	134	113	8	133	70	9	84	78
175	Milano	158	129**	109	36	140	74	28	71	66*
176	Bergamo	29	107	91	10	171	90	15	138	129
177	Brescia	42	137	115	4	61	32*	6	51	48
178	Pavia	20	131	110	3	105	56	0	0*	0*
179	Cremona	14	140	118	6	306*	161	1	32	30
180	Mantova	16	143	121	2	91	48	3	87	81
181	Bolzano	4	32*	27**	1	38	20	8	144	134
182	Trento	14	107	91	7	256*	135	4	83	77
183	Verona	21	91	77	6	125	66	1	12**	11**
184	Vicenza	20	93	78	4	87	46	6	72	67
185	Belluno	10	157	132	1	77	41	3	144	134
186	Treviso	20	93	79	4	88	46	6	75	70
187	Venezia	36	143*	121	6	114	60	5	60	56
188	Padova	47	195***	164**	3	59	31*	8	90	84
189	Rovigo	13	173	146	2	137	72	1	40	37
190	Udine/Gorizia	22	110	93	5	121	64	7	116	108
191	Trieste	12	148	125	6	392**	208	1	54	51
192	Pordenone	9	112	94	1	58	31	4	144	135
193	Piacenza	12	144	121	1	65	34	0	0	0
194	Parma	22	184*	155	4	176	93	3	92	86
195	Reggio Emilia	17	137	115	1	41	22	3	78	73
196	Modena	32	176**	148*	6	164	86	3	55	52
197	Bologna	25	87	74	8	145	76	7	102	95
198	Ferrara	13	113	95	2	92	49	0	0	0
199	Ravenna	11	102	86	1	49	26	2	69	65
200	Forli	24	132	111	2	54	29	5	82	77
201	Pesaro	14	142	119	3	154	81	3	86	80
202	Ancona	12	92	78	0	0	0*	2	46	43
203	Macerata	9	103	86	4	243	128	1	34	31
204	Ascoli Piceno	11	103	86	4	196	103	1	26	24
205	Massa-Carrara	6	98	83	1	85	45	2	101	94
206	Lucca	14	123	104	2	90	47	2	55	52
207	Pistoia	9	114	96	1	63	33	2	80	75
208	Firenze	49	135	114	8	110	58	2	19**	18**
209	Livorno	21	204**	172*	2	97	52	2	64	60
210	Pisa	16	138	116	1	43	23	1	27	25
211	Arezzo	9	96	81	2	110	58	2	66	62
212	Siena	5	65	55	1	71	38	1	48	45
213	Grosseto	4	60	50	1	78	41	0	0	0
214	Perugia	27	152*	128	5	147	77	4	66	62
215	Terni	15	219**	184*	4	308	163	2	94	87
216	Viterbo/Rieti	14	113	95	4	168	88	5	106	99
217	Roma	127	112	95	53	226***	119	40	97	90
218	Latina	16	122	103	6	210	111	4	62	58
219	Frosinone	21	156	131	6	218	115	4	62	58
220	Caserta	32	149*	126	17	368***	194*	13	97	90
221	Benevento	6	73	61	10	644***	339**	4	98	91
222	Napoli	93	113	96	67	365***	192***	81	156***	145**
223	Avellino	18	146	123	4	165	87	14	226**	210*
224	Salerno	36	123	104	17	289***	152	23	147	136
225	L'Aquila	9	105	89	6	366*	192	3	85	79
226	Teramo	8	100	84	3	190	100	4	115	107
227	Pescara	4	47	40	4	239	126	5	145	135
228	Chieti	19	173*	146	3	139	73	4	87	81
229	Isernia/Campobasso	15	159	134	8	445**	234*	5	122	114
230	Foggia	17	92	78	7	181	95	18	165	154
231	Bari	32	78	66*	31	346***	182**	26	114	106

Table 8.2(b)

Area		HODG			CRHD			RESP		
		Deaths	SMR to EC std	SMR to own std	Deaths	SMR to EC std	SMR to own std	Deaths	SMR to EC std	SMR to own std
232	Taranto	12	74	63	12	334***	176	14	152	142
233	Brindisi	11	100	84	6	257	135	6	96	90
234	Lecce	33	148*	125	10	216*	114	20	170*	159
235	Potenza/Matera	21	123	103	8	240*	126	14	161	150
236	Cosenza	15	71	60*	13	297**	156	8	71	66
237	Catanzaro	14	69	58*	15	351***	184*	10	83	77
238	Reggio Calabria	24	153	129	9	282*	148	12	136	126
239	Trapani	10	84	71	4	164	86	5	82	76
240	Palermo	32	94	80	13	180	95	36	189***	176**
241	Messina	15	78	66	12	315**	166	20	221**	206**
242	Agrigento	19	144	121	9	341**	179	13	178	166
243	Caltanisetta	5	63	53	7	438**	230	5	113	105
244	Enna	7	131	110	0	0	0	9	310**	287*
245	Catania	35	120	102	16	264**	139	35	214***	198***
246	Ragusa	6	75	64	3	185	97	9	218	202
247	Siracusa	11	98	83	3	124	66	5	83	77
248	Sassari	17	137	116	3	110	58	9	153	143
249	Nuoro	8	107	90	1	63	33	11	287**	267**
250	Cagliari/Oristano	34	135	114	6	107	56	14	108	101
IRELAND		96	113	100	14	71	100	87	127*	100
251	Eastern	20	66	59*	6	83	118	31	135	107
252	Midland	10	204	179	0	0	0	7	163	129
253	Mid-Western	8	107	94	0	0	0	4	64	51
254	North-Eastern	11	155	136	2	119	167	7	110	87
255	North-Western	5	102	89	2	181	251	5	119	94
256	South-Eastern	12	131	115	2	95	134	14	185*	146
257	Southern	20	156	137	1	34	48	12	115	91
258	Western	10	123	108	1	55	77	7	104	82
THE NETHERLANDS		324	98	100	35	44***	100	115	78**	100
259	Groningen	10	81	83	2	69	155	2	38	49
260	Friesland	12	94	96	1	33	75	8	121	157
261	Drenthe	11	113	115	0	0	0	1	22	29
262	Overijssel	23	104	106	0	0*	0	9	83	106
263	Gelderland	46	115	118	1	11**	24	18	99	128
264	Utrecht	21	97	99	2	38	85	6	61	77
265	Noord Holland	41	76	78	7	54	121	19	89	112
266	Zuid Holland	72	100	103	9	53	119	22	70	88
267	Zeeland	11	142	145	0	0	0	2	55	70
268	Noord Brabant	42	85	87	7	59	133	16	73	94
269	Limburg	28	108	110	4	67	150	10	98	126
270	Flevoland	7	173	179	2	184	404	2	72	88
UK: ENGLAND AND WALES		1395	101	100	222	72***	100	690	107	100
271	Northern	92	107	107	20	108	149	41	103	96
	Hartlepool	7	279*	279*	1	188	260	1	80	75
	North Tees	7	141	140	2	180	250	2	80	74
	South Tees	10	125	125	1	57	79	4	96	89
	East Cumbria	7	140	140	1	93	129	2	93	87
	South Cumbria	7	147	147	1	98	135	1	51	47
	West Cumbria	5	129	128	1	118	163	1	57	53
	Darlington	1	29	29	0	0	0	2	130	121
	Durham	5	75	75	2	138	191	5	167	156
	North-West Durham	5	207	208	0	0	0	1	95	89
	South-West Durham	2	46	46	1	106	146	1	51	47
	Northumberland	6	71	71	1	54	74	1	26	25
	Gateshead	4	68	68	0	0	0	3	119	111
	Newcastle	7	91	90	3	182	255	7	202	188
	North Tyneside	6	110	111	1	87	120	5	209	195
	South Tyneside	3	68	68	0	0	0	0	0	0

Table 8.2(b)

Area		HODG			CRHD			RESP		
		Deaths	SMR to EC std	SMR to own std	Deaths	SMR to EC std	SMR to own std	Deaths	SMR to EC std	SMR to own std
	Sunderland	10	121	120	5	278	385*	5	120	112
272	Yorkshire	96	97	96	17	78	108	58	123	114
	Hull	13	159	159	1	57	79	5	121	112
	East Yorkshire	3	55	55	2	169	232	1	44	42
	Grimsby	7	160	160	2	210	291	0	0	0
	Scunthorpe	8	146	145	2	166	228	3	114	107
	Northallerton	2	63	62	0	0	0	1	72	67
	York	7	95	95	1	61	85	5	157	146
	Scarborough	1	26	26	0	0	0	2	123	115
	Harrogate	7	186	186	0	0	0	1	66	62
	Bradford	7	79	78	4	205	285	6	112	104
	Airedale	5	104	104	0	0	0	2	90	84
	Calderdale	4	76	75	2	168	231	2	77	72
	Huddersfield	5	86	86	2	154	212	3	109	102
	Dewsbury	5	112	111	0	0	0	4	167	156
	Leeds Western	9	90	89	0	0	0	12	264**	246**
	Leeds Eastern	3	31*	31*	1	48	67	2	45	42
	Wakefield	7	172	170	0	0	0	5	271	253
	Pontefract	3	64	64	0	0	0	4	181	169
273	Trent	138	107	106	23	80	111	61	103	96
	North Derbyshire	9	88	88	5	220	302	2	45	42
	Southern Derbyshire	21	143	143	1	31	42	11	162	151
	Leicestershire	24	99	98	3	54	75	16	135	126
	North Lincolnshire	11	146	145	0	0	0	4	119	112
	South Lincolnshire	11	130	130	0	0	0	1	27	26
	Bassetlaw	6	201	201	0	0	0	2	154	144
	Central Nottinghamshire	6	74	74	1	56	77	5	133	124
	Nottingham	12	70	70	5	133	185	8	103	96
	Barnsley	7	113	112	0	0	0	2	70	65
	Doncaster	8	98	98	1	57	79	1	26	24
	Rotherham	6	85	84	3	191	263	3	87	81
	Sheffield	17	115	115	4	126	174	6	99	93
274	East Anglian	52	95	95	3	25**	34*	25	96	90
	Cambridge	10	134	132	1	58	81	2	60	56
	Peterborough	5	90	89	0	0	0	5	169	157
	West Suffolk	4	66	65	0	0	0	5	153	142
	East Suffolk	6	70	69	1	53	73	1	23	22
	Norwich	12	93	93	1	36	50	5	92	86
	Great Yarmouth and Waveney	6	112	112	0	0	0	0	0	0
	West Norfolk and Wisbech	8	155	155	0	0	0	2	88	82
	Huntingdon	1	28	27	0	0	0	5	252	235
275	North-West Thames	79	81	80*	23	103	143	47	106	98
	North Bedfordshire	3	43	43	0	0	0	2	59	55
	South Bedfordshire	5	65	64	1	56	78	4	98	91
	North Hertfordshire	4	76	76	0	0	0	1	40	37
	East Hartfordshire	10	119	118	1	53	73	2	54	51
	North-West Hertfordshire	9	121	120	1	60	82	2	59	55
	South-West Hertfordshire	4	58	58	2	132	182	6	196	183
	Barnet	10	119	118	2	104	145	3	78	72
	Harrow	8	146	145	0	0	0	2	78	73
	Hillingdon	1	15*	15*	1	70	97	1	34	31
	Hounslow and Spelthorne	7	88	88	1	57	78	9	251*	234*
	Ealing	11	133	131	6	312*	435**	5	129	120
	Riverside	2	25*	24*	3	157	222	0	0	0
	Parkside	5	47	46	5	205	287	10	209*	193
276	North-East Thames	103	99	98	23	98	136	55	113	106
	Basildon and Thurrock	11	139	137	0	0	0	6	152	142
	Mid Essex	9	112	111	1	52	71	1	26	24
	North-East Essex	10	123	122	1	56	78	3	83	77
	West Essex	9	125	125	0	0	0	0	0	0
	Southend	6	68	68	1	51	70	6	149	139

Table 8.2(b)

	Area	HODG			CRHD			RESP		
		Deaths	SMR to EC std	SMR to own std	Deaths	SMR to EC std	SMR to own std	Deaths	SMR to EC std	SMR to own std
	Barking, Havering, and Brentwood	16	123	124	2	73	100	7	125	116
	Hampstead	2	65	64	1	139	195	1	90	83
	Bloomsbury	3	81	80	3	370	526*	0	0	0
	Islington	5	105	103	1	92	130	3	145	134
	City and Hackney	1	19	19	1	85	119	7	251*	232
	Newham	5	90	89	3	241	338	2	64	59
	Tower Hamlets	5	119	117	2	224	318	3	129	119
	Enfield	6	82	82	3	180	248	7	209	194
	Haringey	5	92	91	1	79	110	1	40	37
	Redbridge	6	93	93	0	0	0	3	108	101
	Waltham Forest	4	69	68	3	224	311	5	174	161
277	South-East Thames	100	101	100	9	41**	57	46	103	96
	Brighton	13	160	160	0	0	0	0	0	0
	Eastbourne	4	67	67	1	80	111	3	122	114
	Hastings	3	71	71	0	0	0	4	221	206
	South-East Kent	8	111	110	0	0	0	5	153	143
	Canterbury and Thanet	12	151	151	1	59	82	2	56	52
	Dartford and Gravesham	8	130	129	1	72	99	6	208	195
	Maidstone	3	53	53	1	77	106	4	159	149
	Medway	6	67	66	0	0	0	7	150	140
	Tunbridge Wells	3	55	55	2	169	232	3	133	124
	Bexley	3	48	48	0	0	0	4	143	134
	Greenwich	7	120	119	1	77	107	3	102	94
	Bromley	8	94	94	1	53	74	2	58	54
	West Lambeth	3	67	65	0	0	0	0	0	0
	Camberwell	7	122	120	1	78	110	1	34	31
	Lewisham and North Southwark	12	139	138	0	0	0	2	49	46
278	South-West Thames	75	91	91	11	60	82	34	95	89
	North-West Surrey	5	85	85	1	77	106	3	119	111
	West Surrey and North-East Hampshire	4	52	51	1	55	75	4	110	102
	South-West Surrey	4	80	80	2	182	251	4	181	170
	Mid Surrey	5	107	108	0	0	0	1	52	49
	East Surrey	7	135	135	0	0	0	1	45	42
	Chichester	5	104	105	0	0	0	0	0	0
	Mid Downs	9	116	115	1	57	79	5	138	129
	Worthing	4	64	65	0	0	0	5	199	186
	Croydon	7	78	77	2	96	133	3	72	67
	Kingston and Esher	6	120	120	0	0	0	0	0	0
	Richmond, Twickenham, and Roehampton	4	61	61	1	67	93	1	39	37
	Wandsworth	6	114	111	1	81	114	4	175	162
	Merton and Sutton	9	97	97	2	95	131	3	73	68
279	Wessex	71	90	89	9	52*	72	30	84	78
	East Dorset	9	75	76	0	0	0	3	62	58
	West Dorset	7	131	131	0	0	0	4	180	168
	Portsmouth and South-East Hampshire	17	118	117	2	63	87	6	89	83
	Southampton and South-West Hampshire	7	61	61	2	80	111	4	76	71
	Winchester	4	68	68	1	76	104	3	114	107
	Basingstoke and North Hampshire	6	99	98	2	141	194	0	0	0
	Salisbury	0	0	0	0	0	0	2	137	128
	Swindon	4	63	62	0	0	0	3	91	85
	Bath	16	146	145	1	41	57	4	83	78
	Isle of Wight	1	29	30	1	142	195	1	70	66
280	Oxford	90	131*	129*	7	44*	60	34	101	94
	East Berkshire	16	158	156	2	85	118	3	61	57
	West Berkshire	14	112	110	0	0	0	4	68	63
	Aylesbury Vale	7	175	172	1	105	145	1	50	47
	Wycombe	13	169	168	1	58	79	4	117	110
	Milton Keynes	5	111	107	0	0	0	3	105	98
	Kettering	9	129	128	2	125	173	2	58	55
	Northampton	12	143	141	0	0	0	8	188	175
	Oxfordshire	14	95	93	1	29	41	9	127	118

Table 8.2(b)

	Area	HODG			CRHD			RESP		
		Deaths	SMR to EC std	SMR to own std	Deaths	SMR to EC std	SMR to own std	Deaths	SMR to EC std	SMR to own std
281	South-Western	96	110	110	10	53*	73	35	91	85
	Bristol and Weston	6	60	60	1	45	63	4	89	83
	Frenchay	9	147	146	2	146	202	2	73	68
	Southmead	6	92	92	0	0	0	8	278*	260*
	Cornwall and Isles of Scilly	18	144	145	1	38	52	5	92	86
	Exeter	6	73	74	1	58	81	2	58	54
	North Devon	6	165	165	1	128	176	0	0	0
	Plymouth	11	123	122	0	0	0	6	145	135
	Torbay	7	110	111	1	77	106	1	39	37
	Cheltenham and District	5	87	86	1	79	110	2	82	76
	Gloucester	7	81	81	1	52	72	2	50	46
	Somerset	15	138	138	1	42	59	3	62	58
282	West Midlands	161	111	111	22	69	95	80	117	109
	Bromsgrove and Redditch	4	87	85	0	0	0	0	0	0
	Herefordshire	3	70	70	1	107	148	1	53	49
	Kidderminster and District	2	70	69	2	298	408	1	75	71
	Worcester and District	5	75	74	0	0	0	4	135	126
	Shropshire	13	119	118	1	41	56	0	0*	0**
	Mid Staffordshire	12	134	132	0	0	0	3	74	69
	North Staffordshire	16	123	123	3	106	146	4	68	64
	South-East Staffordshire	4	56	55	1	59	81	7	203	189
	Rugby	0	0	0	1	190	261	0	0	0
	North Warwickshire	5	101	101	0	0	0	1	44	41
	South Warwickshire	7	111	110	0	0	0	1	38	36
	Central Birmingham	7	146	145	1	95	132	10	387***	361**
	East Birmingham	6	113	113	2	182	254	6	211	196
	North Birmingham	2	43	43	1	99	137	3	151	141
	South Birmingham	8	118	117	1	67	93	5	156	146
	West Birmingham	13	240**	237**	1	85	118	4	117	108
	Coventry	4	48	47	1	55	77	3	72	67
	Dudley	11	126	126	3	155	213	5	133	124
	Sandwell	8	97	97	1	58	80	3	75	70
	Solihull	9	154	154	0	0	0	4	154	145
	Walsall	7	94	94	1	63	87	10	286**	267*
	Wolverhampton	15	218*	218*	1	70	97	5	149	139
283	Mersey	60	90	90	10	69	95	34	107	100
	Chester	9	181	180	1	92	127	2	90	84
	Crewe	8	114	114	0	0	0	6	186	174
	Halton	1	26	25	2	223	307	1	46	43
	Macclesfield	1	19	19	0	0	0	3	141	132
	Warrington	4	78	77	1	85	117	4	159	149
	Liverpool	14	108	108	2	74	103	5	79	74
	St Helens and Knowsley	6	62	62	3	142	197	6	122	114
	North Sefton	5	151	152	0	0	0	1	75	70
	South Sefton	3	60	60	0	0	0	1	42	39
	Wirral	9	93	92	1	47	65	5	108	101
284	North-Western	112	102	102	18	74	103	74	139**	130*
	Lancaster	3	86	86	0	0	0	3	197	184
	Blackpool Wyre and Fylde	6	68	69	1	56	78	4	117	109
	Preston	4	117	117	1	138	192	1	57	53
	Blackburn, Hyndburn, and Ribble Valley	4	55	55	1	62	86	2	53	49
	Burnley, Pendle, and Rossendale	5	81	80	1	72	99	8	242*	225
	West Lancashire	2	67	67	1	146	200	3	211	198
	Chorley and South Ribble	4	73	72	1	77	106	1	37	35
	Bolton	10	140	138	3	184	254	8	217	203
	Bury	3	62	62	0	0	0	5	218	204
	North Manchester	4	106	105	0	0	0	0	0	0
	Central Manchester	3	92	90	2	290	414	5	309*	286
	South Manchester	5	103	101	1	95	134	1	42	39
	Oldham	10	167	166	2	147	203	3	97	90
	Rochdale	6	103	102	1	76	105	4	128	119

Table 8.2(b)

	Area	HODG			CRHD			RESP		
		Deaths	SMR to EC std	SMR to own std	Deaths	SMR to EC std	SMR to own std	Deaths	SMR to EC std	SMR to own std
	Salford	5	77	77	1	72	100	6	196	183
	Stockport	8	98	97	1	55	76	3	80	75
	Tameside and Glossop	11	162	161	1	66	91	5	151	141
	Trafford	13	215*	215*	0	0	0	5	183	170
	Wigan	6	70	69	0	0	0	7	170	159
285	Wales	70	90	90	17	101	140	36	98	92
	Clwyd	9	82	82	0	0	0	10	194	182
	East Dyfed	3	47	47	4	303	419*	4	145	135
	Pembrokeshire	2	65	65	1	152	209	0	0	0
	Gwent	5	41*	41*	2	75	103	7	121	113
	Gwynedd	7	111	111	0	0	0	5	172	161
	Mid Glamorgan	13	88	88	6	184	254	6	82	77
	Powys	6	191	191	0	0	0	1	73	68
	South Glamorgan	14	129	128	2	85	119	3	56	52
	West Glamorgan	11	110	110	2	94	130	0	0*	0*
UK: NORTHERN IRELAND		55	138*	100	7	79	100	37	136	100
286	Northern Ireland	55	138*	100	7	79	100	37	136	100
UK: SCOTLAND		147	104	100	27	89	100	104	158***	100
287	Highlands and Islands	11	147	142	0	0	0	8	211	134
288	Grampian	14	101	97	1	32	36	6	92	58
289	Tayside	17	157	151	3	131	147	5	103	65
290	Fife	14	148	143	2	95	106	5	110	70
291	Lothian	16	77	74	1	22	25	13	147	93
292	Borders	2	71	69	1	167	184	2	165	104
293	Forth Valley	11	145	139	0	0	0	8	228	144
294	Argyll and Clyde	12	97	94	4	151	170	8	136	86
295	Greater Glasgow	21	80	77	11	208*	242*	24	200**	127
296	Lanarkshire	11	70	67	2	58	66	12	153	97
297	Ayrshire and Arran	10	96	93	2	89	98	10	201	127
298	Dumfries and Galloway	8	194	188	0	0	0	3	165	104
PORTUGAL		205	73***	100	173	296***	100	398	268***	100
299	Viana do Castelo	3	44	61	4	306	102	8	204	76
300	Braga	14	73	105	13	311***	103	50	362***	135*
301	Vila Real	4	59	82	3	238	78	13	325***	121
302	Bragança	3	61	84	3	346	114	8	322**	120
303	Guarda	4	78	106	1	108	36	7	276*	103
304	Viseu	14	131	179	7	343*	114	23	350***	130
305	Porto	25	56**	78	32	316***	106	81	306***	114
306	Aveiro	7	40**	55	15	392***	132	23	224***	83
307	Coimbra	10	81	110	6	244	83	11	186	69
308	Castelo Branco	0	0**	0*	8	738***	248*	7	265*	99
309	Portalegre	3	79	104	4	612**	206	1	62	23
310	Santarem	6	46	62	1	41	14*	14	242**	90
311	Leiria	14	117	159	8	331**	112	13	211*	79
312	Lisboa	55	88	118	29	214***	73	82	298***	111
313	Setubal	17	75	100	10	196	67	20	185*	69
314	Evora	6	121	159	0	0	0	3	136	51
315	Beja	6	122	162	6	700***	235	3	136	51
316	Faro	5	53	71	6	323*	110	8	178	66
317	Madeira	3	46	64	7	521***	173	8	180	67
318	Azores	6	101	139	10	816***	273**	15	325***	121
SPAIN		817	98	100	327	204***	100	496	95	100
319	La Coruña	29	121	124	8	173	84	9	63	67
320	Lugo	9	102	104	4	274	132	3	83	88
321	Orense	4	42	43	2	115	55	6	147	153
322	Pontevedra	18	94	96	1	26	13**	13	95	101
323	Asturias	30	115	117	2	46	22*	9	68	72

Table 8.2(b)

Area		HODG			CRHD			RESP		
		Deaths	SMR to EC std	SMR to own std	Deaths	SMR to EC std	SMR to own std	Deaths	SMR to EC std	SMR to own std
324	Cantabria	10	87	88	2	97	48	10	150	160
325	Alava	5	80	82	2	148	72	1	25	26
326	Guipuzcoa	9	57	58	3	95	46	9	98	102
327	Vizcaya	31	110	113	9	169	83	8	52	54
328	Navarra	14	123	125	4	182	89	7	110	115
329	Rioja	5	86	88	2	193	94	0	0	0
330	Huesca	6	126	128	1	139	69	2	94	100
331	Teruel	2	64	65	3	649*	320	3	229	243
332	Zaragoza	32	167**	170**	9	260*	127	11	113	118
333	Madrid Centro	89	81*	82	20	87	42***	49	68**	71*
334	Avila	3	81	82	0	0	0	6	342*	360*
335	Burgos	8	101	102	1	73	36	3	77	81
336	Leon	12	106	108	10	571***	281**	7	139	147
337	Palencia	5	126	128	1	156	78	2	105	112
338	Salamanca	9	121	123	5	399*	197	5	141	146
339	Segovia	6	194	198	0	0	0	0	0	0
340	Soria	0	0	0	1	333	165	1	122	129
341	Valladolid	8	74	75	5	226	110	3	42	44
342	Zamora	4	85	87	2	280	137	1	54	57
343	Albacete	5	73	74	3	244	121	3	69	72
344	Ciudad Real	8	83	85	8	506***	251*	8	152	159
345	Cuenca	2	48	49	3	455	225	1	51	53
346	Guadalajara	3	103	105	3	642*	320	1	63	67
347	Toledo	5	50	51	5	300	148	10	175	185
348	Badajoz	18	144	147	11	508***	252*	16	211*	221**
349	Caceres	7	85	86	1	73	36	6	136	143
350	Barcelona	94	87	89	44	203***	99	38	57***	60***
351	Gerona	10	93	95	1	53	26	4	63	67
352	Lerida	9	113	115	4	313	154	5	130	138
353	Tarragona	7	59	60	9	409***	201	2	27*	28
354	Alicante	19	72	73	11	210*	103	16	87	92
355	Castellon de la Plana	8	83	85	2	111	54	6	102	108
356	Valencia	49	105	107	30	319***	156*	27	88	93
357	Baleares	20	131	133	6	198	96	8	86	90
358	Almeria	7	82	84	5	304	150	3	47	50
359	Cadiz	28	139	141	9	215	106	18	105	111
360	Cordoba	23	158*	160*	9	347**	172	13	140	148
361	Granada	25	161*	163*	4	142	70	16	159	166
362	Huelva	10	120	122	4	253	125	10	160	168
363	Jaen	12	95	96	7	313*	155	7	88	92
364	Malaga	22	97	98	14	303***	148	21	128	134
365	Sevilla	35	114	116	16	258**	126	42	175**	184***
366	Murcia	16	78	80	10	253*	124	18	117	123
367	Las Palmas	13	84	85	7	202	100	13	107	110
368	Sta Cruz de Tenerife	14	103	104	4	137	67	16	152	159
EC		8849	100	-	1863	100	-	4038	100	-

Table 8.2(c)

Area		ASTH Deaths	ASTH SMR to EC std	ASTH SMR to own std	APP Deaths	APP SMR to EC std	APP SMR to own std	HERN Deaths	HERN SMR to EC std	HERN SMR to own std
BELGIUM		222	131***	100	12	40***	100	29	50***	100
1	Antwerpen	27	99	76	0	0*	0	0	0***	0*
2	Brabant	59	155**	118	4	59	147	7	52	105
3	West-Vlaanderen	21	113	87	1	30	76	1	16*	31
4	Oost-Vlaanderen	14	62	47**	1	25	63	7	90	182
5	Hainaut	45	208***	158**	4	102	249	9	115	233*
6	Liege	22	131	100	0	0	0	1	16*	33
7	Limburg	11	81	62	0	0	0	3	77	152
8	Luxembourg (province)	7	184	142	0	0	0	1	77	156
9	Namur	16	225**	172	2	161	393	0	0	0
LUXEMBOURG		10	153	100	0	0	0	2	93	100
10	Luxembourg	10	153	100	0	0	0	2	93	100
FEDERAL REPUBLIC OF GERMANY		1384	135***	100	223	122**	100	238	65***	100
11	Schleswig-Holstein	65	150**	111	10	133	110	13	88	135
12	Hamburg	30	114	84	7	147	120	8	83	127
13	Braunschweig	41	158**	117	11	229*	187	9	93	142
14	Hannover	45	138*	102	3	49	40	6	49	75
15	Lüneburg	34	140	104	6	139	115	1	12**	18
16	Weser-Ems	46	128	95	10	163	135	9	76	116
17	Bremen	24	220***	163*	9	456***	373**	2	50	77
18	Düsseldorf	107	129*	96	10	63	52*	16	50**	76
19	Köln	91	137**	101	11	93	77	9	38**	59
20	Munster	54	133	98	7	97	80	8	56	86
21	Detmold	48	165**	122	4	74	61	5	46	71
22	Arnsberg	90	154***	114	14	125	102	12	53*	81
23	Darmstadt	75	128*	95	12	117	96	7	34**	52
24	Giessen	25	155*	115	3	105	87	5	88	135
25	Kassel	20	107	79	5	141	116	6	84	128
26	Koblenz	38	175**	130	2	48	39	6	71	109
27	Trier	6	80	59	4	277	228	2	69	105
28	Rheinhessen-Pfalz	52	173***	128	6	109	89	9	81	124
29	Stuttgart	57	96	71**	7	68	56	11	54*	84
30	Karlsruhe	53	129	95	9	125	103	15	105	161
31	Freiburg	34	107	79	1	18	15*	10	93	143
32	Tübingen	19	72	53**	8	183	152	4	47	73
33	Oberbayern	82	127*	94	16	149	123	13	61	95
34	Niederbayern	26	152	113	5	166	138	8	135	208
35	Oberpfalz	19	118	88	6	207	171	4	70	107
36	Oberfranken	28	169*	125	5	157	129	11	171	262**
37	Mittelfranken	42	164**	122	5	110	90	6	66	101
38	Unterfranken	22	109	81	5	140	116	5	71	109
39	Schwaben	40	155*	115	9	199	165	4	45	69
40	Saarland	20	116	86	3	91	74	9	134	205
41	Berlin (West)	51	152**	112	10	186	153	5	47	73
DENMARK		73	80	100	29	203***	100	29	106	100
42	Kobenhavn andFrederiksberg (M)	6	62	84	4	276	137	3	104	101
43	Kobenhavns County	13	120	150	5	274	134	1	28	26
44	Frederiksborg County	1	15*	19	2	211	103	1	57	52
45	Roskilde County	3	71	87	0	0	0	2	189	171
46	Vestsjællands County	4	80	99	4	505*	246	1	66	62
47	Storstroms County	2	46	57	1	133	64	2	135	127
48	Bornholms County	0	0	0	0	0	0	0	0	0
49	Fyns County	4	50	62	2	157	77	3	123	116
50	Sonderjyllands County	2	47	57	0	0	0	2	147	138
51	Ribe County	4	103	128	2	336	167	0	0	0
52	Vejle County	7	120	149	3	328	161	5	288	271
53	Ringkobing County	5	105	129	0	0	0	0	0	0
54	Århus County	10	91	114	4	254	127	2	69	65

Table 8.2(c)—*cont.*

	Area	ASTH			APP			HERN		
		Deaths	SMR to EC std	SMR to own std	Deaths	SMR to EC std	SMR to own std	Deaths	SMR to EC std	SMR to own std
55	Viborg County	6	153	189	1	156	77	2	163	155
56	Nordjyllands County	6	71	89	1	74	36	5	194	183
FRANCE		1049	109**	100	148	94	100	430	143***	100
57	Ain	13	162	147	5	403*	430*	4	175	122
58	Aisne	18	198*	182*	1	65	70	10	345**	242*
59	Allier	6	106	97	2	178	192	5	220	154
60	Alpes-de-Haute-Provence	1	49	44	0	0	0	0	0	0
61	Hautes-Alpes	3	161	147	0	0	0	0	0	0
62	Alpes-Maritimes	20	137	125	1	36	38	4	70	49
63	Ardèche	7	159	145	0	0	0	1	62	43
64	Ardennes	8	159	146	1	117	126	3	187	130
65	Ariège	0	0	0	0	0	0	3	342	240
66	Aube	4	81	74	0	0	0	2	130	91
67	Aude	4	90	82	1	112	121	3	165	115
68	Aveyron	5	121	111	1	118	127	5	288	202
69	Bouches-du-Rhône	32	105	96	1	20	21	10	105	73
70	Calvados	7	66	60	0	0	0	0	0	0*
71	Cantal	2	80	73	0	0	0	1	103	72
72	Charente	6	109	100	1	99	106	3	151	106
73	Charente-Maritime	12	145	132	3	191	205	4	128	89
74	Cher	4	76	70	2	213	229	2	109	76
75	Corrèze	5	137	125	1	133	143	0	0	0
76	Corse	4	98	89	0	0	0	1	69	48
77	Côte-d'Or	5	58	53	0	0	0	4	162	113
78	Côtes-du-Nord	12	142	130	3	181	195	2	60	42
79	Creuse	0	0	0	1	229	248	2	217	152
80	Dordogne	5	87	79	1	82	89	2	80	56
81	Doubs	5	58	53	0	0	0	2	84	58
82	Drôme	12	172	157	2	169	181	3	132	93
83	Eure	16	184*	168	3	225	240	3	123	86
84	Eure-et-Loir	5	76	69	1	96	102	0	0	0
85	Finistère	24	177*	163*	2	81	87	10	207	145
86	Gard	8	86	78	1	60	64	4	122	85
87	Haute-Garonne	13	81	74	2	81	86	2	43	30
88	Gers	1	38	35	0	0	0	1	87	61
89	Gironde	28	135	124	7	209	222	5	78	55
90	Hérault	9	70	64	4	181	193	2	47	33
91	Ille-et-Vilaine	14	103	95	2	92	98	8	198	139
92	Indre	5	135	123	2	276	297	3	205	144
93	Indre-et-Loire	4	45	41	1	69	73	2	73	51
94	Isère	9	50*	46*	2	74	79	13	260**	181
95	Jura	5	123	112	0	0	0	5	360*	252
96	Landes	4	82	75	1	106	114	1	53	37
97	Loir-et-Cher	6	124	113	0	0	0	1	58	41
98	Loire	9	72	66	1	46	50	5	120	84
99	Haute-Loire	0	0	0	1	160	172	4	320	224
100	Loire-Atlantique	23	127	117	2	69	74	4	75	52
101	Loiret	16	164	150	3	193	206	3	103	72
102	Lot	2	86	79	0	0	0	2	196	138
103	Lot-et-Garonne	2	42	39	0	0	0	5	266	186
104	Lozère	1	87	79	0	0	0	1	230	161
105	Maine-et-Loire	16	135	124	1	53	57	7	201	141
106	Manche	9	118	109	1	71	77	0	0	0*
107	Marne	7	70	65	3	202	215	11	409***	285**
108	Haute-Marne	3	87	80	1	170	183	1	90	63
109	Mayenne	6	133	123	1	127	136	1	67	47
110	Meurthe-et-Moselle	3	24**	22**	4	197	211	6	158	110
111	Meuse	3	92	85	1	172	185	3	269	188
112	Morbihan	14	141	129	3	167	180	5	144	101
113	Moselle	19	106	98	7	241	259*	3	55	38

Table 8.2(c)—*cont.*

Area		ASTH			APP			HERN		
		Deaths	SMR to EC std	SMR to own std	Deaths	SMR to EC std	SMR to own std	Deaths	SMR to EC std	SMR to own std
114	Nièvre	4	111	102	1	140	151	3	209	146
115	Nord	104	236***	218***	12	173	185	33	260***	181**
116	Oise	18	140	128	0	0	0	2	61	43
117	Orne	2	42	38	0	0	0	1	59	42
118	Pas-de-Calais	48	199***	184***	4	99	107	20	265***	185*
119	Puy-de-dôme	12	115	105	3	172	184	4	119	83
120	Pyrénées-Atlantiques	16	173	159	2	118	127	4	120	84
121	Hautes-Pyrénées	4	111	101	0	0	0	3	212	148
122	Pyrénées-Orientales	8	150	138	0	0	0	2	90	63
123	Bas-Rhin	10	59	55	1	39	41	9	188	131
124	Haut-Rhin	13	111	102	2	107	115	6	171	119
125	Rhône	17	65	59*	5	123	131	7	92	64
126	Haute-Saône	5	130	119	0	0	0	1	80	56
127	Saône-et-Loire	7	77	70	1	60	64	5	152	106
128	Sarthe	5	58	54	1	69	74	4	146	102
129	Savoie	4	67	61	0	0	0	2	110	77
130	Haute-Savoie	5	49	45	1	68	72	4	150	104
131	Paris	28	70	64*	7	116	121	17	145	102
132	Seine-Maritime	22	103	95	4	121	129	15	246**	172
133	Seine-et-Marne	17	91	82	0	0	0	11	252*	175
134	Yvelines	30	126	114	3	89	95	7	118	82
135	Deux-Sèvres	7	126	115	0	0	0	2	103	72
136	Somme	7	74	68	1	66	70	4	141	98
137	Tarn	6	113	103	0	0	0	0	0	0
138	Tarn-et-Garonne	1	32	29	0	0	0	1	85	59
139	Var	18	145	132	0	0	0	6	128	90
140	Vaucluse	8	104	95	0	0	0	2	80	56
141	Vendée	5	62	57	0	0	0	0	0	0*
142	Vienne	5	79	73	0	0	0	0	0	0
143	Haute-Vienne	3	52	48	1	93	100	3	140	98
144	Vosges	5	77	71	1	90	97	1	47	33
145	Yonne	6	119	108	3	326	350	3	167	117
146	Territoire-de-Belfort	1	43	39	0	0	0	1	144	100
147	Essonne	23	116	106	1	36	39	6	124	86
148	Hauts-de-Seine	25	99	91	4	100	106	14	184*	128
149	Seine-Saint-Denis	30	119	109	2	54	58	13	196*	136
150	Val-de-Marne	16	72	66	2	60	63	10	160	111
151	Val-d'Oise	20	106	97	2	77	82	7	154	107
GREECE		22	14***	100	2	7***	100	12	23***	100
152	Greater Athens	4	8***	56	2	23*	321	4	25***	108
153	Rest of Central Greece and Eubea	2	11***	80	0	0	0	1	16*	70
154	Peloponnisos	2	13***	96	0	0	0	1	18*	75
155	Ionian Islands	0	0	0	0	0	0	0	0	0
156	Epirus	3	59	436	0	0	0	2	116	494
157	Thessaly	0	0***	0	0	0	0	1	26	113
158	Macedonia	8	22***	160	0	0**	0	1	9***	41
159	Thrace	1	18*	128	0	0	0	0	0	0
160	Aegean Islands	0	0**	0	0	0	0	1	43	182
161	Crete	2	25*	190	0	0	0	1	37	156
ITALY		346	36***	100	142	82*	100	379	111*	100
162	Torino	19	49***	136	10	138	168	24	166*	149
163	Vercelli	1	17*	47	1	79	97	5	190	171
164	Novara	2	24*	68	0	0	0	5	158	142
165	Cuneo	4	46	129	1	58	70	8	225	203
166	Asti	1	31	88	0	0	0	2	140	127
167	Alessandria	6	89	249	0	0	0	7	225	203
168	Aosta	4	206	575*	0	0	0	2	277	249
169	Imperia	3	89	249	0	0	0	5	329*	296
170	Savona	1	23	63	2	206	251	1	49	44

Table 8.2(c)—*cont.*

	Area	ASTH			APP			HERN		
		Deaths	SMR to EC std	SMR to own std	Deaths	SMR to EC std	SMR to own std	Deaths	SMR to EC std	SMR to own std
171	Genova	9	58	163	4	120	147	7	100	90
172	La Spezia	2	56	156	0	0	0	0	0	0
173	Varese	5	36*	102	1	41	50	6	127	114
174	Como/Sondrio	4	24***	67	1	34	42	7	124	111
175	Milano	10	14***	40**	3	24**	29*	26	105	94
176	Bergamo	2	12***	34	2	74	90	3	58	52
177	Brescia	4	22***	61	5	159	194	4	66	59
178	Pavia	6	77	216	3	181	221	1	29	26
179	Cremona	3	56	156	0	0	0	5	228	206
180	Mantova	2	33	93	0	0	0	4	163	147
181	Bolzano	2	26*	73	1	80	98	3	127	114
182	Trento	2	26*	73	3	222	274	3	112	101
183	Verona	4	30**	83	2	83	102	1	21	19
184	Vicenza	2	15***	43	0	0	0	7	165	148
185	Belluno	2	56	156	0	0	0	0	0	0
186	Treviso	3	23**	65	2	91	112	3	70	63
187	Venezia	9	61	171	1	39	47	0	0*	0**
188	Padova	6	42*	117	1	41	50	3	63	56
189	Rovigo	1	24	68	2	248	305	1	61	55
190	Udine/Gorizia	4	36*	101	1	48	59	2	47	42
191	Trieste	2	50	140	0	0	0	1	53	48
192	Pordenone	0	0*	0	0	0	0	2	122	110
193	Piacenza	0	0*	0	1	110	135	1	52	47
194	Parma	2	33	91	2	154	190	6	221	199
195	Reggio Emilia	2	30	84	0	0	0	0	0	0
196	Modena	1	10**	28	3	156	192	0	0*	0*
197	Bologna	6	41*	115	2	65	80	5	78	70
198	Ferrara	1	17*	47	1	80	99	0	0	0
199	Ravenna	0	0**	0	1	86	106	3	125	113
200	Forli	1	10***	28	1	52	64	2	52	47
201	Pesaro	0	0**	0	2	189	232	0	0	0
202	Ancona	2	29	80	0	0	0	3	104	94
203	Macerata	0	0*	0	0	0	0	1	51	46
204	Ascoli Piceno	1	17*	48	2	174	214	2	86	77
205	Massa-Carrara	0	0	0	0	0	0	2	147	133
206	Lucca	1	16*	46	1	82	101	1	40	36
207	Pistoia	0	0*	0	0	0	0	2	117	106
208	Firenze	6	31***	86	1	26	32	7	89	80
209	Livorno	5	90	251	3	272	335	4	177	160
210	Pisa	6	96	269	3	242	297	1	39	36
211	Arezzo	2	40	113	1	98	121	2	95	86
212	Siena	4	107	298	0	0	0	1	55	50
213	Grosseto	4	115	322	2	273	336	0	0	0
214	Perugia	2	21**	60	0	0	0	5	126	114
215	Terni	0	0	0	1	133	163	1	63	57
216	Viterbo/Rieti	5	75	209	1	74	91	0	0	0
217	Roma	30	46***	128	11	95	116	23	101	91
218	Latina	1	12**	34	1	75	91	2	80	72
219	Frosinone	3	38	105	0	0	0	7	251*	227
220	Caserta	2	14***	40	0	0	0	6	148	134
221	Benevento	1	21	60	0	0	0	6	336*	304*
222	Napoli	28	50***	141	6	72	88	32	215***	194***
223	Avellino	1	14*	38	1	76	93	3	117	106
224	Salerno	5	28***	78	5	162	199	11	188	170
225	L'Aquila	0	0*	0	2	215	265	0	0	0
226	Teramo	2	44	122	3	355	435	1	60	54
227	Pescara	1	21	58	0	0	0	3	167	151
228	Chieti	3	49	136	0	0	0	3	127	115
229	Isernia/Campobasso	0	0*	0	1	98	121	2	99	89
230	Foggia	5	42*	118	2	103	126	5	139	125
231	Bari	8	30***	84	2	48	59	13	171	154

Table 8.2(c)—*cont.*

Area		ASTH			APP			HERN		
		Deaths	SMR to EC std	SMR to own std	Deaths	SMR to EC std	SMR to own std	Deaths	SMR to EC std	SMR to own std
232	Taranto	7	66	185	3	180	221	4	132	119
233	Brindisi	0	0**	0	0	0	0	3	139	126
234	Lecce	2	15***	41	1	43	52	3	68	61
235	Potenza/Matera	7	69	192	0	0	0	4	114	103
236	Cosenza	4	30**	84	2	90	111	6	145	131
237	Catanzaro	1	8***	21	2	94	116	3	77	70
238	Reggio Calabria	8	83	231	2	120	148	2	63	57
239	Trapani	4	56	156	1	79	97	3	123	111
240	Palermo	13	61	170	5	141	174	6	91	82
241	Messina	11	98	275**	3	146	180	4	99	90
242	Agrigento	1	12**	35	1	71	87	2	75	67
243	Caltanisetta	1	20	57	1	119	147	2	127	115
244	Enna	2	63	176	1	174	214	1	91	82
245	Catania	4	22***	62	6	197	242	7	122	110
246	Ragusa	1	21	59	0	0	0	3	185	167
247	Siracusa	2	28	79	2	172	212	5	230	208
248	Sassari	7	88	246	1	79	97	2	86	77
249	Nuoro	0	0*	0	0	0	0	0	0	0
250	Cagliari/Oristano	5	30**	84	3	119	146	5	109	98
IRELAND		98	163***	100	9	103	100	13	86	100
251	Eastern	28	126	78	3	100	100	1	20	23
252	Midland	11	325**	198	1	190	182	1	109	127
253	Mid-Western	12	227*	139	0	0	0	1	74	85
254	North-Eastern	12	237*	144	2	268	256	1	79	92
255	North-Western	3	90	55	0	0	0	3	321	376
256	South-Eastern	9	141	86	0	0	0	1	60	69
257	Southern	10	112	69	2	149	144	0	0	0
258	Western	13	236**	144	1	115	110	5	324*	377*
THE NETHERLANDS		92	42***	100	45	141*	100	52	88	100
259	Groningen	1	12**	29	1	84	60	2	91	104
260	Friesland	5	58	139	3	237	167	1	43	49
261	Drenthe	3	48	114	4	410*	296	3	164	187
262	Overijssel	6	41*	98	6	274*	195	8	198	225
263	Gelderland	12	45**	108	5	129	91	6	84	95
264	Utrecht	6	41*	96	2	98	68	1	27	30
265	Noord Holland	17	48***	114	5	98	70	8	84	96
266	Zuid Holland	24	51***	121	11	159	114	11	85	98
267	Zeeland	0	0*	0	2	258	185	2	136	157
268	Noord Brabant	8	24***	58	2	42	30	7	81	91
269	Limburg	9	55	131	4	158	115	2	42	48
270	Flevoland	1	33	78	0	0	0	1	160	178
UK: ENGLAND AND WALES		1438	168***	100	174	123**	100	356	130***	100
271	Northern	80	155***	92	13	146	119	12	69	53*
	Hartlepool	1	67	39	0	0	0	0	0	0
	North Tees	5	160	95	0	0	0	2	212	163
	South Tees	10	202	120	5	607**	488**	1	63	49
	East Cumbria	2	68	40	1	192	157	0	0	0
	South Cumbria	5	178	105	1	201	163	1	101	77
	West Cumbria	3	129	77	0	0	0	0	0	0
	Darlington	1	49	29	1	275	224	0	0	0
	Durham	7	174	103	1	146	119	0	0	0
	North-West Durham	1	71	42	0	0	0	0	0	0
	South-West Durham	8	310*	185	1	223	181	1	113	87
	Northumberland	9	179	106	1	114	93	2	117	89
	Gateshead	7	204	121	0	0	0	0	0	0
	Newcastle	3	63	38	1	128	104	2	131	101
	North Tyneside	4	128	76	0	0	0	1	86	66
	South Tyneside	5	199	118	0	0	0	0	0	0

Table 8.2(c)—*cont.*

	Area	ASTH			APP			HERN		
		Deaths	SMR to EC std	SMR to own std	Deaths	SMR to EC std	SMR to own std	Deaths	SMR to EC std	SMR to own std
	Sunderland	9	177	105	1	118	95	2	123	94
272	Yorkshire	107	175***	104	7	69	56	26	133	102
	Hull	12	239*	141	1	118	95	4	245	188
	East Yorkshire	3	94	56	0	0	0	2	178	136
	Grimsby	6	225	133	0	0	0	1	115	88
	Scunthorpe	6	181	108	0	0	0	0	0	0
	Northallerton	1	48	28	0	0	0	0	0	0
	York	8	175	104	0	0	0	0	0	0
	Scarborough	3	133	79	0	0	0	1	121	93
	Harrogate	0	0	0*	1	261	212	1	134	103
	Bradford	19	335***	197**	0	0	0	0	0	0
	Airedale	4	138	82	0	0	0	2	207	159
	Calderdale	4	122	72	0	0	0	2	193	148
	Huddersfield	3	83	49	3	506*	409	2	175	134
	Dewsbury	7	248	147	0	0	0	0	0	0
	Leeds Western	6	97	58	1	98	80	4	203	156
	Leeds Eastern	9	154	91	0	0	0	4	211	162
	Wakefield	8	312**	186	0	0	0	2	258	198
	Pontefract	8	281*	167	1	208	169	1	107	82
273	Trent	153	192***	114	25	189**	154	27	106	81
	North Derbyshire	10	164	98	0	0	0	0	0	0
	Southern Derbyshire	15	167	99	7	466**	378**	2	69	53
	Leicestershire	40	260***	154*	2	82	67	4	87	67
	North Lincolnshire	8	174	103	2	260	211	0	0	0
	South Lincolnshire	9	177	106	4	457*	372*	1	58	44
	Bassetlaw	2	110	65	0	0	0	1	171	131
	Central Nottinghamshire	16	325***	193*	1	121	98	2	124	96
	Nottingham	19	179*	106	3	173	141	2	60	46
	Barnsley	3	80	48	0	0	0	1	80	61
	Doncaster	10	202	120	1	120	97	0	0	0
	Rotherham	7	161	96	3	416	337	2	144	111
	Sheffield	14	156	93	2	133	109	12	408***	313**
274	East Anglian	65	192***	114	7	125	102	12	111	85
	Cambridge	8	165	97	1	136	110	1	72	55
	Peterborough	8	228	135	0	0	0	1	94	72
	West Suffolk	9	226*	134	0	0	0	1	90	69
	East Suffolk	11	210*	124	1	112	91	3	173	132
	Norwich	15	198*	118	3	222	181	3	112	86
	Great Yarmouth and Waveney	5	160	95	0	0	0	2	177	135
	West Norfolk and Wisbech	5	165	98	2	371	302	1	93	72
	Huntingdon	4	160	95	0	0	0	0	0	0
275	North-West Thames	98	159***	95	5	52	42*	23	125	96
	North Bedfordshire	3	67	40	0	0	0	1	78	60
	South Bedfordshire	14	282**	168	0	0	0	1	71	55
	North Hertfordshire	7	216	128	0	0	0	2	197	152
	East Hartfordshire	10	195	116	1	117	95	0	0	0
	North-West Hertfordshire	5	111	66	1	131	107	2	135	104
	South-West Hertfordshire	6	145	86	0	0	0	4	288	221
	Barnet	7	132	79	0	0	0	0	0	0
	Harrow	5	147	87	0	0	0	1	97	75
	Hillingdon	2	50	30	0	0	0	1	80	61
	Hounslow and Spelthorne	9	186	111	1	125	102	3	193	148
	Ealing	9	168	100	0	0	0	2	135	103
	Riverside	9	167	100	0	0	0	2	142	109
	Parkside	12	175	104	2	199	164	4	212	163
276	North-East Thames	109	167***	100	14	134	109	26	129	99
	Basildon and Thurrock	13	260**	155	1	125	101	0	0	0
	Mid Essex	9	173	103	2	255	206	2	136	105
	North-East Essex	14	284**	169	1	118	96	0	0	0
	West Essex	6	141	84	1	133	109	3	203	156
	Southend	6	113	67	2	220	179	2	112	86

Table 8.2(c)—*cont.*

	Area	ASTH			APP			HERN		
		Deaths	SMR to EC std	SMR to own std	Deaths	SMR to EC std	SMR to own std	Deaths	SMR to EC std	SMR to own std
	Barking, Havering, and Brentwood	14	187*	111	2	146	120	3	110	84
	Hampstead	3	145	86	0	0	0	1	192	147
	Bloomsbury	0	0	0*	0	0	0	0	0	0
	Islington	3	97	58	1	222	183	0	0	0
	City and Hackney	4	116	69	0	0	0	2	217	167
	Newham	6	166	98	1	184	149	4	396*	304
	Tower Hamlets	6	222	131	0	0	0	2	256	196
	Enfield	6	133	80	1	137	112	1	71	55
	Haringey	7	199	118	1	193	158	2	206	158
	Redbridge	8	206	123	0	0	0	3	235	181
	Waltham Forest	4	108	64	1	178	145	1	94	73
277	South-East Thames	103	170***	101	14	139	113	22	112	86
	Brighton	7	145	86	3	359	295	2	120	92
	Eastbourne	8	236*	140	0	0	0	3	228	174
	Hastings	2	85	50	2	431	352	0	0	0
	South-East Kent	7	160	95	0	0	0	3	205	157
	Canterbury and Thanet	10	212*	126	1	118	96	4	237	181
	Dartford and Gravesham	3	79	47	2	319	258	1	83	64
	Maidstone	4	114	68	2	360	293	1	94	73
	Medway	11	187	111	0	0	0	1	61	47
	Tunbridge Wells	3	93	55	0	0	0	2	179	138
	Bexley	5	131	78	1	161	131	1	83	64
	Greenwich	5	134	80	1	171	138	2	180	138
	Bromley	10	200	120	1	114	93	0	0	0
	West Lambeth	6	202	120	0	0	0	0	0	0
	Camberwell	10	269*	159	1	178	145	2	189	145
	Lewisham and North Southwark	12	223*	132	0	0	0	0	0	0
278	South-West Thames	89	178***	106	13	156	128	15	92	71
	North-West Surrey	3	85	51	1	167	136	0	0	0
	West Surrey and North-East Hampshire	4	78	46	2	268	215	2	146	113
	South-West Surrey	7	232	137	1	193	156	1	99	76
	Mid Surrey	3	113	67	0	0	0	2	201	155
	East Surrey	1	33	19	0	0	0	2	188	145
	Chichester	6	224	133	0	0	0	0	0	0
	Mid Downs	11	230*	137	1	128	103	0	0	0
	Worthing	11	322**	192	1	147	121	1	71	55
	Croydon	14	246**	147	2	228	186	4	240	184
	Kingston and Esher	4	133	80	2	397	327	0	0	0
	Richmond, Twickenham, and Roehampton	5	126	75	2	310	257	1	79	61
	Wandsworth	12	340***	203*	0	0	0	0	0	0
	Merton and Sutton	8	141	85	1	108	88	2	111	85
279	Wessex	86	177***	105	6	74	60	22	140	108
	East Dorset	12	178	106	0	0	0	2	77	59
	West Dorset	3	94	55	0	0	0	2	180	138
	Portsmouth and South-East Hampshire	26	282***	167*	2	140	113	6	222	171
	Southampton and South-West Hampshire	6	86	51	3	254	206	3	130	99
	Winchester	9	245*	145	0	0	0	2	177	136
	Basingstoke and North Hampshire	9	228*	135	0	0	0	4	363	279
	Salisbury	5	250	147	0	0	0	0	0	0
	Swindon	5	123	73	0	0	0	1	85	65
	Bath	9	132	78	1	90	73	1	47	36
	Isle of Wight	2	105	62	0	0	0	1	134	103
280	Oxford	76	169***	100	11	163	131	20	159	122
	East Berkshire	17	263***	156	2	199	161	5	262	202
	West Berkshire	9	109	65	2	166	134	3	134	103
	Aylesbury Vale	2	76	45	2	516	414	0	0	0
	Wycombe	4	86	51	1	127	103	2	131	101
	Milton Keynes	7	211	125	1	248	196	2	295	226
	Kettering	11	249*	148	1	142	114	0	0	0
	Northampton	12	220*	131	0	0	0	5	324*	249
	Oxfordshire	14	142	83	2	140	113	3	114	88

Table 8.2(c)—*cont.*

Area		ASTH			APP			HERN		
		Deaths	SMR to EC std	SMR to own std	Deaths	SMR to EC std	SMR to own std	Deaths	SMR to EC std	SMR to own std
281	South-Western	73	139**	82	9	99	81	28	157*	120
	Bristol and Weston	6	97	58	2	196	159	5	252	194
	Frenchay	4	106	63	1	162	132	2	168	129
	Southmead	9	225*	134	2	304	247	3	234	180
	Cornwall and Isles of Scilly	14	195*	116	1	75	62	8	301*	231
	Exeter	6	126	75	0	0	0	2	115	88
	North Devon	5	232	138	0	0	0	0	0	0
	Plymouth	9	158	93	0	0	0	0	0	0
	Torbay	5	142	84	0	0	0	2	142	109
	Cheltenham and District	1	29	17*	0	0	0	1	86	66
	Gloucester	7	133	79	2	226	183	1	58	45
	Somerset	7	108	64	1	88	71	4	178	136
282	West Midlands	134	151***	89	17	115	93	53	185***	142*
	Bromsgrove and Redditch	1	33	20	0	0	0	2	235	181
	Herefordshire	3	117	69	0	0	0	3	345	265
	Kidderminster and District	1	56	34	1	345	280	1	179	138
	Worcester and District	6	147	87	1	146	118	2	150	115
	Shropshire	8	117	69	1	91	73	1	47	36
	Mid Staffordshire	6	107	64	0	0	0	4	237	182
	North Staffordshire	16	206*	123	1	74	61	9	339**	260*
	South-East Staffordshire	6	129	77	2	283	228	1	75	58
	Rugby	1	68	40	0	0	0	1	208	160
	North Warwickshire	3	98	58	0	0	0	2	209	161
	South Warwickshire	4	104	62	0	0	0	1	80	61
	Central Birmingham	8	264*	155	0	0	0	3	324	248
	East Birmingham	4	125	73	2	356	287	2	182	139
	North Birmingham	3	107	63	1	210	171	0	0	0
	South Birmingham	6	142	84	0	0	0	3	225	173
	West Birmingham	4	114	67	0	0	0	4	387*	297
	Coventry	13	250**	148	1	115	93	1	59	46
	Dudley	9	173	103	1	113	92	5	288	221
	Sandwell	11	226*	134	2	230	186	5	291	224
	Solihull	5	141	84	2	333	269	2	171	132
	Walsall	7	158	94	1	129	105	0	0	0
	Wolverhampton	9	218	128	1	138	111	1	70	54
283	Mersey	72	177***	105	4	58	47	13	98	75
	Chester	4	133	79	1	196	159	2	201	155
	Crewe	12	280**	167	0	0	0	3	218	167
	Halton	4	159	94	0	0	0	0	0	0
	Macclesfield	2	65	39	0	0	0	1	97	75
	Warrington	6	182	108	0	0	0	0	0	0
	Liverpool	12	153	90	1	75	60	3	115	88
	St Helens and Knowsley	12	200*	118	1	100	81	0	0	0
	North Sefton	4	211	126	0	0	0	1	144	111
	South Sefton	7	236	140	0	0	0	0	0	0
	Wirral	9	154	92	1	99	80	3	153	117
284	North Western	117	173***	103	20	179*	145	35	163**	125
	Lancaster	2	96	57	0	0	0	2	277	213
	Blackpool Wyre and Fylde	18	374***	223**	0	0	0	4	204	157
	Preston	6	288*	170	0	0	0	0	0	0
	Blackburn, Hyndburn, and Ribble Valley	10	224*	132	1	134	108	3	210	161
	Burnley, Pendle, and Rossendale	9	237*	141	0	0	0	5	404*	310*
	West Lancashire	9	476***	282*	0	0	0	1	177	136
	Chorley and South Ribble	2	57	34	1	185	150	0	0	0
	Bolton	5	110	66	0	0	0	2	146	112
	Bury	1	33	20	1	207	168	2	217	166
	North Manchester	8	339**	199	1	257	208	1	133	102
	Central Manchester	1	45	26	0	0	0	2	343	263
	South Manchester	3	96	56	4	816**	659**	0	0	0
	Oldham	6	160	95	0	0	0	1	87	67
	Rochdale	8	217	129	0	0	0	2	180	138

Table 8.2(c)—*cont.*

	Area	ASTH			APP			HERN		
		Deaths	SMR to EC std	SMR to own std	Deaths	SMR to EC std	SMR to own std	Deaths	SMR to EC std	SMR to own std
	Salford	4	102	60	2	298	241	3	229	176
	Stockport	9	181	108	2	241	196	1	62	48
	Tameside and Glossop	7	166	99	4	582*	472*	2	151	116
	Trafford	1	27	16*	1	162	132	0	0	0
	Wigan	8	148	88	3	350	282	4	245	188
285	Wales	76	162***	96	9	111	90	22	138	106
	Clwyd	10	150	89	0	0	0	6	273*	209
	East Dyfed	4	109	64	0	0	0	1	73	56
	Pembrokeshire	3	164	97	0	0	0	1	157	121
	Gwent	15	202*	120	0	0	0	0	0	0
	Gwynedd	10	265*	157	2	298	241	1	76	58
	Mid Glamorgan	18	200*	119	4	262	212	5	169	129
	Powys	0	0	0	0	0	0	2	301	231
	South Glamorgan	7	103	61	2	180	145	5	233	179
	West Glamorgan	9	153	91	1	94	77	1	48	36
UK: NORTHERN IRELAND		43	162**	100	6	147	100	5	68	100
286	Northern Ireland	43	162**	100	6	147	100	5	68	100
UK: SCOTLAND		136	156***	100	17	117	100	26	93	100
287	Highlands and Islands	12	259**	167	1	131	114	3	206	224
288	Grampian	11	124	80	1	72	63	2	77	83
289	Tayside	16	247**	158	3	265	222	1	45	48
290	Fife	10	170	109	1	104	89	0	0	0
291	Lothian	20	153	98	0	0	0	2	50	54
292	Borders	1	61	39	0	0	0	1	171	184
293	Forth Valley	11	235*	150	1	129	110	4	268	290
294	Argyll and Clyde	6	80	51	0	0	0	4	166	179
295	Greater Glasgow	22	140	89	5	183	153	6	112	119
296	Lanarkshire	16	162	103	4	250	216	2	66	72
297	Ayrshire and Arran	8	127	81	1	93	79	1	48	52
298	Dumfries and Galloway	3	127	82	0	0	0	0	0	0
PORTUGAL		145	84*	100	29	99	100	47	86	100
299	Viana do Castelo	6	141	168	1	136	136	2	145	172
300	Braga	13	94	112	2	105	100	5	156	184
301	Vila Real	5	117	139	0	0	0	1	73	87
302	Bragança	0	0	0	1	187	191	0	0	0
303	Guarda	2	68	81	1	177	182	2	180	214
304	Viseu	0	0**	0**	0	0	0	2	92	109
305	Porto	19	62*	74	4	90	89	7	89	104
306	Aveiro	10	85	102	6	335*	332*	2	62	72
307	Coimbra	7	97	116	2	152	155	1	39	46
308	Castelo Branco	1	30	36	1	149	154	0	0	0
309	Portalegre	0	0	0	0	0	0	0	0	0
310	Santarem	2	28	33	2	142	147	6	215	252
311	Leiria	7	97	116	0	0	0	2	83	97
312	Lisboa	43	117	140*	4	62	63	7	56	65
313	Setubal	12	87	105	1	43	43	3	68	78
314	Evora	1	39	46	0	0	0	1	88	104
315	Beja	3	116	138	1	182	188	0	0	0
316	Faro	4	76	91	1	98	101	3	148	174
317	Madeira	4	90	107	1	146	144	1	83	98
318	Azores	6	154	184	1	157	151	2	174	207
SPAIN		244	49***	100	70	79	100	128	79**	100
319	La Coruña	8	58	118	3	120	151	7	149	185
320	Lugo	1	24	48	0	0	0	2	98	120
321	Orense	2	41	82	1	97	119	3	145	179
322	Pontevedra	7	59	121	2	100	128	0	0	0
323	Asturias	4	29**	60	1	36	43	0	0**	0*

Table 8.2(c)—*cont.*

Area		ASTH			APP			HERN		
		Deaths	SMR to EC std	SMR to own std	Deaths	SMR to EC std	SMR to own std	Deaths	SMR to EC std	SMR to own std
324	Cantabria	7	106	219	1	83	102	3	132	166
325	Alava	2	49	100	1	163	209	1	94	120
326	Guipuzcoa	4	41	84	0	0	0	3	103	131
327	Vizcaya	14	84	172	3	104	129	3	57	73
328	Navarra	4	59	120	1	84	104	0	0	0
329	Rioja	2	62	127	0	0	0	0	0	0
330	Huesca	3	129	267	1	186	223	0	0	0
331	Teruel	0	0	0	0	0	0	1	141	179
332	Zaragoza	5	48	97	2	96	119	5	124	156
333	Madrid Centro	11	16***	32***	5	44	56	7	35**	44*
334	Avila	2	108	222	0	0	0	0	0	0
335	Burgos	1	23	46	1	117	144	0	0	0
336	Leon	2	36	74	1	79	96	1	40	51
337	Palencia	0	0	0	1	233	281	0	0	0
338	Salamanca	5	123	253	0	0	0	1	63	79
339	Segovia	0	0	0	0	0	0	0	0	0
340	Soria	1	103	212	0	0	0	0	0	0
341	Valladolid	1	15*	30	1	90	113	3	152	194
342	Zamora	0	0	0	0	0	0	1	93	118
343	Albacete	3	75	153	1	131	164	2	141	179
344	Ciudad Real	3	57	117	0	0	0	0	0	0
345	Cuenca	1	47	96	0	0	0	2	213	268
346	Guadalajara	0	0	0	0	0	0	0	0	0
347	Toledo	1	19	38	0	0	0	0	0	0
348	Badajoz	5	70	143	2	146	183	5	195	248
349	Caceres	1	22	45	0	0	0	1	59	76
350	Barcelona	39	60***	122	6	53	67	12	58	74
351	Gerona	9	151	310**	1	86	106	4	180	225
352	Lerida	3	74	151	1	114	138	1	57	71
353	Tarragona	2	29	60	2	157	195	1	42	53
354	Alicante	7	43*	87	2	71	90	2	40	51
355	Castellon de la Plana	3	55	111	2	193	239	6	305*	384*
356	Valencia	9	31***	64	11	224*	282**	15	167	212*
357	Baleares	3	32*	66	2	124	156	1	33	42
358	Almeria	4	76	155	0	0	0	1	63	81
359	Cadiz	13	95	194*	4	191	251	8	227	288*
360	Cordoba	1	12**	24	0	0	0	4	136	172
361	Granada	1	11**	22	0	0	0	4	129	164
362	Huelva	2	39	81	0	0	0	2	123	155
363	Jaen	4	54	111	2	144	181	4	156	201
364	Malaga	12	82	168	2	83	107	1	24	30
365	Sevilla	15	76	155	3	91	118	7	121	152
366	Murcia	5	39*	81	1	46	58	2	51	67
367	Las Palmas	6	53	109	1	65	87	1	41	53
368	Sta Cruz de Tenerife	6	65	132	2	143	189	1	43	54
EC		5302	100	-	906	100	-	1746	100	-

Table 8.2(d)

Area	CHOLY Deaths	CHOLY SMR to EC std	CHOLY SMR to own std	HYP/S Deaths	HYP/S SMR to EC std	HYP/S SMR to own std	MAT Deaths	MAT SMR to EC std	MAT SMR to own std
BELGIUM	48	48***	100	5828	88***	100	27	62*	100
1 Antwerpen	6	37**	78	886	84***	95	4	58	94
2 Brabant	9	39**	82	1217	80***	91***	9	92	147
3 West-Vlaanderen	6	54	113	447	61***	70***	2	42	68
4 Oost-Vlaanderen	9	67	141	669	76***	86***	3	56	90
5 Hainaut	10	74	157	914	103	118***	2	35	57
6 Liege	0	0***	0*	895	129***	147***	5	113	182
7 Limburg	5	74	153	343	78***	88*	1	30	48
8 Luxembourg (province)	0	0	0	136	93	106	0	0	0
9 Namur	3	72	152	321	118**	134***	1	51	81
LUXEMBOURG	5	135	100	325	134***	100	1	62	100
10 Luxembourg	5	135	100	325	134***	100	1	62	100
FEDERAL REPUBLIC OF GERMANY	618	98	100	37225	90***	100	264	112	100
11 Schleswig-Holstein	34	133	136	1360	81***	90***	15	159	142
12 Hamburg	11	66	67	869	79***	88***	5	96	86
13 Braunschweig	9	54	55	976	89***	99	4	71	64
14 Hannover	15	71	72	1149	82***	92**	4	59	53
15 Lüneburg	11	75	76	779	80***	89**	4	75	67
16 Weser-Ems	25	122	125	1148	86***	95	5	56	50
17 Bremen	2	29	30	366	81***	90*	3	138	123
18 Düsseldorf	41	74	75	3464	95**	105**	23	122	109
19 Köln	38	94	96	2225	84***	93***	13	87	78
20 Munster	25	102	103	1506	93**	104	10	99	88
21 Detmold	16	86	88	1098	90***	100	3	43	38
22 Arnsberg	43	110	112	2602	101	112***	18	131	117
23 Darmstadt	28	79	81	2065	89***	99	15	123	110
24 Giessen	10	102	104	573	90**	100	5	136	121
25 Kassel	15	122	124	719	89***	99	2	48	43
26 Koblenz	14	96	98	923	97	107*	7	136	121
27 Trier	3	60	61	332	101	112*	1	54	48
28 Rheinhessen-Pfalz	9	47*	48*	1378	110***	122***	10	145	130
29 Stuttgart	42	121	123	1734	76***	84***	8	56	50*
30 Karlsruhe	29	118	120	1392	86***	96	8	86	77
31 Freiburg	30	162*	165*	1058	87***	97	2	26*	23*
32 Tübingen	17	117	120	712	75***	84***	1	15*	13**
33 Oberbayern	36	99	100	1797	75***	83***	25	178*	159*
34 Niederbayern	9	89	90	670	101	112**	6	141	125
35 Oberpfalz	11	112	114	690	107	119***	10	246*	219*
36 Oberfranken	13	117	120	823	113***	126***	8	199	177
37 Mittelfranken	14	89	91	933	91**	101	13	216*	193*
38 Unterfranken	9	74	76	711	90**	100	6	116	103
39 Schwaben	20	130	133	885	88***	98	10	151	135
40 Saarland	21	181*	185*	911	120***	133***	8	209	186
41 Berlin (West)	18	99	101	1377	116***	128***	12	167	149
DENMARK	63	134*	100	2774	90***	100	15	72	100
42 Kobenhavn and Frederiksberg (M)	10	201	149	391	121***	136***	2	92	129
43 Kobenhavns County	7	113	84	371	91	101	0	0	0
44 Frederiksborg County	4	131	100	158	79**	86	0	0	0
45 Roskilde County	0	0	0	101	84	92	2	238	332
46 Vestsjællands County	3	114	85	167	97	108	1	88	123
47 Storstroms County	6	233	172	142	84*	94	1	105	147
48 Bornholms County	0	0	0	30	102	114	0	0	0
49 Fyns County	6	142	106	188	68***	76***	2	111	155
50 Sonderjyllands County	3	128	95	139	90	100	1	93	130
51 Ribe County	4	209	156	100	80*	88	2	203	284
52 Vejle County	3	100	75	185	94	105	1	73	103
53 Ringkobing County	1	43	33	134	89	98	0	0	0
54 Århus County	5	100	75	282	86*	96	2	79	110

Table 8.2(d)—*cont.*

	Area	CHOLY			HYP/S			MAT		
		Deaths	SMR to EC std	SMR to own std	Deaths	SMR to EC std	SMR to own std	Deaths	SMR to EC std	SMR to own std
55	Viborg County	3	142	106	111	80*	89	1	100	140
56	Nordjyllands County	8	180	134	275	94	105	0	0	0
FRANCE		426	82***	100	26579	79***	100	380	134***	100
57	Ain	3	76	92	182	71***	89	2	89	66
58	Aisne	8	161	195	275	85**	108	3	103	76
59	Allier	4	102	124	209	81**	104	2	150	111
60	Alpes-de-Haute-Provence	0	0	0	61	71**	91	0	0	0
61	Hautes-Alpes	2	186	226	48	68**	87	1	191	142
62	Alpes-Maritimes	5	51	62	395	61***	78***	6	153	114
63	Ardèche	2	72	87	154	84*	107	3	255	190
64	Ardennes	3	109	132	157	87	111	2	123	91
65	Ariège	0	0	0	74	74**	96	0	0	0
66	Aube	1	38	46	151	87	111	2	141	104
67	Aude	2	64	77	142	69***	88	3	257	191
68	Aveyron	3	100	121	147	75***	96	0	0	0
69	Bouches-du-Rhône	7	43*	52	778	72***	92*	12	139	104
70	Calvados	2	38	46	286	82***	105	2	62	46
71	Cantal	3	179	217	113	102	131**	2	327	243
72	Charente	3	88	106	201	90	115	3	202	151
73	Charente-Maritime	10	185	224*	257	72***	93	1	45	34
74	Cher	3	95	115	178	86*	109	1	72	54
75	Corrèze	4	150	182	144	82*	106	0	0	0
76	Corse	5	199	242	141	86	109	1	92	68
77	Côte-d'Or	3	70	85	178	64***	81**	4	162	121
78	Côtes-du-Nord	5	88	106	343	91	117**	2	85	63
79	Creuse	1	63	76	72	68***	88	0	0	0
80	Dordogne	5	115	140	200	70***	90	3	211	157
81	Doubs	2	49	59	216	81**	102	4	158	117
82	Drôme	4	102	124	173	68***	86*	0	0	0
83	Eure	6	143	174	240	88*	112	3	110	82
84	Eure-et-Loir	2	60	73	132	61***	77**	2	99	73
85	Finistère	8	96	117	497	91*	117***	5	129	96
86	Gard	5	89	107	284	77***	98	7	268*	199
87	Haute-Garonne	2	25*	30	315	60***	77***	2	50	37
88	Gers	0	0	0	87	66***	86	1	164	122
89	Gironde	10	91	110	519	72***	92	3	56	42
90	Hérault	7	94	114	283	58***	74***	8	231	172
91	Ille-et-Vilaine	1	14*	18*	394	87**	111*	7	177	132
92	Indre	1	40	48	119	72***	92	0	0	0
93	Indre-et-Loire	3	64	77	189	61***	78***	3	121	90
94	Isère	5	58	71	353	63***	80***	4	77	57
95	Jura	1	42	51	97	62***	79*	0	0	0
96	Landes	4	122	148	171	79**	102	1	83	62
97	Loir-et-Cher	1	34	41	141	73***	93	0	0	0
98	Loire	10	139	169	354	75***	96	2	57	42
99	Haute-Loire	3	139	169	124	88	112	4	472*	351
100	Loire-Atlantique	10	109	133	510	85***	108	3	57	42
101	Loiret	6	120	146	220	67***	86*	7	242	180
102	Lot	0	0	0	96	83	107	1	180	134
103	Lot-et-Garonne	1	31	37	140	65***	84*	1	80	59
104	Lozère	0	0	0	41	83	107	0	0	0
105	Maine-et-Loire	6	100	122	296	76***	97	4	107	79
106	Manche	1	21	26	256	83**	107	2	81	60
107	Marne	6	130	158	276	92	116*	4	132	98
108	Haute-Marne	3	156	190	110	88	112	3	285	212
109	Mayenne	2	78	94	121	72***	92	4	290	216
110	Meurthe-et-Moselle	3	46	56	333	78***	99	7	187	139
111	Meuse	2	104	126	112	89	114	4	395*	293
112	Morbihan	5	84	101	476	121***	155***	8	269*	200
113	Moselle	15	161	196*	648	106	135***	5	92	69

Table 8.2(d)—*cont.*

	Area	CHOLY			HYP/S			MAT		
		Deaths	SMR to EC std	SMR to own std	Deaths	SMR to EC std	SMR to own std	Deaths	SMR to EC std	SMR to own std
114	Nièvre	4	161	196	153	94	120*	2	211	157
115	Nord	31	142	173**	1598	113***	143***	21	137	102
116	Oise	3	53	65	331	91	114*	3	76	56
117	Orne	0	0	0	157	83*	106	0	0	0
118	Pas-de-Calais	17	131	159	969	114***	146***	11	133	99
119	Puy-de-dôme	8	138	168	312	82***	105	8	315**	234*
120	Pyrénées-Atlantiques	2	35	42	308	82***	104	2	85	63
121	Hautes-Pyrénées	4	164	198	121	75**	96	0	0	0
122	Pyrénées-Orientales	3	78	95	177	70***	90	2	137	102
123	Bas-Rhin	10	122	148	471	88**	112*	5	104	77
124	Haut-Rhin	8	133	162	377	96	122***	5	142	106
125	Rhône	7	54	65	554	65***	82***	10	123	91
126	Haute-Saône	3	140	170	120	86	109	5	448*	333*
127	Saône-et-Loire	2	35	43	281	75***	96	2	81	60
128	Sarthe	2	42	52	191	62***	79***	4	162	120
129	Savoie	2	64	77	143	70***	88	0	0	0
130	Haute-Savoie	0	0*	0*	222	74***	93	5	177	132
131	Paris	10	49*	60	859	65***	83***	21	179*	133
132	Seine-Maritime	7	67	81	615	90**	114**	4	58	43
133	Seine-et-Marne	4	53	65	405	83***	104	7	123	92
134	Yvelines	10	98	119	427	64***	80***	9	123	91
135	Deux-Sèvres	1	30	36	128	58***	74***	0	0	0
136	Somme	5	102	124	288	90	115*	8	276*	205
137	Tarn	2	54	65	150	62***	79**	3	222	165
138	Tarn-et-Garonne	2	98	119	83	62***	79*	0	0	0
139	Var	5	62	75	358	67***	86**	5	138	103
140	Vaucluse	3	70	84	205	72***	92	5	218	162
141	Vendée	2	41	50	258	81***	104	4	170	127
142	Vienne	3	85	103	130	56***	72***	2	124	92
143	Haute-Vienne	5	135	164	177	73***	93	1	78	58
144	Vosges	2	55	67	202	85*	108	6	309*	230
145	Yonne	1	32	39	177	87	112	0	0	0
146	Territoire-de-Belfort	1	84	102	54	69**	88	2	289	215
147	Essonne	5	60	73	372	69***	86**	5	85	63
148	Hauts-de-Seine	11	84	102	550	64***	81***	6	76	56
149	Seine-Saint-Denis	6	53	64	611	83***	104	19	216**	160
150	Val-de-Marne	10	93	113	490	70***	88**	14	206*	153
151	Val-d'Oise	6	77	94	346	68***	85**	10	163	121
	GREECE	37	42***	100	6926	120***	100	32	80	100
152	Greater Athens	15	55*	130	2188	123***	102	9	72	90
153	Rest of Central Greece and Eubea	2	19**	45	782	114***	95	4	90	113
154	Peloponnisos	5	52	120	625	98	81***	2	50	62
155	Ionian Islands	0	0	0	140	112	91	0	0	0
156	Epirus	0	0	0	196	100	84*	1	83	104
157	Thessaly	2	31	73	498	117***	97	2	68	85
158	Macedonia	8	44*	112	1592	134***	115***	5	58	72
159	Thrace	1	37	94	343	193***	164***	4	265	332
160	Aegean Islands	0	0*	0	295	112	91	2	111	139
161	Crete	4	86	196	267	88*	72***	3	130	163
	ITALY	884	151***	100	42700	111***	100	172	83*	100
162	Torino	45	181***	120	1813	111***	100	4	61	73
163	Vercelli	6	132	88	436	145***	131***	1	103	124
164	Novara	7	129	85	466	130***	117***	1	72	86
165	Cuneo	11	180	120	526	130***	118***	2	119	143
166	Asti	7	285*	190	189	116*	105	1	188	226
167	Alessandria	10	186	124	407	114**	103	2	202	243
168	Aosta	4	321	213	94	114	103	1	293	351
169	Imperia	5	191	127	159	92	83*	0	0	0
170	Savona	5	141	94	251	107	97	0	0	0

Table 8.2(d)—*cont.*

	Area	CHOLY			HYP/S			MAT		
		Deaths	SMR to EC std	SMR to own std	Deaths	SMR to EC std	SMR to own std	Deaths	SMR to EC std	SMR to own std
171	Genova	27	222***	148	766	95	86***	5	219	263
172	La Spezia	5	177	118	162	87	78**	0	0	0
173	Varese	16	197*	130	574	107	97	3	119	143
174	Como/Sondrio	12	124	82	729	114***	103	2	62	75
175	Milano	43	101	67**	2872	103	93***	7	60	72
176	Bergamo	12	135	89	639	109*	99	1	30	36
177	Brescia	13	124	82	788	114***	103	0	0	0
178	Pavia	6	101	67	567	144***	130***	0	0	0
179	Cremona	6	159	106	368	148***	133***	1	108	130
180	Mantova	5	118	79	325	116**	105	0	0	0
181	Bolzano	2	49	33	223	84**	76***	0	0	0
182	Trento	8	173	115	320	106	95	0	0	0
183	Verona	7	86	57	536	100	90*	1	39	47
184	Vicenza	8	110	73	523	109*	99	0	0	0
185	Belluno	3	128	85	181	117*	106	1	167	200
186	Treviso	10	136	90	465	96	87**	1	43	51
187	Venezia	5	57	38*	534	93	84***	2	85	102
188	Padova	7	85	56	486	90*	81***	2	76	92
189	Rovigo	2	71	47	204	110	99	1	137	165
190	Udine/Gorizia	9	122	81	541	111*	101	3	174	209
191	Trieste	9	278*	185	197	92	83**	0	0	0
192	Pordenone	4	141	94	201	108	98	0	0	0
193	Piacenza	7	212	142	266	122**	110	1	165	198
194	Parma	5	107	71	305	98	89*	1	107	129
195	Reggio Emilia	5	106	70	268	86*	77***	0	0	0
196	Modena	7	104	69	481	108	98	0	0	0
197	Bologna	11	99	66	658	90**	81***	2	101	121
198	Ferrara	10	223*	149	324	109	99	2	258	309
199	Ravenna	2	48	32	216	79***	71***	0	0	0
200	Forli	8	120	80	313	71***	65***	1	59	71
201	Pesaro	4	108	72	189	77***	70***	0	0	0
202	Ancona	4	81	54	284	87*	78***	0	0	0
203	Macerata	3	89	59	225	101	91	0	0	0
204	Ascoli Piceno	5	125	83	246	93	84**	0	0	0
205	Massa-Carrara	3	128	85	153	99	89	0	0	0
206	Lucca	1	23	15*	307	108	97	0	0	0
207	Pistoia	2	68	45	159	82*	74***	0	0	0
208	Firenze	24	177*	118	755	84***	76***	2	63	76
209	Livorno	3	77	51	240	93	84**	0	0	0
210	Pisa	8	183	122	240	83**	75***	0	0	0
211	Arezzo	4	110	73	216	90	81**	1	109	130
212	Siena	6	192	128	189	91	82**	0	0	0
213	Grosseto	7	265*	177	152	87	79**	0	0	0
214	Perugia	14	204*	136	414	91	83***	1	55	66
215	Terni	6	220	147	171	95	86*	0	0	0
216	Viterbo/Rieti	5	105	70	330	105	95	2	140	168
217	Roma	73	186***	123	2626	102	92***	11	87	104
218	Latina	7	163	108	319	114*	103	3	149	179
219	Frosinone	3	63	42	385	122***	110	1	50	60
220	Caserta	17	245**	163	731	162***	146***	4	89	107
221	Benevento	4	130	87	266	132***	119**	2	144	172
222	Napoli	45	177***	117	2720	164***	149***	16	94	113
223	Avellino	11	249*	166	371	128***	116**	1	51	62
224	Salerno	20	199**	133	933	142***	128***	2	39	46
225	L'Aquila	2	61	41	247	115*	104	0	0	0
226	Teramo	3	105	70	180	96	87	0	0	0
227	Pescara	4	130	86	221	109	98	2	189	227
228	Chieti	9	221*	148	257	96	87*	1	73	88
229	Isernia/Campobasso	7	201	134	282	123***	111	0	0	0
230	Foggia	12	195*	129	481	119***	108	1	29	35
231	Bari	24	185**	122	836	99	89***	7	96	115

Table 8.2(d)—*cont.*

Area		CHOLY			HYP/S			MAT		
		Deaths	SMR to EC std	SMR to own std	Deaths	SMR to EC std	SMR to own std	Deaths	SMR to EC std	SMR to own std
232	Taranto	6	115	76	370	109	99	5	177	212
233	Brindisi	4	108	72	289	120**	108	2	108	129
234	Lecce	17	224**	149	509	102	92	3	90	109
235	Potenza/Matera	4	67	44	480	122***	110*	6	221	265
236	Cosenza	9	127	84	594	128***	116***	3	88	106
237	Catanzaro	6	90	60	540	125***	113**	4	105	126
238	Reggio Calabria	10	185	123	414	117**	106	3	101	121
239	Trapani	3	72	48	289	105	95	0	0	0
240	Palermo	23	202**	134	884	119***	108*	3	46	56
241	Messina	11	159	106	566	125***	112**	6	205	246
242	Agrigento	9	196	131	346	115*	104	6	267	320*
243	Caltanisetta	8	297*	197	258	146***	132***	3	209	251
244	Enna	2	106	70	188	152***	137***	4	459*	551*
245	Catania	13	132	88	952	148***	134***	7	128	154
246	Ragusa	6	216	143	225	123**	111	2	148	178
247	Siracusa	7	188	125	344	141***	128***	3	158	189
248	Sassari	10	249*	165	291	111	101	1	60	72
249	Nuoro	10	405***	269*	162	100	91	0	0	0
250	Cagliari/Oristano	12	152	101	501	98	88**	5	147	177
IRELAND		23	89	100	1718	103	100	12	56*	100
251	Eastern	4	47	51	561	102	99	3	40	70
252	Midland	1	64	72	117	115	111	3	237	420
253	Mid-Western	1	43	49	160	106	103	3	160	284
254	North-Eastern	5	230	258	171	121*	117*	0	0	0
255	North-Western	0	0	0	91	87	84	0	0	0
256	South-Eastern	1	35	39	202	109	105	0	0	0
257	Southern	7	175	197	262	101	98	2	65	115
258	Western	4	151	174	154	90	87	1	49	88
THE NETHERLANDS		126	123*	100	4741	71***	100	55	102	100
259	Groningen	2	53	43	168	68***	96	1	53	52
260	Friesland	5	126	102	174	67***	94	1	44	43
261	Drenthe	4	127	103	144	70***	98	0	0	0
262	Overijssel	15	216*	175	331	73***	103	8	200	197
263	Gelderland	22	179*	145	632	79***	111*	8	123	120
264	Utrecht	6	93	75	322	77***	108	5	136	134
265	Noord Holland	21	127	103	660	62***	86***	5	60	59
266	Zuid Holland	21	94	76	998	69***	97	15	124	122
267	Zeeland	2	79	64	97	59***	83	0	0	0
268	Noord Brabant	21	141	114	760	78***	109*	6	76	75
269	Limburg	6	72	59	414	76***	107	6	160	157
270	Flevoland	1	93	75	41	60***	84	0	0	0
UK: ENGLAND AND WALES		422	90*	100	32508	105***	100	231	93	100
271	Northern	31	103	115	2588	131***	124***	13	88	95
	Hartlepool	1	115	128	82	143**	136**	0	0	0
	North Tees	2	123	138	137	129**	123*	0	0	0
	South Tees	1	37	41	249	140***	133***	1	62	66
	East Cumbria	4	226	252	122	105	100	2	271	291
	South Cumbria	1	58	65	116	103	98	2	274	294
	West Cumbria	1	74	83	97	110	104	0	0	0
	Darlington	1	80	90	113	138**	131**	0	0	0
	Durham	4	175	195	221	147***	140***	2	187	200
	North-West Durham	2	231	257	90	158***	150***	0	0	0
	South-West Durham	1	66	73	147	147***	140***	0	0	0
	Northumberland	3	101	113	255	131***	124***	1	77	83
	Gateshead	0	0	0	188	136***	129***	1	104	112
	Newcastle	2	76	85	208	121**	115	1	74	79
	North Tyneside	2	100	111	169	129**	122*	1	113	121
	South Tyneside	1	61	68	150	139***	132**	1	128	138

Table 8.2(d)—*cont.*

	Area	CHOLY			HYP/S			MAT		
		Deaths	SMR to EC std	SMR to own std	Deaths	SMR to EC std	SMR to own std	Deaths	SMR to EC std	SMR to own std
	Sunderland	5	178	200	244	133***	126***	1	65	70
272	Yorkshire	27	80	89	2533	114***	109***	18	100	107
	Hull	2	71	79	227	123**	117*	1	58	62
	East Yorkshire	1	51	58	112	88	83*	0	0	0
	Grimsby	4	267	298	86	88	83	0	0	0
	Scunthorpe	0	0	0	136	109	104	1	106	114
	Northallerton	0	0	0	84	128*	121	0	0	0
	York	2	81	91	154	96	91	0	0	0
	Scarborough	1	70	78	113	120	114	1	170	182
	Harrogate	0	0	0	88	104	99	1	183	196
	Bradford	1	34	38	275	143***	136***	1	47	50
	Airedale	1	60	67	97	88	84	1	125	134
	Calderdale	1	56	62	148	126**	120*	2	203	218
	Huddersfield	5	254	283	171	133***	126**	1	98	106
	Dewsbury	2	137	153	121	127*	120	2	215	230
	Leeds Western	1	29	33	261	118*	112	2	116	124
	Leeds Eastern	2	61	68	252	118*	112	2	114	122
	Wakefield	1	75	84	86	98	93	2	287	309
	Pontefract	3	187	208	122	116	110	1	113	122
273	Trent	36	82	91	3160	109***	104*	20	90	97
	North Derbyshire	0	0	0	259	109	104	0	0	0
	Southern Derbyshire	1	20	22	367	111*	106	2	78	84
	Leicestershire	9	113	127	491	95	90*	2	45	48
	North Lincolnshire	4	155	173	177	105	99	2	163	175
	South Lincolnshire	2	67	75	200	102	97	2	157	169
	Bassetlaw	1	99	111	77	116	110	0	0	0
	Central Nottinghamshire	2	72	81	206	113	108	3	217	233
	Nottingham	2	35	39	475	126***	120***	1	33	35
	Barnsley	4	185	206	157	110	105	1	95	102
	Doncaster	5	179	200	212	116*	110	4	266	285
	Rotherham	4	167	187	176	112	107	0	0	0
	Sheffield	2	39	44	363	109	104	3	126	135
274	East Anglian	16	86	96	1010	83***	79***	12	128	138
	Cambridge	1	42	47	115	73***	70***	2	161	173
	Peterborough	5	273	305	121	101	96	3	273	293
	West Suffolk	0	0	0	111	89	85	0	0	0
	East Suffolk	2	67	74	145	74***	70***	1	64	69
	Norwich	2	43	48	246	81***	77***	3	154	165
	Great Yarmouth and Waveney	2	102	114	121	94	89	1	113	121
	West Norfolk and Wisbech	3	163	181	107	88	84	2	247	265
	Huntingdon	1	97	109	44	66**	63**	0	0	0
275	North-West Thames	15	47**	53**	1911	92***	88***	21	117	125
	North Bedfordshire	0	0	0	136	95	90	4	320	343
	South Bedfordshire	4	166	186	135	86	82*	1	57	62
	North Hertfordshire	1	57	64	119	104	99	3	308	331
	East Hartfordshire	1	35	40	153	82*	78**	1	74	80
	North-West Hertfordshire	1	39	44	127	75**	72***	0	0	0
	South-West Hertfordshire	0	0	0	136	87	82*	2	176	189
	Barnet	2	73	82	126	71***	67***	2	137	147
	Harrow	2	112	126	80	69***	65***	1	98	105
	Hillingdon	0	0	0	135	95	90	0	0	0
	Hounslow and Spelthorne	0	0	0	169	96	91	2	129	138
	Ealing	2	78	87	171	103	98	1	64	69
	Riverside	1	41	46	163	103	98	2	146	157
	Parkside	1	31	35	261	124**	117*	2	92	99
276	North-East Thames	24	69	77	2256	99	94**	17	85	91
	Basildon and Thurrock	4	153	171	149	87	83*	0	0	0
	Mid Essex	1	39	44	116	70***	67***	2	139	149
	North-East Essex	1	35	39	160	85*	81**	0	0	0
	West Essex	1	39	44	154	92	87	1	83	89
	Southend	2	65	72	165	82**	77***	1	68	73

Table 8.2(d)—*cont.*

	Area	CHOLY			HYP/S			MAT		
		Deaths	SMR to EC std	SMR to own std	Deaths	SMR to EC std	SMR to own std	Deaths	SMR to EC std	SMR to own std
	Barking, Havering, and Brentwood	2	42	47	267	86*	82***	2	93	100
	Hampstead	1	111	124	51	87	83	0	0	0
	Bloomsbury	2	170	190	81	106	101	3	512*	549*
	Islington	2	136	152	126	132**	125*	1	107	115
	City and Hackney	0	0	0	179	175***	166***	1	75	81
	Newham	1	58	64	136	121*	114	2	132	141
	Tower Hamlets	3	224	250	137	157***	149***	0	0	0
	Enfield	1	41	46	150	94	90	1	75	80
	Haringey	0	0	0	113	104	98	1	83	89
	Redbridge	1	45	51	135	94	89	2	182	196
	Waltham Forest	2	110	123	137	115	109	0	0	0
277	South-East Thames	33	97	108	2187	98	93**	15	83	89
	Brighton	3	104	116	158	84*	80**	1	74	79
	Eastbourne	3	132	146	114	76**	72***	0	0	0
	Hastings	3	182	202	103	95	90	0	0	0
	South-East Kent	2	79	88	149	90	85	3	242	259
	Canterbury and Thanet	2	69	76	204	106	101	2	154	165
	Dartford and Gravesham	0	0	0	131	96	91	0	0	0
	Maidstone	2	109	123	103	86	82*	1	107	115
	Medway	6	212	238	172	93	89	0	0	0
	Tunbridge Wells	0	0	0	90	71***	67***	0	0	0
	Bexley	0	0	0	112	82*	78**	1	90	96
	Greenwich	1	52	58	150	120*	114	2	160	172
	Bromley	2	66	74	151	76***	72***	0	0	0
	West Lambeth	0	0	0	119	137**	130**	1	102	109
	Camberwell	2	110	122	196	166***	157***	1	71	76
	Lewisham and North Southwark	7	241	268*	235	124**	118*	3	164	176
278	South-West Thames	21	75	84	1483	81***	77***	11	79	85
	North-West Surrey	2	99	111	90	68***	64***	2	203	218
	West Surrey and North-East Hampshire	2	85	96	87	57***	54***	1	73	78
	South-West Surrey	2	115	128	74	65***	61***	2	263	283
	Mid Surrey	2	116	130	77	68***	64***	0	0	0
	East Surrey	0	0	0	106	88	83	1	122	131
	Chichester	1	54	60	87	71***	67***	0	0	0
	Mid Downs	1	39	43	128	75***	72***	0	0	0
	Worthing	0	0	0	132	82*	78**	1	106	114
	Croydon	2	69	78	216	115*	109	1	58	62
	Kingston and Esher	1	58	65	79	70***	67***	0	0	0
	Richmond, Twickenham, and Roehampton	2	91	102	130	91	86	2	190	204
	Wandsworth	3	194	217	122	122*	116	0	0	0
	Merton and Sutton	3	96	107	155	76***	72***	1	58	62
279	Wessex	15	55*	62	1549	87***	83***	8	59	64
	East Dorset	3	67	74	246	84**	79***	1	57	61
	West Dorset	1	52	58	123	98	93	2	244	262
	Portsmouth and South-East Hampshire	6	129	144	301	99	94	1	37	40
	Southampton and South-West Hampshire	0	0*	0	213	81**	77***	2	99	107
	Winchester	0	0	0	102	80*	76**	0	0	0
	Basingstoke and North Hampshire	0	0	0	107	86	82*	0	0	0
	Salisbury	1	89	99	71	96	91	0	0	0
	Swindon	0	0	0	111	84	80*	0	0	0
	Bath	0	0*	0	195	80**	76***	1	54	58
	Isle of Wight	4	310	344	80	94	89	1	203	218
280	Oxford	20	92	104	1163	82***	78***	12	95	102
	East Berkshire	0	0	0	173	81**	77***	2	105	112
	West Berkshire	1	26	29	216	86*	82**	0	0	0
	Aylesbury Vale	0	0	0	59	73*	70**	0	0	0
	Wycombe	9	343**	386**	133	77**	73***	2	167	179
	Milton Keynes	1	86	96	68	91	87	1	95	102
	Kettering	3	130	145	166	110	104	3	228	245
	Northampton	3	113	126	168	97	92	3	188	202
	Oxfordshire	3	66	74	180	61***	58***	1	38	41

Table 8.2(d)—*cont.*

Area		CHOLY			HYP/S			MAT		
		Deaths	SMR to EC std	SMR to own std	Deaths	SMR to EC std	SMR to own std	Deaths	SMR to EC std	SMR to own std
281	South-Western	31	101	112	1767	87***	83***	12	83	89
	Bristol and Weston	4	117	130	231	103	98	2	114	122
	Frenchay	3	146	164	123	91	87	0	0	0
	Southmead	4	181	202	110	76**	72***	0	0	0
	Cornwall and Isles of Scilly	6	131	146	254	84**	80***	2	99	106
	Exeter	1	33	37	165	84*	79**	1	78	84
	North Devon	3	231	257	57	67**	63***	1	176	189
	Plymouth	1	34	38	179	94	89	1	63	67
	Torbay	3	123	137	134	83*	79**	1	107	115
	Cheltenham and District	2	99	111	128	97	92	1	109	117
	Gloucester	1	34	38	173	89	84*	3	201	216
	Somerset	3	77	86	213	83**	79***	0	0	0
282	West Midlands	57	115	129	3781	117***	111***	30	114	122
	Bromsgrove and Redditch	1	68	77	83	87	83	1	121	130
	Herefordshire	1	67	74	93	95	90	2	285	306
	Kidderminster and District	0	0	0	67	106	101	1	216	232
	Worcester and District	3	130	146	138	91	87	4	383*	411*
	Shropshire	3	82	92	253	106	101	4	212	228
	Mid Staffordshire	6	206	231	186	98	93	1	66	71
	North Staffordshire	8	175	195	381	127***	120***	1	45	48
	South-East Staffordshire	1	44	49	166	111	106	0	0	0
	Rugby	3	362	404	67	123	117	0	0	0
	North Warwickshire	2	121	136	153	142***	134***	0	0	0
	South Warwickshire	2	92	103	103	72***	69***	3	322	346
	Central Birmingham	2	126	140	140	135***	128**	3	276	297
	East Birmingham	4	211	235	183	148***	140***	1	79	84
	North Birmingham	2	125	140	119	113	107	1	133	142
	South Birmingham	1	44	48	177	118*	112	2	150	161
	West Birmingham	3	169	189	214	185***	176***	1	69	74
	Coventry	2	69	77	252	133***	126***	1	59	63
	Dudley	3	100	112	224	114	108	1	69	74
	Sandwell	5	169	189	269	138***	131***	1	63	67
	Solihull	1	50	56	88	66***	63***	0	0	0
	Walsall	3	116	129	187	110	104	1	74	80
	Wolverhampton	1	41	46	238	149***	141***	1	77	83
283	Mersey	23	101	112	1803	120***	114***	8	66	71
	Chester	1	58	66	99	88	84	1	113	122
	Crewe	2	84	94	159	102	97	2	167	180
	Halton	2	158	176	105	127*	121	1	125	134
	Macclesfield	2	113	127	111	95	90	0	0	0
	Warrington	1	60	68	151	140***	133***	0	0	0
	Liverpool	9	200	223*	438	149***	141***	1	38	41
	St Helens and Knowsley	4	122	137	296	138***	131***	2	110	118
	North Sefton	1	84	93	94	119	113	0	0	0
	South Sefton	1	57	64	135	118	112	1	110	118
	Wirral	0	0	0	215	97	92	0	0	0
284	North-Western	42	113	126	3199	132***	125***	21	101	109
	Lancaster	4	322	358	79	97	92	0	0	0
	Blackpool Wyre and Fylde	8	236*	263*	283	127***	120**	1	75	80
	Preston	3	257	287	124	162***	154***	0	0	0
	Blackburn, Hyndburn, and Ribble Valley	2	81	91	217	134***	128***	4	270	290
	Burnley, Pendle, and Rossendale	1	47	52	185	132***	126**	2	155	167
	West Lancashire	1	103	115	67	105	100	0	0	0
	Chorley and South Ribble	2	115	128	140	123*	117	0	0	0
	Bolton	1	42	47	230	149***	142***	2	144	154
	Bury	2	126	141	132	126*	120*	2	218	235
	North Manchester	0	0	0	154	183***	174***	0	0	0
	Central Manchester	2	200	223	104	161***	152***	1	129	138
	South Manchester	0	0	0	135	129**	122*	1	105	113
	Oldham	1	50	56	174	134***	127**	2	164	177
	Rochdale	2	104	116	162	129**	123*	0	0	0

Table 8.2(d)—*cont.*

	Area	CHOLY			HYP/S			MAT		
		Deaths	SMR to EC std	SMR to own std	Deaths	SMR to EC std	SMR to own std	Deaths	SMR to EC std	SMR to own std
	Salford	1	44	49	209	141***	134***	3	242	260
	Stockport	4	144	162	176	97	92	0	0	0
	Tameside and Glossop	2	88	98	204	137***	130***	1	76	81
	Trafford	2	97	108	143	105	100	1	95	102
	Wigan	4	142	159	281	153***	145***	1	65	70
285	Wales	31	113	126	2118	118***	112***	13	94	101
	Clwyd	0	0*	0	256	103	98	3	159	171
	East Dyfed	3	126	140	203	130***	123**	0	0	0
	Pembrokeshire	1	91	102	90	125*	119	0	0	0
	Gwent	7	162	180	355	125***	119**	2	89	95
	Gwynedd	1	44	49	160	107	101	2	191	205
	Mid Glamorgan	9	176	196	441	132***	125***	1	36	38
	Powys	1	87	97	107	142***	135**	0	0	0
	South Glamorgan	5	135	151	222	92	87*	3	141	151
	West Glamorgan	4	110	123	284	119**	113*	2	116	124
UK: NORTHERN IRELAND		7	55	100	1035	126***	100	1	10***	100
286	Northern Ireland	7	55	100	1035	126***	100	1	10***	100
UK: SCOTLAND		43	90	100	4601	146***	100	30	124	100
287	Highlands and Islands	2	80	88	226	138***	94	1	78	62
288	Grampian	1	22	24	338	116*	79***	5	210	169
289	Tayside	4	104	118	313	124***	85**	3	173	139
290	Fife	1	31	35	297	142***	97	2	121	97
291	Lothian	6	88	97	648	145***	99	4	115	92
292	Borders	0	0	0	68	103	70**	1	241	194
293	Forth Valley	4	156	173	253	150***	103	1	82	66
294	Argyll and Clyde	5	121	134	412	152***	104	3	139	112
295	Greater Glasgow	8	87	99	1023	170***	116***	5	107	86
296	Lanarkshire	4	77	85	553	163***	111*	2	74	60
297	Ayrshire and Arran	7	196	219	327	140***	96	1	57	46
298	Dumfries and Galloway	1	67	76	143	145***	99	2	311	250
PORTUGAL		107	114	100	12055	196***	100	58	127	100
299	Viana do Castelo	1	42	38	337	219***	111	0	0	0
300	Braga	5	92	82	764	218***	112**	9	203	160
301	Vila Real	1	43	38	393	259***	132***	0	0	0
302	Bragança	0	0	0	243	210***	106	2	273	215
303	Guarda	1	52	46	290	232***	118**	0	0	0
304	Viseu	5	135	119	614	253***	129***	1	49	39
305	Porto	15	112	99	1839	212***	109***	11	129	102
306	Aveiro	4	72	64	629	175***	90**	1	31	25
307	Coimbra	1	23	20	563	196***	100	2	114	90
308	Castelo Branco	0	0	0	262	170***	86*	1	120	95
309	Portalegre	5	324*	284	220	216***	109	1	192	152
310	Santarem	1	21	18	594	188***	96	1	58	46
311	Leiria	4	96	85	618	227***	116***	3	160	126
312	Lisboa	33	153*	134	2264	160***	82***	8	98	77
313	Setubal	12	158	138	784	157***	80***	5	171	135
314	Evora	5	256	223	241	187***	95	0	0	0
315	Beja	2	104	91	245	194***	98	1	147	116
316	Faro	6	172	151	415	181***	92	5	343*	271
317	Madeira	3	146	129	391	294***	150***	3	209	165
318	Azores	3	153	136	349	274***	140***	4	248	196
SPAIN		193	70***	100	17866	99	100	83	65***	100
319	La Coruña	5	62	88	584	111*	111*	1	32	50
320	Lugo	2	57	80	224	96	97	0	0	0
321	Orense	1	28	40	235	100	100	1	118	181
322	Pontevedra	3	49	69	460	114**	115**	3	107	165
323	Asturias	8	85	122	536	87***	88**	1	35	54

Table 8.2(d)—*cont.*

	Area	CHOLY			HYP/S			MAT		
		Deaths	SMR to EC std	SMR to own std	Deaths	SMR to EC std	SMR to own std	Deaths	SMR to EC std	SMR to own std
324	Cantabria	0	0*	0	231	91	92	1	64	99
325	Alava	0	0	0	82	70***	71**	0	0	0
326	Guipuzcoa	2	40	58	283	87*	88*	1	56	85
327	Vizcaya	4	44	64	531	90*	92*	1	32	49
328	Navarra	2	53	75	165	66***	67***	0	0	0
329	Rioja	4	200	285	137	104	105	0	0	0
330	Huesca	2	107	152	102	82*	83	0	0	0
331	Teruel	1	83	118	65	81	82	0	0	0
332	Zaragoza	8	117	166	401	88*	89*	4	174	268
333	Madrid Centro	12	35***	50*	1553	70***	70***	6	38**	58
334	Avila	0	0	0	78	80	81	0	0	0
335	Burgos	4	144	205	151	82*	84*	0	0	0
336	Leon	2	47	67	261	92	94	1	68	104
337	Palencia	0	0	0	71	75*	77*	0	0	0
338	Salamanca	1	37	52	149	83*	84*	0	0	0
339	Segovia	0	0	0	62	82	84	0	0	0
340	Soria	0	0	0	33	67*	68*	0	0	0
341	Valladolid	1	30	43	153	70***	71***	1	72	111
342	Zamora	1	54	78	115	94	95	0	0	0
343	Albacete	4	166	236	202	127**	129***	1	78	120
344	Ciudad Real	3	85	120	261	111	113	1	55	85
345	Cuenca	0	0	0	123	116	117	0	0	0
346	Guadalajara	1	94	134	45	64**	65**	0	0	0
347	Toledo	0	0	0	233	96	98	0	0	0
348	Badajoz	2	46	65	412	143***	145***	2	77	118
349	Caceres	2	70	100	224	118*	121**	2	131	202
350	Barcelona	27	77	110	1895	82***	83***	10	73	113
351	Gerona	4	106	150	199	80**	81**	3	199	305
352	Lerida	3	100	142	189	95	96	0	0	0
353	Tarragona	9	221*	316**	231	87*	87*	3	179	274
354	Alicante	7	82	117	673	119***	121***	2	45	68
355	Castellon de la Plana	4	119	170	242	109	111	1	73	112
356	Valencia	17	111	159	1275	127***	129***	7	106	162
357	Baleares	7	137	195	346	104	104	4	156	239
358	Almeria	0	0	0	202	114	117*	0	0	0
359	Cadiz	4	67	95	566	146***	148***	7	147	226
360	Cordoba	2	40	57	419	127***	129***	1	33	51
361	Granada	7	133	189	356	103	104	5	160	245
362	Huelva	0	0	0	271	150***	152***	0	0	0
363	Jaen	2	46	66	358	124***	127***	3	114	174
364	Malaga	12	166	236*	592	125***	126***	2	47	71
365	Sevilla	6	61	87	743	115***	116***	1	16*	24
366	Murcia	3	46	66	491	113**	116**	2	48	74
367	Las Palmas	2	49	69	369	140***	142***	2	62	95
368	Sta Cruz de Tenerife	2	50	71	287	111	112	3	107	164
EC		3002	100	-	196881	100	-	1361	100	-

Table 8.2(e)

Area	PER			BREAST			ISHD		
	Deaths	SMR to EC std	SMR to own std	Deaths	SMR to EC std	SMR to own std	Deaths	SMR to EC std	SMR to own std
BELGIUM	6066	103	100	5276	118***	100	14019	83***	100
1 Antwerpen	905	97	94	839	118***	100	2097	78***	94**
2 Brabant	1555	116***	113***	1306	126***	107*	2825	73***	88***
3 West-Vlaanderen	631	98	95	648	131***	111**	1266	68***	82***
4 Oost-Vlaanderen	783	107	104	761	128***	108*	1894	85***	102
5 Hainaut	771	100	98	657	111**	95	2152	95*	115***
6 Liege	604	100	98	463	99	84***	1702	96	116***
7 Limburg	423	93	91*	307	102	87*	1028	92**	110**
8 Luxembourg (province)	147	92	90	99	102	86	344	93	111*
9 Namur	247	92	90	196	107	91	711	103	124***
LUXEMBOURG	185	84*	100	204	120*	100	664	107	100
10 Luxembourg	185	84*	100	204	120*	100	664	107	100
FEDERAL REPUBLIC OF GERMANY	22912	71***	100	29924	102***	100	112034	106***	100
11 Schleswig-Holstein	901	70***	98	1373	114***	111***	4968	116***	110***
12 Hamburg	517	73***	102	895	112***	110**	2479	88***	83***
13 Braunschweig	483	63***	89**	756	98	96	3173	113***	106***
14 Hannover	621	67***	95	1033	105	102	3906	110***	103*
15 Lüneburg	476	65***	91*	700	103	100	2621	106**	100
16 Weser-Ems	952	77***	109*	974	102	100	3829	112***	106***
17 Bremen	219	73***	103	334	102	100	1226	106*	100
18 Düsseldorf	2013	78***	110***	2743	107***	105*	10896	117***	110***
19 Köln	1451	71***	100	1956	105*	102	7411	109***	103*
20 Munster	1111	81***	113***	1208	107*	105	4791	116***	109***
21 Detmold	737	77***	108	847	99	97	3248	104*	98
22 Arnsberg	1526	82***	115***	1830	103	100	8251	125***	118***
23 Darmstadt	1091	65***	92**	1714	105	102	5807	98	92***
24 Giessen	378	75***	105	438	99	97	1717	105*	99
25 Kassel	432	76***	107	527	94	92*	2049	99	93**
26 Koblenz	516	73***	103	697	106	103	2757	113***	106**
27 Trier	188	75***	105	211	93	91	877	104	98
28 Rheinhessen-Pfalz	664	71***	99	892	102	100	3472	108***	102
29 Stuttgart	1261	64***	90***	1600	99	96	5313	91***	86***
30 Karlsruhe	871	69***	96	1026	90***	88***	4379	106***	100
31 Freiburg	623	59***	83***	828	96	94	2694	87***	82***
32 Tübingen	579	62***	87***	623	92*	90**	2153	89***	84***
33 Oberbayern	1326	69***	97	1733	100	98	5089	84***	79***
34 Niederbayern	372	64***	90*	428	91*	89*	1807	106**	100
35 Oberpfalz	403	72***	102	441	97	95	1912	116***	109***
36 Oberfranken	372	68***	95	486	95	93	2232	120***	113***
37 Mittelfranken	542	66***	93	748	102	100	2944	112***	106**
38 Unterfranken	484	68***	96	508	92	90*	1909	94**	89***
39 Schwaben	594	66***	92*	735	103	101	2460	96*	90***
40 Saarland	447	85***	120***	560	105	103	2458	126***	119***
41 Berlin (West)	762	77***	109*	1080	120***	117***	3206	106**	100
DENMARK	2470	86***	100	2674	125***	100	10976	141***	100
42 Kobenhavn and Frederiksberg (M)	236	80***	92	316	144***	115*	1248	153***	108**
43 Kobenhavns County	230	73***	84**	384	133***	106	1247	120***	85***
44 Frederiksborg County	148	81**	93	209	145***	117*	644	128***	91*
45 Roskilde County	112	97	113	114	130**	105	423	141***	101
46 Vestsjællands County	143	92	107	148	126**	101	667	153***	109*
47 Storstroms County	104	80*	93	141	125*	99	694	162***	115***
48 Bornholms County	25	98	114	18	91	73	135	181***	128**
49 Fyns County	193	78***	91	204	107	86*	961	137***	97
50 Sonderjyllands County	117	80*	93	113	107	86	596	152***	108
51 Ribe County	133	99	115	78	91	73**	488	153***	109
52 Vejle County	163	88	102	163	120*	96	614	124***	88**
53 Ringkobing County	167	100	116	131	125*	100	575	151***	107
54 Århus County	294	85**	98	293	126***	102	1084	131***	94*

Table 8.2(e)—*cont.*

Area		PER			BREAST			ISHD		
		Deaths	SMR to EC std	SMR to own std	Deaths	SMR to EC std	SMR to own std	Deaths	SMR to EC std	SMR to own std
55	Viborg County	128	94	108	112	119	95	499	142***	101
56	Nordjyllands County	277	100	116*	250	125***	100	1101	149***	106
FRANCE		37777	98***	100	19911	86***	100	43448	51***	100
57	Ain	286	93	95	119	68***	80*	316	48***	95
58	Aisne	393	98	101	191	88	102	532	64***	128***
59	Allier	196	107	110	132	78**	90	361	55***	109
60	Alpes-de-Haute-Provence	66	86	88	39	69*	80	88	40***	80*
61	Hautes-Alpes	70	98	100	38	83	96	83	46***	92
62	Alpes-Maritimes	550	103	105	384	86**	100	623	38***	75***
63	Ardèche	166	103	106	83	70***	81	206	44***	88
64	Ardennes	229	103	105	85	70***	82	291	63***	126***
65	Ariège	70	103	106	44	70*	81	108	42***	85
66	Aube	192	99	101	85	72**	84	245	56***	110
67	Aude	177	111	113	100	75**	87	242	46***	92
68	Aveyron	109	81*	82*	113	89	104	217	43***	86*
69	Bouches-du-Rhône	1248	106*	108**	614	82***	96	1143	42***	82***
70	Calvados	386	87**	89*	189	78***	91	425	48***	95
71	Cantal	119	143***	146***	54	76*	89	173	61***	123**
72	Charente	204	101	103	123	83*	96	223	39***	78***
73	Charente-Maritime	270	90	92	213	91	106	383	42***	84***
74	Cher	170	90	92	118	86	100	291	55***	109
75	Corrèze	139	120*	123*	76	67***	78*	248	55***	111
76	Corse	181	122*	124**	78	73**	85	230	55***	109
77	Côte-d'Or	308	91	93	182	95	111	343	49***	96
78	Côtes-du-Nord	287	89	91	186	75***	88	467	49***	97
79	Creuse	58	97	100	37	57***	66**	132	49***	99
80	Dordogne	216	111	114	155	84*	98	397	54***	109
81	Doubs	356	103	105	169	91	106	399	59***	115**
82	Drôme	249	90	92	137	79**	92	307	47***	93
83	Eure	340	91	93	160	86	100	378	55***	108
84	Eure-et-Loir	279	101	103	108	74**	86	273	50***	98
85	Finistère	396	74***	76***	278	75***	87*	669	48***	96
86	Gard	374	105	107	206	83**	96	461	49***	97
87	Haute-Garonne	568	104	106	294	80***	94	572	43***	85***
88	Gers	105	126*	129*	65	79	92	119	36***	71***
89	Gironde	664	90**	92*	401	81***	94	877	48***	95
90	Hérault	561	118***	121***	355	107	125***	543	44***	87**
91	Ille-et-Vilaine	473	88**	90*	287	92	107	467	41***	80***
92	Indre	111	90	92	79	73**	85	218	51***	103
93	Indre-et-Loire	292	86*	88*	172	82**	95	311	40***	79***
94	Isère	621	88**	90**	298	77***	89*	706	50***	98
95	Jura	155	99	101	81	78*	90	235	59***	117*
96	Landes	155	94	96	113	80*	93	263	48***	95
97	Loir-et-Cher	173	96	98	101	79*	92	185	37***	74***
98	Loire	444	93	95	263	82***	95	605	50***	100
99	Haute-Loire	101	87	89	68	74*	86	200	55***	111
100	Loire-Atlantique	573	80***	81***	374	89*	104	693	46***	90**
101	Loiret	391	99	101	199	89	104	373	45***	89*
102	Lot	89	117	120	51	69**	80	141	48***	95
103	Lot-et-Garonne	163	95	97	105	75**	87	237	43***	87*
104	Lozère	44	116	118	17	56*	65	76	60***	121
105	Maine-et-Loire	450	88**	90*	228	85*	99	362	37***	72***
106	Manche	263	78***	80***	167	82**	95	389	50***	99
107	Marne	438	106	108	166	79**	93	424	56***	110
108	Haute-Marne	142	99	101	57	68**	80	150	47***	93
109	Mayenne	155	82*	84*	93	82	96	161	37***	75***
110	Meurthe-et-Moselle	510	100	102	231	78***	91	679	63***	124***
111	Meuse	146	105	108	61	74*	86	206	64***	128***
112	Morbihan	329	81***	83***	233	88	103	505	50***	101
113	Moselle	713	96	98	342	82***	96	1194	77***	152***

Table 8.2(e)—*cont.*

	Area	PER			BREAST			ISHD		
		Deaths	SMR to EC std	SMR to own std	Deaths	SMR to EC std	SMR to own std	Deaths	SMR to EC std	SMR to own std
114	Nièvre	125	96	99	87	82	95	282	68***	135***
115	Nord	2313	110***	113***	971	98	115***	2630	73***	144***
116	Oise	561	104	106	214	84*	99	523	57***	111*
117	Orne	159	84*	85*	95	75**	88	254	52***	104
118	Pas-de-Calais	1265	112***	114***	616	106	123***	1618	75***	149***
119	Puy-de-dôme	375	108	110	206	80**	93	571	59***	117***
120	Pyrénées-Atlantiques	335	105	107	200	78***	91	434	45***	90*
121	Hautes-Pyrénées	128	110	112	79	74**	86	189	46***	92
122	Pyrénées-Orientales	195	98	100	114	68***	79**	315	49***	97
123	Bas-Rhin	606	92	94	289	76***	89*	905	67***	131***
124	Haut-Rhin	461	96	98	226	83**	96	695	70***	137***
125	Rhône	1032	93*	95	561	94	109*	997	46***	91**
126	Haute-Saône	152	100	102	58	62***	72*	198	56***	110
127	Saône-et-Loire	323	95	97	197	80**	93	503	53***	105
128	Sarthe	269	80***	81***	199	95	111	332	42***	84**
129	Savoie	184	82**	84*	114	81*	95	243	47***	92
130	Haute-Savoie	339	88*	90	208	99	115*	429	57***	111*
131	Paris	1689	106*	108**	949	99	115***	1293	39***	76***
132	Seine-Maritime	990	105	107*	474	99	116**	892	51***	101
133	Seine-et-Marne	727	94	96	314	89*	104	672	55***	106
134	Yvelines	894	89***	91**	432	89*	104	728	43***	84***
135	Deux-Sèvres	193	93	95	117	81*	94	206	37***	73***
136	Somme	457	115**	118***	189	88	102	495	61***	121***
137	Tarn	195	105	108	125	78**	91	282	45***	91
138	Tarn-et-Garonne	107	97	99	80	91	106	132	39***	77**
139	Var	516	104	107	252	71***	82**	598	44***	88**
140	Vaucluse	303	97	99	147	76***	88	319	44***	88*
141	Vendée	255	79***	81***	204	97	113	311	38***	76***
142	Vienne	222	100	103	116	76**	88	247	42***	83**
143	Haute-Vienne	152	86	88	152	94	109	282	46***	91
144	Vosges	253	95	97	139	86	100	297	49***	97
145	Yonne	199	98	100	115	87	101	282	55***	109
146	Territoire-de-Belfort	101	107	109	40	75	87	104	53***	104
147	Essonne	737	92*	94	356	90*	105	657	48***	93
148	Hauts-de-Seine	1060	98	100	557	92	107	988	45***	89***
149	Seine-Saint-Denis	1347	112***	114***	483	92	107	1029	55***	107*
150	Val-de-Marne	846	91**	93*	483	96	112*	810	46***	89**
151	Val-d'Oise	799	95	97	356	97	113*	561	44***	85***
GREECE		7680	140***	100	3427	80***	100	14191	96***	100
152	Greater Athens	2551	149***	106**	1286	93*	117***	5701	125***	130***
153	Rest of Central Greece and Eubea	776	128***	92*	334	68***	86**	1354	77***	80***
154	Peloponnisos	730	133***	95	285	65***	81***	1190	73***	76***
155	Ionian Islands	109	116	83	53	60***	75*	218	68***	70***
156	Epirus	235	142***	102	75	52***	65***	357	72***	74***
157	Thessaly	541	134***	96	232	75***	94	912	84***	87***
158	Macedonia	1700	144***	102	788	87***	109*	3036	100	105**
159	Thrace	361	175***	125***	97	71***	90	464	102	106
160	Aegean Islands	333	135***	96	132	74***	91	501	74***	77***
161	Crete	344	109	78***	145	67***	84*	458	59***	61***
ITALY		34496	122***	100	24734	92***	100	72287	73***	100
162	Torino	1063	118***	96	1162	101	109**	3079	73***	100
163	Vercelli	177	134***	109	204	100	108	674	88***	120***
164	Novara	202	106	87*	283	113*	122**	742	81***	110**
165	Cuneo	243	106	87*	264	99	108	737	71***	97
166	Asti	86	118	97	87	81*	87	287	69***	94
167	Alessandria	173	128**	105	259	109	118*	664	73***	100
168	Aosta	43	92	75	69	124	134*	146	70***	95
169	Imperia	60	82	67**	98	82	89	317	71***	97
170	Savona	89	101	83	134	84*	91	448	75***	102

Table 8.2(e)—*cont.*

Area		PER			BREAST			ISHD		
		Deaths	SMR to EC std	SMR to own std	Deaths	SMR to EC std	SMR to own std	Deaths	SMR to EC std	SMR to own std
171	Genova	301	96	79***	611	111*	120***	1388	67***	92**
172	La Spezia	97	128*	105	117	93	101	319	67***	91
173	Varese	331	96	79***	416	109	118**	1045	77***	104
174	Como/Sondrio	381	87**	71***	481	107	116**	1480	91***	124***
175	Milano	1515	95*	77***	2257	112***	121***	5639	79***	107***
176	Bergamo	461	102	84***	437	106	114**	1272	85***	116***
177	Brescia	407	87**	71***	519	107	115**	1494	85***	116***
178	Pavia	170	101	83*	269	100	109	886	88***	120***
179	Cremona	113	90	73***	161	95	103	602	95	129***
180	Mantova	131	99	81*	167	88	96	641	90**	123***
181	Bolzano	200	80**	65***	185	99	107	509	75***	102
182	Trento	199	95	78***	212	102	111	587	76***	104
183	Verona	386	110	90*	395	106	115**	1050	77***	105
184	Vicenza	341	97	80***	298	88*	96	987	81***	110**
185	Belluno	78	95	78*	118	111	121	335	85**	116**
186	Treviso	244	76***	63***	322	96	104	819	66***	91**
187	Venezia	285	89*	73***	412	102	111*	953	65***	88***
188	Padova	325	91	74***	377	99	107	1030	75***	102
189	Rovigo	97	97	80*	122	98	106	357	75***	103
190	Udine/Gorizia	187	80**	65***	325	97	106	996	80***	110**
191	Trieste	52	66**	54***	138	93	101	352	64***	88*
192	Pordenone	79	73**	59***	123	96	104	301	63***	86*
193	Piacenza	130	157***	128**	140	97	105	476	85***	116**
194	Parma	127	100	82*	211	102	110	649	82***	112**
195	Reggio Emilia	125	84*	68***	240	115*	125***	551	69***	94
196	Modena	239	110	90	260	86*	94	911	80***	109**
197	Bologna	258	95	78***	527	106	114**	1410	75***	102
198	Ferrara	104	98	80*	202	101	109	623	82***	112**
199	Ravenna	121	110	90	168	91	99	416	60***	81***
200	Forli	276	119**	97	244	82**	89	670	60***	82***
201	Pesaro	150	106	87	139	86	93	367	59***	80***
202	Ancona	190	111	91	195	88	95	503	60***	82***
203	Macerata	132	104	85	117	79**	85	338	59***	81***
204	Ascoli Piceno	184	110	90	130	73***	79**	396	59***	80***
205	Massa-Carrara	79	102	84	87	84	91	287	73***	99
206	Lucca	149	105	86	195	101	109	458	63***	86***
207	Pistoia	127	129**	105	101	76**	83	338	68***	93
208	Firenze	434	100	82***	550	90**	97	1393	61***	83***
209	Livorno	120	100	82*	193	110	119*	414	63***	86**
210	Pisa	204	139***	114	186	95	103	479	65***	89**
211	Arezzo	119	95	77**	128	81*	88	358	58***	80***
212	Siena	95	112	91	117	87	94	289	55***	75***
213	Grosseto	74	101	83	99	85	92	286	64***	88*
214	Perugia	287	115*	94	242	80***	87*	815	70***	96
215	Terni	102	123*	101	92	77*	83	295	64***	88*
216	Viterbo/Rieti	217	111	91	182	88	95	611	76***	104
217	Roma	1855	107**	87***	1813	98	106**	4915	75***	102
218	Latina	295	107	88*	160	82**	88	466	65***	89**
219	Frosinone	343	126***	103	139	66***	71***	551	69***	94
220	Caserta	884	144***	118***	220	69***	75***	1080	94*	128***
221	Benevento	279	147***	120**	86	63***	69***	390	75***	103
222	Napoli	3415	147***	120***	983	83***	89***	4264	101	138***
223	Avellino	373	140***	115**	114	58***	63***	551	74***	102
224	Salerno	1072	151***	124***	320	71***	77***	1262	75***	103
225	L'Aquila	221	139***	114	90	62***	68***	368	67***	92
226	Teramo	164	113	92	89	71***	77**	279	58***	79***
227	Pescara	214	148***	121**	110	79*	85	349	67***	92
228	Chieti	192	103	84*	97	54***	59***	426	62***	85***
229	Isernia/Campobasso	230	133***	109	101	66***	71***	412	70***	96
230	Foggia	644	136***	111**	233	83**	90	714	70***	95
231	Bari	1266	127***	104	546	90*	97	1292	60***	81***

Table 8.2(e)—*cont.*

Area		PER			BREAST			ISHD		
		Deaths	SMR to EC std	SMR to own std	Deaths	SMR to EC std	SMR to own std	Deaths	SMR to EC std	SMR to own std
232	Taranto	556	144***	117***	186	77***	83**	529	61***	83***
233	Brindisi	357	141***	115*	155	90	98	390	63***	86**
234	Lecce	702	155***	127***	327	92	99	646	51***	69***
235	Potenza/Matera	502	135***	111*	195	73***	79***	678	67***	92*
236	Cosenza	673	145***	118***	207	65***	70***	794	67***	92*
237	Catanzaro	748	144***	118***	163	54***	59***	754	68***	93*
238	Reggio Calabria	623	154***	126***	206	85*	92	554	61***	84***
239	Trapani	329	122***	100	175	92	100	499	71***	97
240	Palermo	1228	139***	114***	405	77***	84***	1255	66***	90***
241	Messina	690	172***	141***	227	73***	79***	750	65***	88***
242	Agrigento	407	133***	108	149	71***	77**	541	70***	96
243	Caltanisetta	335	171***	140***	88	71**	77*	299	66***	90
244	Enna	210	176***	144***	55	64***	69**	242	76***	104
245	Catania	1207	162***	132***	407	92	99	1228	75***	102
246	Ragusa	280	152***	124***	138	109	119	267	57***	78***
247	Siracusa	398	153***	125***	144	85*	92	468	75***	103
248	Sassari	318	139***	113*	195	105	113	479	72***	98
249	Nuoro	226	146***	119*	81	72**	78*	311	76***	103
250	Cagliari/Oristano	701	151***	123***	363	99	107	815	63***	85***
IRELAND		3284	113***	100	1486	130***	100	8625	204***	100
251	Eastern	1179	114***	101	546	134***	103	2812	202***	99
252	Midland	217	125**	111	77	117	90	545	211***	103
253	Mid-Western	281	110	97	140	140***	107	812	213***	104
254	North-Eastern	268	108	96	113	120	93	711	199***	98
255	North-Western	202	116*	103	89	133*	103	518	196***	96
256	South-Eastern	390	121***	107	139	112	87	1029	218***	107*
257	Southern	539	127***	113**	220	125**	96	1407	213***	104
258	Western	208	75***	67***	162	147***	113	791	181***	88***
THE NETHERLANDS		7052	95***	100	5370	115***	100	19810	118***	100
259	Groningen	289	111	116*	192	112	97	963	155***	132***
260	Friesland	271	88*	92	191	106	92	885	135***	115***
261	Drenthe	195	92	97	156	109	95	752	143***	122***
262	Overijssel	563	103	108	383	122***	106	1466	128***	109**
263	Gelderland	884	99	104	649	115***	100	2367	117***	99
264	Utrecht	458	91	96	366	123***	107	1080	102	87***
265	Noord Holland	1142	101	106	887	118***	102	2958	109***	93***
266	Zuid Holland	1472	89***	94**	1203	119***	103	3999	109***	93***
267	Zeeland	153	88	92	136	120*	104	380	91	77***
268	Noord Brabant	1017	95	99	738	107	93	2830	115***	97
269	Limburg	487	95	100	429	114**	99	1947	142***	120***
270	Flevoland	121	94	98	40	81	71*	183	106	91
UK: ENGLAND AND WALES		30739	91***	100	27179	130***	100	143527	183***	100
271	Northern	1879	93**	103	1650	124***	96	11955	238***	130***
	Hartlepool	55	82	91	49	129	99	383	262***	143***
	North Tees	111	86	95	93	128*	99	605	224***	123***
	South Tees	208	94	103	140	116	89	1105	244***	133***
	East Cumbria	95	94	104	90	115	89	596	202***	110*
	South Cumbria	93	93	103	85	112	86	491	172***	94
	West Cumbria	86	97	107	83	140**	108	582	259***	142***
	Darlington	66	85	94	62	115	89	464	223***	122***
	Durham	141	96	106	114	112	86	978	256***	140***
	North-West Durham	54	104	115	44	116	89	380	262***	143***
	South-West Durham	74	74**	82	83	124	95	670	264***	144***
	Northumberland	149	84*	92	168	129**	99	1068	216***	118***
	Gateshead	159	121*	134***	113	124*	95	945	269***	147***
	Newcastle	164	88	98	153	133***	102	1062	243***	133***
	North Tyneside	110	91	100	133	152***	117	677	202***	110*
	South Tyneside	111	104	115	92	130*	100	732	267***	145***

Table 8.2(e)—*cont.*

	Area	PER			BREAST			ISHD		
		Deaths	SMR to EC std	SMR to own std	Deaths	SMR to EC std	SMR to own std	Deaths	SMR to EC std	SMR to own std
	Sunderland	203	97	107	148	118	91	1217	261***	142***
272	Yorkshire	2364	96	106**	1802	120***	93***	12160	216***	118***
	Hull	222	94	104	154	124*	96	1043	223***	122***
	East Yorkshire	88	88	98	123	140***	108	558	171***	94
	Grimsby	114	95	105	103	158***	121	496	198***	108
	Scunthorpe	151	117	129**	129	155***	119	716	226***	123***
	Northallerton	49	74*	82	59	130	100	275	165***	90
	York	134	84*	92	118	107	82*	775	190***	104
	Scarborough	86	107	118	74	116	89	471	197***	107
	Harrogate	66	88	97	73	124	96	330	153***	84**
	Bradford	361	124***	136***	128	99	76**	1395	286***	156***
	Airedale	80	73**	81	82	110	84	565	203***	111*
	Calderdale	136	101	112	93	117	90	713	240***	131***
	Huddersfield	145	104	115	73	83	64***	722	220***	121***
	Dewsbury	152	119*	132**	75	115	89	632	261***	143***
	Leeds Western	195	82**	91	175	117*	90	1247	221***	121***
	Leeds Eastern	193	80**	88	183	127**	98	1156	212***	116***
	Wakefield	88	93	102	71	119	92	456	206***	113*
	Pontefract	104	86	95	89	125*	96	610	227***	124***
273	Trent	2832	93***	103	2593	134***	103	14587	199***	109***
	North Derbyshire	179	83*	92	202	128***	98	1174	195***	106*
	Southern Derbyshire	314	90	99	297	136***	104	1711	204***	111***
	Leicestershire	593	98	108	439	125***	96	2416	183***	100
	North Lincolnshire	152	90	100	150	132**	101	811	189***	103
	South Lincolnshire	165	95	104	181	138***	106	913	184***	100
	Bassetlaw	51	80	88	80	181***	139**	308	183***	100
	Central Nottinghamshire	179	95	104	180	148***	114	894	193***	106
	Nottingham	331	80***	88*	354	141***	108	1794	188***	103
	Barnsley	160	111	122*	140	147***	113	891	247***	135***
	Doncaster	206	100	110	154	126**	97	920	198***	108*
	Rotherham	185	106	116*	123	116	89	919	231***	126***
	Sheffield	317	97	107	293	132***	102	1836	217***	119***
274	East Anglian	992	78***	86***	1002	122***	94*	4199	136***	74***
	Cambridge	110	65***	72***	128	119	92	475	120***	65***
	Peterborough	125	83*	92	112	138**	106	558	184***	100
	West Suffolk	118	77**	85	98	115	89	456	144***	79***
	East Suffolk	164	77***	85*	163	125**	96	647	130***	71***
	Norwich	207	78***	86*	247	121**	93	948	122***	67***
	Great Yarmouth and Waveney	99	82*	90	94	109	84	437	134***	73***
	West Norfolk and Wisbech	113	102	113	113	140***	107	451	146***	80***
	Huntingdon	56	59***	65***	47	99	76	227	135***	74***
275	North-West Thames	2105	85***	94**	1833	129***	100	7873	149***	82***
	North Bedfordshire	151	88	97	133	135***	104	516	142***	78***
	South Bedfordshire	226	95	104	131	124*	96	613	154***	84***
	North Hertfordshire	109	82*	90	112	143***	110	461	159***	87**
	East Hartfordshire	126	68***	75**	166	131***	101	657	139***	76***
	North-West Hertfordshire	142	86	94	145	127**	98	566	132***	72***
	South-West Hertfordshire	105	68***	74**	128	121*	93	549	137***	75***
	Barnet	167	84*	92	151	122*	94	589	130***	71***
	Harrow	121	87	96	104	127*	98	443	150***	82***
	Hillingdon	138	83*	92	143	148***	114	567	157***	86***
	Hounslow and Spelthorne	201	95	104	167	142***	109	700	157***	86***
	Ealing	172	81**	89	149	131**	101	734	174***	95
	Riverside	148	79**	87	133	120*	92	608	152***	83***
	Parkside	299	101	111	171	119*	91	870	162***	89***
276	North-East Thames	2510	92***	101	2111	137***	106*	9351	162***	89***
	Basildon and Thurrock	171	80**	88	190	162***	125**	839	193***	106
	Mid Essex	189	96	106	162	141***	109	577	138***	75***
	North-East Essex	140	77**	85	167	131***	101	682	143***	78***
	West Essex	122	74***	82*	160	141***	109	607	142***	78***
	Southend	182	90	99	190	138***	107	724	141***	77***

Table 8.2(e)—*cont.*

	Area	PER			BREAST			ISHD		
		Deaths	SMR to EC std	SMR to own std	Deaths	SMR to EC std	SMR to own std	Deaths	SMR to EC std	SMR to own std
	Barking, Havering, and Brentwood	272	93	102	290	140***	107	1310	166***	91***
	Hampstead	50	79	87	74	174***	134*	219	148***	81**
	Bloomsbury	67	84	92	64	125	96	330	170***	93
	Islington	113	89	98	83	127*	98	425	176***	96
	City and Hackney	201	111	122**	89	130*	100	446	171***	94
	Newham	225	108	119*	99	131*	101	627	219***	120***
	Tower Hamlets	151	99	109	84	154***	118	507	229***	125***
	Enfield	131	72***	79**	135	124*	95	589	146***	80***
	Haringey	154	94	103	97	128*	99	433	156***	86**
	Redbridge	146	97	107	117	119	92	541	148***	81***
	Waltham Forest	196	112	124**	110	135**	104	495	164***	90*
277	South-East Thames	2186	88***	97	1940	128***	98	8464	150***	82***
	Brighton	181	98	108	169	132***	101	567	118***	65***
	Eastbourne	95	81*	89	127	123*	95	446	117**	64***
	Hastings	82	88	97	100	136**	105	365	132***	72***
	South-East Kent	151	89	98	138	122*	94	639	152***	83***
	Canterbury and Thanet	149	84*	92	150	115	88	760	156***	85***
	Dartford and Gravesham	134	87	95	104	112	87	605	175***	96
	Maidstone	117	91	101	101	123	95	435	143***	78***
	Medway	241	94	103	169	133***	103	832	178***	98
	Tunbridge Wells	86	76**	83	113	129**	100	400	124***	68***
	Bexley	115	76**	83	112	120	93	473	137***	75***
	Greenwich	161	94	104	108	126*	97	539	170***	93
	Bromley	125	70***	78**	181	133***	103	617	122***	67***
	West Lambeth	127	95	104	79	137**	105	411	186***	102
	Camberwell	185	96	105	106	132**	102	554	184***	101
	Lewisham and North Southwark	237	95	104	183	145***	111	821	170***	93*
278	South-West Thames	1514	80***	88***	1626	128***	99	6228	133***	73***
	North-West Surrey	108	80*	89	113	125*	96	355	105	57***
	West Surrey and North-East Hampshire	133	71***	78**	131	119	92	512	131***	72***
	South-West Surrey	71	68***	75*	105	133**	102	353	121***	66***
	Mid Surrey	61	70**	78*	105	136**	104	338	117**	64***
	East Surrey	100	89	99	128	155***	119	414	135***	73***
	Chichester	67	76*	84	113	136**	104	349	112*	61***
	Mid Downs	144	80**	88	161	138***	106	571	132***	72***
	Worthing	107	83	92	140	128**	98	550	135***	74***
	Croydon	219	93	102	156	120*	92	707	148***	81***
	Kingston and Esher	85	75**	82	100	129*	99	352	123***	67***
	Richmond, Twickenham, and Roehampton	114	79*	87	119	120	92	504	138***	76***
	Wandsworth	120	81*	90	76	111	86	466	185***	101
	Merton and Sutton	185	78***	86*	179	127**	98	757	146***	80***
279	Wessex	1619	88***	97	1559	128***	99	6661	148***	81***
	East Dorset	222	93	102	262	132***	101	978	130***	71***
	West Dorset	83	74**	82	108	126*	97	443	138***	75***
	Portsmouth and South-East Hampshire	357	98	108	279	131***	101	1258	163***	89***
	Southampton and South-West Hampshire	213	77***	85*	234	133***	102	1011	152***	83***
	Winchester	95	74**	81*	117	131**	101	458	141***	77***
	Basingstoke and North Hampshire	120	81*	89	120	138***	107	461	147***	81***
	Salisbury	73	97	106	62	122	94	273	145***	79***
	Swindon	156	88	97	94	104	80*	593	177***	97
	Bath	222	88	97	215	129***	100	848	138***	75***
	Isle of Wight	78	116	128*	68	117	90	338	156***	85**
280	Oxford	1365	79***	87***	1229	126***	98	5064	142***	78***
	East Berkshire	207	79***	87*	195	133***	103	857	157***	86***
	West Berkshire	244	79***	88*	213	123**	95	855	135***	74***
	Aylesbury Vale	73	74**	81	68	121	94	263	129***	71***
	Wycombe	137	84*	92	149	126**	97	521	119***	65***
	Milton Keynes	117	81*	90	61	114	88	281	150***	83**
	Kettering	188	105	115	126	122*	94	679	177***	97
	Northampton	193	88	97	135	113	88	655	149***	82***
	Oxfordshire	206	58***	64***	282	139***	107	953	128***	70***

Table 8.2(e)—*cont.*

	Area	PER			BREAST			ISHD		
		Deaths	SMR to EC std	SMR to own std	Deaths	SMR to EC std	SMR to own std	Deaths	SMR to EC std	SMR to own std
281	South-Western	1605	81***	89***	1772	129***	99	8128	158***	86***
	Bristol and Weston	194	81**	89	185	122**	94	949	167***	91**
	Frenchay	141	94	104	115	126*	97	563	165***	90*
	Southmead	109	74**	82*	126	128**	99	579	158***	86***
	Cornwall and Isles of Scilly	235	85*	94	282	138***	106	1250	162***	89***
	Exeter	157	90	99	141	106	81*	735	146***	80***
	North Devon	65	84	92	75	131*	101	315	145***	79***
	Plymouth	177	81**	89	140	106	81*	973	200***	110**
	Torbay	105	82*	90	166	153***	118*	635	155***	85***
	Cheltenham and District	97	78*	85	113	126*	97	485	144***	79***
	Gloucester	157	77***	85*	180	137***	105	728	147***	80***
	Somerset	168	71***	78***	249	143***	110	916	141***	77***
282	West Midlands	3790	105**	116***	2930	135***	104*	16210	197***	108***
	Bromsgrove and Redditch	110	97	107	87	131*	101	403	166***	91
	Herefordshire	86	90	99	93	141**	108	401	160***	88**
	Kidderminster and District	59	93	103	56	129	99	271	169***	93
	Worcester and District	131	92	101	137	133**	103	616	160***	88***
	Shropshire	267	104	114*	193	119*	92	1131	187***	102
	Mid Staffordshire	173	84*	92	155	118*	91	812	168***	92*
	North Staffordshire	344	112*	124***	303	152***	117**	1826	239***	130***
	South-East Staffordshire	197	110	122**	146	142***	109	737	195***	107
	Rugby	51	97	107	46	127	98	222	160***	88*
	North Warwickshire	125	103	113	85	117	90	523	190***	104
	South Warwickshire	75	59***	65***	142	147***	113	544	150***	82***
	Central Birmingham	166	112	123**	72	105	81	589	223***	122***
	East Birmingham	221	127***	140***	101	128*	98	725	230***	125***
	North Birmingham	120	116	128**	117	166***	127*	466	174***	95
	South Birmingham	183	101	111	154	154***	118*	831	218***	119***
	West Birmingham	220	111	122**	102	135**	104	704	239***	131***
	Coventry	240	103	113	139	111	85	979	203***	111**
	Dudley	203	103	113	152	116	89	954	191***	104
	Sandwell	260	119**	132***	194	153***	117*	1114	225***	123***
	Solihull	126	101	112	142	156***	120*	531	158***	86***
	Walsall	220	120**	132***	176	155***	119*	983	226***	123***
	Wolverhampton	213	120**	133***	138	133**	102	848	208***	113***
283	Mersey	1455	88***	97	1359	133***	102	8785	230***	126***
	Chester	115	95	105	120	155***	119	578	202***	110*
	Crewe	142	87	96	138	130**	100	829	209***	114***
	Halton	93	85	93	91	161***	124	502	239***	131***
	Macclesfield	82	80*	88	103	129*	100	474	160***	87**
	Warrington	100	80*	88	99	134**	104	675	246***	135***
	Liverpool	319	89*	98	254	128***	98	1951	260***	142***
	St Helens and Knowsley	219	88	97	175	120*	92	1515	278***	152***
	North Sefton	57	96	106	77	141**	109	378	188***	103
	South Sefton	97	78*	86	111	142***	109	702	241***	132***
	Wirral	231	96	106	191	125**	96	1181	209***	114***
284	North-Western	2758	98	107***	2135	130***	100	14368	233***	127***
	Lancaster	84	107	118	65	118	90	416	200***	109
	Blackpool Wyre and Fylde	160	88	97	175	116	89	1205	211***	115***
	Preston	103	108	119	79	156***	120	447	229***	125***
	Blackburn, Hyndburn, and Ribble Valley	189	93	103	130	121*	93	984	240***	131***
	Burnley, Pendle, and Rossendale	213	121**	133***	94	100	77**	873	246***	134***
	West Lancashire	84	115	127*	58	131	101	332	205***	112*
	Chorley and South Ribble	132	100	111	128	162***	125*	612	212***	116***
	Bolton	180	95	104	144	138***	106	1018	260***	142***
	Bury	133	106	117	107	149***	115	581	219***	120***
	North Manchester	119	104	115	73	134*	103	678	316***	173***
	Central Manchester	105	99	109	59	141*	108	462	280***	153***
	South Manchester	122	94	104	79	111	86	594	223***	122***
	Oldham	157	94	104	130	147***	113	831	252***	138***
	Rochdale	194	118*	130***	91	107	82	813	255***	140***

Table 8.2(e)—*cont.*

	Area	PER			BREAST			ISHD		
		Deaths	SMR to EC std	SMR to own std	Deaths	SMR to EC std	SMR to own std	Deaths	SMR to EC std	SMR to own std
	Salford	162	96	106	130	132**	102	968	257***	140***
	Stockport	167	88	97	159	127**	98	885	192***	105
	Tameside and Glossop	170	94	104	130	129**	99	905	239***	130***
	Trafford	123	86	94	137	147***	113	623	180***	98
	Wigan	161	77***	84*	167	132***	102	1141	244***	134***
285	Wales	1765	93**	103	1638	136***	104	9494	207***	113***
	Clwyd	237	92	101	247	145***	112	1277	202***	110***
	East Dyfed	131	98	109	150	146***	113	742	186***	102
	Pembrokeshire	67	95	105	67	139*	107	381	208***	114*
	Gwent	293	95	105	233	123**	94	1627	225***	123***
	Gwynedd	135	94	104	122	120	92	713	187***	102
	Mid Glamorgan	341	89*	98	311	139***	107	2031	239***	130***
	Powys	69	103	114	64	129	99	310	162***	88*
	South Glamorgan	273	94	103	232	142***	110	1108	181***	99
	West Glamorgan	219	93	102	212	134***	103	1305	215***	117***
	UK: NORTHERN IRELAND	1325	96	100	748	128***	100	4894	234***	100
286	Northern Ireland	1325	96	100	748	128***	100	4894	234***	100
	UK: SCOTLAND	3068	93***	100	2739	125***	100	19811	247***	100
287	Highlands and Islands	145	82*	89	179	159***	127**	985	237***	96
288	Grampian	300	92	99	212	103	83**	1445	194***	79***
289	Tayside	180	76***	81**	229	132***	105	1448	226***	91***
290	Fife	233	103	111	166	115	92	1274	239***	97
291	Lothian	410	86**	93	347	111	89*	2394	211***	85***
292	Borders	35	62**	66*	49	109	87	350	208***	84***
293	Forth Valley	166	100	107	175	149***	119*	1012	236***	96
294	Argyll and Clyde	292	99	106	238	125***	100	1896	274***	111***
295	Greater Glasgow	611	95	102	520	125***	100	4241	276***	111***
296	Lanarkshire	374	101	109	318	132***	105	2492	288***	116***
297	Ayrshire and Arran	246	103	110	218	133***	107	1650	277***	112***
298	Dumfries and Galloway	76	87	93	88	132*	105	624	248***	100
	PORTUGAL	11528	184***	100	3561	81***	100	9729	62***	100
299	Viana do Castelo	318	203***	110	71	61***	77*	228	58***	94
300	Braga	1175	194***	105	149	57***	70***	552	62***	100
301	Vila Real	368	220***	119**	43	42***	52***	168	43***	70***
302	Bragança	213	213***	115*	50	66**	83	147	50***	81**
303	Guarda	197	180***	98	52	61***	78	164	51***	83*
304	Viseu	485	175***	95	113	67***	84	310	50***	81***
305	Porto	2293	197***	107**	479	74***	91*	1386	63***	101
306	Aveiro	760	174***	95	167	64***	79**	468	51***	82***
307	Coimbra	392	163***	89*	154	75***	93	333	45***	73***
308	Castelo Branco	242	212***	115*	76	73**	92	191	48***	79***
309	Portalegre	130	183***	99	52	78	99	155	59***	97
310	Santarem	381	163***	88*	191	88	109	384	47***	77***
311	Leiria	374	146***	79***	151	80**	99	358	52***	83***
312	Lisboa	1967	176***	95*	996	96	118***	2670	74***	119***
313	Setubal	630	157***	85***	349	98	119**	768	60***	97
314	Evora	177	190***	103	70	81	101	206	62***	101
315	Beja	131	141***	77**	74	92	115	240	74***	121**
316	Faro	373	187***	102	147	96	120*	342	58***	95
317	Madeira	407	208***	113*	80	79*	97	196	58***	93
318	Azores	515	233***	127***	97	113	140**	463	142***	231***
	SPAIN	17415	100	100	9889	76***	100	27819	60***	100
319	La Coruña	432	102	102	275	71***	93	804	59***	99
320	Lugo	173	129**	129**	121	75**	100	322	54***	90
321	Orense	158	137***	137***	104	64***	84	240	40***	66***
322	Pontevedra	313	82***	82***	223	74***	97	515	50***	83***
323	Asturias	434	111*	111*	318	75***	99	1050	66***	111**

Table 8.2(e)—*cont.*

Area		PER			BREAST			ISHD		
		Deaths	SMR to EC std	SMR to own std	Deaths	SMR to EC std	SMR to own std	Deaths	SMR to EC std	SMR to own std
324	Cantabria	215	101	101	121	68***	90	371	57***	95
325	Alava	110	100	100	65	77*	100	128	43***	71***
326	Guipuzcoa	247	101	100	172	74***	96	522	63***	105
327	Vizcaya	524	122***	122***	371	87**	115**	658	43***	73***
328	Navarra	159	79**	78**	143	84*	109	363	57***	95
329	Rioja	146	144***	144***	65	72**	95	180	53***	89
330	Huesca	67	89	89	76	95	126	151	47***	79**
331	Teruel	36	63**	63**	42	80	107	108	52***	88
332	Zaragoza	276	88*	88*	287	91	120**	640	55***	92*
333	Madrid Centro	1699	78***	78***	1181	70***	92**	2700	47***	79***
334	Avila	69	98	98	39	61***	81	112	45***	75**
335	Burgos	87	64***	64***	85	67***	88	217	46***	77***
336	Leon	337	167***	166***	157	79**	106	385	52***	88*
337	Palencia	59	78	78	64	99	131*	130	53***	90
338	Salamanca	187	131***	131***	101	80*	106	241	52***	87*
339	Segovia	53	92	92	41	79	105	76	39***	66***
340	Soria	31	88	87	18	54**	72	56	44***	74*
341	Valladolid	41	22***	22***	143	90	117	258	46***	77***
342	Zamora	84	106	106	48	57***	76	138	43***	73***
343	Albacete	195	111	111	64	57***	76*	227	55***	93
344	Ciudad Real	289	117*	117*	123	77**	102	363	60***	101
345	Cuenca	98	112	112	50	69**	92	150	55***	92
346	Guadalajara	21	35***	35***	28	60**	79	72	40***	67***
347	Toledo	239	102	102	104	64***	84	328	53***	88*
348	Badajoz	403	113*	113*	162	81**	107	605	81***	137***
349	Caceres	228	110	110	93	69***	92	366	74***	126***
350	Barcelona	1473	79***	79***	1342	80***	105	3109	53***	88***
351	Gerona	177	86*	86*	154	90	119*	384	60***	100
352	Lerida	135	101	101	102	78*	103	246	48***	81***
353	Tarragona	206	90	90	127	69***	91	334	49***	81***
354	Alicante	515	84***	84***	312	77***	100	1141	79***	132***
355	Castellon de la Plana	200	107	106	103	67***	88	350	62***	103
356	Valencia	741	82***	82***	593	81***	106	1702	66***	110***
357	Baleares	328	94	93	190	81**	106	797	93	155***
358	Almeria	309	119**	118**	62	49***	64***	312	69***	116*
359	Cadiz	987	152***	152***	217	77***	100	910	92**	152***
360	Cordoba	442	108	108	151	65***	85	540	64***	107
361	Granada	527	123***	123***	173	69***	91	543	61***	102
362	Huelva	293	124***	124***	100	78*	103	353	76***	127***
363	Jaen	465	129***	129***	120	59***	77**	366	49***	83***
364	Malaga	724	123***	123***	277	81***	105	989	82***	136***
365	Sevilla	1117	128***	128***	382	82***	107	1301	79***	131***
366	Murcia	543	96	96	256	81***	106	752	67***	113***
367	Las Palmas	430	97	97	199	98	126**	669	99	164***
368	Sta Cruz de Tenerife	393	103	103	145	73***	95	545	82***	136***
EC		185997	100	-	137122	100	-	501834	100	-

Table 8.2(f)

Area	PEPTIC			ALL (age 5–64)			ALL (all ages)		
	Deaths	SMR to EC std	SMR to own std	Deaths	SMR to EC std	SMR to own std	Deaths	SMR to EC std	SMR to own std
BELGIUM	237	61***	100	116013	103***	100	540361	104***	100
1 Antwerpen	18	29***	47***	16691	93***	90***	80901	99**	95***
2 Brabant	64	72**	118	25155	98**	95***	123320	100	96***
3 West-Vlaanderen	16	38***	62*	11569	93***	90***	56682	97***	93***
4 Oost-Vlaanderen	24	47***	76	14930	100	96***	73923	104***	99*
5 Hainaut	52	101	165***	18469	124***	121***	80710	116***	111***
6 Liege	33	82	134	13542	116***	113***	60743	114***	109***
7 Limburg	9	35***	56	7074	91***	88***	26664	100	95***
8 Luxembourg (province)	7	82	135	2846	115***	111***	13077	110***	105***
9 Namur	14	88	144	5737	124***	120***	24341	115***	110***
LUXEMBOURG	11	77	100	4788	114***	100	20090	111***	100
10 Luxembourg	11	77	100	4788	114***	100	20090	111***	100
FEDERAL REPUBLIC OF GERMANY	2498	103	100	724614	102***	100	3478836	102***	100
11 Schleswig-Holstein	105	106	103	29718	103***	100	154163	103***	101***
12 Hamburg	102	158***	153***	21197	113***	111***	108182	103***	101**
13 Braunschweig	65	101	99	18979	102*	99	98036	101***	100
14 Hannover	67	82	80	24749	105***	102***	126182	102***	100
15 Lüneburg	42	74*	72*	16827	101	99	84424	103***	102***
16 Weser-Ems	66	84	81	23581	101*	99	109690	101***	100
17 Bremen	40	150*	146*	9045	117***	115***	42911	103***	101*
18 Düsseldorf	213	99	97	66786	108***	106***	300328	104***	103***
19 Köln	121	77**	75**	44771	98***	96***	205655	102***	101***
20 Munster	103	109	106	29471	106***	104***	124268	105***	103***
21 Detmold	58	81	79	20541	99	97***	102387	97***	95***
22 Arnsberg	164	108	106	47836	110***	107***	212583	106***	104***
23 Darmstadt	150	109	106	39437	99*	97***	187047	99***	98***
24 Giessen	37	98	96	10712	98*	96***	54337	103***	101**
25 Kassel	37	78	76	13191	96***	94***	72060	101	99*
26 Koblenz	48	86	84	16227	101	99	81534	103***	101***
27 Trier	13	68	67	5776	104**	102	27295	103***	102**
28 Rheinhessen-Pfalz	78	106	103	22195	104***	102*	103406	104***	102***
29 Stuttgart	139	103	100	35417	89***	87***	169360	93***	91***
30 Karlsruhe	136	143***	139***	27318	98**	96***	130115	99*	98***
31 Freiburg	64	89	87	19320	92***	90***	93312	92***	91***
32 Tübingen	57	102	99	14565	88***	86***	71778	92***	90***
33 Oberbayern	144	101	98	38315	92***	90***	187195	94***	92***
34 Niederbayern	39	100	98	12267	107***	105***	56587	106***	105***
35 Oberpfalz	51	135*	132	12297	112***	109***	53914	109***	107***
36 Oberfranken	62	145**	143**	13659	111***	109***	64549	106***	105***
37 Mittelfranken	69	114	111	18378	104***	102**	88869	103***	102***
38 Unterfranken	43	92	90	13071	96***	94***	64536	101**	100
39 Schwaben	45	76	74*	16898	98**	96***	86235	100	98***
40 Saarland	50	112	110	14414	112***	110***	62775	110***	109***
41 Berlin (West)	90	127*	122	27656	132***	129***	155123	114***	113***
DENMARK	303	167***	100	63304	118***	100	291354	107***	100
42 Kobenhavn and Frederiksberg (M)	49	258***	155**	9316	166***	141***	50382	117***	111***
43 Kobenhavns County	34	142	85	7975	115***	97**	29706	105***	97***
44 Frederiksborg County	16	135	80	3887	110***	93***	14241	104***	97***
45 Roskilde County	17	238**	142	2442	113***	96*	8677	109***	101
46 Vestsjællands County	10	99	59	3502	118***	100	16563	110***	103***
47 Storstroms County	26	263***	158*	3614	127***	107***	17175	111***	104***
48 Bornholms County	2	116	69	511	102	86***	2908	104*	98
49 Fyns County	21	129	77	5317	111***	94***	26241	103***	97***
50 Sonderjyllands County	14	154	92	2919	110***	93***	13875	105***	98*
51 Ribe County	8	108	65	2325	106**	89***	10680	99	92***
52 Vejle County	25	216***	130	3829	112***	95**	17746	104***	97***
53 Ringkobing County	10	112	67	2911	110***	93***	12769	102	95***
54 Århus County	26	134	81	6403	110***	93***	29835	104***	97***

Table 8.2(f)—*cont.*

	Area	PEPTIC			ALL (age 5–64)			ALL (all ages)		
		Deaths	SMR to EC std	SMR to own std	Deaths	SMR to EC std	SMR to own std	Deaths	SMR to EC std	SMR to own std
55	Viborg County	14	172	103	2564	108***	91***	13052	101	95***
56	Nordjyllands County	31	181**	108	5789	115***	97*	27504	107***	100
FRANCE		1617	81***	100	611368	105***	100	2667420	95***	100
57	Ain	11	72	89	4306	95**	91***	19576	92***	96***
58	Aisne	20	105	129	6933	124***	119***	28001	109***	114***
59	Allier	19	127	157	4517	106***	103	23840	97***	103***
60	Alpes-de-Haute-Provence	3	60	74	1337	93**	89***	6809	88***	92***
61	Hautes-Alpes	5	121	150	1139	95	92**	5434	89***	93***
62	Alpes-Maritimes	25	66*	82	10005	93***	90***	57198	84***	89***
63	Ardèche	3	28*	35	2867	93***	90***	15316	92***	97***
64	Ardennes	8	76	93	3852	124***	118***	15074	106***	111***
65	Ariège	4	69	86	1368	84***	82***	9329	90***	95***
66	Aube	11	108	133	3242	108***	103	14879	95***	100
67	Aude	9	75	93	2872	85***	82***	18213	90***	95***
68	Aveyron	7	61	76	2509	78***	76***	16837	88***	93***
69	Bouches-du-Rhône	36	57***	70*	18469	99	95***	82728	95***	100
70	Calvados	13	64	78	6629	109***	104**	26405	98***	102***
71	Cantal	6	94	116	1909	104	101	9894	97*	103**
72	Charente	9	69	85	3720	98	95**	19141	92***	97***
73	Charente-Maritime	14	68	84	5594	95***	92***	28813	89***	94***
74	Cher	7	58	71	3753	107***	103	19108	97***	102**
75	Corrèze	4	39	49	2693	94**	92***	16029	94***	99
76	Corse	4	42	51	2795	101	97	13671	97**	102**
77	Côte-d'Or	23	141	172*	4940	101	96*	21560	90***	94***
78	Côtes-du-Nord	12	55*	68	7365	119***	115***	32292	102**	107***
79	Creuse	3	49	62	1739	103	101	11395	98*	103***
80	Dordogne	8	48*	60	4418	95***	93***	24896	92***	98***
81	Doubs	10	63	77	4653	98	93***	18588	93***	97***
82	Drôme	9	60	74	3981	91***	87***	19036	88***	93***
83	Eure	16	99	122	5721	119***	113***	22061	103***	107***
84	Eure-et-Loir	8	63	77	3930	104*	99	17230	91***	96***
85	Finistère	28	88	109	11375	123***	119***	48005	104***	110***
86	Gard	18	83	103	6005	96**	93***	29989	94***	99
87	Haute-Garonne	11	36***	44**	7477	82***	78***	37713	87***	91***
88	Gers	6	79	98	1737	81***	79***	10829	87***	92***
89	Gironde	24	57**	70	12006	97***	93***	57826	93***	98***
90	Hérault	13	46**	57*	7241	88***	84***	38637	89***	94***
91	Ille-et-Vilaine	14	53*	65	8112	103*	98	33860	97***	102***
92	Indre	9	93	116	2728	99	96	15756	94***	99
93	Indre-et-Loire	7	39**	48*	4937	92***	88***	23958	86***	90***
94	Isère	31	94	114	9325	94***	89***	38449	91***	95***
95	Jura	5	55	67	2588	97	94***	12811	92***	97***
96	Landes	11	88	108	3377	94***	91***	18054	93***	98**
97	Loir-et-Cher	7	62	76	3156	96*	93***	16635	88***	93***
98	Loire	28	101	125	7877	98	94***	36747	94***	98**
99	Haute-Loire	11	134	166	2487	106**	102	12953	99	105***
100	Loire-Atlantique	23	65*	80	11800	113***	108***	45352	98***	103***
101	Loiret	15	78	96	5638	99	95***	25571	91***	96***
102	Lot	2	30	37	1580	84***	82***	9911	90***	95***
103	Lot-et-Garonne	4	32*	40	2991	85***	82***	17128	89***	94***
104	Lozère	2	70	86	777	95	92*	4583	92***	97
105	Maine-et-Loire	11	48**	59	6402	94***	90***	29072	88***	92***
106	Manche	10	56	69	5343	103*	100	24213	99	104***
107	Marne	19	107	131	6169	115***	109***	24432	100	104***
108	Haute-Marne	5	68	84	2383	110***	106**	10417	98*	102*
109	Mayenne	5	51	63	2705	94***	90***	12736	90***	95***
110	Meurthe-et-Moselle	34	136	166**	8294	111***	106***	32101	101	105***
111	Meuse	9	123	151	2426	114***	110***	10543	101	106***
112	Morbihan	14	61	76	8510	128***	124***	33289	108***	114***
113	Moselle	48	134	163**	12226	114***	109***	43177	109***	113***

Table 8.2(f)—*cont.*

Area	PEPTIC			ALL (age 5–64)			ALL (all ages)		
	Deaths	SMR to EC std	SMR to own std	Deaths	SMR to EC std	SMR to own std	Deaths	SMR to EC std	SMR to own std
114 Nièvre	8	84	105	3244	120***	117***	16476	99	104***
115 Nord	123	147***	181***	34378	138***	131***	121183	114***	119***
116 Oise	20	92	112	7626	116***	109***	28710	104***	108***
117 Orne	3	27**	33*	3336	104*	100	14994	95***	100
118 Pas-de-Calais	90	181***	223***	20483	140***	134***	72759	116***	121***
119 Puy-de-dôme	22	99	122	7133	110***	105***	30458	100	105***
120 Pyrénées-Atlantiques	15	68	84	5901	93***	89***	31785	92***	97***
121 Hautes-Pyrénées	7	75	92	2429	91***	88***	13061	92***	96***
122 Pyrénées-Orientales	14	96	119	3632	88***	85***	20985	89***	94***
123 Bas-Rhin	34	108	131	10395	110***	104***	43751	104***	108***
124 Haut-Rhin	33	142	174**	7734	112***	107***	31338	105***	110***
125 Rhône	46	91	112	14382	96***	91***	59497	91***	94***
126 Haute-Saône	7	85	105	2547	106**	102	12183	98*	103**
127 Saône-et-Loire	22	101	125	6235	100	96**	31518	95***	100
128 Sarthe	14	78	95	5066	95***	92***	23770	88***	92***
129 Savoie	8	66	81	3659	103	98	15396	94***	99
130 Haute-Savoie	15	84	103	5484	102	97*	20499	94***	97***
131 Paris	45	58***	71*	24857	108***	102***	108154	86***	90***
132 Seine-Maritime	45	112	137	14390	120***	114***	55391	101**	106***
133 Seine-et-Marne	21	72	87	9823	109***	102*	37960	100	104***
134 Yvelines	24	60**	73	11296	93***	87***	39018	90***	92***
135 Deux-Sèvres	8	62	77	3039	82***	79***	17240	87***	92***
136 Somme	29	155*	191**	6795	123***	118***	28642	108***	113***
137 Tarn	6	42*	53	3159	79***	76***	19215	86***	91***
138 Tarn-et-Garonne	4	51	64	1874	84***	81***	10935	88***	93***
139 Var	19	61*	76	8390	95***	92***	41713	91***	96***
140 Vaucluse	11	66	82	4696	97*	93***	21553	92***	97***
141 Vendée	7	38**	47*	5080	94***	91***	24590	92***	97***
142 Vienne	7	52	64	3433	87***	83***	18763	86***	91***
143 Haute-Vienne	3	21***	26**	3762	93***	90***	21943	91***	96***
144 Vosges	16	115	141	4733	116***	111***	20861	102**	107***
145 Yonne	11	93	115	3960	116***	112***	20276	99	105***
146 Territoire-de-Belfort	6	131	160	1431	105	100	5914	100	104**
147 Essonne	19	59*	71	9560	96***	90***	32696	91***	94***
148 Hauts-de-Seine	32	63**	77	15030	100	95***	57218	89***	93***
149 Seine-Saint-Denis	38	86	104	15508	116***	109***	48396	99**	102***
150 Val-de-Marne	33	79	96	12460	100	94***	47875	93***	96***
151 Val-d'Oise	21	69	84	9500	102*	96***	32604	97***	100
GREECE	96	28***	100	93157	92***	100	465451	107***	100
152 Greater Athens	40	38***	134	30538	96***	105***	133951	116***	110***
153 Rest of Central Greece and Eubea	14	35***	124	9986	84***	91***	52519	99**	92***
154 Peloponnisos	5	13***	48	8876	82***	89***	56112	98***	90***
155 Ionian Islands	1	14*	48	1680	80***	87***	11700	103**	94***
156 Epirus	0	0***	0	2741	81***	88***	15023	97***	90***
157 Thessaly	5	20***	71	6724	91***	99	33405	108***	101
158 Macedonia	18	25***	92	21008	98*	109***	97238	111***	105***
159 Thrace	4	38*	136	3764	117***	128***	16309	125***	118***
160 Aegean Islands	6	39*	136	3736	82***	89***	24992	101	93***
161 Crete	3	17***	60	4104	78***	85***	24202	93***	86***
ITALY	1947	86***	100	599820	91***	100	2684453	95***	100
162 Torino	104	108	125*	25848	93***	102**	109190	95***	101
163 Vercelli	15	86	100	5197	106***	115***	26619	103***	109***
164 Novara	19	90	105	6496	108***	118***	29619	100	106***
165 Cuneo	26	111	128	6730	100	110***	33904	100	106***
166 Asti	4	42	49	2353	89***	97	15156	98**	103***
167 Alessandria	10	48*	56	5631	97*	106***	32772	95***	101
168 Aosta	7	146	169	1651	119***	130***	6144	102	108***
169 Imperia	8	79	92	2583	91***	99	14515	94***	99
170 Savona	8	59	68	3455	90***	99	19087	94***	99

Table 8.2(f)—*cont.*

	Area	PEPTIC			ALL (age 5–64)			ALL (all ages)		
		Deaths	SMR to EC std	SMR to own std	Deaths	SMR to EC std	SMR to own std	Deaths	SMR to EC std	SMR to own std
171	Genova	27	58**	67*	12252	93***	102*	65627	96***	101***
172	La Spezia	4	37*	43	2571	84***	92***	14695	91***	96***
173	Varese	32	102	118	8424	92***	101	36338	94***	99
174	Como/Sondrio	27	72	83	11235	102**	112***	45499	98***	104***
175	Milano	114	69***	80*	46218	97***	106***	173137	94***	100
176	Bergamo	19	55**	64*	11221	110***	121***	38553	103***	109***
177	Brescia	39	96	112	13321	112***	123***	46141	102***	108***
178	Pavia	14	61	71	7226	112***	122***	34618	104***	110***
179	Cremona	11	76	88	4839	117***	128***	20152	109***	115***
180	Mantova	14	86	100	4497	97	106***	21914	98**	104***
181	Bolzano	14	89	104	4507	97*	106***	17474	91***	97***
182	Trento	19	107	125	5478	107***	117***	23026	96***	102**
183	Verona	24	76	89	9007	99	108***	37255	94***	100
184	Vicenza	25	89	103	8322	101	110***	32900	96***	102**
185	Belluno	10	111	129	3135	121***	133***	13117	101	107***
186	Treviso	18	63	74	7797	94***	103**	32890	89***	95***
187	Venezia	30	89	103	9794	100	109***	37235	95***	100
188	Padova	33	104	121	9043	97**	107***	36143	95***	101
189	Rovigo	15	139	161	3134	102	111***	13444	97**	103***
190	Udine/Gorizia	32	113	131	8966	111***	121***	39826	100	106***
191	Trieste	16	129	150	3624	104*	114***	20523	98*	104***
192	Pordenone	12	110	128	3281	104*	114***	14609	95***	101
193	Piacenza	7	55	64	3640	102	111***	17552	96***	101
194	Parma	21	117	136	4685	92***	101	24340	91***	96***
195	Reggio Emilia	12	66	77	4580	89***	97*	22313	88***	93***
196	Modena	22	85	98	6671	90***	98	30140	90***	95***
197	Bologna	37	87	101	10485	87***	95***	51214	88***	93***
198	Ferrara	21	122	142	4734	97	106***	21635	95***	100
199	Ravenna	9	57	66	3667	81***	89***	18266	81***	86***
200	Forli	10	39***	45**	6047	82***	90***	28030	86***	91***
201	Pesaro	8	56	65	3212	79***	86***	16495	86***	91***
202	Ancona	13	68	79	4124	76***	83***	21658	85***	89***
203	Macerata	3	23**	27**	2751	75***	82***	14990	84***	89***
204	Ascoli Piceno	9	58	68	3226	73***	80***	16525	86***	91***
205	Massa-Carrara	4	44	52	2461	96	105*	11931	95***	100
206	Lucca	8	48*	56	4398	93***	102	23145	96***	101*
207	Pistoia	9	80	92	2607	81***	88***	14396	87***	92***
208	Firenze	25	48***	56**	11706	79***	86***	63318	87***	92***
209	Livorno	7	47*	54	3641	85***	93***	19154	92***	97***
210	Pisa	8	48*	55	3967	83***	91***	21931	91***	96***
211	Arezzo	4	29**	33*	3170	80***	88***	17052	87***	92***
212	Siena	10	83	97	2611	78***	85***	15766	87***	92***
213	Grosseto	8	79	92	2351	83***	90***	12573	92***	97***
214	Perugia	19	72	84	5993	81***	88***	29983	88***	93***
215	Terni	10	96	111	2211	75***	82***	12173	89***	94***
216	Viterbo/Rieti	10	55	64	4526	87***	95**	23064	97***	102**
217	Roma	129	85	99	38517	87***	96***	155395	94***	100
218	Latina	7	42*	49	4133	84***	92***	16365	92***	97***
219	Frosinone	13	71	82	4562	85***	93***	21914	93***	99
220	Caserta	40	150*	174**	8251	103**	113***	30623	108***	114***
221	Benevento	16	136	158	2756	81***	89***	14115	91***	96***
222	Napoli	114	117	135**	31369	106***	116***	113406	114***	121***
223	Avellino	19	112	131	3834	78***	85***	19359	86***	91***
224	Salerno	33	86	99	9409	83***	91***	40510	92***	97***
225	L'Aquila	17	137	159	3178	90***	98	16028	93***	98*
226	Teramo	8	73	84	2396	75***	82***	12209	85***	90***
227	Pescara	12	101	117	2744	80***	88***	13152	88***	93***
228	Chieti	11	71	82	3297	74***	80***	17830	85***	90***
229	Isernia/Campobasso	12	90	105	3134	82***	89***	16488	87***	91***
230	Foggia	20	85	98	5924	84***	92***	27543	93***	99*
231	Bari	36	72*	83	12070	80***	88***	55973	93***	98***

Table 8.2(f)—*cont.*

Area		PEPTIC			ALL (age 5–64)			ALL (all ages)		
		Deaths	SMR to EC std	SMR to own std	Deaths	SMR to EC std	SMR to own std	Deaths	SMR to EC std	SMR to own std
232	Taranto	16	80	93	5090	85***	93***	20252	95***	100
233	Brindisi	19	134	156	3594	85***	94***	15493	96***	101
234	Lecce	24	82	95	6699	78***	85***	30375	90***	95***
235	Potenza/Matera	27	117	136	5416	80***	88***	26255	90***	95***
236	Cosenza	38	140	162**	6108	76***	83***	28856	87***	92***
237	Catanzaro	34	133	155*	6383	84***	92***	29368	91***	96***
238	Reggio Calabria	19	92	107	5633	92***	101	26716	95***	100
239	Trapani	9	56	65	3528	75***	82***	20211	95***	100
240	Palermo	45	103	120	11327	88***	96***	53333	101	106***
241	Messina	38	143*	167**	6028	78***	86***	31825	89***	94***
242	Agrigento	11	62	73	4049	78***	86***	20743	92***	97***
243	Caltanisetta	18	174*	202**	2738	90***	98	12764	101	106***
244	Enna	12	166	192	1756	83***	91***	9361	98	104***
245	Catania	33	88	102	9729	87***	96***	43976	103***	109***
246	Ragusa	7	66	76	2435	78***	85***	12857	95***	101
247	Siracusa	12	84	97	3618	85***	93***	16861	99	105***
248	Sassari	17	110	128	4144	90***	99	18676	95***	100
249	Nuoro	8	84	98	2621	93***	102	11962	92***	97**
250	Cagliari/Oristano	29	96	111	8050	88***	97**	33893	93***	98***
IRELAND		134	136***	100	33442	111***	100	161943	123***	100
251	Eastern	46	140*	104	11165	108***	99	46490	118***	97***
252	Midland	9	150	109	2099	116***	104	10172	130***	106***
253	Mid-Western	14	157	116	3118	115***	104*	15547	130***	106***
254	North-Eastern	11	132	97	2842	112***	101	13412	124***	101
255	North-Western	10	163	119	2034	111***	99	12171	122***	99
256	South-Eastern	13	118	87	3705	111***	100	18086	124***	101
257	Southern	22	143	105	5224	112***	101	26927	126***	102**
258	Western	9	89	65	3255	107***	96*	19138	119***	96***
THE NETHERLANDS		227	58***	100	104522	88***	100	494338	95***	100
259	Groningen	12	83	143	4074	93***	105**	21396	98***	102***
260	Friesland	13	85	147	4021	87***	99	21976	96***	100
261	Drenthe	7	57	100	3423	95**	107***	15182	96***	101
262	Overijssel	15	56*	98	7272	91***	102*	34439	98***	103***
263	Gelderland	25	53***	92	12551	88***	100	59204	96***	101**
264	Utrecht	12	48**	84	6419	85***	97**	30727	93***	98***
265	Noord Holland	31	49***	85	17098	90***	102*	84565	95***	100
266	Zuid Holland	59	69**	119	22448	87***	99	112833	93***	97***
267	Zeeland	5	51	89	2370	82***	93***	13565	90***	94***
268	Noord Brabant	30	52***	90	15053	86***	98**	61535	95***	101
269	Limburg	18	56*	98	8869	93***	105***	35976	101*	107***
270	Flevoland	0	0*	0	924	71***	82***	2940	75***	80***
UK: ENGLAND AND WALES		2886	159***	100	543378	102***	100	2877484	106***	100
271	Northern	231	200***	125**	40692	121***	118***	190815	118***	112***
	Hartlepool	6	179	112	1336	137***	133***	5622	127***	120***
	North Tees	7	112	71	2161	117***	115***	8543	115***	108***
	South Tees	21	201**	126	3916	128***	125***	16129	123***	116***
	East Cumbria	13	191*	120	2125	108***	105*	11409	112***	106***
	South Cumbria	4	61	38*	1887	100	97	11187	105***	99
	West Cumbria	9	174	109	1840	122***	119***	8131	119***	112***
	Darlington	13	273**	170	1551	112***	109***	8261	120***	113***
	Durham	19	216**	135	3104	121***	118***	13714	119***	112***
	North-West Durham	7	211	131	1186	124***	120***	5849	119***	112***
	South-West Durham	17	291***	182*	2155	127***	124***	9810	124***	117***
	Northumberland	17	149	94	3767	114***	111***	19622	120***	113***
	Gateshead	17	211**	132	2984	128***	124***	13482	121***	114***
	Newcastle	19	189*	118	3741	127***	124***	18454	115***	108***
	North Tyneside	18	235**	146	2623	119***	116***	12751	117***	110***
	South Tyneside	22	351***	218**	2418	135***	130***	10810	124***	117***

Table 8.2(f)—*cont.*

	Area	PEPTIC			ALL (age 5–64)			ALL (all ages)		
		Deaths	SMR to EC std	SMR to own std	Deaths	SMR to EC std	SMR to own std	Deaths	SMR to EC std	SMR to own std
	Sunderland	22	204**	128	3898	123***	120***	17041	122***	115***
272	Yorkshire	204	157***	99	41701	110***	107***	215069	111***	104***
	Hull	16	149	93	3724	118***	115***	18172	113***	106***
	East Yorkshire	8	107	67	1948	90***	88***	11807	103***	97**
	Grimsby	7	122	76	1882	112***	109***	8775	109***	102*
	Scunthorpe	11	151	94	2377	112***	109***	10685	111***	104***
	Northallerton	6	155	98	1113	96	94	5701	100	94***
	York	7	74	47*	2699	97	95**	14813	106***	100
	Scarborough	4	73	46	1598	102	98	10624	104***	98*
	Harrogate	4	81	51	1249	86***	84***	8749	107***	101
	Bradford	32	284***	178**	4375	131***	128***	19947	122***	115***
	Airedale	10	156	98	1875	101	98	11253	109***	102*
	Calderdale	17	247**	155	2386	118***	116***	12626	116***	109***
	Huddersfield	15	198*	124	2471	111***	109***	13316	116***	109***
	Dewsbury	9	160	101	1909	115***	112***	9318	118***	112***
	Leeds Western	10	77	48*	4273	112***	109***	21287	104***	98**
	Leeds Eastern	23	183*	115	4101	111***	109***	20277	109***	103***
	Wakefield	9	175	110	1599	105*	103	7915	115***	109***
	Pontefract	16	259**	162	2122	118***	115***	9804	119***	112***
273	Trent	285	168***	106	52084	105***	102***	265271	109***	103***
	North Derbyshire	31	224***	140	4147	103*	100	21814	110***	104***
	Southern Derbyshire	34	176**	110	6037	107***	104**	31281	112***	106***
	Leicestershire	35	115	72	8649	96***	94***	44696	102***	96***
	North Lincolnshire	12	121	76	2911	101	98	16317	113***	107***
	South Lincolnshire	13	114	71	3263	98	96*	17881	103***	97***
	Bassetlaw	8	206	129	1199	105	103	5612	109***	102
	Central Nottinghamshire	14	131	82	3258	105*	102	15592	107***	101
	Nottingham	53	240***	151**	6918	107***	104***	34404	108***	102**
	Barnsley	18	216**	135	2847	118***	115***	13224	117***	110***
	Doncaster	16	149	94	3660	117***	114***	16181	116***	109***
	Rotherham	14	152	96	3004	111***	109***	13596	114***	108***
	Sheffield	37	190***	119	6191	109***	106***	34673	111***	104***
274	East Anglian	85	119	75**	18101	87***	84***	110665	98***	92***
	Cambridge	12	130	82	2236	81***	80***	13458	94***	89***
	Peterborough	15	213*	134	2170	104*	102	10260	107***	101
	West Suffolk	4	54	34*	1953	89***	87***	11567	103**	97**
	East Suffolk	15	131	82	2725	81***	79***	18009	96***	90***
	Norwich	17	96	60*	4217	82***	80***	28348	95***	89***
	Great Yarmouth and Waveney	8	107	66	1960	91***	88***	12352	98	92***
	West Norfolk and Wisbech	5	71	44	1826	89***	87***	11483	102*	96***
	Huntingdon	9	227*	145	1014	83***	83***	5188	100	95***
275	North-West Thames	181	148***	93	34047	94***	92***	171925	99***	93***
	North Bedfordshire	11	130	82	2260	89***	88***	11716	105***	99
	South Bedfordshire	14	150	95	2656	95*	94**	11857	102*	96***
	North Hertfordshire	7	104	66	1847	93**	91***	8961	102*	97***
	East Hartfordshire	10	91	57	2641	82***	80***	12691	90***	85***
	North-West Hertfordshire	6	61	38**	2391	83***	81***	12464	97**	92***
	South-West Hertfordshire	4	43	27**	2261	85***	82***	13083	100	94***
	Barnet	6	57	36**	2533	82***	80***	16506	97***	92***
	Harrow	8	116	74	1618	80***	78***	10204	90***	85***
	Hillingdon	11	132	83	2254	92***	90***	11709	95***	90***
	Hounslow and Spelthorne	19	184*	116	3038	100	98	14796	101	96***
	Ealing	22	223**	141	3022	102	101	14601	102*	96***
	Riverside	35	374***	237***	3382	119***	118***	15374	100	95***
	Parkside	28	224***	142	4144	110***	109***	17963	100	95***
276	North-East Thames	235	176***	111	39168	100	98***	203744	102***	96***
	Basildon and Thurrock	16	159	100	3013	101	99	12771	107***	101
	Mid Essex	8	82	52	2436	84***	82***	13116	97***	92***
	North-East Essex	9	82	51*	2838	89***	87***	19329	97***	91***
	West Essex	13	133	83	2499	88***	85***	12534	101	95***
	Southend	19	161	101	2988	87***	85***	19567	100	94***

Table 8.2(f)—*cont.*

	Area	PEPTIC Deaths	PEPTIC SMR to EC std	PEPTIC SMR to own std	ALL (age 5–64) Deaths	ALL (age 5–64) SMR to EC std	ALL (age 5–64) SMR to own std	ALL (all ages) Deaths	ALL (all ages) SMR to EC std	ALL (all ages) SMR to own std
	Barking, Havering, and Brentwood	18	100	62*	4981	96**	93***	25281	103***	97***
	Hampstead	11	318**	202*	1137	108*	107*	5788	96**	91***
	Bloomsbury	14	311***	195*	1688	126***	124***	7745	101	96***
	Islington	17	301***	190*	2198	130***	128***	8960	105***	100
	City and Hackney	12	198*	125	2272	124***	122***	9896	108***	102
	Newham	21	315***	198**	2370	119***	117***	11050	113***	107***
	Tower Hamlets	18	351***	220**	2232	145***	142***	9161	119***	113***
	Enfield	15	160	101	2391	87***	85***	14032	95***	89***
	Haringey	17	263***	167	2014	104	102	10282	109***	103***
	Redbridge	11	130	82	2123	86***	84***	12144	92***	87***
	Waltham Forest	16	228**	144	1988	95*	93**	12088	100	94***
277	South-East Thames	216	166***	104	37124	97***	95***	220644	102***	96***
	Brighton	16	146	91	3060	96*	93***	22621	104***	98**
	Eastbourne	12	138	86	1952	79***	76***	17891	91***	86***
	Hastings	11	175	108	1593	90***	86***	14446	101	95***
	South-East Kent	13	134	84	2699	96*	93***	17139	104***	98**
	Canterbury and Thanet	10	90	56	3095	96*	93***	22738	105***	99
	Dartford and Gravesham	13	163	102	2302	98	96*	11506	112***	106***
	Maidstone	5	71	45	1889	91***	89***	9728	103***	98*
	Medway	13	120	76	3157	97	96*	15350	104***	98
	Tunbridge Wells	6	81	51	1765	82***	80***	11650	100	94***
	Bexley	12	150	95	1981	84***	83***	10620	94***	89***
	Greenwich	21	287***	180*	2334	108***	105*	11954	107***	101
	Bromley	15	129	81	2653	79***	77***	15874	93***	88***
	West Lambeth	16	310***	196*	2036	130***	129***	8800	107***	101
	Camberwell	22	315***	198**	2734	131***	129***	11619	109***	103***
	Lewisham and North Southwark	31	279***	174**	3874	119***	116***	18708	105***	99
278	South-West Thames	109	101	64***	27427	87***	85***	170508	98***	92***
	North-West Surrey	9	115	72	1823	80***	78***	10919	98**	92***
	West Surrey and North-East Hampshire	6	66	42*	2130	77***	77***	10868	96***	91***
	South-West Surrey	3	45	28*	1589	81***	79***	9626	89***	84***
	Mid Surrey	10	151	94	1581	83***	81***	10814	104***	98
	East Surrey	5	71	44	1853	90***	88***	10720	101	95***
	Chichester	10	141	87	1656	82***	79***	13705	98*	92***
	Mid Downs	9	90	57	2481	84***	83***	13445	99	94***
	Worthing	6	65	40*	2250	86***	83***	21072	96***	90***
	Croydon	11	99	63	3006	91***	90***	16472	105***	99
	Kingston and Esher	7	106	67	1572	82***	80***	9833	90***	85***
	Richmond, Twickenham, and Roehampton	10	119	75	2333	95**	93***	13447	94***	89***
	Wandsworth	11	185	118	2019	112***	111***	10971	114***	108***
	Merton and Sutton	12	100	63	3134	89***	87***	18616	94***	89***
279	Wessex	114	110	69***	27044	89***	87***	165775	98***	92***
	East Dorset	16	94	58*	4154	85***	82***	31162	91***	86***
	West Dorset	7	95	59	1865	88***	85***	12807	94***	89***
	Portsmouth and South-East Hampshire	25	140	88	5067	95***	94***	28137	102***	97***
	Southampton and South-West Hampshire	21	137	86	4005	90***	87***	23919	99	93***
	Winchester	3	40	25**	1902	86***	84***	10910	101	95***
	Basingstoke and North Hampshire	6	82	52	1920	88***	86***	9023	96***	91***
	Salisbury	1	23	14*	1117	88***	86***	7336	100	94***
	Swindon	9	116	73	2207	95*	93**	10957	105***	99
	Bath	21	148	93	3541	85***	83***	22244	97***	91***
	Isle of Wight	5	101	63	1266	90***	87***	9280	99	93***
280	Oxford	96	115	73**	21836	88***	86***	113238	100	94***
	East Berkshire	17	134	85	3450	92***	90***	16743	102**	97***
	West Berkshire	17	115	73	3720	83***	82***	19309	99	93***
	Aylesbury Vale	5	105	67	1226	86***	85***	6335	103*	97*
	Wycombe	10	99	62	2361	80***	78***	12362	93***	88***
	Milton Keynes	3	67	43	1270	89***	90***	5734	105***	100
	Kettering	11	124	78	2754	105*	103	13809	105***	99
	Northampton	13	127	80	2823	93***	91***	15402	105***	99
	Oxfordshire	20	115	73	4232	81***	80***	23544	94***	89***

Table 8.2(f)—*cont.*

	Area	PEPTIC			ALL (age 5–64)			ALL (all ages)		
		Deaths	SMR to EC std	SMR to own std	Deaths	SMR to EC std	SMR to own std	Deaths	SMR to EC std	SMR to own std
281	South-Western	119	101	63***	31442	92***	89***	194750	99***	93***
	Bristol and Weston	20	153	96	3669	96**	93***	21165	100	95***
	Frenchay	11	139	88	2031	87***	86***	11126	95***	89***
	Southmead	11	130	81	2299	93***	90***	12794	102**	97***
	Cornwall and Isles of Scilly	9	51*	32***	4649	92***	89***	29265	101	95***
	Exeter	8	70	43*	2885	87***	85***	20704	95***	89***
	North Devon	5	100	62	1302	90***	88***	8729	101	95***
	Plymouth	12	107	67	3318	100	98	18374	102**	97***
	Torbay	11	118	73	2423	92***	88***	18310	94***	89***
	Cheltenham and District	8	104	65	2022	90***	88***	12218	96***	90***
	Gloucester	8	70	44*	3010	90***	88***	16801	100	95***
	Somerset	16	107	67	3834	89***	86***	25264	102*	96***
282	West Midlands	297	157***	98	59050	106***	104***	286757	110***	104***
	Bromsgrove and Redditch	10	177	112	1500	89***	88***	7399	109***	103*
	Herefordshire	3	52	33*	1584	95*	92**	9325	101	95***
	Kidderminster and District	2	54	34	1044	96	94*	5689	110***	104**
	Worcester and District	12	135	85	2352	91***	89***	13702	106***	100
	Shropshire	15	107	67	4055	98	96*	21387	106***	100
	Mid Staffordshire	19	169*	107	3170	95**	94***	14906	110***	104***
	North Staffordshire	34	193***	121	6038	118***	115***	28074	115***	108***
	South-East Staffordshire	9	102	65	2660	101	100	12663	117***	110***
	Rugby	3	94	59	873	94	91**	4574	108***	102
	North Warwickshire	9	142	89	1999	107**	105*	8961	111***	105***
	South Warwickshire	9	108	68	2234	92***	89***	12465	107***	101
	Central Birmingham	15	246**	154	2070	115***	112***	10003	107***	101
	East Birmingham	15	208*	129	2514	120***	116***	11770	112***	105***
	North Birmingham	9	146	92	1786	99	97	9432	113***	106***
	South Birmingham	24	273***	171*	2901	113***	110***	15205	116***	109***
	West Birmingham	20	294***	184*	2647	131***	128***	12307	125***	117***
	Coventry	19	171*	107	3710	114***	111***	17422	112***	106***
	Dudley	17	147	93	3444	102	100	16318	109***	103***
	Sandwell	22	194**	121	4009	122***	118***	18012	112***	105***
	Solihull	4	51	32*	1942	86***	84***	8527	90***	85***
	Walsall	14	140	88	3386	116***	113***	14108	115***	108***
	Wolverhampton	13	139	87	3132	115***	112***	14508	111***	105***
283	Mersey	178	202***	127**	30352	118***	115***	143068	114***	108***
	Chester	12	182	114	2085	108***	106*	9586	107***	101
	Crewe	19	208**	131	2746	103	100	13820	112***	105***
	Halton	7	144	91	1664	115***	113***	7082	115***	109***
	Macclesfield	15	219**	138	1861	94**	91***	9893	104***	98*
	Warrington	10	157	99	2159	114***	112***	10146	122***	115***
	Liverpool	41	238***	148*	7182	143***	139***	32360	121***	114***
	St Helens and Knowsley	32	255***	160*	4826	130***	127***	18588	117***	111***
	North Sefton	4	87	54	1349	102	99	8915	111***	105***
	South Sefton	12	179	112	2357	121***	118***	10264	112***	106***
	Wirral	26	200**	125	4123	109***	106***	22414	111***	105***
284	North-Western	328	230***	144***	49825	119***	116***	251973	118***	111***
	Lancaster	2	42	26*	1513	110***	106*	9359	107***	101
	Blackpool Wyre and Fylde	32	247***	153*	4280	116***	112***	26206	114***	107***
	Preston	15	335***	209*	1658	126***	123***	8240	120***	113***
	Blackburn, Hyndburn, and Ribble Valley	26	275***	172*	3434	124***	121***	17610	123***	116***
	Burnley, Pendle, and Rossendale	14	171	107	2817	118***	115***	15245	120***	113***
	West Lancashire	5	133	84	1203	108**	106*	5623	123***	116***
	Chorley and South Ribble	12	178	113	2136	107**	105*	10106	116***	110***
	Bolton	18	198*	125	3284	123***	120***	15783	119***	113***
	Bury	9	147	92	1951	108***	106*	10561	116***	109***
	North Manchester	23	468***	291***	2298	159***	154***	10570	136***	128***
	Central Manchester	17	446***	279***	1744	149***	147***	7218	120***	114***
	South Manchester	16	261**	163	2228	122***	120***	11386	116***	109***
	Oldham	24	314***	197**	2792	124***	121***	13572	121***	114***
	Rochdale	16	217**	136	2621	120***	118***	12304	119***	112***

Table 8.2(f)—*cont.*

Area		PEPTIC			ALL (age 5–64)			ALL (all ages)		
		Deaths	SMR to EC std	SMR to own std	Deaths	SMR to EC std	SMR to own std	Deaths	SMR to EC std	SMR to own std
	Salford	30	347***	216***	3419	135***	132***	16190	121***	114***
	Stockport	16	150	94	3129	100	98	16906	112***	106***
	Tameside and Glossop	17	194*	122	3096	120***	118***	14836	117***	110***
	Trafford	13	163	102	2394	103	100	12353	106***	100
	Wigan	23	212**	134	3828	120***	117***	17905	123***	116***
285	Wales	208	198***	123**	33485	110***	106***	173282	110***	103***
	Clwyd	31	213***	133	4483	106***	103	25568	109***	102***
	East Dyfed	18	198*	123	2822	108***	105*	15449	107***	101
	Pembrokeshire	7	167	104	1330	109**	106*	6496	110***	103*
	Gwent	27	163*	102	5427	112***	109***	25897	112***	106***
	Gwynedd	12	138	86	2654	105*	102	15500	102**	96***
	Mid Glamorgan	49	250***	156**	6851	120***	117***	32209	119***	112***
	Powys	8	182	114	1198	95	92**	7338	107***	101
	South Glamorgan	29	205***	128	4277	103	100	21963	105***	99*
	West Glamorgan	27	194**	121	4443	111***	107***	22862	110***	104***
UK: NORTHERN IRELAND		81	167***	100	17406	119***	100	79011	118***	100
286	Northern Ireland	81	167***	100	17406	119***	100	79011	118***	100
UK: SCOTLAND		330	206***	100	70602	130***	100	316975	122***	100
287	Highlands and Islands	13	135	66	3730	132***	101	17091	119***	98**
288	Grampian	31	180**	88	5826	114***	88***	28305	114***	94***
289	Tayside	21	143	69	5120	120***	92***	26295	116***	96***
290	Fife	15	122	59*	4261	118***	91***	20630	117***	96***
291	Lothian	48	183***	89	9090	117***	90***	44699	116***	95***
292	Borders	6	155	75	1195	107*	82***	7165	110***	91***
293	Forth Valley	16	162	79	3677	127***	97	16124	122***	100
294	Argyll and Clyde	37	232***	113	6514	139***	107***	27547	128***	105***
295	Greater Glasgow	109	310***	150***	15798	154***	117***	65470	130***	107***
296	Lanarkshire	45	225***	110	7855	132***	102	29950	128***	104***
297	Ayrshire and Arran	32	233***	113	5226	130***	100	23594	125***	102**
298	Dumfries and Galloway	7	122	59	2310	139***	106**	10105	121***	99
PORTUGAL		418	115**	100	120737	113***	100	481295	106***	100
299	Viana do Castelo	16	178*	155	3175	119***	106**	14495	108***	103**
300	Braga	16	77	66	7655	117***	101	28481	113***	105***
301	Vila Real	10	113	98	3490	132***	117***	13942	123***	116***
302	Bragança	7	104	90	2262	115***	103	10230	108***	102*
303	Guarda	7	96	84	2545	121***	109***	13068	106***	101
304	Viseu	17	120	104	5098	121***	108***	23202	112***	106***
305	Porto	43	83	72*	18048	115***	100	63784	112***	105***
306	Aveiro	16	75	65	7098	110***	97**	27372	107***	101
307	Coimbra	11	65	57	5003	102	92***	23857	103***	97***
308	Castelo Branco	14	157	137	2954	116***	105**	14821	101	97***
309	Portalegre	7	119	104	1704	103	93**	9207	101	97***
310	Santarem	10	54*	47*	5703	108***	97*	25155	101	96***
311	Leiria	17	107	92	5580	119***	106***	21666	112***	106***
312	Lisboa	120	144***	125*	25930	107***	95***	95412	106***	100
313	Setubal	26	88	76	8524	98	87***	28664	98***	92***
314	Evora	12	160	140	2206	104	94**	10515	108***	103**
315	Beja	18	246**	214**	2504	120***	109***	11859	109***	104***
316	Faro	17	127	110	4535	118***	106***	19962	100	95***
317	Madeira	16	204*	176*	3473	145***	127***	12309	88***	83***
318	Azores	18	240**	208**	3250	145***	128***	13294	94***	89***
SPAIN		738	69***	100	292573	92***	100	1242935	92***	100
319	La Coruña	17	54**	79	9357	102	111***	40168	92***	100
320	Lugo	2	15***	21**	3482	91***	100	19055	89***	97***
321	Orense	4	29**	42	3139	80***	87***	16607	80***	87***
322	Pontevedra	15	63	90	7151	100	108***	29203	94***	102***
323	Asturias	28	77	112	10242	97**	106***	43131	93***	101*

Table 8.2(f)—*cont.*

	Area	PEPTIC			ALL (age 5–64)			ALL (all ages)		
		Deaths	SMR to EC std	SMR to own std	Deaths	SMR to EC std	SMR to own std	Deaths	SMR to EC std	SMR to own std
324	Cantabria	16	107	155	4103	92***	101	17709	90***	98**
325	Alava	5	71	102	1733	80***	87***	6589	85***	92***
326	Guipuzcoa	15	77	112	5585	96***	104**	20247	92***	101
327	Vizcaya	14	40***	58*	9856	93***	102*	34878	93***	102**
328	Navarra	12	82	118	3625	83***	90***	16555	86***	94***
329	Rioja	3	39	56	2031	89***	97	9314	93***	102
330	Huesca	6	83	121	1690	82***	90***	8652	85***	92***
331	Teruel	2	43	63	1046	78***	86***	6506	81***	88***
332	Zaragoza	32	120	175**	6347	82***	90***	30189	89***	96***
333	Madrid Centro	47	35***	51***	34068	84***	92***	125774	83***	91***
334	Avila	1	18*	26	1214	75***	83***	6689	78***	85***
335	Burgos	8	74	108	2801	88***	97	12120	81***	89***
336	Leon	9	54	80	4593	96**	106***	19705	88***	95***
337	Palencia	4	72	106	1647	102	112***	7146	88***	95***
338	Salamanca	9	86	125	2503	81***	90***	13263	79***	86***
339	Segovia	0	0*	0	1041	81***	89***	5438	83***	90***
340	Soria	0	0	0	648	77***	86***	3989	73***	79***
341	Valladolid	12	92	132	3146	79***	86***	13241	81***	88***
342	Zamora	1	14*	21	1646	81***	89***	9480	82***	89***
343	Albacete	9	96	141	2323	84***	92***	11729	93***	101
344	Ciudad Real	14	102	150	3647	91***	100	17926	97***	105***
345	Cuenca	3	48	71	1499	84***	92**	8734	84***	91***
346	Guadalajara	2	49	71	975	81***	89***	5563	82***	89***
347	Toledo	7	49	72	3267	79***	87***	17542	89***	97***
348	Badajoz	28	165*	242***	5224	104**	114***	24541	100	109***
349	Caceres	12	107	158	3185	96*	106**	15940	91***	99
350	Barcelona	91	67***	96	34538	85***	92***	141639	88***	96***
351	Gerona	12	82	119	3811	89***	97	16958	93***	102*
352	Lerida	9	78	113	2761	83***	91***	13570	89***	96***
353	Tarragona	6	38**	55	3797	82***	89***	18508	93***	101
354	Alicante	21	63*	91	9164	91***	99	38746	96***	104***
355	Castellon de la Plana	10	77	111	3273	86***	94***	17074	95***	103***
356	Valencia	42	71*	102	17043	96***	104***	72990	102***	111***
357	Baleares	10	51*	73	5974	102	111***	25714	98**	107***
358	Almeria	7	67	98	3095	97	106***	13231	100	109***
359	Cadiz	23	99	143	8164	114***	123***	28952	109***	118***
360	Cordoba	8	41**	60	5312	92***	101	24888	96***	105***
361	Granada	26	127	186**	5663	93***	101	25140	98***	107***
362	Huelva	10	93	136	3256	102	111***	15181	101	110***
363	Jaen	15	89	130	4535	90***	99	22208	96***	104***
364	Malaga	22	78	113	9181	108***	117***	33929	104***	113***
365	Sevilla	49	129	185***	11844	103**	111***	47124	104***	113***
366	Murcia	16	62	91	7122	91***	100	31151	97***	106***
367	Las Palmas	17	106	152	5884	114***	123***	18993	105***	115***
368	Sta Cruz de Tenerife	7	45*	65	5342	111***	120***	19316	98*	107***
EC		11573	100	-	3395724	100	-	15801946	100	-

Table 8.3. Observed numbers of 'avoidable deaths', age-standardized mortality rates, range and heterogeneity of SMRs (chi-square) by disease and country.

Notes on the use of this table

1. This table shows observed numbers of deaths (totals for years in 2, below), age-standardized mortality rates (based on the EC standard), and range and heterogeneity of SMRs (based on the country's own standard).

2. The mortality data are for 1985–89 and cover five years, except for The Netherlands (four years, 1985–88) and Spain (four years, 1985–88). The population data are for 1985–89, except for France (1987), Greece (1987), Ireland (1986), and Spain (1986).

3. All countries supplied data according to the 9th revision of the International Classification of Diseases except for Denmark where 8th revision coding rules applied.

4. The maximum and minimum SMRs (based on the country's own standard) show the range of SMRs found in the small areas of a particular country. The chi-square value provides a test of whether the degree of heterogeneity between different small areas within one country is greater than could be expected by chance. The p-values achieved are indicated as follows: *$p<0.05$; **$p<0.01$.

Table 8.3(a) Tuberculosis (ages 5–64).

Country	Total deaths	Rates and SMRs based on EC standard		Within-country variation of SMRs based on own country standard			
		Age-standardized mortality rate (100 000)	National SMR	Minimum	Maximum	Heterogeneity	df
Belgium	205	0.49	62	22	210	71.5**	8
Luxembourg	8	0.51	65	-	-	-	-
Federal Republic of Germany	1855	0.70	89	55	210	192.3**	30
Denmark	79	0.40	50	0	214	26.2*	14
France	1661	0.77	97	12	213	225.5**	94
Greece	298	0.79	99	57	313	54.4**	9
Italy	1580	0.65	82	11	387	294.6**	88
Ireland	118	1.08	136	70	140	8.4	7
The Netherlands	131	0.30	38	0	123	5.5	11
UK: England and Wales	973	0.50	62	0	644	627.1**	198
UK: Northern Ireland	19	0.36	45	-	-	-	-
UK: Scotland	132	0.66	83	58	182	23.9*	11
Portugal	1110	2.83	356	32	144	114.4**	19
Spain	1806	1.54	194	14	208	225.7**	49
EC	9975	0.79	-	-	-	-	-

*p=<0.05 **p=<0.01

Table 8.3(b) Malignant neoplasm of the cervix uteri (ages 15–64).

Country	Total deaths	Rates and SMRs based on EC standard		Within-country variation of SMRs based on own country standard			
		Age-standardized mortality rate (100000)	National SMR	Minimum	Maximum	Heterogeneity	df
Belgium	507	2.97	93	52	133	32.9**	8
Luxembourg	26	3.97	125	-	-	-	-
Federal Republic of Germany	4297	3.88	122	71	182	214.7**	30
Denmark	578	6.89	216	60	125	25.1*	14
France	2141	2.38	75	0	181	172.7**	94
Greece	289	1.76	55	21	133	33.8**	9
Italy	1010	1.00	31	0	275	168.4**	88
Ireland	183	4.01	126	80	117	2.1	7
The Netherlands	541	2.92	92	67	119	13.5	11
UK: England and Wales	5054	6.24	196	37	242	598.0**	198
UK: Northern Ireland	98	4.31	135	-	-	-	-
UK: Scotland	552	6.57	206	81	133	13.0	11
Portugal	489	2.91	91	34	147	31.9*	19
Spain	956	1.95	61	0	220	160.7**	49
EC	16721	3.18	-	-	-	-	-

**p*=<0.05 ***p*=<0.01

Table 8.3(c) Malignant neoplasm of the cervix and body of the uterus (ages 15–54).

Country	Total deaths	Rates and SMRs based on EC standard		Within-country variation of SMRs based on own country standard			
		Age-standardized mortality rate (100000)	National SMR	Minimum	Maximum	Heterogeneity	df
Belgium	440	3.23	88	75	112	4.9	8
Luxembourg	21	3.90	106	-	-	-	-
Federal Republic of Germany	3392	3.66	100	64	164	129.3**	30
Denmark	334	4.65	127	59	139	19.5	14
France	2514	3.45	94	15	207	162.1**	94
Greece	439	2.91	79	63	145	10.5	9
Italy	2193	2.66	72	11	188	244.3**	88
Ireland	157	4.05	110	69	135	5.9	7
The Netherlands	382	2.40	65	61	124	13.2	11
UK: England and Wales	3624	5.45	148	10	240	451.2**	198
UK: Northern Ireland	75	3.93	107	-	-	-	-
UK: Scotland	390	5.68	155	71	126	9.3	11
Portugal	719	5.21	142	62	165	30.5*	19
Spain	1311	3.10	84	26	165	103.0**	49
EC	15991	3.67	-	-	-	-	-

**p*=<0.05 ***p*=<0.01

Table 8.3(d) Hodgkin's disease (ages 5–64).

Country	Total deaths	Rates and SMRs based on EC standard		Within-country variation of SMRs based on own country standard			
		Age-standardized mortality rate (100000)	National SMR	Minimum	Maximum	Heterogeneity	df
Belgium	276	0.67	96	35	177	33.2**	8
Luxembourg	14	0.89	126	-	-	-	-
Federal Republic of Germany	1908	0.73	104	65	153	83.6**	30
Denmark	118	0.58	82	0	141	11.0	14
France	1189	0.54	77	0	218	123.6*	94
Greece	333	0.87	124	71	142	9.5	9
Italy	1972	0.84	119	27	184	128.9**	88
Ireland	96	0.80	113	59	179	12.7	7
The Netherlands	324	0.69	98	78	179	9.6	11
UK: England and Wales	1395	0.71	101	0	279	216.3	198
UK: Northern Ireland	55	0.97	138	-	-	-	-
UK: Scotland	147	0.73	104	67	188	15.7	11
Portugal	205	0.52	73	0	179	25.3	19
Spain	817	0.69	98	0	198	60.8	49
EC	8849	0.71	-	-	-	-	-

*p=<0.05 **p=<0.01

Table 8.3(e) Chronic rheumatic heart disease (ages 5–44).

Country	Total deaths	Rates and SMRs based on EC standard		Within-country variation of SMRs based on own country standard			
		Age-standardized mortality rate (100000)	National SMR	Minimum	Maximum	Heterogeneity	df
Belgium	8	0.03	13	0	604	12.2	8
Luxembourg	1	0.09	42	-	-	-	-
Federal Republic of Germany	156	0.09	43	0	265	42.8	30
Denmark	16	0.10	47	0	458	14.4	14
France	207	0.13	61	0	448	120.1	94
Greece	24	0.09	41	0	263	5.3	9
Italy	646	0.39	190	0	339	194.4**	88
Ireland	14	0.15	71	0	251	5.4	7
The Netherlands	35	0.09	44	0	404	13.4	11
UK: England and Wales	222	0.15	72	0	526	210.6	198
UK: Northern Ireland	7	0.16	79	-	-	-	-
UK: Scotland	27	0.18	89	0	242	18.7	11
Portugal	173	0.62	296	0	273	42.6**	19
Spain	327	0.43	204	0	320	105.2**	49
EC	1863	0.21	-	-	-	-	-

*p=<0.05 **p=<0.01

Table 8.3(f) All respiratory diseases (ages 1–14).

Country	Total deaths	Rates and SMRs based on EC standard		Within-country variation of SMRs based on own country standard			
		Age-standardized mortality rate (100000)	National SMR	Minimum	Maximum	Heterogeneity	df
Belgium	127	1.47	103	30	151	11.3	8
Luxembourg	4	1.32	93	-	-	-	-
Federal Republic of Germany	512	1.18	83	0	159	49.7*	30
Denmark	46	1.11	77	31	225	10.9	14
France	574	1.05	74	0	431	132.4*	94
Greece	125	1.13	79	70	173	12.7	9
Italy	723	1.53	107	0	287	181.4**	88
Ireland	87	1.81	127	51	146	5.1	7
The Netherlands	115	1.12	78	29	157	7.5	11
UK: England and Wales	690	1.53	107	0	361	261.4**	198
UK: Northern Ireland	37	1.95	136	-	-	-	-
UK: Scotland	104	2.26	158	58	144	7.4	11
Portugal	398	3.82	268	23	135	24.3	19
Spain	496	1.36	95	0	360	106.5**	49
EC	4038	1.43	-	-	-	-	-

*p=<0.05 **p=<0.01

Table 8.3(g) Asthma (ages 5–44).

Country	Total deaths	Rates and SMRs based on EC standard		Within-country variation of SMRs based on own country standard			
		Age-standardized mortality rate (100000)	National SMR	Minimum	Maximum	Heterogeneity	df
Belgium	222	0.78	131	47	172	30.5**	8
Luxembourg	10	0.91	153	-	-	-	-
Federal Republic of Germany	1384	0.80	135	53	163	45.6*	30
Denmark	73	0.47	80	0	189	13.1	14
France	1049	0.65	109	0	218	205.8**	94
Greece	22	0.08	14	0	436	14.7	9
Italy	346	0.21	36	0	575	159.3**	88
Ireland	98	0.97	163	55	198	14.5*	7
The Netherlands	92	0.25	42	0	139	8.8	11
UK: England and Wales	1438	1.00	168	0	282	242.1*	198
UK: Northern Ireland	43	0.96	162	-	-	-	-
UK: Scotland	136	0.93	156	39	167	13.7	11
Portugal	145	0.50	84	0	184	26.4	19
Spain	244	0.29	49	0	310	83.7**	49
EC	5302	0.59	-	-	-	-	-

*p=<0.05 **p=<0.01

Table 8.3(h) Appendicitis (ages 5–64).

Country	Total deaths	Rates and SMRs based on EC standard		Within-country variation of SMRs based on own country standard			
		Age-standardized mortality rate (100 000)	National SMR	Minimum	Maximum	Heterogeneity	df
Belgium	12	0.03	40	0	393	13.1	8
Luxembourg	0	0.00	0	-	-	-	-
Federal Republic of Germany	223	0.09	122	15	373	54.8**	30
Denmark	29	0.15	203	0	246	11.6	14
France	148	0.07	94	0	430	95.8	94
Greece	2	0.01	7	0	321	4.4	9
Italy	142	0.06	82	0	435	94.6	88
Ireland	9	0.07	103	0	256	4.9	7
The Netherlands	45	0.10	141	0	296	14.9	11
UK: England and Wales	174	0.09	123	0	659	209.6	198
UK: Northern Ireland	6	0.11	147	-	-	-	-
UK: Scotland	17	0.08	117	0	222	10.5	11
Portugal	29	0.07	99	0	332	18.0	19
Spain	70	0.06	79	0	282	41.5	49
EC	906	0.07	-	-	-	-	-

*p=<0.05 **p=<0.01

Table 8.3(i) Abdominal hernia (ages 5–64).

Country	Total deaths	Rates and SMRs based on EC standard		Within-country variation of SMRs based on own country standard			
		Age-standardized mortality rate (100 000)	National SMR	Minimum	Maximum	Heterogeneity	df
Belgium	29	0.07	50	0	233	18.9*	8
Luxembourg	2	0.13	93	-	-	-	-
Federal Republic of Germany	238	0.09	65	18	262	43.7	30
Denmark	29	0.15	106	0	271	14.7	14
France	430	0.20	143	0	285	137.8**	94
Greece	12	0.03	23	0	494	8.6	9
Italy	379	0.15	111	0	304	123.5*	88
Ireland	13	0.12	86	0	377	21.1*	7
The Netherlands	52	0.12	88	30	225	10.9	11
UK: England and Wales	356	0.18	130	0	313	212.8	198
UK: Northern Ireland	5	0.09	68	-	-	-	-
UK: Scotland	26	0.13	93	0	290	13.6	11
Portugal	47	0.12	86	0	252	17.4	19
Spain	128	0.11	79	0	384	85.2**	49
EC	1746	0.14	-	-	-	-	-

*p=<0.05 **p=<0.01

Table 8.3(j) Cholelithiasis and cholecystitis (ages 5–64).

Country	Total deaths	Rates and SMRs based on EC standard		Within-country variation of SMRs based on own country standard			
		Age-standardized mortality rate (100000)	National SMR	Minimum	Maximum	Heterogeneity	df
Belgium	48	0.11	48	0	157	11.5	8
Luxembourg	5	0.32	135	-	-	-	-
Federal Republic of Germany	618	0.23	98	30	185	49.7*	30
Denmark	63	0.32	134	0	172	10.2	14
France	426	0.20	82	0	242	114.0	94
Greece	37	0.10	42	0	196	8.6	9
Italy	884	0.36	151	15	269	122.5**	88
Ireland	23	0.21	89	0	258	14.3	7
The Netherlands	126	0.29	123	43	175	14.1	11
UK: England and Wales	422	0.21	90	0	404	252.4*	198
UK: Northern Ireland	7	0.13	55	-	-	-	-
UK: Scotland	43	0.21	90	0	219	11.0	11
Portugal	107	0.27	114	0	284	30.4	19
Spain	193	0.17	70	0	316	76.4*	49
EC	3002	0.24	-	-	-	-	-

*p=<0.05 **p=<0.01

Table 8.3(k) Hypertensive and cerebrovascular diseases (ages 35–64).

Country	Total deaths	Rates and SMRs based on EC standard		Within-country variation of SMRs based on own country standard			
		Age-standardized mortality rate (100000)	National SMR	Minimum	Maximum	Heterogeneity	df
Belgium	5828	30.61	88	70	147	278.6**	8
Luxembourg	325	46.54	134	-	-	-	-
Federal Republic of Germany	37225	31.26	90	83	133	550.1**	30
Denmark	2774	31.28	90	76	136	63.7**	14
France	26579	27.31	79	72	155	974.4**	94
Greece	6926	41.56	120	72	164	184.2**	9
Italy	42700	38.40	111	65	149	1461.0**	88
Ireland	1718	35.82	103	84	117	12.3	7
The Netherlands	4741	24.76	71	83	111	37.7**	11
UK: England and Wales	32508	36.57	105	54	176	1731.6**	198
UK: Northern Ireland	1035	43.63	126	-	-	-	-
UK: Scotland	4601	50.81	146	70	116	67.3**	11
Portugal	12055	67.92	196	80	150	369.7**	19
Spain	17866	34.27	99	65	152	900.6**	49
EC	196881	34.72	-	-	-	-	-

*p=<0.05 **p=<0.01

Table 8.3(l) Maternal deaths (all ages)

Country	Total deaths	Rates and SMRs based on EC standard		Within-country variation of SMRs based on own country standard			
		Age-standardized mortality rate (per 100000) live and still births)	National SMR	Minimum	Maximum	Heterogeneity	df
Belgium	27	4.55	62	0	182	5.5	8
Luxembourg	1	4.54	62	-	-	-	-
Federal Republic of Germany	264	8.19	112	13	219	58.2**	30
Denmark	15	5.23	72	0	332	11.6	14
France	380	9.82	134	0	351	120.4	94
Greece	32	5.83	80	0	332	9.2	9
Italy	172	6.08	83	0	551	103.8	88
Ireland	12	4.12	56	0	420	14.4	7
The Netherlands	55	7.43	102	0	197	13.3	11
UK: England and Wales	231	6.80	93	0	549	179.5	198
UK: Northern Ireland	1	0.72	10	-	-	-	-
UK: Scotland	30	9.09	124	46	250	5.8	11
Portugal	58	9.25	127	0	271	21.5	19
Spain	83	4.76	65	0	305	47.7	49
EC	1361	7.30	-	-	-	-	-

**p*=<0.05 ***p*=<0.01

Table 8.3(m) Perinatal deaths.

Country	Total deaths	Rates and SMRs based on EC standard		Within-country variation of SMRs based on own country standard			
		Age-standardized mortality rate (per 1000 live and still birth)	National SMR	Minimum	Maximum	Heterogeneity	df
Belgium	6066	10.23	103	90	113	38.4**	8
Luxembourg	185	8.40	84	-	-	-	-
Federal Republic of Germany	22912	7.10	71	83	120	182.0**	30
Denmark	2470	8.61	86	84	116	28.2*	14
France	37777	9.76	98	76	146	406.3**	94
Greece	7680	13.99	140	78	125	62.7**	9
Italy	34496	12.20	122	54	144	1432.6**	88
Ireland	3284	11.28	113	67	113	47.6**	7
The Netherlands	7052	9.53	95	92	116	25.8**	11
UK: England and Wales	30739	9.05	91	64	140	635.4**	198
UK: Northern Ireland	1325	9.58	96	-	-	-	-
UK: Scotland	3068	9.29	93	66	111	28.4**	11
Portugal	11528	18.38	184	77	127	137.2**	19
Spain	17415	9.99	100	22	166	988.2**	49
EC	185997	9.98	-	-	-	-	-

**p*=<0.05 ***p*=<0.01

Table 8.3(n) Cancer of the breast (ages 25–64).

Country	Total deaths	Rates and SMRs based on EC standard		Within-country variation of SMRs based on own country standard			
		Age-standardized mortality rate (100000)	National SMR	Minimum	Maximum	Heterogeneity	df
Belgium	5276	40.22	118	84	111	43.8**	8
Luxembourg	204	41.01	120	-	-	-	-
Federal Republic of Germany	29924	34.92	102	88	117	116.8**	30
Denmark	2674	42.59	125	73	117	30.8**	14
France	19911	29.29	86	65	125	255.0**	94
Greece	3427	27.25	80	65	117	84.8**	9
Italy	24734	31.50	92	59	134	616.7**	88
Ireland	1486	44.30	130	87	113	8.5	7
The Netherlands	5370	39.34	115	71	107	14.9	11
UK: England and Wales	27179	44.30	130	64	139	282.0**	198
UK: Northern Ireland	748	43.70	128	-	-	-	-
UK: Scotland	2739	42.68	125	83	127	33.2**	11
Portugal	3561	27.60	81	52	140	122.9**	19
Spain	9889	25.99	76	64	131	121.5**	49
EC	137122	34.10	-	-	-	-	-

**p*=<0.05 ***p*=<0.01

Table 8.3(o) Ischaemic heart disease (ages 35–64).

Country	Total deaths	Rates and SMRs based on EC standard		Within-country variation of SMRs based on own country standard			
		Age-standardized mortality rate (100000)	National SMR	Minimum	Maximum	Heterogeneity	df
Belgium	14019	73.62	83	82	124	232.6**	8
Luxembourg	664	95.08	107	-	-	-	-
Federal Republic of Germany	112034	93.98	106	79	119	1339.8**	30
Denmark	10976	124.50	141	85	128	98.3**	14
France	43448	44.74	51	71	152	1768.1**	94
Greece	14191	84.97	96	61	130	779.7**	9
Italy	72287	64.95	73	69	138	1474.8**	88
Ireland	8625	180.85	204	88	107	21.9**	7
The Netherlands	19810	104.11	118	77	132	288.4**	11
UK: England and Wales	143527	161.91	183	57	173	7792.6**	198
UK: Northern Ireland	4894	206.85	234	-	-	-	-
UK: Scotland	19811	219.00	247	79	116	322.3**	11
Portugal	9729	54.77	62	70	231	581.2**	19
Spain	27819	52.98	60	66	164	1487.8**	49
EC	501834	88.51	-	-	-	-	-

**p*=<0.05 ***p*=<0.01

Table 8.3(p) Peptic ulcers (ages 25–64).

Country	Total deaths	Rates and SMRs based on EC standard		Within-country variation of SMRs based on own country standard			
		Age-standardized mortality rate (100000)	National SMR	Minimum	Maximum	Heterogeneity	df
Belgium	237	0.89	61	47	165	39.8**	8
Luxembourg	11	1.11	77	-	-	-	-
Federal Republic of Germany	2498	1.49	103	67	153	94.3**	30
Denmark	303	2.42	167	59	158	29.7**	14
France	1617	1.18	81	26	223	282.3**	94
Greece	96	0.41	28	0	136	13.2	9
Italy	1947	1.25	86	27	202	193.3**	88
Ireland	134	1.97	136	65	119	2.8	7
The Netherlands	227	0.84	58	0	147	9.6	11
UK: England and Wales	2886	2.31	159	14	291	577.7**	198
UK: Northern Ireland	81	2.42	167	-	-	-	-
UK: Scotland	380	2.99	206	59	150	33.4**	11
Portugal	418	1.67	115	47	214	60.9**	19
Spain	738	1.00	69	0	242	140.8**	49
EC	11573	1.45	-	-	-	-	-

**p*=<0.05 ***p*=<0.01

Table 8.3(q) All causes (ages 5–64).

Country	Total deaths	Rates and SMRs based on EC standard		Within-country variation of SMRs based on own country standard			
		Age-standardized mortality rate (100000)	National SMR	Minimum	Maximum	Heterogeneity	df
Belgium	116013	279.03	103	88	121	1602.8**	8
Luxembourg	4788	309.45	114	-	-	-	-
Federal Republic of Germany	724614	276.77	102	86	129	5044.0**	30
Denmark	63304	320.05	118	86	141	1337.2**	14
France	611368	283.01	105	76	134	10710.6**	94
Greece	93157	247.59	92	85	128	918.4**	9
Italy	599820	247.22	91	80	133	7768.6**	88
Ireland	33442	299.07	111	96	104	14.0	7
The Netherlands	104522	239.08	88	82	107	129.9**	11
UK: England and Wales	543378	277.19	102	76	154	12436.3**	198
UK: Northern Ireland	17406	321.49	119	-	-	-	-
UK: Scotland	70602	352.26	130	82	117	781.8**	11
Portugal	120737	305.43	113	87	128	899.0**	19
Spain	292573	247.81	92	83	123	2753.6**	49
EC	3395724	270.58	-	-	-	-	-

**p*=<0.05 ***p*=<0.01

Table 8.3(r) All causes (all ages).

Country	Total deaths	Rates and SMRs based on EC standard		Within-country variation of SMRs based on own country standard			
		Age-standardized mortality rate (100000)	National SMR	Minimum	Maximum	Heterogeneity	df
Belgium	540361	1049.22	104	93	111	2427.5**	8
Luxembourg	20090	1115.93	111	-	-	-	-
Federal Republic of Germany	3478836	1021.27	102	90	113	8881.7**	30
Denmark	291354	1072.87	107	92	111	827.1**	14
France	2667420	960.12	95	89	121	17022.3**	94
Greece	465451	1075.77	107	86	118	3730.6**	9
Italy	2684453	950.67	95	86	121	11697.7**	88
Ireland	161943	1235.37	123	96	106	157.6**	7
The Netherlands	494338	955.70	95	80	107	503.8**	11
UK: England and Wales	2877484	1066.42	106	84	128	19871.1**	198
UK: Northern Ireland	79011	1189.67	118	-	-	-	-
UK: Scotland	316975	1224.23	122	91	107	774.6**	11
Portugal	481295	1066.59	106	83	116	1641.6**	19
Spain	1242935	924.34	92	79	118	7957.6**	49
EC	15801946	1005.63	-	-	-	-	-

*p=<0.05 **p=<0.01

9. TABLES OF CHANGES BETWEEN 1980–84 AND 1985–89

Table 9.1. Observed numbers of 'avoidable deaths' and age-standardized mortality rates for 1980–84 and 1985–89, and annual percentage changes in mortality rates between 1980–84 and 1985–89, by disease and country.

Table 9.2. Population of countries in 1980–84 and 1985–89, by sex and 10-year age groups.

Table 9.3. Observed numbers of 'avoidable deaths' and age-specific mortality rates for 1980–84 and 1985–89, and annual percentage changes in age-specific mortality rates between 1980–84 and 1985–89, by disease and country.

Table 9.4. Age-standardized mortality rates for 1980–84 and 1985–89, and annual percentage changes in mortality rates between 1980–84 and 1985–89, by disease, small area and country.

Table 9.1. Observed numbers of 'avoidable deaths' and age-standardized mortality rates for 1980–84 and 1985–89, and annual percentage changes in mortality rates between 1980–84 and 1985–89, by disease and country.

Notes on the use of this table

1. This table shows observed numbers of deaths (totals for years in 2 and 3, below) and age-standardized mortality rates (based on the EC standard) for 1980–84 and 1985–89, and annual percentage changes in age-standardized mortality rates between 1980–84 and 1985–89.

2. The mortality data for the later period are for 1985–89 and cover five years, except for The Netherlands (four years, 1985–88) and Spain (four years, 1985–88). The population data are for 1985-89, except for France (1987), Greece (1987), Ireland (1986), and Spain (1986).

3. The mortality data for the earlier period are for 1980–84 and cover five years, except for Greece (three years, 1980–82), Spain (five years, 1979–83), Italy (five years, 1979–83) and England and Wales (Cancer of the breast, Ischaemic heart disease and Peptic ulcers only: three years, 1982–84). The population data are for 1980–84, except for France (1982), Greece (1981), Ireland (1981), Spain (1981), Italy (1979–83), and England and Wales (1982–84).

4. All countries supplied data according to the 9th revision of the International Classification of Diseases except for Denmark where 8th revision coding rules applied.

Table 9.1(a) Tuberculosis (ages 5–64).

Country	Total deaths		Age-standardized mortality rate (per 100000)		Annual % change in rate 1980–84 to 1985–89
	1980–84	1985–89	1980–84	1985–89	
Belgium	331	205	0.84	0.49	–10.0
Luxembourg	5	8	0.35	0.51	7.7
Federal Republic of Germany	2828	1855	1.15	0.70	–9.4
Denmark	97	79	0.49	0.40	–4.1
France	2732	1661	1.33	0.77	–10.3
Greece	367	298	1.67	0.79	–11.8
Italy	3132	1580	1.42	0.65	–12.2
Ireland	232	118	2.17	1.08	–13.1
The Netherlands	188	131	0.36	0.30	–4.2
UK: England and Wales	1417	973	0.71	0.50	–7.0
UK: Northern Ireland	37	19	0.70	0.36	–12.7
UK: Scotland	220	132	1.10	0.66	–9.6
Portugal	1580	1110	4.26	2.83	–7.9
Spain	3442	1806	2.49	1.54	–8.4
EC	16608	9975	1.37	0.79	–9.4

Table 9.1(b) Malignant neoplasm of the cervix uteri (ages 15–64).

Country	Total deaths		Age-standardized mortality rate (per 100000)		Annual % change in rate 1980–84 to 1985–89
	1980–84	1985–89	1980–84	1985–89	
Belgium	524	507	3.20	2.97	−1.5
Luxembourg	19	26	3.13	3.97	4.9
Federal Republic of Germany	4980	4297	4.62	3.88	−3.4
Denmark	753	578	9.14	6.89	−5.5
France	2352	2141	2.75	2.38	−2.8
Greece	165	289	1.73	1.76	0.3
Italy	1161	1010	1.23	1.00	−3.4
Ireland	167	183	3.83	4.01	0.9
The Netherlands	780	541	3.59	2.92	−4.5
UK: England and Wales	5333	5054	6.57	6.24	−1.0
UK: Northern Ireland	124	98	5.57	4.31	−5.0
UK: Scotland	576	552	6.85	6.57	−0.8
Portugal	485	489	3.04	2.91	−0.9
Spain	908	956	1.55	1.95	4.3
EC	18327	16721	3.56	3.18	−1.9

Table 9.1(c) Malignant neoplasm of the cervix and body of the uterus (ages 15–54).

Country	Total deaths		Age-standardized mortality rate (per 100000)		Annual % change in rate 1980–84 to 1985–89
	1980–84	1985–89	1980–84	1985–89	
Belgium	471	440	3.48	3.23	−1.5
Luxembourg	23	21	4.32	3.90	−2.0
Federal Republic of Germany	3763	3392	4.22	3.66	−2.8
Denmark	462	334	6.86	4.65	−7.5
France	2882	2514	4.02	3.45	−3.0
Greece	323	439	3.68	2.91	−3.9
Italy	3588	2193	4.38	2.66	−8.0
Ireland	114	157	3.17	4.05	5.0
The Netherlands	538	382	2.92	2.40	−4.2
UK: England and Wales	3455	3624	5.36	5.45	0.3
UK: Northern Ireland	89	75	4.85	3.93	−4.2
UK: Scotland	373	390	5.49	5.68	0.7
Portugal	759	719	5.63	5.21	−1.5
Spain	1949	1311	3.86	3.10	−3.9
EC	18789	15991	4.36	3.67	−2.8

Table 9.1(d) Hodgkin's disease (ages 5–64).

Country	Total deaths		Age-standardized mortality rate (per 100 000)		Annual % change in rate 1980–84 to 1985–89
	1980–84	1985–89	1980–84	1985–89	
Belgium	428	276	1.09	0.67	–9.1
Luxembourg	10	14	0.68	0.89	5.5
Federal Republic of Germany	2617	1908	1.06	0.73	–7.0
Denmark	165	118	0.82	0.58	–6.9
France	1487	1189	0.71	0.54	–5.1
Greece	214	333	0.96	0.87	–1.6
Italy	2845	1972	1.29	0.84	–6.9
Ireland	149	96	1.30	0.80	–9.3
The Netherlands	428	324	0.77	0.69	–2.5
UK: England and Wales	1657	1395	0.85	0.71	–3.6
UK: Northern Ireland	67	55	1.23	0.97	–4.5
UK: Scotland	170	147	0.86	0.73	–3.1
Portugal	269	205	0.72	0.52	–6.4
Spain	1128	817	0.81	0.69	–2.8
EC	11634	8849	0.95	0.71	–5.3

Table 9.1(e) Chronic rheumatic heart disease (ages 5–44).

Country	Total deaths		Age-standardized mortality rate (per 100 000)		Annual % change in rate 1980–84 to 1985–89
	1980–84	1985–89	1980–84	1985–89	
Belgium	11	8	0.04	0.03	–7.6
Luxembourg	5	1	0.46	0.09	–28.5
Federal Republic of Germany	314	156	0.17	0.09	–11.7
Denmark	25	16	0.17	0.10	–10.2
France	263	207	0.18	0.13	–6.5
Greece	51	24	0.31	0.09	–19.4
Italy	1515	646	0.94	0.39	–13.4
Ireland	24	14	0.28	0.15	–12.2
The Netherlands	75	35	0.18	0.09	–13.5
UK: England and Wales	391	222	0.29	0.15	–12.0
UK: Northern Ireland	11	7	0.28	0.16	–9.9
UK: Scotland	49	27	0.35	0.18	–12.2
Portugal	421	173	1.62	0.62	–17.6
Spain	992	327	1.03	0.43	–14.8
EC	4147	1863	0.47	0.21	–12.9

Table 9.1(f) All respiratory diseases (ages 1–14).

Country	Total deaths		Age-standardized mortality rate (per 100000)		Annual % change in rate 1980–84 to 1985–89
	1980–84	1985–89	1980–84	1985–89	
Belgium	159	127	1.77	1.47	–3.7
Luxembourg	4	4	1.29	1.32	0.6
Federal Republic of Germany	829	512	1.76	1.18	–7.6
Denmark	62	46	1.34	1.11	–3.8
France	683	574	1.20	1.05	–2.7
Greece	157	125	2.37	1.13	–11.6
Italy	1416	723	2.55	1.53	–8.1
Ireland	130	87	2.63	1.81	–7.2
The Netherlands	177	115	1.28	1.12	–3.0
UK: England and Wales	1275	690	2.79	1.53	–11.3
UK: Northern Ireland	59	37	3.07	1.95	–8.7
UK: Scotland	121	104	2.45	2.26	–1.7
Portugal	710	398	6.25	3.82	–9.4
Spain	1213	496	2.67	1.36	–11.6
EC	6995	4038	2.27	1.43	–8.0

Table 9.1(g) Asthma (ages 5–44).

Country	Total deaths		Age-standardized mortality rate (per 100000)		Annual % change in rate 1980–84 to 1985–89
	1980–84	1985–89	1980–84	1985–89	
Belgium	261	222	0.95	0.78	–4.0
Luxembourg	8	10	0.75	0.91	3.9
Federal Republic of Germany	1886	1384	1.04	0.80	–5.1
Denmark	62	73	0.42	0.47	2.6
France	581	1049	0.38	0.65	11.3
Greece	–	22	–	0.08	-
Italy	245	346	0.15	0.21	5.6
Ireland	95	98	1.01	0.97	–0.9
The Netherlands	151	92	0.35	0.25	–7.1
UK: England and Wales	1312	1438	0.95	1.00	1.1
UK: Northern Ireland	45	43	1.05	0.96	–1.8
UK: Scotland	119	136	0.83	0.93	2.3
Portugal	–	145	–	0.50	-
Spain	233	244	0.23	0.29	4.4
EC	4998	5302	0.54	0.59	1.6

Table 9.1(h) Appendicitis(ages 5–64).

Country	Total deaths		Age-standardized mortality rate (per 100000)		Annual % change in rate 1980–84 to 1985–89
	1980–84	1985–89	1980–84	1985–89	
Belgium	29	12	0.07	0.03	−16.8
Luxembourg	4	0	0.28	0.00	−100.0
Federal Republic of Germany	465	223	0.19	0.09	−14.5
Denmark	31	29	0.15	0.15	−1.0
France	353	148	0.17	0.07	−16.6
Greece	14	2	0.06	0.01	−33.9
Italy	324	142	0.15	0.06	−14.0
Ireland	17	9	0.14	0.07	−12.3
The Netherlands	67	45	0.12	0.10	−4.4
UK: England and Wales	201	174	0.10	0.09	−2.4
UK: Northern Ireland	8	6	0.14	0.11	−5.6
UK: Scotland	24	17	0.12	0.08	−6.3
Portugal	79	29	0.20	0.07	−19.0
Spain	235	70	0.16	0.06	−17.3
EC	1851	906	0.15	0.07	−11.6

Table 9.1(i) Abdominal hernia (ages 5–64).

.Country	Total deaths		Age-standardized mortality rate (per 100000)		Annual % change in rate 1980–84 to 1985–89
	1980–84	1985–89	1980–84	1985–89	
Belgium	41	29	0.10	0.07	−7.8
Luxembourg	2	2	0.15	0.13	−2.4
Federal Republic of Germany	398	238	0.17	0.09	−11.3
Denmark	27	29	0.14	0.15	1.7
France	558	430	0.27	0.20	−6.1
Greece	19	12	0.09	0.03	−15.4
Italy	558	379	0.26	0.15	−8.2
Ireland	14	13	0.13	0.12	−1.7
The Netherlands	78	52	0.15	0.12	−5.0
UK: England and Wales	420	356	0.21	0.18	−2.7
UK: Northern Ireland	13	5	0.25	0.09	−17.4
UK: Scotland	41	26	0.20	0.13	−8.5
Portugal	70	47	0.19	0.12	−8.8
Spain	290	128	0.21	0.11	−11.3
EC	2529	1746	0.21	0.14	−7.0

Table 9.1(j) Cholelithiasis and cholecystitis (ages 5–64).

Country	Total deaths		Age-standardized mortality rate (per 100000)		Annual % change in rate 1980–84 to 1985–89
	1980–84	1985–89	1980–84	1985–89	
Belgium	139	48	0.35	0.11	–20.2
Luxembourg	7	5	0.51	0.32	–8.8
Federal Republic of Germany	1080	618	0.45	0.23	–12.2
Denmark	52	63	0.26	0.32	4.1
France	730	426	0.36	0.20	–11.3
Greece	40	37	0.19	0.10	–9.8
Italy	1476	884	0.69	0.36	–10.2
Ireland	39	23	0.37	0.21	–10.3
The Netherlands	220	126	0.43	0.29	–8.3
UK: England and Wales	498	422	0.25	0.21	–2.7
UK: Northern Ireland	20	7	0.38	0.13	–19.0
UK: Scotland	60	43	0.30	0.21	–6.3
Portugal	123	107	0.33	0.27	–4.0
Spain	512	193	0.38	0.17	–13.7
EC	4996	3002	0.42	0.24	–9.4

Table 9.1(k) Hypertensive and cerebrovascular diseases (ages 35–64).

Country	Total deaths		Age-standardized mortality rate (per 100000)		Annual % change in rate 1980–84 to 1985–89
	1980–84	1985–89	1980–84	1985–89	
Belgium	6385	5828	35.74	30.61	–3.0
Luxembourg	322	325	52.22	46.54	–2.3
Federal Republic of Germany	43928	37225	40.28	31.26	–4.9
Denmark	2991	2774	33.44	31.28	–1.3
France	31290	26579	34.14	27.31	–4.4
Greece	4558	6926	47.04	41.56	–2.0
Italy	50342	42700	51.55	38.40	–4.8
Ireland	2406	1718	50.78	35.82	–6.7
The Netherlands	6509	4741	28.75	24.76	–3.3
UK: England and Wales	40556	32508	44.37	36.57	–3.8
UK: Northern Ireland	1287	1035	54.30	43.63	–4.3
UK: Scotland	5713	4601	62.55	50.81	–4.1
Portugal	14457	12055	86.72	67.92	–4.8
Spain	26728	17866	43.55	34.27	–4.3
EC	237472	196881	43.67	34.72	–4.3

Table 9.1(l) Maternal deaths (all ages).

Country	Total deaths		Age-standardized mortality rate (per 100000 live and still births)		Annual % change in rate 1980–84 to 1985–89
	1980–84	1985–89	1980–84	1985–89	
Belgium	44	27	7.27	4.55	–8.9
Luxembourg	0	1	0.00	4.54	–0.6
Federal Republic of Germany	487	264	15.97	8.19	–12.5
Denmark	15	15	5.62	5.23	–1.4
France	545	380	13.85	9.82	–6.6
Greece	58	32	8.40	5.83	–5.9
Italy	355	172	11.39	6.08	–9.9
Ireland	24	12	6.83	4.12	–9.6
The Netherlands	67	55	7.60	7.43	–0.5
UK: England and Wales	271	231	8.52	6.80	–4.4
UK: Northern Ireland	12	1	8.64	0.72	–39.1
UK: Scotland	45	30	13.38	9.09	–7.4
Portugal	134	58	17.71	9.25	–12.2
Spain	273	83	10.64	4.76	–13.6
EC	2330	1361	11.71	7.30	–8.2

Table 9.1(m) Perinatal deaths.

Country	Total deaths		Age-standardized mortality rate (per 1000 live and still births)		Annual % change in rate 1980–84 to 1985–89
	1980–84	1985–89	1980–84	1985–89	
Belgium	7713	6066	12.74	10.23	–4.3
Luxembourg	236	185	11.04	8.40	–5.3
Federal Republic of Germany	30320	22912	9.94	7.10	–6.5
Denmark	2357	2470	8.83	8.61	–0.5
France	46876	37777	11.92	9.76	–3.9
Greece	12251	7680	17.73	13.99	–3.9
Italy	49514	34496	15.89	12.20	–4.3
Ireland	4857	3284	13.83	11.28	–4.0
The Netherlands	9159	7052	10.39	9.53	–1.9
UK: England and Wales	36429	30739	11.45	9.05	–4.6
UK: Northern Ireland	1895	1325	13.64	9.58	–6.8
UK: Scotland	3897	3068	11.59	9.29	–4.3
Portugal	16418	11528	21.70	18.38	–3.3
Spain	33771	17415	13.16	9.99	–4.9
EC	255693	185997	12.85	9.98	–4.4

Table 9.1(n) Cancer of the breast (ages 25–64).

Country	Total deaths		Age-standardized mortality rate (per 100000)		Annual % change in rate 1980–84 to 1985–89
	1980–84	1985–89	1980–84	1985–89	
Belgium	5091	5276	40.24	40.22	–0.0
Luxembourg	184	204	39.66	41.01	0.7
Federal Republic of Germany	27319	29924	32.79	34.92	1.3
Denmark	2383	2674	38.33	42.59	2.1
France	18908	19911	28.94	29.29	0.2
Greece	1924	3427	26.33	27.25	0.6
Italy	22981	24734	31.52	31.50	–0.0
Ireland	1418	1486	43.42	44.30	0.4
The Netherlands	6305	5370	38.93	39.34	0.2
UK: England and Wales	16643	27179	44.51	44.30	–0.1
UK: Northern Ireland	741	748	43.68	43.70	0.0
UK: Scotland	2904	2739	44.72	42.68	–0.9
Portugal	3206	3561	26.07	27.60	1.2
Spain	10702	9889	23.73	25.99	2.0
EC	120709	137122	32.57	34.10	0.4

Table 9.1(o) Ischaemic heart disease (ages 35–64).

Country	Total deaths		Age-standardized mortality rate (per 100000)		Annual % change in rate 1980–84 to 1985–89
	1980–84	1985–89	1980–84	1985–89	
Belgium	17316	14019	96.57	73.62	–5.3
Luxembourg	822	664	133.07	95.08	–6.5
Federal Republic of Germany	118150	112034	108.33	93.98	–2.8
Denmark	13041	10976	146.34	124.50	–3.2
France	45463	43448	49.48	44.74	–2.0
Greece	7239	14191	74.55	84.97	2.2
Italy	81674	72287	83.36	64.95	–4.9
Ireland	9903	8625	209.26	180.85	–2.9
The Netherlands	26994	19810	119.56	104.11	–3.0
UK: England and Wales	98953	143527	180.62	161.91	–2.7
UK: Northern Ireland	5930	4894	250.45	206.85	–3.8
UK: Scotland	22583	19811	246.93	219.00	–2.4
Portugal	10107	9729	60.48	54.77	–2.0
Spain	35795	27819	58.11	52.98	–2.0
EC	493970	501834	97.24	88.51	–2.8

Table 9.1(p) Peptic ulcers (ages 25–64).

Country	Total deaths		Age-standardized mortality rate (per 100000)		Annual % change in rate 1980–84 to 1985–89
	1980–84	1985–89	1980–84	1985–89	
Belgium	327	237	1.30	0.89	−7.3
Luxembourg	25	11	2.85	1.11	−17.1
Federal Republic of Germany	3561	2498	2.31	1.49	−8.4
Denmark	259	303	2.06	2.42	3.3
France	2123	1617	1.64	1.18	−6.3
Greece	127	96	0.92	0.41	−12.8
Italy	2712	1947	1.96	1.25	−8.6
Ireland	183	134	2.73	1.97	−6.3
The Netherlands	376	227	1.17	0.84	−7.2
UK: England and Wales	2011	2886	2.62	2.31	−3.1
UK: Northern Ireland	90	81	2.70	2.42	−2.2
UK: Scotland	472	380	3.68	2.99	−4.1
Portugal	595	418	2.53	1.67	−7.9
Spain	1489	738	1.71	1.00	−11.3
EC	14350	11573	2.00	1.45	−5.9

Table 9.1(q) All causes (ages 5–64).

Country	Total deaths		Age-standardized mortality rate (per 100000)		Annual % change in rate 1980–84 to 1985–89
	1980–84	1985–89	1980–84	1985–89	
Belgium	123752	116013	312.51	279.03	−2.2
Luxembourg	5096	4788	363.16	309.45	−3.2
Federal Republic of Germany	753470	724614	308.76	276.77	−2.2
Denmark	64659	63304	326.40	320.05	−0.4
France	633730	611368	307.14	283.01	−1.6
Greece	51676	93157	236.21	247.59	0.8
Italy	625425	599820	284.89	247.22	−2.3
Ireland	37293	33442	340.70	299.07	−2.6
The Netherlands	131427	104522	252.90	239.08	−1.2
UK: England and Wales	602565	543378	302.22	277.19	−1.7
UK: Northern Ireland	19434	17406	362.43	321.49	−2.4
UK: Scotland	77203	70602	382.67	352.26	−1.6
Portugal	125142	120737	334.96	305.43	−1.8
Spain	360103	292573	259.52	247.81	−0.8
EC	3610975	3395724	296.83	270.58	−1.7

Table 9.1(r) All causes (all ages).

Country	Total deaths		Age-standardized mortality rate (per 100000)		Annual % change in rate 1980–84 to 1985–89
	1980–84	1985–89	1980–84	1985–89	
Belgium	563017	540361	1148.57	1049.22	−1.8
Luxembourg	20704	20090	1250.91	1115.93	−2.3
Federal Republic of Germany	3566537	3478836	1121.41	1021.27	−1.9
Denmark	280635	291354	1101.17	1072.87	−0.5
France	2728240	2667420	983.39	960.12	−0.5
Greece	258776	465451	1032.19	1075.77	0.7
Italy	2718889	2684453	1101.92	950.67	−2.4
Ireland	163916	161943	1321.11	1235.37	−1.3
The Netherlands	584573	494338	988.19	955.70	−0.7
UK: England and Wales	2878384	2877484	1117.99	1066.42	−0.9
UK: Northern Ireland	80740	79011	1285.29	1189.67	−1.5
UK: Scotland	317948	316975	1285.72	1224.23	−1.0
Portugal	476055	481295	1196.53	1066.59	−2.3
Spain	1440845	1242935	969.14	924.34	−0.9
EC	16079259	15801946	1077.74	1005.63	−1.3

Table 9.2. Population of countries in 1980–84 and 1985–89, by sex and 10-year age groups.

Notes on the use of this table

1. This table shows average yearly populations in 100s (based on years in 2 and 3, below) in the two time periods 1980–84 and 1985–89.

2. The population data in the later period are for 1985–89, except for France (1987), Greece (1987), Ireland (1986), and Spain (1986).

3. The population data in the earlier period are for 1980–84, except for France (1982), Greece (1981), Ireland (1981), Spain (1981), Italy (1979–83), and England and Wales (1982–84).

Table 9.2 Population in 100s for the two time periods 1980–84 and 1985–89, by country and sex and 10-year age group.

Country	Sex	Age group								
		<1	1–4	5–14	15–24	25–34	35–44	45–54	55–64	65+
1980–84										
Belgium	M	611	2487	6725	7982	7610	6087	5981	5226	5409
Belgium	F	579	2367	6420	7655	7281	5932	6100	5711	8386
Belgium	T	1190	4854	13146	15638	14891	12019	12081	10938	13795
Luxembourg	M	22	84	239	286	296	253	246	157	194
Luxembourg	F	22	81	227	285	282	236	238	196	301
Luxembourg	T	44	165	466	570	578	489	484	353	495
Federal Republic of Germany	M	3102	12166	37840	52480	44169	44864	39929	26757	32674
Federal Republic of Germany	F	2948	11578	36116	49362	41903	42538	39191	37347	59989
Federal Republic of Germany	T	6050	23743	73956	101841	86072	87403	79120	64103	92663
Denmark	M	275	1208	3684	4004	3896	3688	2716	2609	3150
Denmark	F	264	1157	3518	3822	3721	3543	2753	2806	4363
Denmark	T	539	2366	7202	7826	7618	7232	5469	5415	7513
France	M	4083	16063	41502	43670	43229	33273	31443	26433	29317
France	F	3872	15314	39504	42485	42418	31743	31483	29144	46020
France	T	7956	31377	81005	86155	85646	65016	62925	55577	75337
Greece	M	791	3216	7853	7223	6527	5880	6566	4241	5498
Greece	F	726	3048	7439	7081	6632	6261	6769	4749	6895
Greece	T	1517	6264	15292	14304	13159	12141	13335	8990	12393
Italy	M	3274	14493	44860	44789	39427	36757	35078	27226	30724
Italy	F	3096	13726	42636	43247	39173	37376	36735	31290	43941
Italy	T	6370	28220	87497	88036	78601	74133	71813	58515	74665
Ireland	M	374	1432	3535	3063	2419	1837	1523	1405	1641
Ireland	F	353	1359	3355	2947	2346	1745	1477	1467	2024
Ireland	T	727	2791	6890	6010	4765	3582	3000	2872	3665
The Netherlands	M	894	3620	10987	12675	12020	9821	7621	6389	6819
The Netherlands	F	853	3459	10498	12151	11454	9198	7543	7041	9938
The Netherlands	T	1747	7079	21485	24827	23474	19020	15165	13430	16757
UK: England and Wales	M	3190	12733	34025	41037	34513	32373	27518	26969	29526
UK: England and Wales	F	3031	12098	32208	39491	34019	31970	27469	29018	45549
UK: England and Wales	T	6220	24834	66235	80527	68530	64346	54989	55985	75075
UK: Northern Ireland	M	139	537	1419	1418	1028	884	738	669	724
UK: Northern Ireland	F	133	518	1341	1316	996	891	784	762	1108
UK: Northern Ireland	T	272	1055	2761	2733	2024	1775	1521	1431	1833
UK: Scotland	M	339	1321	3836	4472	3622	3082	2817	2607	2772
UK: Scotland	F	323	1253	3646	4299	3564	3131	2995	2984	4530
UK: Scotland	T	662	2574	7482	8771	7186	6212	5812	5591	7301
Portugal	M	742	3100	8683	8415	6724	5469	5447	4657	4716
Portugal	F	698	2950	8340	8275	6865	6006	6101	5400	6895
Portugal	T	1440	6050	17023	16690	13589	11475	11547	10056	11610
Spain	M	3000	12762	33948	31511	25153	21323	22851	17127	17343
Spain	F	2825	12007	32052	30638	24874	21439	23552	19294	25282
Spain	T	5825	24769	66000	62149	50027	42762	46403	36421	42625
EC	M	20836	85223	239137	263024	230633	205592	190472	152472	170508
EC	F	19722	80915	227302	253054	225529	202010	193190	177208	265221
EC	T	40558	166140	466441	516076	456159	407605	383664	329678	435728
1985–89										
Belgium	M	596	2430	6392	7654	7959	6837	5712	5614	5558
Belgium	F	564	2307	6104	7346	7655	6597	5784	6106	8638

Table 9.2—*cont.*

Country	Sex	Age group								
		<1	1–4	5–14	15–24	25–34	35–44	45–54	55–64	65+
Belgium	T	1160	4737	12496	15000	15613	13434	11496	11720	14196
Luxembourg	M	22	88	215	272	311	279	234	200	186
Luxembourg	F	21	83	204	265	311	260	229	224	309
Luxembourg	T	43	171	418	537	622	539	463	424	495
Federal Republic of Germany	M	3243	12458	30979	49563	48242	40998	45362	31905	31917
Federal Republic of Germany	F	3077	11832	29536	47000	45841	39374	43676	37575	61438
Federal Republic of Germany	T	6320	24290	60515	96562	94083	80372	89038	69480	93355
Denmark	M	288	1098	3273	4037	3851	4024	2936	2484	3279
Denmark	F	274	1050	3136	3825	3660	3862	2919	2662	4605
Denmark	T	562	2148	6409	7862	7510	7887	5855	5146	7885
France	M	3925	15478	39999	43728	42692	39097	29470	28200	28806
France	F	3739	14763	38127	42554	42561	37887	29442	31161	45321
France	T	7662	30241	78126	86280	85253	76985	58913	59359	74126
Greece	M	1006	3122	8104	7438	6720	6060	6770	4375	5676
Greece	F	928	2974	7692	7311	6843	6464	6992	4904	7122
Greece	T	1934	6096	15796	14749	13563	12524	13762	9279	12798
Italy	M	2932	12207	38276	47041	41023	37792	35545	31763	32037
Italy	F	2766	11547	36315	45332	40564	38158	37024	35708	47422
Italy	T	5697	23754	74592	92372	81587	75951	72570	67471	79458
Ireland	M	319	1345	3592	3140	2513	2144	1579	1377	1688
Ireland	F	298	1279	3414	3035	2498	2071	1513	1445	2157
Ireland	T	616	2625	7006	6175	5011	4215	3093	2822	3844
The Netherlands	M	941	3608	9459	12635	12341	11402	8103	6708	7290
The Netherlands	F	899	3458	9039	12122	11862	10794	7819	7234	10934
The Netherlands	T	1840	7066	18499	24757	24202	22196	15922	13942	18224
UK: England and Wales	M	3419	13181	31844	40603	36486	34625	27633	25984	31182
UK: England and Wales	F	3254	12541	30148	38998	35918	34431	27509	27456	47212
UK: England and Wales	T	6673	25722	61992	79601	72404	69056	55142	53440	78394
UK: Northern Ireland	M	142	557	1333	1456	1115	939	765	658	748
UK: Northern Ireland	F	133	528	1274	1320	1101	950	797	748	1157
UK: Northern Ireland	T	275	1085	2607	2776	2216	1889	1562	1407	1905
UK: Scotland	M	337	1322	3322	4327	3823	3352	2780	2575	2862
UK: Scotland	F	319	1260	3154	4138	3722	3355	2931	2901	4630
UK: Scotland	T	655	2582	6476	8465	7545	6707	5711	5476	7492
Portugal	M	632	2772	8233	8749	7574	6031	5332	4967	5289
Portugal	F	595	2596	7843	8490	7616	6452	5985	5832	7670
Portugal	T	1227	5368	16076	17239	15190	12483	11317	10799	12959
Spain	M	2844	12597	35140	34168	27062	20503	25274	18587	19494
Spain	F	2686	11789	32996	33115	26568	20479	25416	20465	28703
Spain	T	5530	24386	68136	67283	53630	40982	50690	39052	48197
EC	M	20645	82263	220161	264811	241710	214084	197495	165398	176013
EC	F	19552	78008	208982	254850	236720	211136	198036	184421	277316
EC	T	40195	160271	429144	519658	478429	425219	395533	349818	453327

Table 9.3. Observed numbers of 'avoidable deaths' and age-specific mortality rates for 1980–84 and 1985–89, and annual percentage changes in age-specific mortality rates between 1980–84 and 1985–89, by disease and country.

Notes on the use of this table

1. This table shows observed numbers of deaths (totals for years in 2 and 3, below) and age-specific mortality rates (per 100 000) for 1980–84 and 1985–89, and annual percentage changes in age-specific mortality rates between 1980–84 and 1985–89, by disease and country.

2. The mortality data for the later period are for 1985–89 and cover five years, except for The Netherlands (four years, 1985–88) and Spain (four years, 1985–88). The population data are for 1985–89, except for France (1987), Greece (1987), Ireland (1986), and Spain (1986).

3. The mortality data for the earlier period are for 1980–84 and cover five years, except for Greece (three years, 1980–82), Spain (five years, 1979–83), Italy (five years, 1979–83) and England and Wales (Cancer of the breast, Ischaemic heart disease and Peptic ulcers only: three years, 1982–84). The population data are for 1980–84, except for France (1982), Greece (1981), Ireland (1981), Spain (1981), Italy (1979–83), and England and Wales (1982–84).

4. All countries supplied data according to the 9th revision of the International Classification of Diseases except for Denmark where 8th revision coding rules applied.

Table 9.3(a) Tuberculosis.

	Age group (years)					
	5–14	15–24	25–34	35–44	45–54	55–64
BELGIUM						
Deaths 1980–84	3	5	13	34	111	165
Deaths 1985–89	0	1	8	24	47	125
Death rate 1980–84	0.05	0.06	0.18	0.57	1.84	3.02
Death rate 1985–89	0.00	0.01	0.10	0.36	0.82	2.13
Ann. % ch. in rate	-	-	−10.1	−8.8	−15.0	−6.7
LUXEMBOURG						
Deaths 1980–84	0	0	0	0	3	2
Deaths 1985–89	0	0	1	1	2	4
Death rate 1980–84	0.00	0.00	0.00	0.00	1.24	1.13
Death rate 1985–89	0.00	0.00	0.32	0.37	0.86	1.89
Ann. % ch. in rate	-	-	-	-	-	-
FEDERAL REPUBLIC OF GERMANY						
Deaths 1980–84	8	37	126	410	864	1383
Deaths 1985–89	2	12	74	225	526	1016
Death rate 1980–84	0.02	0.07	0.29	0.94	2.18	4.32
Death rate 1985–89	0.01	0.03	0.16	0.56	1.18	2.93
Ann. % ch. in rate	−21.1	−19.3	−11.7	−9.8	−11.6	−7.5
DENMARK						
Deaths 1980–84	2	0	2	7	17	69
Deaths 1985–89	1	0	5	3	15	55
Death rate 1980–84	0.06	0.00	0.05	0.19	0.62	2.55
Death rate 1985–89	0.03	0.00	0.13	0.08	0.51	2.14
Ann. % ch. in rate	-	-	-	−17.0	−3.8	−3.5
FRANCE						
Deaths 1980–84	10	28	120	290	843	1441
Deaths 1985–89	1	21	68	227	419	925
Death rate 1980–84	0.03	0.07	0.28	0.89	2.68	5.19
Death rate 1985–89	0.00	0.05	0.16	0.59	1.42	3.12
Ann. % ch. in rate	−36.4	−5.6	−10.7	−7.9	−11.9	−9.7
GREECE						
Deaths 1980–84	6	11	16	25	124	185
Deaths 1985–89	3	5	25	30	74	161
Death rate 1980–84	0.13	0.26	0.41	0.69	3.10	6.86
Death rate 1985–89	0.04	0.07	0.37	0.48	1.08	3.47
Ann. % ch. in rate	−18.6	−19.9	−1.6	−5.8	−16.2	−10.7
ITALY						
Deaths 1980–84	9	63	133	328	949	1650
Deaths 1985–89	7	18	51	140	414	950

Table 9.3(a)—*cont.*

	Age group (years)					
	5–14	15–24	25–34	35–44	45–54	55–64
Death rate 1980–84	0.02	0.14	0.34	0.89	2.64	5.64
Death rate 1985–89	0.02	0.04	0.13	0.37	1.14	2.82
Ann. % ch. in rate	–1.5	–19.5	–15.3	–13.6	–13.1	–10.9
IRELAND						
Deaths 1980–84	0	2	9	14	52	155
Deaths 1985–89	0	1	3	5	28	81
Death rate 1980–84	0.00	0.07	0.38	0.78	3.47	10.79
Death rate 1985–89	0.00	0.03	0.12	0.24	1.81	5.74
Ann. % ch. in rate	-	-	–20.5	–21.2	–12.2	–11.9
THE NETHERLANDS						
Deaths 1980–84	2	2	12	13	34	125
Deaths 1985–89	2	4	2	8	18	97
Death rate 1980–84	0.02	0.02	0.10	0.14	0.45	1.86
Death rate 1985–89	0.03	0.04	0.02	0.09	0.28	1.74
Ann. % ch. in rate	-	-	–29.9	–8.8	–9.7	–1.5
UK: ENGLAND AND WALES						
Deaths 1980–84	11	26	54	119	358	849
Deaths 1985–89	4	28	38	82	195	626
Death rate 1980–84	0.03	0.07	0.16	0.37	1.30	3.03
Death rate 1985–89	0.01	0.07	0.11	0.24	0.71	2.34
Ann. % ch. in rate	–17.2	1.7	–7.8	–8.5	–11.5	–5.0
UK: N. IRELAND						
Deaths 1980–84	0	0	2	2	11	22
Deaths 1985–89	0	0	0	2	5	12
Death rate 1980–84	0.00	0.00	0.20	0.23	1.45	3.08
Death rate 1985–89	0.00	0.00	0.00	0.21	0.64	1.71
Ann. % ch. in rate	-	-	-	-	–15.0	–11.1
UK: SCOTLAND						
Deaths 1980–84	0	2	2	18	74	124
Deaths 1985–89	0	0	5	6	34	87
Death rate 1980–84	0.00	0.05	0.06	0.58	2.55	4.44
Death rate 1985–89	0.00	0.00	0.13	0.18	1.19	3.18
Ann. % ch. in rate	-	-	-	–20.9	–14.1	–6.5
PORTUGAL						
Deaths 1980–84	10	33	110	244	499	690
Deaths 1985–89	2	27	80	176	314	511
Death rate 1980–84	0.12	0.40	1.62	4.25	8.64	13.72
Death rate 1985–89	0.03	0.31	1.05	2.82	5.55	9.46
Ann. % ch. in rate	–26.7	–4.6	–8.2	–7.9	–8.5	–7.2
SPAIN						
Deaths 1980–84	37	63	204	474	1095	1569
Deaths 1985–89	14	52	179	280	463	818
Death rate 1980–84	0.11	0.20	0.82	2.22	4.72	8.62
Death rate 1985–89	0.05	0.19	0.83	1.71	2.28	5.24
Ann. % ch. in rate	–13.2	–0.9	0.4	–4.6	–12.4	–8.7
EC						
Deaths 1980–84	97	264	777	1910	4886	8186
Deaths 1985–89	39	180	575	1267	2651	5653
Death rate 1980–84	0.04	0.10	0.34	0.94	2.55	4.97
Death rate 1985–89	0.02	0.07	0.24	0.60	1.34	3.23
Ann. % ch. in rate	–15.1	–7.5	–6.7	–8.7	–12.1	–8.2

Table 9.3(b) Malignant neoplasm of the cervix uteri.

	Age group (years)					
	5–14	15–24	25–34	35–44	45–54	55–64
BELGIUM						
Deaths 1980–84	0	2	24	68	173	257
Deaths 1985–89	0	0	20	89	146	252
Death rate 1980–84	0.00	0.05	0.66	2.29	5.67	9.00
Death rate 1985–89	0.00	0.00	0.52	2.70	5.05	8.25
Ann. % ch. in rate	-	-	–4.5	3.3	–2.3	–1.7
LUXEMBOURG						
Deaths 1980–84	0	0	0	5	8	6
Deaths 1985–89	0	0	2	3	10	11
Death rate 1980–84	0.00	0.00	0.00	4.24	6.72	6.12
Death rate 1985–89	0.00	0.00	1.29	2.31	8.73	9.82
Ann. % ch. in rate	-	-	-	-	5.4	9.9
FEDERAL REPUBLIC OF GERMANY						
Deaths 1980–84	0	13	277	886	1423	2381
Deaths 1985–89	1	14	304	782	1388	1809
Death rate 1980–84	0.00	0.05	1.32	4.17	7.26	12.75
Death rate 1985–89	0.01	0.06	1.33	3.97	6.36	9.63
Ann. % ch. in rate	-	2.5	0.1	–0.9	–2.6	–5.5
DENMARK						
Deaths 1980–84	0	6	58	120	214	355
Deaths 1985–89	0	5	51	88	146	288
Death rate 1980–84	0.00	0.31	3.12	6.77	15.55	25.30
Death rate 1985–89	0.00	0.26	2.79	4.56	10.00	21.64
Ann. % ch. in rate	-	–3.6	–2.2	–7.6	–8.4	–3.1
FRANCE						
Deaths 1980–84	0	5	120	367	797	1063
Deaths 1985–89	0	4	157	461	608	911
Death rate 1980–84	0.00	0.02	0.57	2.31	5.06	7.30
Death rate 1985–89	0.00	0.02	0.74	2.43	4.13	5.85
Ann. % ch. in rate	-	-	5.5	1.0	–4.0	–4.3
GREECE						
Deaths 1980–84	0	0	12	33	70	50
Deaths 1985–89	0	3	21	69	89	107
Death rate 1980–84	0.00	0.00	0.63	1.76	3.45	3.51
Death rate 1985–89	0.00	0.08	0.61	2.14	2.55	4.36
Ann. % ch. in rate	-	-	0.3	3.3	–4.9	3.7
ITALY						
Deaths 1980–84	1	2	44	155	359	601
Deaths 1985–89	0	1	58	179	324	448
Death rate 1980–84	0.01	0.01	0.23	0.83	1.96	3.84
Death rate 1985–89	0.00	0.00	0.29	0.94	1.75	2.51
Ann. % ch. in rate	-	-	4.1	2.1	–1.8	–6.9
IRELAND						
Deaths 1980–84	0	0	19	21	40	87
Deaths 1985–89	0	1	15	49	45	73
Death rate 1980–84	0.00	0.00	1.52	2.41	5.42	11.86
Death rate 1985–89	0.00	0.07	1.20	4.73	5.95	10.10
Ann. % ch. in rate	-	-	–5.8	14.5	1.9	–3.2
THE NETHERLANDS						
Deaths 1980–84	0	3	42	127	241	367

Table 9.3(b)—*cont.*

	Age group (years)					
	5–14	15–24	25–34	35–44	45–54	55–64
Deaths 1985–89	0	5	43	102	148	243
Death rate 1980–84	0.00	0.05	0.73	2.76	6.39	10.43
Death rate 1985–89	0.00	0.10	0.91	2.36	4.73	8.40
Ann. % ch. in rate	-	-	4.8	–3.4	–6.5	–4.7
UK: ENGLAND AND WALES						
Deaths 1980–84	0	32	539	963	1350	2449
Deaths 1985–89	0	33	566	1251	1290	1914
Death rate 1980–84	0.00	0.16	3.17	6.02	9.83	16.88
Death rate 1985–89	0.00	0.17	3.15	7.27	9.38	13.94
Ann. % ch. in rate	-	0.9	–0.1	3.8	–0.9	–3.8
UK: N. IRELAND						
Deaths 1980–84	0	3	13	22	35	51
Deaths 1985–89	0	0	11	26	21	40
Death rate 1980–84	0.00	0.46	2.61	4.94	8.93	13.39
Death rate 1985–89	0.00	0.00	2.00	5.47	5.27	10.70
Ann. % ch. in rate	-	-	–5.2	2.1	–10.0	–4.4
UK: SCOTLAND						
Deaths 1980–84	0	6	45	110	157	258
Deaths 1985–89	0	1	74	134	131	212
Death rate 1980–84	0.00	0.28	2.53	7.03	10.48	17.29
Death rate 1985–89	0.00	0.05	3.98	7.99	8.94	14.62
Ann. % ch. in rate	-	–29.6	9.5	2.6	–3.1	–3.3
PORTUGAL						
Deaths 1980–84	1	1	34	79	183	189
Deaths 1985–89	0	0	28	113	169	179
Death rate 1980–84	0.02	0.02	0.99	2.63	6.00	7.00
Death rate 1985–89	0.00	0.00	0.74	3.50	5.65	6.14
Ann. % ch. in rate	-	-	–5.8	5.9	–1.2	–2.6
SPAIN						
Deaths 1980–84	0	6	43	145	303	411
Deaths 1985–89	1	6	43	157	338	412
Death rate 1980–84	0.00	0.04	0.35	1.35	2.57	4.26
Death rate 1985–89	0.01	0.05	0.41	1.92	3.33	5.03
Ann. % ch. in rate	-	2.7	2.9	6.5	4.8	3.1
EC						
Deaths 1980–84	2	79	1278	3124	5401	8556
Deaths 1985–89	2	76	1414	3569	4980	7067
Death rate 1980–84	0.00	0.06	1.13	3.09	5.59	9.66
Death rate 1985–89	0.00	0.06	1.20	3.38	5.03	7.66
Ann. % ch. in rate	-	–1.0	1.1	1.8	–2.1	–4.5

Table 9.3(c) Malignant neoplasm of the cervix and body of the uterus.

	Age group (years)					
	5–14	15–24	25–34	35–44	45–54	55–64
BELGIUM						
Deaths 1980–84	0	2	32	106	331	676
Deaths 1985–89	0	1	27	148	264	596
Death rate 1980–84	0.00	0.05	0.88	3.57	10.85	23.67
Death rate 1985–89	0.00	0.03	0.71	4.49	9.13	19.52
Ann. % ch. in rate	-	-	–4.3	4.7	–3.4	–3.8
LUXEMBOURG						
Deaths 1980–84	0	0	0	6	17	23
Deaths 1985–89	0	0	2	4	15	29
Death rate 1980–84	0.00	0.00	0.00	5.09	14.29	23.47
Death rate 1985–89	0.00	0.00	1.29	3.08	13.10	25.89
Ann. % ch. in rate	-	-	-	–9.6	–1.7	2.0
FEDERAL REPUBLIC OF GERMANY						
Deaths 1980–84	0	17	351	1164	2231	4850
Deaths 1985–89	1	17	357	976	2042	3829
Death rate 1980–84	0.00	0.07	1.68	5.47	11.39	25.97
Death rate 1985–89	0.01	0.07	1.56	4.96	9.35	20.38
Ann. % ch. in rate	-	1.0	–1.4	–2.0	–3.9	–4.7
DENMARK						
Deaths 1980–84	0	6	59	133	264	548
Deaths 1985–89	0	5	53	92	184	498
Death rate 1980–84	0.00	0.31	3.17	7.51	19.18	39.06
Death rate 1985–89	0.00	0.26	2.90	4.76	12.61	37.42
Ann. % ch. in rate	-	–3.6	–1.8	–8.7	–8.0	–0.9
FRANCE						
Deaths 1980–84	3	13	217	690	1962	3669
Deaths 1985–89	1	10	261	815	1428	3086
Death rate 1980–84	0.02	0.06	1.02	4.35	12.46	25.18
Death rate 1985–89	0.01	0.05	1.23	4.30	9.70	19.81
Ann. % ch. in rate	-	–5.1	3.7	–0.2	–4.9	–4.7
GREECE						
Deaths 1980–84	0	1	29	76	217	241
Deaths 1985–89	1	5	40	125	269	440
Death rate 1980–84	0.00	0.05	1.46	4.05	10.69	16.92
Death rate 1985–89	0.03	0.14	1.17	3.87	7.70	17.95
Ann. % ch. in rate	-	-	–3.6	–0.7	–5.3	1.0
ITALY						
Deaths 1980–84	5	21	227	882	2458	4518
Deaths 1985–89	0	21	142	535	1495	3160
Death rate 1980–84	0.02	0.10	1.16	4.72	13.38	28.88
Death rate 1985–89	0.00	0.09	0.70	2.80	8.08	17.70
Ann. % ch. in rate	-	–0.8	–8.1	–8.3	–8.1	–7.8
IRELAND						
Deaths 1980–84	0	1	19	25	69	190
Deaths 1985–89	0	1	15	56	85	154
Death rate 1980–84	0.00	0.07	1.62	2.87	9.34	25.90
Death rate 1985–89	0.00	0.07	1.20	5.41	11.24	21.32
Ann. % ch. in rate	-	-	–5.8	13.5	3.8	–3.8
THE NETHERLANDS						
Deaths 1980–84	0	4	45	142	347	691

Table 9.3(c)—*cont.*

	Age group (years)					
	5–14	15–24	25–34	35–44	45–54	55–64
Deaths 1985–89	0	6	46	112	218	472
Death rate 1980–84	0.00	0.07	0.79	3.09	9.20	19.63
Death rate 1985–89	0.00	0.12	0.97	2.59	6.97	16.31
Ann. % ch. in rate	-	15.1	4.8	–3.8	–6.0	–4.0
UK: ENGLAND AND WALES						
Deaths 1980–84	1	35	558	1049	1813	4020
Deaths 1985–89	0	37	578	1345	1664	3194
Death rate 1980–84	0.01	0.18	3.28	6.56	13.20	27.71
Death rate 1985–89	0.00	0.19	3.22	7.81	12.10	23.27
Ann. % ch. in rate	-	1.4	–0.4	3.5	–1.7	–3.4
UK: N. IRELAND						
Deaths 1980–84	0	3	14	25	47	95
Deaths 1985–89	0	0	12	29	34	73
Death rate 1980–84	0.00	0.46	2.81	5.61	11.99	24.93
Death rate 1985–89	0.00	0.00	2.18	6.11	8.53	19.52
Ann. % ch. in rate	-	-	–5.0	1.7	–6.6	–4.8
UK: SCOTLAND						
Deaths 1980–84	0	6	47	118	202	392
Deaths 1985–89	0	2	76	141	171	336
Death rate 1980–84	0.00	0.28	2.64	7.54	13.49	26.27
Death rate 1985–89	0.00	0.10	4.08	8.41	11.67	23.16
Ann. % ch. in rate	-	–19.1	9.1	2.2	–2.9	–2.5
PORTUGAL						
Deaths 1980–84	1	3	69	191	497	690
Deaths 1985–89	0	3	53	233	430	687
Death rate 1980–84	0.02	0.07	2.01	6.36	16.29	25.56
Death rate 1985–89	0.00	0.07	1.39	7.22	14.37	23.56
Ann. % ch. in rate	-	-	–7.1	2.6	–2.5	–1.6
SPAIN						
Deaths 1980–84	2	20	109	461	1359	2294
Deaths 1985–89	3	11	84	326	890	1646
Death rate 1980–84	0.01	0.13	0.88	4.30	11.54	23.78
Death rate 1985–89	0.02	0.08	0.79	3.98	8.75	20.11
Ann. % ch. in rate	-	–7.9	–1.9	–1.4	–4.9	–3.0
EC						
Deaths 1980–84	12	130	1771	5025	11695	22592
Deaths 1985–89	7	123	1775	5036	9439	18678
Death rate 1980–84	0.01	0.10	1.57	4.98	12.11	25.50
Death rate 1985–89	0.01	0.10	1.50	4.77	9.53	20.26
Ann. % ch. in rate	–8.8	–1.3	–0.9	–0.8	–4.7	–4.5

Table 9.3(d) Hodgkin's disease.

	Age group (years)					
	5–14	15–24	25–34	35–44	45–54	55–64
BELGIUM						
Deaths 1980–84	6	40	87	78	92	125
Deaths 1985–89	1	28	53	52	52	90
Death rate 1980–84	0.09	0.51	1.17	1.30	1.52	2.29
Death rate 1985–89	0.02	0.37	0.68	0.77	0.91	1.54
Ann. % ch. in rate	−29.4	−6.1	−10.3	−9.8	−9.9	−7.6
LUXEMBOURG						
Deaths 1980–84	0	0	4	0	3	3
Deaths 1985–89	0	1	7	2	2	2
Death rate 1980–84	0.00	0.00	1.38	0.00	1.24	1.70
Death rate 1985–89	0.00	0.37	2.25	0.74	0.86	0.94
Ann. % ch. in rate	-	-	10.2	-	-	-
FEDERAL REPUBLIC OF GERMANY						
Deaths 1980–84	33	284	412	485	583	820
Deaths 1985–89	14	177	382	353	449	533
Death rate 1980–84	0.09	0.56	0.96	1.11	1.47	2.56
Death rate 1985–89	0.05	0.37	0.81	0.88	1.01	1.53
Ann. % ch. in rate	−12.3	−8.0	−3.2	−4.6	−7.3	−9.7
DENMARK						
Deaths 1980–84	4	21	33	33	31	43
Deaths 1985–89	1	7	25	27	20	38
Death rate 1980–84	0.11	0.54	0.87	0.91	1.13	1.59
Death rate 1985–89	0.03	0.18	0.67	0.69	0.68	1.48
Ann. % ch. in rate	-	−19.8	−5.1	−5.6	−9.6	−1.4
FRANCE						
Deaths 1980–84	11	161	345	289	327	354
Deaths 1985–89	9	104	300	273	220	283
Death rate 1980–84	0.03	0.37	0.81	0.89	1.04	1.27
Death rate 1985–89	0.02	0.24	0.70	0.71	0.75	0.95
Ann. % ch. in rate	−3.2	−8.4	−2.7	−4.4	−6.4	−5.6
GREECE						
Deaths 1980–84	2	21	30	32	55	74
Deaths 1985–89	3	19	44	43	90	134
Death rate 1980–84	0.04	0.49	0.76	0.88	1.38	2.74
Death rate 1985–89	0.04	0.26	0.65	0.69	1.31	2.89
Ann. % ch. in rate	-	−10.1	−2.6	−4.0	−0.8	0.9
ITALY						
Deaths 1980–84	50	261	459	536	688	851
Deaths 1985–89	26	216	340	340	450	600
Death rate 1980–84	0.11	0.59	1.17	1.45	1.92	2.91
Death rate 1985–89	0.07	0.47	0.83	0.90	1.24	1.78
Ann. % ch. in rate	−7.9	−3.9	−5.5	−7.7	−7.0	−7.9
IRELAND						
Deaths 1980–84	5	21	26	23	29	45
Deaths 1985–89	4	8	15	25	17	27
Death rate 1980–84	0.15	0.70	1.09	1.28	1.93	3.13
Death rate 1985–89	0.11	0.26	0.60	1.19	1.10	1.91
Ann. % ch. in rate	-	−18.0	−11.3	−1.6	−10.7	−9.4
THE NETHERLANDS						
Deaths 1980–84	1	45	98	86	85	113

Table 9.3(d)—*cont.*

	Age group (years)					
	5–14	15–24	25–34	35–44	45–54	55–64
Deaths 1985–89	1	38	69	69	64	83
Death rate 1980–84	0.01	0.36	0.84	0.90	1.12	1.68
Death rate 1985–89	0.01	0.38	0.71	0.78	1.01	1.49
Ann. % ch. in rate	-	1.3	–3.5	–3.3	–2.4	–2.7
UK: ENGLAND AND WALES						
Deaths 1980–84	12	204	348	319	287	487
Deaths 1985–89	13	183	316	305	257	321
Death rate 1980–84	0.04	0.51	1.02	0.99	1.04	1.74
Death rate 1985–89	0.04	0.46	0.87	0.88	0.93	1.20
Ann. % ch. in rate	3.0	–1.9	–3.0	–2.3	–2.2	–7.1
UK: N. IRELAND						
Deaths 1980–84	1	11	14	8	13	20
Deaths 1985–89	2	8	11	17	7	10
Death rate 1980–84	0.07	0.81	1.38	0.90	1.71	2.80
Death rate 1985–89	0.15	0.58	0.99	1.80	0.90	1.42
Ann. % ch. in rate	-	–6.5	–6.4	14.8	–12.1	–12.6
UK: SCOTLAND						
Deaths 1980–84	1	23	42	36	34	34
Deaths 1985–89	1	20	28	30	32	36
Death rate 1980–84	0.03	0.52	1.17	1.16	1.17	1.22
Death rate 1985–89	0.03	0.47	0.74	0.90	1.12	1.32
Ann. % ch. in rate	-	–2.1	–8.7	–5.0	–0.9	1.6
PORTUGAL						
Deaths 1980–84	7	25	55	46	61	75
Deaths 1985–89	6	17	23	47	41	71
Death rate 1980–84	0.08	0.30	0.81	0.80	1.06	1.49
Death rate 1985–89	0.08	0.20	0.30	0.75	0.73	1.32
Ann. % ch. in rate	–1.9	–8.0	–17.9	–1.2	–7.3	–2.5
SPAIN						
Deaths 1980–84	39	121	218	178	265	307
Deaths 1985–89	9	107	165	142	160	234
Death rate 1980–84	0.12	0.39	0.87	0.83	1.14	1.69
Death rate 1985–89	0.03	0.40	0.77	0.87	0.79	1.50
Ann. % ch. in rate	–20.7	0.4	–2.2	0.7	–6.5	–2.1
EC						
Deaths 1980–84	169	1230	2152	2128	2533	3331
Deaths 1985–89	92	967	1833	1774	1913	2536
Death rate 1980–84	0.07	0.48	0.94	1.04	1.32	2.02
Death rate 1985–89	0.04	0.37	0.77	0.84	0.97	1.45
Ann. % ch. in rate	–9.9	–4.8	–4.1	–4.4	–6.0	–6.4

Table 9.3(e) Chronic rheumatic heart disease.

	Age group (years)					
	5–14	15–24	25–34	35–44	45–54	55–64
BELGIUM						
Deaths 1980–84	1	1	4	5	35	103
Deaths 1985–89	0	1	0	7	13	39
Death rate 1980–84	0.02	0.01	0.05	0.08	0.58	1.88
Death rate 1985–89	0.00	0.01	0.00	0.10	0.23	0.67
Ann. % ch. in rate	-	-	-	4.6	−17.2	−18.8
LUXEMBOURG						
Deaths 1980–84	0	0	0	5	4	6
Deaths 1985–89	0	0	0	1	2	1
Death rate 1980–84	0.00	0.00	0.00	2.05	1.65	3.40
Death rate 1985–89	0.00	0.00	0.00	0.37	0.86	0.47
Ann. % ch. in rate	-	-	-	-	-	−32.6
FEDERAL REPUBLIC OF GERMANY						
Deaths 1980–84	2	22	60	230	718	1759
Deaths 1985–89	3	24	36	93	532	1678
Death rate 1980–84	0.01	0.04	0.14	0.53	1.82	5.49
Death rate 1985–89	0.01	0.05	0.08	0.23	1.20	4.83
Ann. % ch. in rate	-	2.8	−11.3	−15.2	−8.0	−2.5
DENMARK						
Deaths 1980–84	2	1	9	13	68	206
Deaths 1985–89	0	2	1	13	56	165
Death rate 1980–84	0.06	0.03	0.24	0.36	2.49	7.61
Death rate 1985–89	0.00	0.05	0.03	0.33	1.91	6.41
Ann. % ch. in rate	-	-	−35.4	−1.7	−5.1	−3.4
FRANCE						
Deaths 1980–84	12	31	59	161	443	1069
Deaths 1985–89	3	24	47	133	315	889
Death rate 1980–84	0.03	0.07	0.14	0.50	1.41	3.85
Death rate 1985–89	0.01	0.06	0.11	0.35	1.07	3.00
Ann. % ch. in rate	−23.7	−5.0	−4.4	−6.9	−5.4	−4.9
GREECE						
Deaths 1980–84	0	3	15	33	86	127
Deaths 1985–89	0	5	6	13	46	78
Death rate 1980–84	0.00	0.07	0.38	0.91	2.15	4.71
Death rate 1985–89	0.00	0.07	0.09	0.21	0.67	1.68
Ann. % ch. in rate	-	-	−21.6	−21.8	−17.7	−15.8
ITALY						
Deaths 1980–84	43	173	382	917	2360	4108
Deaths 1985–89	9	60	161	416	998	2585
Death rate 1980–84	0.10	0.39	0.97	2.47	6.57	14.04
Death rate 1985–89	0.02	0.13	0.40	1.10	2.75	7.66
Ann. % ch. in rate	−20.9	−16.8	−13.9	−12.7	−13.5	−9.6
IRELAND						
Deaths 1980–84	0	1	6	17	66	135
Deaths 1985–89	0	2	1	11	34	76
Death rate 1980–84	0.00	0.03	0.25	0.95	4.40	9.40
Death rate 1985–89	0.00	0.07	0.04	0.52	2.20	5.39
Ann. % ch. in rate	-	-	−30.8	−11.3	−13.0	−10.5
THE NETHERLANDS						
Deaths 1980–84	0	7	19	49	139	293

Table 9.3(e)—*cont.*

	Age group (years)					
	5–14	15–24	25–34	35–44	45–54	55–64
Deaths 1985–89	0	1	11	23	64	148
Death rate 1980–84	0.00	0.06	0.16	0.52	1.83	4.36
Death rate 1985–89	0.00	0.01	0.11	0.26	1.01	2.65
Ann. % ch. in rate	-	–31.8	–7.6	–14.2	–12.5	–10.5
UK: ENGLAND AND WALES						
Deaths 1980–84	7	16	68	300	1161	3191
Deaths 1985–89	9	16	36	161	655	2106
Death rate 1980–84	0.02	0.04	0.20	0.93	4.22	11.40
Death rate 1985–89	0.03	0.04	0.10	0.47	2.38	7.88
Ann. % ch. in rate	6.6	0.2	–12.9	–12.9	–10.9	–7.1
UK: N. IRELAND						
Deaths 1980–84	0	0	2	9	27	84
Deaths 1985–89	0	0	1	6	16	61
Death rate 1980–84	0.00	0.00	0.20	1.01	3.55	11.74
Death rate 1985–89	0.00	0.00	0.09	0.64	2.05	8.67
Ann. % ch. in rate	-	-	-	–8.9	–10.4	–5.9
UK: SCOTLAND						
Deaths 1980–84	1	0	13	35	188	448
Deaths 1985–89	0	2	2	23	94	302
Death rate 1980–84	0.03	0.00	0.36	1.13	6.47	16.03
Death rate 1985–89	0.00	0.05	0.05	0.69	3.29	11.03
Ann. % ch. in rate	-	-	–31.9	–9.5	–12.6	–7.2
PORTUGAL						
Deaths 1980–84	12	63	122	225	344	427
Deaths 1985–89	4	24	45	100	233	362
Death rate 1980–84	0.14	0.76	1.80	3.92	5.96	8.49
Death rate 1985–89	0.05	0.28	0.59	1.60	4.12	6.70
Ann. % ch. in rate	–18.8	–18.1	–19.9	–16.4	–7.1	–4.6
SPAIN						
Deaths 1980–84	33	108	271	580	1680	2591
Deaths 1985–89	5	27	75	220	577	1347
Death rate 1980–84	0.10	0.35	1.08	2.71	7.24	14.23
Death rate 1985–89	0.02	0.10	0.35	1.34	2.85	8.62
Ann. % ch. in rate	–26.5	–20.2	–18.6	–12.0	–15.6	–8.7
EC						
Deaths 1980–84	105	397	968	2434	6932	13890
Deaths 1985–89	34	194	439	1269	3765	10139
Death rate 1980–84	0.05	0.15	0.42	1.20	3.61	8.43
Death rate 1985–89	0.02	0.08	0.18	0.60	1.90	5.80
Ann. % ch. in rate	–18.8	–13.5	–15.4	–13.0	–12.0	–7.2

Table 9.3(f) Asthma.

	Age group (years)					
	5–14	15–24	25–34	35–44	45–54	55–64
BELGIUM						
Deaths 1980–84	11	58	78	114	249	497
Deaths 1985–89	14	42	73	93	172	426
Death rate 1980–84	0.17	0.74	1.05	1.90	4.12	9.09
Death rate 1985–89	0.22	0.56	0.94	1.39	2.99	7.27
Ann. % ch. in rate	6.0	–5.5	–2.2	–6.1	–6.2	–4.4
LUXEMBOURG						
Deaths 1980–84	0	3	3	2	12	17
Deaths 1985–89	1	1	2	6	9	19
Death rate 1980–84	0.00	1.05	1.04	0.82	4.96	9.63
Death rate 1985–89	0.48	0.37	0.64	2.23	3.89	8.96
Ann. % ch. in rate	-	-	-	22.2	–4.7	–1.4
FEDERAL REPUBLIC OF GERMANY						
Deaths 1980–84	137	524	428	797	2120	3893
Deaths 1985–89	67	399	400	518	1753	4158
Death rate 1980–84	0.37	1.03	1.00	1.82	5.36	12.15
Death rate 1985–89	0.22	0.83	0.85	1.29	3.94	11.97
Ann. % ch. in rate	–9.8	–4.3	–3.1	–6.7	–6.0	–0.3
DENMARK						
Deaths 1980–84	5	15	18	24	71	136
Deaths 1985–89	8	23	12	30	78	217
Death rate 1980–84	0.14	0.38	0.47	0.66	2.60	5.02
Death rate 1985–89	0.25	0.59	0.32	0.76	2.66	8.43
Ann. % ch. in rate	12.4	8.8	–7.5	2.8	0.5	10.9
FRANCE						
Deaths 1980–84	30	159	171	221	582	1065
Deaths 1985–89	75	212	294	468	786	1573
Death rate 1980–84	0.07	0.37	0.40	0.68	1.85	3.83
Death rate 1985–89	0.19	0.49	0.69	1.22	2.67	5.30
Ann. % ch. in rate	21.0	5.9	11.6	12.3	7.6	6.7
GREECE						
Deaths 1980–84	-	-	-	-	-	-
Deaths 1985–89	1	7	5	9	37	75
Death rate 1980–84	-	-	-	-	-	-
Death rate 1985–89	0.01	0.10	0.07	0.14	0.54	1.62
Ann. % ch. in rate	-	-	-	-	-	-
ITALY						
Deaths 1980–84	32	60	50	103	257	699
Deaths 1985–89	26	84	104	132	313	1116
Death rate 1980–84	0.07	0.14	0.13	0.28	0.72	2.39
Death rate 1985–89	0.07	0.18	0.26	0.35	0.86	3.31
Ann. % ch. in rate	–0.8	4.9	12.3	3.8	3.2	5.6
IRELAND						
Deaths 1980–84	10	25	19	41	72	128
Deaths 1985–89	15	24	26	33	62	143
Death rate 1980–84	0.29	0.83	0.80	2.29	4.80	8.91
Death rate 1985–89	0.43	0.78	1.04	1.57	4.01	10.14
Ann. % ch. in rate	8.1	–1.3	5.4	–7.3	–3.5	2.6
THE NETHERLANDS						
Deaths 1980–84	9	39	53	50	95	168

Table 9.3(f)—*cont.*

	Age group (years)					
	5–14	15–24	25–34	35–44	45–54	55–64
Deaths 1985–89	4	22	35	31	69	154
Death rate 1980–84	0.08	0.31	0.45	0.53	1.25	2.50
Death rate 1985–89	0.05	0.22	0.36	0.35	1.08	2.76
Ann. % ch. in rate	–9.3	–7.4	–4.8	–8.7	–3.2	2.2
UK: ENGLAND AND WALES						
Deaths 1980–84	166	391	341	414	923	1582
Deaths 1985–89	106	440	382	510	970	1768
Death rate 1980–84	0.50	0.97	1.00	1.29	3.36	5.65
Death rate 1985–89	0.34	1.11	1.06	1.48	3.52	6.62
Ann. % ch. in rate	–7.4	2.6	1.2	2.8	0.9	3.2
UK: N. IRELAND						
Deaths 1980–84	5	14	9	17	38	50
Deaths 1985–89	0	12	9	22	29	72
Death rate 1980–84	0.36	1.03	0.89	1.92	5.00	6.99
Death rate 1985–89	0.00	0.87	0.81	2.33	3.71	10.24
Ann. % ch. in rate	-	–3.3	–1.8	4.0	–5.8	7.9
UK: SCOTLAND						
Deaths 1980–84	16	35	22	46	113	165
Deaths 1985–89	13	47	31	45	86	158
Death rate 1980–84	0.43	0.80	0.61	1.48	3.89	5.90
Death rate 1985–89	0.40	1.11	0.82	1.34	3.01	5.77
Ann. % ch. in rate	–1.3	6.8	6.1	–2.0	–5.0	–0.5
PORTUGAL						
Deaths 1980–84	-	-	-	-	-	-
Deaths 1985–89	8	40	47	50	138	273
Death rate 1980–84	-	-	-	-	-	-
Death rate 1985–89	0.10	0.46	0.62	0.80	2.44	5.06
Ann. % ch. in rate	-	-	-	-	-	-
SPAIN						
Deaths 1980–84	21	45	48	119	339	841
Deaths 1985–89	23	74	56	91	206	608
Death rate 1980–84	0.06	0.15	0.19	0.56	1.46	4.62
Death rate 1985–89	0.08	0.28	0.26	0.56	1.02	3.89
Ann. % ch. in rate	5.3	12.4	5.8	0.0	–6.4	–3.1
EC						
Deaths 1980–84	445	1373	1245	1959	4900	9317
Deaths 1985–89	368	1452	1499	2070	4780	10961
Death rate 1980–84	0.19	0.53	0.55	0.96	2.55	5.65
Death rate 1985–89	0.17	0.56	0.63	0.97	2.42	6.27
Ann. % ch. in rate	–2.1	1.0	2.8	0.3	–1.1	2.1

Table 9.3(g) Appendicitis.

	Age group (years)					
	5–14	15–24	25–34	35–44	45–54	55–64
BELGIUM						
Deaths 1980–84	2	3	2	2	4	16
Deaths 1985–89	3	0	1	1	0	7
Death rate 1980–84	0.03	0.04	0.03	0.03	0.07	0.29
Death rate 1985–89	0.05	0.00	0.01	0.02	0.00	0.12
Ann. % ch. in rate	-	-	-	-	-	–16.4
LUXEMBOURG						
Deaths 1980–84	0	1	1	0	1	1
Deaths 1985–89	0	0	0	0	0	0
Death rate 1980–84	0.00	0.35	0.35	0.00	0.41	0.57
Death rate 1985–89	0.00	0.00	0.00	0.00	0.00	0.00
Ann. % ch. in rate	-	-	-	-	-	-
FEDERAL REPUBLIC OF GERMANY						
Deaths 1980–84	34	39	30	55	103	204
Deaths 1985–89	7	14	15	14	57	116
Death rate 1980–84	0.09	0.08	0.07	0.13	0.26	0.64
Death rate 1985–89	0.02	0.03	0.03	0.04	0.13	0.33
Ann. % ch. in rate	–24.1	–17.7	–14.5	–22.7	–13.2	–12.1
DENMARK						
Deaths 1980–84	3	3	1	4	8	12
Deaths 1985–89	2	2	1	4	5	15
Death rate 1980–84	0.08	0.08	0.03	0.11	0.29	0.44
Death rate 1985–89	0.06	0.05	0.03	0.10	0.17	0.58
Ann. % ch. in rate	-	-	-	-	–10.2	5.6
FRANCE						
Deaths 1980–84	36	42	38	39	76	122
Deaths 1985–89	11	11	15	22	21	68
Death rate 1980–84	0.09	0.10	0.09	0.12	0.24	0.44
Death rate 1985–89	0.03	0.03	0.04	0.06	0.07	0.23
Ann. % ch. in rate	–20.5	–23.5	–16.9	–13.8	–21.7	–12.2
GREECE						
Deaths 1980–84	1	1	4	3	1	4
Deaths 1985–89	0	0	0	0	0	2
Death rate 1980–84	0.02	0.02	0.10	0.08	0.03	0.15
Death rate 1985–89	0.00	0.00	0.00	0.00	0.00	0.04
Ann. % ch. in rate	-	-	-	-	-	-
ITALY						
Deaths 1980–84	49	24	30	22	82	117
Deaths 1985–89	12	9	5	15	32	69
Death rate 1980–84	0.11	0.06	0.08	0.06	0.23	0.40
Death rate 1985–89	0.03	0.02	0.01	0.04	0.09	0.21
Ann. % ch. in rate	–18.8	–15.8	–26.3	–6.6	–14.7	–10.6
IRELAND						
Deaths 1980–84	6	1	1	1	2	6
Deaths 1985–89	2	0	0	2	0	5
Death rate 1980–84	0.17	0.03	0.04	0.06	0.13	0.42
Death rate 1985–89	0.06	0.00	0.00	0.10	0.00	0.35
Ann. % ch. in rate	–20.0	-	-	-	-	–3.2
THE NETHERLANDS						
Deaths 1980–84	8	6	8	7	13	25

Table 9.3(g)—*cont.*

	Age group (years)					
	5–14	15–24	25–34	35–44	45–54	55–64
Deaths 1985–89	7	5	5	9	6	13
Death rate 1980–84	0.07	0.05	0.07	0.07	0.17	0.37
Death rate 1985–89	0.10	0.05	0.05	0.10	0.09	0.23
Ann. % ch. in rate	5.5	1.0	–6.0	7.4	–12.5	–9.9
UK: ENGLAND AND WALES						
Deaths 1980–84	26	9	12	8	48	98
Deaths 1985–89	25	17	12	12	27	81
Death rate 1980–84	0.08	0.02	0.04	0.03	0.18	0.35
Death rate 1985–89	0.08	0.04	0.03	0.04	0.10	0.30
Ann. % ch. in rate	0.5	13.8	–1.1	6.9	–10.9	–2.8
UK: N. IRELAND						
Deaths 1980–84	1	1	0	0	1	5
Deaths 1985–89	0	0	0	1	0	5
Death rate 1980–84	0.07	0.07	0.00	0.00	0.13	0.70
Death rate 1985–89	0.00	0.00	0.00	0.11	0.00	0.71
Ann. % ch. in rate	-	-	-	-	-	-
UK: SCOTLAND						
Deaths 1980–84	2	4	1	4	3	10
Deaths 1985–89	1	1	0	0	4	11
Death rate 1980–84	0.05	0.09	0.03	0.13	0.10	0.36
Death rate 1985–89	0.03	0.02	0.00	0.00	0.14	0.40
Ann. % ch. in rate	-	-	-	-	-	2.3
PORTUGAL						
Deaths 1980–84	20	7	4	8	17	23
Deaths 1985–89	6	2	2	3	2	14
Death rate 1980–84	0.24	0.08	0.06	0.14	0.29	0.46
Death rate 1985–89	0.08	0.02	0.03	0.05	0.04	0.26
Ann. % ch. in rate	–20.5	–22.7	-	–19.2	–34.6	–10.7
SPAIN						
Deaths 1980–84	23	27	16	22	56	91
Deaths 1985–89	3	4	7	4	16	36
Death rate 1980–84	0.07	0.09	0.06	0.10	0.24	0.50
Death rate 1985–89	0.01	0.02	0.03	0.02	0.08	0.23
Ann. % ch. in rate	–28.5	–27.5	–11.5	–23.0	–18.4	–13.1
EC						
Deaths 1980–84	200	160	142	169	394	703
Deaths 1985–89	81	67	65	90	174	450
Death rate 1980–84	0.09	0.06	0.06	0.08	0.21	0.43
Death rate 1985–89	0.04	0.03	0.03	0.04	0.09	0.26
Ann. % ch. in rate	–15.2	–16.2	–15.2	–12.6	–15.6	–9.6

Table 9.3(h) Abdominal hernia.

	Age group (years)					
	5–14	15–24	25–34	35–44	45–54	55–64
BELGIUM						
Deaths 1980–84	0	2	2	3	8	26
Deaths 1985–89	1	0	2	2	5	19
Death rate 1980–84	0.00	0.03	0.03	0.05	0.13	0.48
Death rate 1985–89	0.02	0.00	0.03	0.03	0.09	0.32
Ann. % ch. in rate	-	-	-	-	–8.1	–7.4
LUXEMBOURG						
Deaths 1980–84	0	0	0	0	1	1
Deaths 1985–89	1	0	0	0	0	1
Death rate 1980–84	0.00	0.00	0.00	0.00	0.41	0.57
Death rate 1985–89	0.48	0.00	0.00	0.00	0.00	0.47
Ann. % ch. in rate	-	-	-	-	-	-
FEDERAL REPUBLIC OF GERMANY						
Deaths 1980–84	2	1	3	30	98	264
Deaths 1985–89	0	1	8	12	52	165
Death rate 1980–84	0.01	0.00	0.01	0.07	0.25	0.82
Death rate 1985–89	0.00	0.00	0.02	0.03	0.12	0.48
Ann. % ch. in rate	-	-	19.5	–15.3	–14.0	–10.4
DENMARK						
Deaths 1980–84	0	1	0	2	7	17
Deaths 1985–89	0	0	0	3	8	18
Death rate 1980–84	0.00	0.03	0.00	0.06	0.26	0.63
Death rate 1985–89	0.00	0.00	0.00	0.08	0.27	0.70
Ann. % ch. in rate	-	-	-	-	1.3	2.2
FRANCE						
Deaths 1980–84	4	5	8	31	131	379
Deaths 1985–89	3	8	9	30	85	295
Death rate 1980–84	0.01	0.01	0.02	0.10	0.42	1.36
Death rate 1985–89	0.01	0.02	0.02	0.08	0.29	0.99
Ann. % ch. in rate	-	9.8	2.5	–4.0	–7.1	–6.1
GREECE						
Deaths 1980–84	0	0	0	0	7	12
Deaths 1985–89	0	0	0	0	4	8
Death rate 1980–84	0.00	0.00	0.00	0.00	0.18	0.45
Death rate 1985–89	0.00	0.00	0.00	0.00	0.06	0.17
Ann. % ch. in rate	-	-	-	-	–16.8	–14.6
ITALY						
Deaths 1980–84	2	6	12	32	130	376
Deaths 1985–89	2	3	11	21	93	249
Death rate 1980–84	0.01	0.01	0.03	0.09	0.36	1.29
Death rate 1985–89	0.01	0.01	0.03	0.06	0.26	0.74
Ann. % ch. in rate	-	–11.6	–2.1	–7.2	–5.6	–8.8
IRELAND						
Deaths 1980–84	0	0	0	1	2	11
Deaths 1985–89	0	0	0	0	6	7
Death rate 1980–84	0.00	0.00	0.00	0.06	0.13	0.77
Death rate 1985–89	0.00	0.00	0.00	0.00	0.39	0.50
Ann. % ch. in rate	-	-	-	-	23.8	–8.3
THE NETHERLANDS						
Deaths 1980–84	2	4	4	4	12	52

Table 9.3(h)—*cont.*

	Age group (years)					
	5–14	15–24	25–34	35–44	45–54	55–64
Deaths 1985–89	2	2	2	4	15	27
Death rate 1980–84	0.02	0.03	0.03	0.04	0.16	0.77
Death rate 1985–89	0.03	0.02	0.02	0.05	0.24	0.48
Ann. % ch. in rate	-	-	-	-	9.2	–9.9
UK: ENGLAND AND WALES						
Deaths 1980–84	6	11	12	14	100	277
Deaths 1985–89	5	4	11	23	67	246
Death rate 1980–84	0.02	0.03	0.04	0.04	0.36	0.99
Death rate 1985–89	0.02	0.01	0.03	0.07	0.24	0.92
Ann. % ch. in rate	–2.3	–18.1	–2.8	8.9	–7.7	–1.4
UK: N. IRELAND						
Deaths 1980–84	0	0	1	1	3	8
Deaths 1985–89	0	1	0	1	0	3
Death rate 1980–84	0.00	0.00	0.10	0.11	0.39	1.12
Death rate 1985–89	0.00	0.07	0.00	0.11	0.00	0.43
Ann. % ch. in rate	-	-	-	-	-	–17.5
UK: SCOTLAND						
Deaths 1980–84	0	1	2	4	11	23
Deaths 1985–89	0	1	2	1	3	19
Death rate 1980–84	0.00	0.02	0.06	0.13	0.38	0.82
Death rate 1985–89	0.00	0.02	0.05	0.03	0.11	0.69
Ann. % ch. in rate	-	-	-	-	–22.6	–3.3
PORTUGAL						
Deaths 1980–84	2	0	3	1	17	47
Deaths 1985–89	0	1	0	3	15	28
Death rate 1980–84	0.02	0.00	0.04	0.02	0.29	0.94
Death rate 1985–89	0.00	0.01	0.00	0.05	0.27	0.52
Ann. % ch. in rate	-	-	-	-	–2.1	–11.1
SPAIN						
Deaths 1980–84	3	2	6	16	63	200
Deaths 1985–89	0	2	5	8	27	86
Death rate 1980–84	0.01	0.01	0.02	0.08	0.27	1.10
Death rate 1985–89	0.00	0.01	0.02	0.05	0.13	0.55
Ann. % ch. in rate	-	-	–0.5	–7.5	–12.2	–11.8
EC						
Deaths 1980–84	20	32	51	135	575	1645
Deaths 1985–89	14	24	51	110	388	1193
Death rate 1980–84	0.01	0.01	0.02	0.07	0.30	1.00
Death rate 1985–89	0.01	0.01	0.02	0.05	0.20	0.68
Ann. % ch. in rate	–5.2	–6.0	–0.9	–4.7	–8.1	–7.3

Table 9.3(i) Cholelithiasis and cholecystitis.

	Age group (years)					
	5–14	15–24	25–34	35–44	45–54	55–64
BELGIUM						
Deaths 1980–84	0	1	3	7	25	103
Deaths 1985–89	0	2	3	2	10	31
Death rate 1980–84	0.00	0.01	0.04	0.12	0.41	1.88
Death rate 1985–89	0.00	0.03	0.04	0.03	0.17	0.53
Ann. % ch. in rate	-	-	-	–23.9	–15.9	–22.4
LUXEMBOURG						
Deaths 1980–84	0	0	1	1	0	5
Deaths 1985–89	0	0	0	1	2	2
Death rate 1980–84	0.00	0.00	0.35	0.41	0.00	2.83
Death rate 1985–89	0.00	0.00	0.00	0.37	0.86	0.94
Ann. % ch. in rate	-	-	-	-	-	-
FEDERAL REPUBLIC OF GERMANY						
Deaths 1980–84	0	10	18	75	229	748
Deaths 1985–89	0	6	11	41	148	412
Death rate 1980–84	0.00	0.02	0.04	0.17	0.58	2.33
Death rate 1985–89	0.00	0.01	0.02	0.10	0.33	1.19
Ann. % ch. in rate	-	–8.7	–11.0	–9.9	–10.5	–12.7
DENMARK						
Deaths 1980–84	0	0	0	2	16	34
Deaths 1985–89	0	0	1	2	13	47
Death rate 1980–84	0.00	0.00	0.00	0.06	0.59	1.26
Death rate 1985–89	0.00	0.00	0.03	0.05	0.44	1.83
Ann. % ch. in rate	-	-	-	-	–5.4	7.8
FRANCE						
Deaths 1980–84	0	2	5	10	34	101
Deaths 1985–89	0	4	12	37	79	294
Death rate 1980–84	0.00	0.01	0.01	0.03	0.11	0.36
Death rate 1985–89	0.00	0.01	0.03	0.10	0.27	0.99
Ann. % ch. in rate	-	-	19.2	25.6	19.9	22.2
GREECE						
Deaths 1980–84	0	2	2	4	6	26
Deaths 1985–89	0	0	1	2	3	31
Death rate 1980–84	0.00	0.05	0.05	0.11	0.15	0.96
Death rate 1985–89	0.00	0.00	0.02	0.03	0.04	0.67
Ann. % ch. in rate	-	-	-	-	–18.6	–5.9
ITALY						
Deaths 1980–84	1	10	46	128	386	905
Deaths 1985–89	1	3	21	71	209	579
Death rate 1980–84	0.00	0.02	0.12	0.35	1.08	3.09
Death rate 1985–89	0.00	0.01	0.05	0.19	0.58	1.72
Ann. % ch. in rate	-	–18.8	–12.8	–9.7	–9.9	–9.4
IRELAND						
Deaths 1980–84	0	0	1	2	13	23
Deaths 1985–89	1	1	2	2	5	12
Death rate 1980–84	0.00	0.00	0.04	0.11	0.87	1.60
Death rate 1985–89	0.03	0.03	0.08	0.10	0.32	0.85
Ann. % ch. in rate	-	-	-	-	–17.9	–11.9
THE NETHERLANDS						
Deaths 1980–84	0	1	6	11	53	149

Table 9.3(i)—*cont.*

	Age group (years)					
	5–14	15–24	25–34	35–44	45–54	55–64
Deaths 1985–89	0	2	5	11	21	87
Death rate 1980–84	0.00	0.01	0.05	0.12	0.70	2.22
Death rate 1985–89	0.00	0.02	0.05	0.12	0.33	1.56
Ann. % ch. in rate	-	-	0.2	1.5	−15.4	−7.5
UK: ENGLAND AND WALES						
Deaths 1980–84	0	2	19	26	122	329
Deaths 1985–89	1	5	8	41	66	301
Death rate 1980–84	0.00	0.01	0.06	0.08	0.44	1.18
Death rate 1985–89	0.00	0.01	0.02	0.12	0.24	1.13
Ann. % ch. in rate	-	-	−16.8	8.0	−11.6	−0.8
UK: N. IRELAND						
Deaths 1980–84	0	0	0	3	1	16
Deaths 1985–89	0	0	0	1	1	5
Death rate 1980–84	0.00	0.00	0.00	0.34	0.13	2.24
Death rate 1985–89	0.00	0.00	0.00	0.11	0.13	0.71
Ann. % ch. in rate	-	-	-	-	-	−20.5
UK: SCOTLAND						
Deaths 1980–84	0	0	0	0	0	4
Deaths 1985–89	0	1	2	7	8	25
Death rate 1980–84	0.00	0.00	0.00	0.00	0.00	0.14
Death rate 1985–89	0.00	0.02	0.05	0.21	0.28	0.91
Ann. % ch. in rate	-	-	-	-	-	44.9
PORTUGAL						
Deaths 1980–84	0	0	2	13	29	79
Deaths 1985–89	0	0	1	7	24	75
Death rate 1980–84	0.00	0.00	0.03	0.23	0.50	1.57
Death rate 1985–89	0.00	0.00	0.01	0.11	0.42	1.39
Ann. % ch. in rate	-	-	-	−13.1	−3.3	−2.4
SPAIN						
Deaths 1980–84	0	4	19	41	146	302
Deaths 1985–89	0	4	4	11	47	127
Death rate 1980–84	0.00	0.01	0.08	0.19	0.63	1.66
Death rate 1985–89	0.00	0.02	0.02	0.07	0.23	0.81
Ann. % ch. in rate	-	-	−22.5	−17.4	−16.6	−12.2
EC						
Deaths 1980–84	1	31	116	306	1004	2704
Deaths 1985–89	3	29	73	240	648	2067
Death rate 1980–84	0.00	0.01	0.05	0.15	0.52	1.64
Death rate 1985–89	0.00	0.01	0.03	0.11	0.33	1.18
Ann. % ch. in rate	-	−1.7	−9.7	−5.6	−8.9	−6.3

Table 9.3(j) Hypertensive and cerebrovascular diseases.

	Age group (years)					
	5–14	15–24	25–34	35–44	45–54	55–64
BELGIUM						
Deaths 1980–84	36	105	237	482	1573	4330
Deaths 1985–89	29	107	249	577	1266	3985
Death rate 1980–84	0.55	1.34	3.18	8.02	26.04	79.17
Death rate 1985–89	0.46	1.43	3.19	8.59	22.03	68.00
Ann. % ch. in rate	–3.3	1.2	0.0	1.4	–3.3	–3.0
LUXEMBOURG						
Deaths 1980–84	1	4	11	17	88	217
Deaths 1985–89	0	3	11	22	69	234
Death rate 1980–84	0.43	1.40	3.81	6.95	36.36	122.95
Death rate 1985–89	0.00	1.12	3.54	8.16	29.81	110.38
Ann. % ch. in rate	-	-	–1.5	3.3	–3.9	–2.1
FEDERAL REPUBLIC OF GERMANY						
Deaths 1980–84	115	465	1211	3952	11383	28593
Deaths 1985–89	78	361	1056	2767	9495	24963
Death rate 1980–84	0.31	0.91	2.81	9.04	28.77	89.21
Death rate 1985–89	0.26	0.75	2.25	6.89	21.33	71.86
Ann. % ch. in rate	–3.7	–3.9	–4.4	–5.3	–5.8	–4.2
DENMARK						
Deaths 1980–84	15	25	111	293	702	1996
Deaths 1985–89	7	27	104	341	675	1758
Death rate 1980–84	0.42	0.64	2.91	8.10	25.67	73.72
Death rate 1985–89	0.22	0.69	2.77	8.65	23.06	68.33
Ann. % ch. in rate	–12.1	1.5	–1.0	1.3	–2.1	–1.5
FRANCE						
Deaths 1980–84	135	503	1293	2671	8453	20166
Deaths 1985–89	119	439	1075	2775	6044	17760
Death rate 1980–84	0.33	1.17	3.02	8.22	26.87	72.57
Death rate 1985–89	0.31	1.02	2.52	7.21	20.52	59.84
Ann. % ch. in rate	–1.8	–2.7	–3.5	–2.6	–5.2	–3.8
GREECE						
Deaths 1980–84	32	84	115	315	1081	3162
Deaths 1985–89	50	151	242	460	1468	4998
Death rate 1980–84	0.70	1.96	2.91	8.65	27.02	117.24
Death rate 1985–89	0.63	2.05	3.57	7.35	21.33	107.73
Ann. % ch. in rate	–1.6	0.8	3.4	–2.7	–3.9	–1.4
ITALY						
Deaths 1980–84	245	549	1150	3630	12785	33927
Deaths 1985–89	238	531	1049	3008	9217	30475
Death rate 1980–84	0.56	1.25	2.93	9.79	35.61	115.96
Death rate 1985–89	0.64	1.15	2.57	7.92	25.40	90.34
Ann. % ch. in rate	2.2	–1.3	–2.1	–3.5	–5.5	–4.1
IRELAND						
Deaths 1980–84	16	49	79	207	517	1682
Deaths 1985–89	10	24	73	156	340	1222
Death rate 1980–84	0.46	1.63	3.32	11.56	34.47	117.13
Death rate 1985–89	0.29	0.78	2.91	7.40	21.99	86.61
Ann. % ch. in rate	–9.3	–13.8	–2.6	–8.5	–8.6	–5.9
THE NETHERLANDS						
Deaths 1980–84	29	126	289	610	1629	4270

Table 9.3(j)—*cont.*

	Age group (years)					
	5–14	15–24	25–34	35–44	45–54	55–64
Deaths 1985–89	27	84	243	495	1149	3097
Death rate 1980–84	0.27	1.02	2.46	6.41	21.48	63.59
Death rate 1985–89	0.37	0.85	2.51	5.58	18.04	55.53
Ann. % ch. in rate	6.9	–3.9	0.4	–3.1	–3.8	–3.0
UK: ENGLAND AND WALES						
Deaths 1980–84	113	427	1053	2780	8906	28870
Deaths 1985–89	90	344	947	2636	6734	23138
Death rate 1980–84	0.34	1.06	3.07	8.64	32.39	103.14
Death rate 1985–89	0.29	0.86	2.62	7.63	24.42	86.59
Ann. % ch. in rate	–3.2	–4.0	–3.2	–2.4	–5.5	–3.4
UK: N. IRELAND						
Deaths 1980–84	6	24	41	83	291	913
Deaths 1985–89	2	22	42	93	207	735
Death rate 1980–84	0.44	1.76	4.05	9.35	38.26	127.60
Death rate 1985–89	0.15	1.59	3.79	9.85	26.50	104.48
Ann. % ch. in rate	–18.8	–2.0	–1.3	1.0	–7.1	–3.9
UK: SCOTLAND						
Deaths 1980–84	13	64	166	434	1266	4013
Deaths 1985–89	6	37	133	347	966	3288
Death rate 1980–84	0.35	1.46	4.62	13.97	43.57	143.55
Death rate 1985–89	0.19	0.87	3.53	10.35	33.83	120.09
Ann. % ch. in rate	–11.8	–9.7	–5.3	–5.8	–4.9	–3.5
PORTUGAL						
Deaths 1980–84	72	137	278	777	3312	10402
Deaths 1985–89	46	134	276	722	2596	8737
Death rate 1980–84	0.85	1.64	4.09	13.54	57.37	206.88
Death rate 1985–89	0.57	1.56	3.63	11.57	45.88	161.81
Ann. % ch. in rate	–7.5	–1.1	–2.3	–3.1	–4.4	–4.8
SPAIN						
Deaths 1980–84	325	588	962	2022	6783	17923
Deaths 1985–89	181	503	747	1509	4062	12295
Death rate 1980–84	0.99	1.89	3.85	9.46	29.24	98.42
Death rate 1985–89	0.66	1.87	3.48	9.21	20.03	78.71
Ann. % ch. in rate	–6.9	–0.2	–1.8	–0.5	–6.6	–4.0
EC						
Deaths 1980–84	1148	3152	6972	18211	58549	160069
Deaths 1985–89	930	2899	6470	16359	45461	140147
Death rate 1980–84	0.49	1.22	3.06	8.94	30.52	97.11
Death rate 1985–89	0.43	1.12	2.71	7.70	22.99	80.13
Ann. % ch. in rate	–2.5	–1.8	–2.4	–2.9	–5.5	–3.8

Table 9.3(k) Cancer of the breast.

	Age group (years)					
	5–14	15–24	25–34	35–44	45–54	55–64
BELGIUM						
Deaths 1980–84	0	3	132	622	1750	2587
Deaths 1985–89	0	4	112	680	1655	2829
Death rate 1980–84	0.00	0.08	3.63	20.97	57.38	90.60
Death rate 1985–89	0.00	0.11	2.93	20.62	57.23	92.66
Ann. % ch. in rate	-	-	–4.2	–0.3	–0.1	0.5
LUXEMBOURG						
Deaths 1980–84	0	0	5	31	58	90
Deaths 1985–89	0	0	3	27	66	108
Death rate 1980–84	0.00	0.00	3.55	26.27	48.74	91.84
Death rate 1985–89	0.00	0.00	1.93	20.77	57.64	96.43
Ann. % ch. in rate	-	-	-	–4.6	3.4	1.0
FEDERAL REPUBLIC OF GERMANY						
Deaths 1980–84	0	19	611	3872	8823	14014
Deaths 1985–89	1	17	687	3733	10579	14925
Death rate 1980–84	0.00	0.08	2.92	18.21	45.03	75.05
Death rate 1985–89	0.01	0.07	3.00	18.96	48.44	79.44
Ann. % ch. in rate	-	–1.2	0.5	0.8	1.5	1.1
DENMARK						
Deaths 1980–84	1	2	56	306	766	1255
Deaths 1985–89	0	1	47	378	887	1362
Death rate 1980–84	0.06	0.11	3.01	17.27	55.65	89.45
Death rate 1985–89	0.00	0.05	2.57	19.58	60.77	102.33
Ann. % ch. in rate	-	-	–3.1	2.5	1.8	2.7
FRANCE						
Deaths 1980–84	2	17	490	2279	6500	9639
Deaths 1985–89	3	19	462	2756	6126	10567
Death rate 1980–84	0.01	0.08	2.31	14.36	41.29	66.15
Death rate 1985–89	0.02	0.09	2.17	14.55	41.61	67.82
Ann. % ch. in rate	-	2.2	–1.2	0.3	0.2	0.5
GREECE						
Deaths 1980–84	0	5	72	304	762	786
Deaths 1985–89	0	7	96	449	1240	1642
Death rate 1980–84	0.00	0.24	3.62	16.19	37.52	55.17
Death rate 1985–89	0.00	0.19	2.81	13.89	35.47	66.97
Ann. % ch. in rate	-	–3.4	–4.2	–2.5	–0.9	3.3
ITALY						
Deaths 1980–84	5	35	598	3232	8028	11123
Deaths 1985–89	0	14	571	3266	8238	12659
Death rate 1980–84	0.02	0.16	3.05	17.30	43.71	71.10
Death rate 1985–89	0.00	0.06	2.82	17.12	44.50	70.90
Ann. % ch. in rate	-	–17.5	–1.6	–0.2	0.4	–0.1
IRELAND						
Deaths 1980–84	0	2	41	217	498	662
Deaths 1985–89	0	2	38	255	504	689
Death rate 1980–84	0.00	0.14	3.50	24.87	67.43	90.25
Death rate 1985–89	0.00	0.13	3.04	24.63	66.62	95.36
Ann. % ch. in rate	-	-	–2.7	–0.2	–0.2	1.1
THE NETHERLANDS						
Deaths 1980–84	0	3	160	865	2071	3209

Table 9.3(k)—*cont.*

	Age group (years)					
	5–14	15–24	25–34	35–44	45–54	55–64
Deaths 1985–89	0	3	136	831	1678	2725
Death rate 1980–84	0.00	0.05	2.79	18.81	54.91	91.15
Death rate 1985–89	0.00	0.06	2.87	19.25	53.65	94.17
Ann. % ch. in rate	-	-	0.6	0.5	–0.5	0.7
UK: ENGLAND AND WALES						
Deaths 1980–84	0	13	405	2071	5378	8789
Deaths 1985–89	0	24	677	3783	8568	14151
Death rate 1980–84	0.00	0.11	3.97	21.59	65.26	100.96
Death rate 1985–89	0.00	0.12	3.77	21.97	62.29	103.08
Ann. % ch. in rate	-	2.9	–1.3	0.4	–1.2	0.5
UK: N. IRELAND						
Deaths 1980–84	0	0	21	104	252	364
Deaths 1985–89	0	1	23	105	269	351
Death rate 1980–84	0.00	0.00	4.22	23.35	64.29	95.54
Death rate 1985–89	0.00	0.15	4.18	22.11	67.50	93.85
Ann. % ch. in rate	-	-	–0.2	–1.1	1.0	–0.4
UK: SCOTLAND						
Deaths 1980–84	0	0	61	393	995	1455
Deaths 1985–89	0	2	54	367	918	1400
Death rate 1980–84	0.00	0.00	3.42	25.10	66.44	97.52
Death rate 1985–89	0.00	0.10	2.90	21.88	62.64	96.52
Ann. % ch. in rate	-	-	–3.3	–2.7	–1.2	–0.2
PORTUGAL						
Deaths 1980–84	*	*	109	547	1173	1377
Deaths 1985–89	0	3	87	602	1236	1636
Death rate 1980–84	*	*	3.18	18.22	38.45	51.00
Death rate 1985–89	0.00	0.07	2.29	18.66	41.30	56.10
Ann. % ch. in rate	*	*	–6.4	0.5	1.4	1.9
SPAIN						
Deaths 1980–84	1	21	373	1641	4025	4663
Deaths 1985–89	0	13	294	1596	3316	4683
Death rate 1980–84	0.01	0.14	3.00	15.31	34.18	48.34
Death rate 1985–89	0.00	0.10	2.77	19.48	32.62	57.21
Ann. % ch. in rate	-	–7.2	–1.8	5.5	–1.0	3.8
EC						
Deaths 1980–84	9	132	3461	18107	45269	66512
Deaths 1985–89	4	114	3398	19456	46572	71642
Death rate 1980–84	0.01	0.11	3.07	17.93	46.87	75.07
Death rate 1985–89	0.00	0.09	2.87	18.43	47.03	77.69
Ann. % ch. in rate	–13.6	–3.1	–1.3	0.6	0.1	0.7

* Portugal did not supply data for this disease for 1980–84 in this age-group.

Table 9.3(l) Ischaemic heart disease.

	Age group (years)					
	5–14	15–24	25–34	35–44	45–54	55–64
BELGIUM						
Deaths 1980–84	0	33	211	1069	4522	11725
Deaths 1985–89	0	29	171	964	3106	9949
Death rate 1980–84	0.00	0.42	2.83	17.79	74.86	214.39
Death rate 1985–89	0.00	0.39	2.19	14.35	54.04	169.78
Ann. % ch. in rate	-	−1.7	−5.0	−4.2	−6.3	−4.6
LUXEMBOURG						
Deaths 1980–84	0	3	7	62	225	535
Deaths 1985–89	0	1	10	62	160	442
Death rate 1980–84	0.00	1.05	2.42	25.36	92.98	303.12
Death rate 1985–89	0.00	0.37	3.22	23.01	69.11	208.49
Ann. % ch. in rate	-	-	5.8	−1.9	−5.8	−7.2
FEDERAL REPUBLIC OF GERMANY						
Deaths 1980–84	0	133	964	8013	32435	77702
Deaths 1985–89	0	109	875	5727	27947	78360
Death rate 1980–84	0.00	0.26	2.24	18.34	81.99	242.43
Death rate 1985–89	0.00	0.23	1.86	14.25	62.78	225.56
Ann. % ch. in rate	-	−2.9	−3.6	−4.9	−5.2	−1.4
DENMARK						
Deaths 1980–84	0	9	83	639	2858	9544
Deaths 1985–89	0	8	61	619	2424	7933
Death rate 1980–84	0.00	0.23	2.18	17.67	104.52	352.50
Death rate 1985–89	0.00	0.20	1.63	15.70	82.80	308.32
Ann. % ch. in rate	-	−2.4	−5.7	−2.3	−4.6	−2.6
FRANCE						
Deaths 1980–84	19	114	771	3152	12429	29882
Deaths 1985–89	25	104	715	3908	10010	29530
Death rate 1980–84	0.05	0.27	1.80	9.70	39.50	107.53
Death rate 1985–89	0.06	0.24	1.68	10.15	33.98	99.50
Ann. % ch. in rate	6.4	−1.8	−1.4	0.9	−3.0	−1.5
GREECE						
Deaths 1980–84	0	21	124	583	2295	4361
Deaths 1985–89	0	61	276	1147	3627	9417
Death rate 1980–84	0.00	0.49	3.14	16.01	57.37	161.70
Death rate 1985–89	0.00	0.83	4.07	18.32	52.71	202.97
Ann. % ch. in rate	-	9.1	4.4	2.3	−1.4	3.9
ITALY						
Deaths 1980–84	36	267	1191	5514	21904	54256
Deaths 1985–89	26	181	849	4596	16755	50936
Death rate 1980–84	0.08	0.61	3.03	14.88	61.00	185.44
Death rate 1985–89	0.07	0.39	2.08	12.10	46.18	150.99
Ann. % ch. in rate	−3.3	−8.4	−7.2	−4.0	−5.4	−4.0
IRELAND						
Deaths 1980–84	0	7	78	551	2316	7036
Deaths 1985–89	0	7	59	480	1956	6189
Death rate 1980–84	0.00	0.23	3.27	30.77	154.40	489.97
Death rate 1985–89	0.00	0.23	2.36	22.78	126.48	438.63
Ann. % ch. in rate	-	−0.5	−6.4	−5.8	−3.9	−2.2
THE NETHERLANDS						
Deaths 1980–84	2	36	314	1824	6873	18297

Table 9.3(l)—*cont.*

	Age group (years)					
	5–14	15–24	25–34	35–44	45–54	55–64
Deaths 1985–89	0	22	219	1529	4672	13609
Death rate 1980–84	0.02	0.29	2.68	19.18	90.64	272.48
Death rate 1985–89	0.00	0.22	2.26	17.22	73.36	244.03
Ann. % ch. in rate	-	–5.8	–3.7	–2.4	–4.6	–2.4
UK: ENGLAND AND WALES						
Deaths 1980–84	5	66	647	4805	22258	71890
Deaths 1985–89	4	69	881	7573	31130	104824
Death rate 1980–84	0.03	0.27	3.15	24.89	134.92	428.03
Death rate 1985–89	0.01	0.17	2.43	21.93	112.91	392.31
Ann. % ch. in rate	-	–10.7	–6.2	–3.1	–4.4	–2.2
UK: N. IRELAND						
Deaths 1980–84	2	3	47	321	1345	4264
Deaths 1985–89	0	2	33	247	1096	3551
Death rate 1980–84	0.15	0.22	4.64	36.17	176.86	595.95
Death rate 1985–89	0.00	0.14	2.98	26.15	140.33	504.76
Ann. % ch. in rate	-	-	–8.5	–6.3	–4.5	–3.3
UK: SCOTLAND						
Deaths 1980–84	1	12	129	1126	5686	15771
Deaths 1985–89	2	9	124	1060	4448	14303
Death rate 1980–84	0.03	0.27	3.59	36.25	195.66	564.16
Death rate 1985–89	0.06	0.21	3.29	31.61	155.77	522.39
Ann. % ch. in rate	-	–4.9	–1.8	–2.7	–4.5	–1.5
PORTUGAL						
Deaths 1980–84	*	*	*	742	2814	6551
Deaths 1985–89	11	42	173	724	2318	6687
Death rate 1980–84	*	*	*	12.93	48.74	130.29
Death rate 1985–89	0.14	0.49	2.28	11.60	40.97	123.85
Ann. % ch. in rate	*	*	*	–2.2	–3.4	–1.0
SPAIN						
Deaths 1980–84	53	223	811	2963	9883	22949
Deaths 1985–89	17	144	552	2241	6909	18669
Death rate 1980–84	0.16	0.72	3.24	13.86	42.60	126.02
Death rate 1985–89	0.06	0.54	2.57	13.67	34.08	119.51
Ann. % ch. in rate	–19.0	–6.3	–5.0	–0.3	–4.8	–1.2
EC						
Deaths 1980–84	119	971	5852	34875	144075	386028
Deaths 1985–89	89	827	5180	31764	119281	361986
Death rate 1980–84	0.05	0.38	2.57	17.11	75.11	234.19
Death rate 1985–89	0.04	0.32	2.17	14.94	60.31	206.96
Ann. % ch. in rate	–4.0	–3.3	–3.3	–2.7	–4.3	–2.4

* Portugal did not supply data for this disease for 1980–84 in this age-group.

Table 9.3(m) Peptic ulcers.

	Age group (years)					
	5–14	15–24	25–34	35–44	45–54	55–64
BELGIUM						
Deaths 1980–84	0	5	11	36	90	190
Deaths 1985–89	1	7	11	37	42	147
Death rate 1980–84	0.00	0.06	0.15	0.60	1.49	3.47
Death rate 1985–89	0.02	0.09	0.14	0.55	0.73	2.51
Ann. % ch. in rate	-	7.9	–0.9	–1.7	–13.3	–6.3
LUXEMBOURG						
Deaths 1980–84	0	0	1	4	7	13
Deaths 1985–89	0	0	0	3	1	7
Death rate 1980–84	0.00	0.00	0.35	1.64	2.89	7.37
Death rate 1985–89	0.00	0.00	0.00	1.11	0.43	3.30
Ann. % ch. in rate	-	-	-	-	–31.6	–14.8
FEDERAL REPUBLIC OF GERMANY						
Deaths 1980–84	5	33	122	476	1137	1826
Deaths 1985–89	4	24	80	220	761	1437
Death rate 1980–84	0.01	0.07	0.28	1.09	2.87	5.70
Death rate 1985–89	0.01	0.05	0.17	0.55	1.71	4.14
Ann. % ch. in rate	-	–5.2	–9.7	–12.9	–9.9	–6.2
DENMARK						
Deaths 1980–84	0	2	1	25	60	173
Deaths 1985–89	1	2	6	27	81	189
Death rate 1980–84	0.00	0.05	0.03	0.69	2.19	6.39
Death rate 1985–89	0.03	0.05	0.16	0.69	2.77	7.35
Ann. % ch. in rate	-	-	43.5	–0.2	4.7	2.8
FRANCE						
Deaths 1980–84	5	17	65	181	625	1252
Deaths 1985–89	1	16	49	159	386	1023
Death rate 1980–84	0.01	0.04	0.15	0.56	1.99	4.51
Death rate 1985–89	0.00	0.04	0.12	0.41	1.31	3.45
Ann. % ch. in rate	-	–1.2	–5.4	–5.8	–8.0	–5.2
GREECE						
Deaths 1980–84	1	2	3	14	38	72
Deaths 1985–89	0	2	4	9	22	61
Death rate 1980–84	0.02	0.05	0.08	0.38	0.95	2.67
Death rate 1985–89	0.00	0.03	0.06	0.14	0.32	1.32
Ann. % ch. in rate	-	-	-	–15.1	–16.6	–11.1
ITALY						
Deaths 1980–84	3	25	74	255	729	1654
Deaths 1985–89	3	12	46	141	473	1287
Death rate 1980–84	0.01	0.06	0.19	0.69	2.03	5.65
Death rate 1985–89	0.01	0.03	0.11	0.37	1.30	3.82
Ann. % ch. in rate	-	–14.5	–9.7	–11.6	–8.5	–7.6
IRELAND						
Deaths 1980–84	1	1	1	8	54	120
Deaths 1985–89	0	3	4	7	29	94
Death rate 1980–84	0.03	0.03	0.04	0.45	3.60	8.36
Death rate 1985–89	0.00	0.10	0.16	0.33	1.88	6.66
Ann. % ch. in rate	-	-	-	–5.8	–12.2	–4.4
THE NETHERLANDS						
Deaths 1980–84	1	5	10	39	99	228

Table 9.3(m)—*cont.*

	Age group (years)					
	5–14	15–24	25–34	35–44	45–54	55–64
Deaths 1985–89	0	4	9	21	56	141
Death rate 1980–84	0.01	0.04	0.09	0.41	1.31	3.40
Death rate 1985–89	0.00	0.04	0.09	0.24	0.88	2.53
Ann. % ch. in rate	-	-	2.0	–11.5	–8.4	–6.3
UK: ENGLAND AND WALES						
Deaths 1980–84	1	14	32	129	393	1457
Deaths 1985–89	6	23	49	198	561	2078
Death rate 1980–84	0.01	0.06	0.16	0.67	2.38	8.68
Death rate 1985–89	0.02	0.06	0.14	0.57	2.04	7.78
Ann. % ch. in rate	40.0	–0.1	–3.4	–3.8	–3.9	–2.7
UK: N. IRELAND						
Deaths 1980–84	1	0	2	8	21	59
Deaths 1985–89	0	0	0	7	14	60
Death rate 1980–84	0.07	0.00	0.20	0.90	2.76	8.25
Death rate 1985–89	0.00	0.00	0.00	0.74	1.79	8.53
Ann. % ch. in rate	-	-	-	–3.8	–8.3	0.7
UK: SCOTLAND						
Deaths 1980–84	0	4	13	37	123	299
Deaths 1985–89	0	4	3	26	75	276
Death rate 1980–84	0.00	0.09	0.36	1.19	4.23	10.70
Death rate 1985–89	0.00	0.10	0.08	0.78	2.63	10.08
Ann. % ch. in rate	-	-	–26.1	–8.2	–9.1	–1.2
PORTUGAL						
Deaths 1980–84	*	*	37	75	167	316
Deaths 1985–89	1	4	18	34	104	262
Death rate 1980–84	*	*	0.55	1.31	2.89	6.29
Death rate 1985–89	0.01	0.05	0.24	0.55	1.84	4.85
Ann. % ch. in rate	*	*	–15.3	–16.1	–8.7	–5.0
SPAIN						
Deaths 1980–84	4	19	65	137	390	897
Deaths 1985–89	2	8	32	75	168	463
Death rate 1980–84	0.01	0.06	0.26	0.64	1.68	4.93
Death rate 1985–89	0.01	0.03	0.15	0.46	0.83	2.96
Ann. % ch. in rate	-	–14.8	–11.6	–7.2	–14.5	–10.7
EC						
Deaths 1980–84	22	134	448	1486	4128	9397
Deaths 1985–89	19	111	319	982	2815	7639
Death rate 1980–84	0.01	0.05	0.20	0.73	2.15	5.70
Death rate 1985–89	0.01	0.04	0.13	0.46	1.42	4.37
Ann. % ch. in rate	–1.3	–3.7	–7.5	–8.7	–7.9	–5.2

* Portugal did not supply data for this disease for 1980–84 in this age-group.

Table 9.3(n) All causes.

	Age group (years)					
	5–14	15–24	25–34	35–44	45–54	55–64
BELGIUM						
Deaths 1980–84	1816	6366	7666	11457	30059	66388
Deaths 1985–89	1380	5582	7341	12170	24398	65142
Death rate 1980–84	27.63	81.42	102.96	190.65	497.62	1213.90
Death rate 1985–89	22.09	74.43	94.04	181.18	424.46	1111.64
Ann. % ch. in rate	–4.4	–1.8	–1.8	–1.0	–3.1	–1.7
LUXEMBOURG						
Deaths 1980–84	66	276	344	566	1357	2487
Deaths 1985–89	45	258	323	515	1127	2520
Death rate 1980–84	28.33	96.84	119.03	231.49	560.74	1409.07
Death rate 1985–89	21.53	96.09	103.86	191.10	486.83	1188.68
Ann. % ch. in rate	–5.3	–0.2	–2.7	–3.8	–2.8	–3.3
FEDERAL REPUBLIC OF GERMANY						
Deaths 1980–84	9638	42337	41620	90294	199955	369626
Deaths 1985–89	6070	30959	38742	69522	196240	383081
Death rate 1980–84	26.06	83.14	96.71	206.62	505.45	1153.23
Death rate 1985–89	20.06	64.12	82.36	173.00	440.80	1102.71
Ann. % ch. in rate	–5.1	–5.1	–3.2	–3.5	–2.7	–0.9
DENMARK						
Deaths 1980–84	802	2578	3855	6874	14558	35992
Deaths 1985–89	640	2369	3623	7679	14729	34264
Death rate 1980–84	22.27	65.88	101.21	190.10	532.38	1329.34
Death rate 1985–89	19.97	60.27	96.49	194.73	503.13	1331.68
Ann. % ch. in rate	–2.2	–1.8	–1.0	0.5	–1.1	0.0
FRANCE						
Deaths 1980–84	10482	39820	47940	66241	167659	301588
Deaths 1985–89	7944	33509	46405	76537	138739	308234
Death rate 1980–84	25.88	92.44	111.95	203.77	532.89	1085.30
Death rate 1985–89	20.34	77.68	108.86	198.84	471.00	1038.54
Ann. % ch. in rate	–4.7	–3.4	–0.6	–0.5	–2.4	–0.9
GREECE						
Deaths 1980–84	1213	2800	2934	4843	13647	26239
Deaths 1985–89	1468	5204	5511	8405	21064	51505
Death rate 1980–84	26.44	65.25	74.32	132.97	341.13	972.90
Death rate 1985–89	18.59	70.57	81.27	134.22	306.12	1110.14
Ann. % ch. in rate	–5.7	1.3	1.5	0.2	–1.8	2.2
ITALY						
Deaths 1980–84	11846	29320	29674	58735	165447	330403
Deaths 1985–89	7332	27239	30089	51520	135792	347848
Death rate 1980–84	27.08	66.61	75.51	158.46	460.77	1129.29
Death rate 1985–89	19.66	58.98	73.76	135.67	374.24	1031.10
Ann. % ch. in rate	–5.2	–2.0	–0.4	–2.6	–3.4	–1.5
IRELAND						
Deaths 1980–84	922	2122	1907	3100	7964	21278
Deaths 1985–89	768	1855	1809	3017	6871	19122
Death rate 1980–84	26.76	70.62	80.04	173.09	530.93	1481.76
Death rate 1985–89	21.92	60.08	72.20	143.16	444.29	1355.21
Ann. % ch. in rate	–3.9	–3.2	–2.0	–3.7	–3.5	–1.8
THE NETHERLANDS						
Deaths 1980–84	2572	6626	7844	12889	30299	71197

Table 9.3(n)—*cont.*

	Age group (years)					
	5–14	15–24	25–34	35–44	45–54	55–64
Deaths 1985–89	1399	4729	6181	11518	23447	57248
Death rate 1980–84	23.94	53.38	66.83	135.53	399.59	1060.27
Death rate 1985–89	18.91	47.75	63.85	129.73	368.15	1026.54
Ann. % ch. in rate	−5.1	−2.4	−1.0	−1.0	−1.8	−0.7
UK: ENGLAND AND WALES						
Deaths 1980–84	7704	22305	23903	45802	130763	372088
Deaths 1985–89	6007	21196	23816	47912	112293	332154
Death rate 1980–84	23.26	55.40	69.76	142.36	475.60	1329.24
Death rate 1985–89	19.38	53.26	65.79	138.76	407.29	1243.09
Ann. % ch. in rate	−3.6	−0.8	−1.2	−0.5	−3.1	−1.3
UK: N. IRELAND						
Deaths 1980–84	370	1026	994	1638	4162	11244
Deaths 1985–89	291	1009	946	1519	3629	10012
Death rate 1980–84	26.80	75.08	98.22	184.56	547.27	1571.49
Death rate 1985–89	22.33	72.70	85.38	160.83	464.66	1423.17
Ann. % ch. in rate	−3.6	−0.6	−2.8	−2.7	−3.2	−2.0
UK: SCOTLAND						
Deaths 1980–84	995	2788	3149	6245	17995	46031
Deaths 1985–89	699	2669	3192	6131	15238	42673
Death rate 1980–84	26.60	63.57	87.64	201.06	619.24	1646.61
Death rate 1985–89	21.59	63.06	84.61	182.82	533.64	1558.55
Ann. % ch. in rate	−4.1	−0.2	−0.7	−1.9	−2.9	−1.1
PORTUGAL						
Deaths 1980–84	4165	8813	9075	13602	31218	58852
Deaths 1985–89	3162	8561	9197	13044	27734	59039
Death rate 1980–84	48.93	105.61	133.56	237.07	540.71	1170.49
Death rate 1985–89	39.34	99.32	121.09	208.99	490.13	1093.42
Ann. % ch. in rate	−4.3	−1.2	−1.9	−2.5	−1.9	−1.4
SPAIN						
Deaths 1980–84	9886	20107	21825	35246	93792	179247
Deaths 1985–89	5877	18712	20258	29769	65822	152135
Death rate 1980–84	29.96	64.71	87.25	164.85	404.25	984.31
Death rate 1985–89	21.56	69.53	94.43	181.60	324.63	973.93
Ann. % ch. in rate	−5.8	1.3	1.4	1.8	−3.9	−0.2
EC						
Deaths 1980–84	62950	188353	203868	359193	913600	1901471
Deaths 1985–89	44861	169583	203896	349346	808938	1916138
Death rate 1980–84	26.99	72.99	89.39	176.25	476.25	1153.54
Death rate 1985–89	20.91	65.27	85.24	164.31	409.04	1095.51
Ann. % ch. in rate	−5.0	−2.2	−0.9	−1.4	−3.0	−1.0

Table 9.4. Age-standardized mortality rates for 1980–84 and 1985–89, and annual percentage changes in mortality rates between 1980–84 and 1985–89, by disease, small area and country.

Notes on the use of this table

1. This table shows age-standardized mortality rates (based on the EC standard) for 1980–84 and 1985–89, and annual percentage changes in age-standardized mortality rates between 1980–84 and 1985–89.

2. The mortality data for the later period are for 1985–89 and cover five years, except for The Netherlands (four years, 1985–88), and Spain (four years, 1985–88). The population data are for 1985–89, except for France (1987), Greece (1987), Ireland (1986), and Spain (1986).

3. The mortality data for the earlier period are for 1980–84 and cover five years, except for Greece (three years, 1980–82), Spain (five years, 1979–83), Italy (five years, 1979–83), and England and Wales (Cancer of the breast, Ischaemic heart disease and Peptic ulcers only: three years, 1982–84). The population data are for 1980–84, except for France (1982), Greece (1981), Ireland (1981), Spain (1981), Italy (1979–83), and England and Wales (1982–84).

4. All countries supplied data according to the 9th revision of the International Classification of Diseases except for Denmark where 8th revision coding rules applied.

Table 9.4(a)

Area		Age-standardized mortality rates (per 100000) and percentage changes TUB			CERV			UTER		
		1980–84	1985–89	Annual % change	1980–84	1985–89	Annual % change	1980–84	1985–89	Annual % change
BELGIUM		0.84	0.49	−10.0	3.20	2.97	−1.5	3.48	3.23	−1.5
1	Antwerpen	0.30	0.18	−9.8	3.54	3.82	1.6	3.11	3.30	1.2
2	Brabant	1.27	0.65	−12.5	2.54	2.68	1.1	3.63	3.38	−1.4
3	West-Vlaanderen	0.54	0.33	−9.7	3.24	1.55	−13.7	3.09	3.39	1.8
4	Oost-Vlaanderen	0.34	0.25	−6.0	3.59	3.96	2.0	3.33	3.62	1.7
5	Hainaut	1.38	1.04	−5.4	4.60	2.36	−12.5	3.61	3.01	−3.5
6	Liege	0.96	0.72	−5.6	2.16	3.46	9.9	4.07	2.43	−9.8
7	Limburg	0.62	0.24	−17.0	3.08	2.80	−1.9	3.51	3.44	−0.4
8	Luxembourg (province)	0.35	0.11	−20.6	2.55	2.43	−0.9	3.21	3.20	−0.1
9	Namur	1.36	0.35	−23.6	2.98	3.13	1.0	3.92	2.58	−8.0
LUXEMBOURG		0.35	0.51	7.7	3.13	3.97	4.9	4.32	3.90	−2.0
10	Luxembourg	0.35	0.51	7.7	3.13	3.97	4.9	4.32	3.90	−2.0
FEDERAL REPUBLIC OF GERMANY		1.15	0.70	−9.4	4.62	3.88	−3.4	4.22	3.66	−2.8
11	Schleswig-Holstein	0.89	0.45	−12.9	5.11	4.49	−2.6	4.56	4.32	−1.1
12	Hamburg	0.96	0.64	−7.7	5.05	4.73	−1.3	4.72	4.09	−2.8
13	Braunschweig	1.04	0.89	−2.9	4.62	4.06	−2.5	4.31	4.19	−0.6
14	Hannover	1.10	0.65	−10.0	5.68	5.20	−1.8	5.11	4.77	−1.4
15	Lüneburg	0.91	0.50	−11.3	4.14	3.68	−2.4	3.65	3.02	−3.7
16	Weser-Ems	0.86	0.70	−4.0	5.28	4.08	−5.0	4.96	3.26	−8.1
17	Bremen	0.93	0.97	0.9	5.48	5.36	−0.4	5.32	4.13	−4.9
18	Düsseldorf	1.05	0.67	−8.5	5.31	4.47	−3.4	4.33	3.91	−2.0
19	Köln	1.18	0.54	−14.5	4.92	3.76	−5.2	4.19	3.35	−4.4
20	Munster	0.91	0.48	−12.1	4.26	3.33	−4.8	4.00	3.33	−3.6
21	Detmold	0.95	0.39	−16.3	4.12	2.77	−7.6	3.69	3.07	−3.6
22	Arnsberg	1.11	0.64	−10.6	4.63	3.94	−3.2	4.30	3.87	−2.1
23	Darmstadt	1.08	0.70	−8.2	3.82	3.62	−1.0	3.48	3.26	−1.3
24	Giessen	1.15	0.59	−12.5	3.11	3.05	−0.3	3.38	4.05	3.6
25	Kassel	0.78	0.65	−3.7	3.86	3.52	−1.8	4.04	3.22	−4.4
26	Koblenz	0.95	0.49	−12.5	3.72	3.70	−0.1	3.28	3.86	3.3
27	Trier	1.10	0.68	−9.1	5.56	3.93	−6.7	6.01	3.86	−8.5
28	Rheinhessen-Pfalz	0.97	0.67	−7.2	4.84	3.57	−5.9	4.41	3.87	−2.6
29	Stuttgart	0.97	0.68	−6.9	3.82	2.91	−5.3	3.55	3.08	−2.8
30	Karlsruhe	1.59	1.01	−8.5	4.25	3.01	−6.7	3.51	2.98	−3.2
31	Freiburg	1.47	0.84	−10.7	3.60	3.56	−0.3	4.16	2.99	−6.3
32	Tübingen	1.02	0.65	−8.6	3.19	2.93	−1.7	2.97	3.12	1.0
33	Oberbayern	1.03	0.72	−6.9	3.82	3.00	−4.7	3.39	3.07	−2.0
34	Niederbayern	1.65	1.47	−2.2	5.21	3.92	−5.5	5.78	4.14	−6.4
35	Oberpfalz	2.14	1.13	−12.0	5.16	4.45	−2.9	5.46	4.60	−3.4
36	Oberfranken	2.97	1.16	−17.1	4.98	4.31	−2.8	4.34	4.63	1.3
37	Mittelfranken	1.86	1.48	−4.4	4.48	4.84	1.6	4.77	4.71	−0.2
38	Unterfranken	1.29	0.56	−15.4	3.99	3.49	−2.7	3.39	2.94	−2.8

Table 9.4(a)—*cont.*

	Area	Age-standardized mortality rates (per 100000) and percentage changes TUB			CERV			UTER		
		1980–84	1985–89	Annual % change	1980–84	1985–89	Annual % change	1980–84	1985–89	Annual % change
39	Schwaben	0.73	0.47	−8.5	4.00	2.84	−6.6	4.03	2.33	−10.4
40	Saarland	1.35	0.80	−10.0	4.33	4.02	−1.5	3.73	3.49	−1.3
41	Berlin (West)	1.57	0.78	−13.1	8.91	7.07	−4.5	7.81	6.01	−5.1
DENMARK		0.49	0.40	−4.1	9.14	6.89	−5.5	6.86	4.65	−7.5
42	Kobenhavn and Frederiksberg (M)	1.08	0.87	−4.2	12.33	8.05	−8.2	9.74	6.72	−7.1
43	Kobenhavns County	0.50	0.42	−3.2	6.71	4.56	−7.5	4.47	2.71	−9.5
44	Frederiksborg County	0.42	0.08	−28.9	5.52	3.97	−6.4	4.35	3.66	−3.4
45	Roskilde County	0.28	0.12	−15.1	8.49	6.14	−6.3	6.41	4.90	−5.2
46	Vestsjællands County	0.46	0.36	−4.8	8.59	7.82	−1.9	6.67	4.61	−7.1
47	Storstroms County	0.28	0.38	6.0	7.91	6.89	−2.7	7.38	3.93	−11.9
48	Bornholms County	0.53	0.00	−100.0	10.66	6.55	−9.3	6.72	6.33	−1.2
49	Fyns County	0.51	0.45	−2.5	10.17	7.67	−5.5	7.96	4.60	−10.4
50	Sonderjyllands County	0.21	0.71	27.2	9.04	8.60	−1.0	6.97	6.30	−2.0
51	Ribe County	0.76	0.74	−0.6	10.20	7.39	−6.2	6.97	5.45	−4.8
52	Vejle County	0.40	0.08	−27.8	10.87	7.53	−7.1	7.28	5.03	−7.1
53	Ringkobing County	0.10	0.20	14.2	7.36	5.33	−6.3	5.07	3.90	−5.1
54	Århus County	0.38	0.37	−0.4	9.21	8.53	−1.5	7.58	5.67	−5.6
55	Viborg County	0.34	0.34	−0.1	11.48	7.69	−7.7	6.21	3.93	−8.8
56	Nordjyllands County	0.43	0.27	−8.9	9.41	7.19	−5.2	8.35	4.41	−12.0
FRANCE		1.33	0.77	−10.3	2.75	2.38	−2.8	4.02	3.45	−3.0
57	Ain	0.71	0.60	−3.3	2.20	1.88	−3.1	2.59	2.60	0.0
58	Aisne	1.62	0.63	−17.2	2.48	2.62	1.1	4.21	3.67	−2.7
59	Allier	0.85	0.63	−5.8	2.10	2.52	3.7	5.56	3.83	−7.2
60	Alpes-de-Haute-Provence	1.03	0.37	−18.4	2.56	2.80	1.8	1.92	1.79	−1.5
61	Hautes-Alpes	1.89	0.90	−13.7	0.59	0.00	−100.0	0.75	1.41	13.4
62	Alpes-Maritimes	1.21	0.75	−9.1	2.30	2.68	3.1	3.81	3.79	−0.1
63	Ardèche	1.58	0.44	−22.6	2.57	2.21	−3.0	4.13	2.03	−13.3
64	Ardennes	1.75	0.79	−14.8	3.83	2.79	−6.1	6.10	4.88	−4.4
65	Ariège	1.19	0.83	−6.9	3.96	2.13	−11.6	3.49	3.58	0.5
66	Aube	1.78	0.72	−16.5	4.99	3.48	−7.0	6.29	5.15	−3.9
67	Aude	0.75	0.64	−3.2	1.47	2.20	8.4	1.93	2.75	7.3
68	Aveyron	0.96	0.75	−4.8	1.77	1.70	−0.7	2.25	3.16	7.0
69	Bouches-du-Rhône	1.34	0.76	−10.8	2.32	1.93	−3.6	3.60	3.10	−2.9
70	Calvados	1.57	0.99	−8.9	3.50	3.60	0.6	4.41	4.42	0.1
71	Cantal	1.51	0.59	−17.2	3.07	1.89	−9.3	3.42	4.05	3.4
72	Charente	0.90	0.50	−11.1	4.45	2.47	−11.1	6.82	4.08	−9.7
73	Charente-Maritime	0.92	0.60	−8.4	2.63	1.58	−9.7	4.58	2.56	−11.0
74	Cher	1.45	0.39	−23.3	3.18	1.15	−18.5	4.18	2.94	−6.8
75	Corrèze	1.16	0.09	−39.4	1.46	1.42	−0.5	4.47	4.58	0.5
76	Corse	1.21	0.10	−39.7	1.28	1.71	5.9	3.27	3.80	3.1
77	Côte-d'Or	0.65	0.78	3.9	4.92	4.26	−2.8	4.52	4.21	−1.4
78	Côtes-du-Nord	1.18	0.74	−8.8	2.36	1.52	−8.5	4.32	2.82	−8.2
79	Creuse	0.83	0.80	−0.8	0.88	2.54	23.6	5.96	3.74	−8.9
80	Dordogne	1.46	0.41	−22.6	2.79	1.90	−7.4	5.34	4.71	−2.5
81	Doubs	1.02	0.57	−10.9	3.16	2.45	−5.0	3.80	2.57	−7.6
82	Drôme	1.01	0.12	−34.3	4.06	2.82	−7.0	4.28	4.59	1.4
83	Eure	1.16	0.96	−3.7	3.82	3.93	0.6	5.53	6.15	2.2
84	Eure-et-Loir	0.93	0.72	−5.0	3.00	1.21	−16.6	6.00	2.54	−15.8
85	Finistère	1.47	1.24	−3.4	2.00	2.51	4.7	3.40	3.33	−0.4
86	Gard	1.20	0.95	−4.5	1.35	2.10	9.2	2.40	4.46	13.2
87	Haute-Garonne	1.02	0.36	−19.0	2.41	2.02	−3.5	5.27	2.51	−13.8
88	Gers	0.41	0.38	−1.5	2.42	2.61	1.5	5.28	5.72	1.6
89	Gironde	1.19	0.50	−15.8	2.41	2.28	−1.1	4.24	3.10	−6.0
90	Hérault	0.81	0.63	−5.1	1.70	2.68	9.5	3.12	3.14	0.1
91	Ille-et-Vilaine	1.54	0.69	−14.8	2.88	2.47	−3.0	3.14	3.46	2.0
92	Indre	0.82	0.69	−3.5	2.32	0.74	−20.3	2.90	2.66	−1.8
93	Indre-et-Loire	0.81	0.71	−2.6	3.12	2.19	−6.8	3.44	4.20	4.1
94	Isère	1.36	0.60	−15.0	3.65	2.92	−4.4	3.29	2.92	−2.3
95	Jura	0.75	0.71	−0.9	2.88	2.01	−6.9	3.27	4.20	5.1

Table 9.4(a)—*cont.*

	Area	TUB 1980–84	TUB 1985–89	TUB Annual % change	CERV 1980–84	CERV 1985–89	CERV Annual % change	UTER 1980–84	UTER 1985–89	UTER Annual % change
96	Landes	0.58	0.53	−1.8	2.04	1.69	−3.7	1.53	2.24	7.9
97	Loir-et-Cher	0.98	0.41	−15.8	4.42	4.30	−0.5	5.77	7.16	4.4
98	Loire	1.37	0.61	−15.0	2.61	2.92	2.3	3.52	3.88	2.0
99	Haute-Loire	0.85	0.57	−7.5	0.61	1.45	19.1	2.31	2.34	0.3
100	Loire-Atlantique	1.89	1.04	−11.3	2.22	1.22	−11.3	3.17	1.95	−9.3
101	Loiret	0.51	0.91	12.1	3.20	1.94	−9.5	3.82	3.49	−1.8
102	Lot	0.60	0.57	−1.1	3.06	0.36	−34.7	5.61	0.51	−38.1
103	Lot-et-Garonne	0.87	0.15	−29.3	2.36	1.52	−8.4	3.99	2.78	−7.0
104	Lozère	2.01	0.33	−30.4	1.77	1.72	−0.5	3.50	4.57	5.5
105	Maine-et-Loire	1.47	0.72	−13.2	2.14	0.96	−14.9	3.28	2.24	−7.3
106	Manche	0.88	0.47	−11.8	2.04	3.25	9.7	3.23	3.93	4.0
107	Marne	1.07	0.92	−3.0	2.92	2.77	−1.0	3.37	4.34	5.2
108	Haute-Marne	1.45	1.64	2.5	1.62	2.50	9.1	4.32	1.99	−14.4
109	Mayenne	1.28	0.76	−10.1	1.93	2.08	1.5	2.36	1.76	−5.7
110	Meurthe-et-Moselle	2.00	0.59	−21.8	4.40	2.54	−10.4	4.35	3.33	−5.2
111	Meuse	0.54	0.64	3.4	2.33	2.85	4.1	3.62	3.75	0.7
112	Morbihan	2.76	0.98	−18.7	1.71	2.40	7.0	2.14	2.76	5.1
113	Moselle	1.45	0.84	−10.3	3.56	2.35	−8.0	4.33	2.47	−10.6
114	Nièvre	1.67	0.70	−15.9	2.08	2.77	5.9	4.78	3.44	−6.4
115	Nord	2.31	1.36	−10.1	3.49	2.86	−3.9	4.70	4.18	−2.3
116	Oise	1.25	0.82	−8.0	3.86	2.64	−7.3	4.84	4.64	−0.9
117	Orne	0.88	0.59	−7.6	2.61	1.67	−8.5	4.30	2.17	−12.8
118	Pas-de-Calais	2.23	1.34	−9.7	3.42	3.08	−2.1	4.43	4.05	−1.8
119	Puy-de-dôme	1.30	0.75	−10.5	1.58	2.21	7.0	2.90	3.42	3.4
120	Pyrénées-Atlantiques	1.36	1.11	−4.0	1.42	2.17	8.8	3.49	3.31	−1.0
121	Hautes-Pyrénées	0.73	0.30	−16.2	2.05	1.98	−0.7	3.85	5.50	7.4
122	Pyrénées-Orientales	0.90	1.11	4.1	1.54	1.44	−1.3	4.29	2.63	−9.4
123	Bas-Rhin	1.71	0.77	−14.6	4.63	3.11	−7.7	5.04	3.62	−6.4
124	Haut-Rhin	1.26	1.10	−2.6	2.98	2.63	−2.4	4.60	4.04	−2.6
125	Rhône	0.95	0.78	−4.0	2.81	2.38	−3.3	3.02	3.23	1.4
126	Haute-Saône	1.41	0.23	−30.7	3.17	3.34	1.0	1.08	3.18	24.0
127	Saône-et-Loire	0.90	0.52	−10.4	3.10	2.25	−6.2	3.71	2.78	−5.6
128	Sarthe	0.65	0.36	−11.2	2.88	2.99	0.7	3.29	3.42	0.8
129	Savoie	1.63	0.46	−22.5	3.54	2.75	−4.9	3.75	2.91	−5.0
130	Haute-Savoie	1.40	0.91	−8.3	3.95	2.36	−9.8	3.77	3.84	0.4
131	Paris	1.74	1.18	−7.5	3.00	2.86	−0.9	4.99	4.20	−3.4
132	Seine-Maritime	2.51	0.95	−17.7	4.24	2.40	−10.7	5.91	3.54	−9.7
133	Seine-et-Marne	1.28	0.72	−10.7	2.17	1.58	−6.1	4.38	3.24	−5.9
134	Yvelines	0.90	0.51	−10.8	2.62	1.73	−8.0	3.99	2.63	−8.0
135	Deux-Sèvres	0.69	0.80	2.9	0.57	2.00	28.4	2.34	2.10	−2.1
136	Somme	1.60	0.84	−12.1	2.37	3.93	10.7	4.78	5.85	4.1
137	Tarn	0.35	0.13	−17.5	1.57	1.00	−8.6	2.84	1.56	−11.3
138	Tarn-et-Garonne	0.77	0.73	−1.2	3.52	0.90	−23.8	4.04	1.60	−16.9
139	Var	1.31	0.88	−7.6	2.64	2.08	−4.7	4.22	3.42	−4.1
140	Vaucluse	0.66	0.56	−3.3	1.73	3.08	12.2	2.96	3.97	6.1
141	Vendée	0.84	0.51	−9.6	1.92	1.00	−12.2	3.43	2.14	−9.0
142	Vienne	1.09	0.76	−7.1	2.51	3.22	5.1	4.87	3.87	−4.5
143	Haute-Vienne	0.84	0.53	−8.6	2.23	0.98	−15.2	4.31	2.37	−11.3
144	Vosges	1.10	0.60	−11.5	2.14	1.61	−5.5	4.19	4.11	−0.4
145	Yonne	0.92	1.11	3.8	3.80	3.58	−1.2	4.88	3.19	−8.2
146	Territoire-de-Belfort	0.84	0.40	−13.8	3.48	2.39	−7.3	6.24	3.48	−11.1
147	Essonne	1.03	0.73	−6.6	2.62	2.30	−2.6	2.73	3.43	4.7
148	Hauts-de-Seine	1.31	0.65	−13.2	2.35	2.66	2.5	3.74	3.74	0.0
149	Seine-Saint-Denis	1.53	0.89	−10.3	2.34	2.81	3.8	4.30	3.90	−2.0
150	Val-de-Marne	1.07	0.78	−6.1	2.79	2.57	−1.7	4.36	3.56	−4.0
151	Val-d'Oise	1.34	0.76	−10.8	2.02	2.06	0.5	4.10	2.56	−9.0
GREECE		1.67	0.79	−11.8	1.73	1.76	0.3	3.68	2.91	−3.9
152	Greater Athens	1.72	0.71	−13.7	2.52	2.35	−1.2	3.90	3.14	−3.6
153	Rest of Central Greece and Eubea	1.37	0.45	−16.9	1.35	1.08	−3.7	2.44	2.49	0.3
154	Peloponnisos	1.41	0.79	−9.2	1.37	1.52	1.7	3.35	2.49	−4.9

Age-standardized mortality rates (per 100000) and percentage changes

Table 9.4(a)—*cont.*

Area		TUB 1980–84	TUB 1985–89	TUB Annual % change	CERV 1980–84	CERV 1985–89	CERV Annual % change	UTER 1980–84	UTER 1985–89	UTER Annual % change
		Age-standardized mortality rates (per 100000) and percentage changes								
155	Ionian Islands	0.66	0.64	–0.5	1.58	2.17	5.4	2.52	1.85	–5.0
156	Epirus	1.49	0.87	–8.5	0.94	0.37	–14.5	1.40	3.26	15.2
157	Thessaly	1.86	0.79	–13.2	1.01	0.93	–1.3	4.44	2.51	–9.1
158	Macedonia	1.76	0.93	–10.1	1.38	2.13	7.5	3.72	3.18	–2.6
159	Thrace	4.26	2.43	–8.9	0.95	0.96	0.2	2.31	4.22	10.6
160	Aegean Islands	1.75	0.54	–17.9	1.77	1.48	–2.9	5.93	2.26	–14.9
161	Crete	0.62	0.62	–0.2	1.70	1.10	–6.9	5.55	2.23	–14.1
ITALY		1.42	0.65	–12.2	1.23	1.00	–3.4	4.38	2.66	–8.0
162	Torino	1.65	0.65	–14.5	2.04	1.36	–6.6	4.40	2.26	–10.5
163	Vercelli	1.12	0.87	–4.1	2.35	0.93	–14.3	4.73	2.59	–9.6
164	Novara	1.76	1.07	–8.0	1.13	1.07	–0.9	4.69	2.26	–11.5
165	Cuneo	1.80	1.40	–4.0	2.12	1.51	–5.5	4.56	3.22	–5.6
166	Asti	1.20	1.21	0.2	1.05	2.76	17.5	4.15	1.67	–14.1
167	Alessandria	1.27	0.46	–15.5	1.17	1.14	–0.4	4.13	2.40	–8.6
168	Aosta	2.99	2.52	–2.8	0.51	1.90	24.7	5.29	4.13	–4.0
169	Imperia	1.83	0.57	–17.8	3.32	2.51	–4.5	7.75	2.67	–16.3
170	Savona	1.41	0.77	–9.6	1.40	0.86	–7.9	2.98	3.29	1.7
171	Genova	1.53	0.84	–9.6	1.47	1.09	–4.9	3.47	3.16	–1.5
172	La Spezia	0.90	0.88	–0.4	1.51	1.73	2.3	4.64	3.48	–4.7
173	Varese	1.06	0.59	–9.4	0.97	1.03	1.0	2.51	2.20	–2.2
174	Como/Sondrio	1.69	0.37	–22.4	1.20	0.93	–4.1	3.43	1.96	–9.0
175	Milano	1.20	0.50	–13.4	0.96	0.94	–0.3	3.34	2.31	–5.9
176	Bergamo	2.72	0.66	–21.0	0.56	0.75	5.2	4.50	2.01	–12.5
177	Brescia	2.97	1.02	–16.3	1.35	1.13	–2.9	2.81	2.61	–1.2
178	Pavia	1.44	0.79	–9.5	1.16	1.62	5.7	5.11	3.42	–6.5
179	Cremona	1.92	0.52	–19.6	2.01	0.32	–26.5	3.58	2.24	–7.5
180	Mantova	1.25	0.47	–15.2	0.59	0.85	6.2	3.40	2.72	–3.6
181	Bolzano	2.23	0.88	–14.4	1.49	2.09	5.8	3.59	1.51	–13.5
182	Trento	3.06	1.58	–10.4	2.33	1.14	–11.2	4.06	1.60	–14.4
183	Verona	1.35	0.44	–16.9	1.22	0.85	–5.9	3.38	2.09	–7.7
184	Vicenza	1.40	0.52	–15.1	1.44	0.93	–7.0	2.92	1.31	–12.5
185	Belluno	3.40	1.25	–15.3	1.29	0.50	–14.5	4.79	1.96	–13.8
186	Treviso	1.37	0.62	–12.4	1.63	1.09	–6.5	3.29	2.00	–7.9
187	Venezia	1.34	0.63	–11.8	2.18	0.39	–24.9	3.40	1.03	–18.0
188	Padova	1.63	0.58	–15.8	1.05	1.31	3.8	2.65	1.50	–9.0
189	Rovigo	1.05	0.44	–13.6	2.04	0.65	–17.5	2.73	1.42	–10.3
190	Udine/Gorizia	1.91	0.60	–17.6	2.57	1.20	–12.0	3.96	2.71	–6.1
191	Trieste	2.12	1.15	–9.6	1.58	1.83	2.5	4.13	2.17	–10.2
192	Pordenone	1.13	0.51	–12.4	2.20	0.82	–15.2	3.15	3.01	–0.7
193	Piacenza	1.04	0.08	–35.4	1.35	1.13	–3.0	3.07	2.23	–5.2
194	Parma	1.45	0.58	–14.2	0.94	1.17	3.8	3.98	2.72	–6.1
195	Reggio Emilia	0.72	0.31	–13.1	1.08	1.03	–0.7	3.12	2.14	–6.1
196	Modena	0.98	0.22	–22.2	0.93	0.79	–2.6	3.34	2.10	–7.5
197	Bologna	1.17	0.49	–13.5	1.10	1.62	6.6	3.33	2.47	–4.9
198	Ferrara	0.87	0.22	–20.4	1.38	2.30	8.9	2.86	1.22	–13.2
199	Ravenna	0.45	0.12	–19.9	0.77	0.73	–0.8	4.33	2.40	–9.4
200	Forli	0.97	0.37	–15.0	1.25	1.07	–2.5	2.92	2.41	–3.1
201	Pesaro	0.58	0.27	–12.1	0.35	0.99	19.0	2.72	1.26	–12.1
202	Ancona	0.91	0.35	–14.9	1.53	0.36	–21.3	3.05	1.84	–8.0
203	Macerata	1.18	0.15	–29.4	0.38	1.09	19.2	3.86	1.62	–13.5
204	Ascoli Piceno	1.41	0.18	–28.8	0.80	0.15	–24.4	4.16	1.71	–13.8
205	Massa-Carrara	2.53	0.63	–20.6	1.64	0.00	–100.0	6.01	4.43	–5.0
206	Lucca	1.96	1.09	–9.4	1.01	1.39	5.4	3.88	1.61	–13.6
207	Pistoia	1.43	0.25	–25.3	0.85	1.21	6.1	3.28	1.25	–14.9
208	Firenze	0.87	0.45	–10.4	1.00	0.65	–6.9	3.60	1.89	–10.2
209	Livorno	0.86	0.50	–8.5	0.63	0.31	–11.4	2.87	2.33	–3.4
210	Pisa	0.54	0.62	2.2	1.72	1.23	–5.4	3.59	2.57	–5.4
211	Arezzo	1.46	0.82	–9.2	1.60	1.70	1.0	4.55	2.42	–10.0
212	Siena	1.26	0.40	–17.4	0.62	0.60	–0.4	4.86	2.14	–12.8
213	Grosseto	1.00	0.38	–15.0	1.70	0.23	–28.2	3.25	4.53	5.7

Table 9.4(a)—*cont.*

Area		TUB 1980–84	TUB 1985–89	TUB Annual % change	CERV 1980–84	CERV 1985–89	CERV Annual % change	UTER 1980–84	UTER 1985–89	UTER Annual % change
		Age-standardized mortality rates (per 100000) and percentage changes								
214	Perugia	0.97	0.76	–4.1	0.57	1.16	12.8	2.28	1.73	–4.4
215	Terni	0.77	0.27	–15.8	2.33	0.68	–18.6	4.57	0.30	–36.6
216	Viterbo/Rieti	1.36	0.42	–17.9	0.69	1.17	9.2	4.42	2.06	–12.0
217	Roma	1.42	0.75	–10.2	1.67	1.07	–7.1	4.69	2.57	–9.5
218	Latina	1.30	0.44	–16.5	1.21	1.31	1.4	6.75	3.85	–8.9
219	Frosinone	1.13	0.96	–2.7	1.22	1.12	–1.5	5.45	4.27	–4.0
220	Caserta	0.83	0.79	–0.9	0.27	0.81	19.9	4.62	3.71	–3.6
221	Benevento	1.69	0.72	–13.2	0.85	0.60	–5.7	4.32	3.15	–5.1
222	Napoli	1.82	0.91	–11.0	0.98	1.12	2.3	6.77	4.02	–8.3
223	Avellino	0.73	0.44	–8.1	0.29	1.09	24.8	4.29	2.29	–9.9
224	Salerno	1.68	0.55	–16.9	0.58	0.53	–1.6	4.57	4.30	–1.0
225	L'Aquila	2.27	1.45	–7.2	1.93	1.31	–6.3	5.30	2.55	–11.5
226	Teramo	1.90	0.60	–17.6	0.23	1.05	29.0	5.06	2.62	–10.4
227	Pescara	1.14	0.87	–4.5	1.03	1.15	1.8	4.27	4.76	1.8
228	Chieti	1.45	0.54	–15.0	0.95	1.04	1.6	3.61	1.53	–13.3
229	Isernia/Campobasso	1.54	0.64	–13.7	1.10	0.52	–11.6	3.06	3.40	1.8
230	Foggia	1.69	0.58	–16.3	1.52	1.02	–6.3	5.11	3.52	–6.0
231	Bari	1.65	0.98	–8.3	1.46	0.76	–10.2	6.21	3.14	–10.7
232	Taranto	1.08	0.91	–2.9	0.59	0.74	3.9	5.23	3.96	–4.5
233	Brindisi	1.51	1.11	–5.1	1.15	1.82	7.9	7.37	3.32	–12.4
234	Lecce	1.65	0.73	–12.8	1.25	1.18	–0.9	4.64	3.32	–5.4
235	Potenza/Matera	1.54	0.69	–12.5	1.17	1.49	4.1	4.63	3.22	–5.9
236	Cosenza	1.17	0.47	–14.0	1.18	0.41	–16.2	6.64	2.89	–12.9
237	Catanzaro	1.38	1.08	–4.0	0.86	0.35	–13.9	4.56	3.29	–5.3
238	Reggio Calabria	1.41	0.81	–8.9	1.15	0.11	–32.5	4.52	4.12	–1.5
239	Trapani	1.16	0.58	–10.9	1.20	0.14	–30.2	9.82	3.62	–15.3
240	Palermo	0.76	0.42	–9.3	0.81	0.84	0.6	6.71	3.24	–11.4
241	Messina	0.73	0.28	–14.6	0.45	0.51	2.1	6.39	3.94	–7.7
242	Agrigento	0.84	0.37	–12.8	0.70	0.63	–1.5	5.86	2.68	–12.2
243	Caltanisetta	1.19	0.72	–8.1	0.23	0.85	24.5	5.55	3.69	–6.6
244	Enna	1.26	0.26	–23.3	0.98	0.31	–17.5	6.92	1.95	–19.0
245	Catania	0.92	0.51	–9.3	1.10	0.59	–10.0	7.15	3.95	–9.4
246	Ragusa	1.35	0.26	–24.0	1.58	1.46	–1.3	8.24	4.89	–8.3
247	Siracusa	1.00	0.26	–20.3	0.50	0.15	–17.9	5.76	4.94	–2.5
248	Sassari	2.23	0.77	–16.3	0.62	1.11	10.1	1.93	1.30	–6.3
249	Nuoro	1.41	1.26	–1.9	0.25	1.15	29.0	1.70	0.83	–11.2
250	Cagliari/Oristano	1.71	0.78	–12.3	1.18	1.12	–1.0	3.60	1.95	–9.7
IRELAND		2.17	1.08	–13.1	3.83	4.01	0.9	3.17	4.05	5.0
251	Eastern	1.83	0.75	–16.2	3.05	3.83	4.6	2.47	3.46	7.0
252	Midland	2.31	0.76	–19.9	4.83	4.61	–0.9	3.46	2.81	–4.1
253	Mid-Western	3.80	1.12	–21.7	3.12	3.50	2.3	3.82	4.75	4.4
254	North-Eastern	1.45	0.97	–7.6	4.51	4.25	–1.2	4.17	3.78	–2.0
255	North-Western	0.88	1.20	6.5	3.47	4.55	5.6	4.00	4.20	1.0
256	South-Eastern	2.38	1.32	–11.1	5.14	4.69	–1.8	3.16	4.62	7.9
257	Southern	2.14	1.42	–7.9	5.19	4.16	–4.3	3.48	5.49	9.5
258	Western	2.93	1.54	–12.0	2.81	3.23	2.8	3.30	3.70	2.3
THE NETHERLANDS		0.36	0.30	–4.2	3.59	2.92	–4.5	2.92	2.40	–4.2
259	Groningen	0.30	0.12	–17.9	3.14	3.24	0.7	1.47	2.61	13.6
260	Friesland	0.30	0.24	–4.9	4.02	2.94	–6.7	3.42	1.97	–11.6
261	Drenthe	0.57	0.37	–8.9	3.67	2.14	–11.3	3.84	1.48	–19.2
262	Overijssel	0.63	0.31	–15.0	2.84	2.60	–2.0	2.73	1.82	–8.6
263	Gelderland	0.26	0.27	0.2	3.27	2.24	–8.1	2.77	1.82	–8.9
264	Utrecht	0.56	0.36	–9.4	3.05	2.67	–3.0	2.80	2.86	0.5
265	Noord Holland	0.28	0.33	3.6	4.11	3.46	–3.7	2.82	2.64	–1.4
266	Zuid Holland	0.29	0.35	4.4	3.93	3.38	–3.3	3.23	2.91	–2.2
267	Zeeland	0.23	0.19	–4.5	5.42	2.92	–12.8	3.45	2.96	–3.4
268	Noord Brabant	0.33	0.28	–3.6	3.28	2.56	–5.4	2.92	2.23	–5.8
269	Limburg	0.63	0.31	–14.6	3.26	3.06	–1.4	2.91	2.23	–5.7
270	Flevoland	0.21	0.00	–100.0	1.47	1.90	5.8	0.83	1.62	16.1

Table 9.4(a)—*cont.*

Area		TUB 1980–84	TUB 1985–89	TUB Annual % change	CERV 1980–84	CERV 1985–89	CERV Annual % change	UTER 1980–84	UTER 1985–89	UTER Annual % change
		Age-standardized mortality rates (per 100000) and percentage changes								
UK: ENGLAND AND WALES		0.71	0.50	−7.0	6.57	6.24	−1.0	5.36	5.45	0.3
271	Northern	0.89	0.68	−5.3	7.82	7.05	−2.1	5.34	6.10	2.7
272	Yorkshire	0.77	0.41	−11.7	7.97	6.95	−2.7	6.28	5.72	−1.8
273	Trent	0.57	0.35	−9.3	6.98	6.99	0.0	5.96	6.01	0.2
274	East Anglian	0.48	0.25	−12.5	5.29	4.57	−2.9	4.03	4.06	0.2
275	North-West Thames	0.89	0.64	−6.5	4.93	5.20	1.1	4.01	4.54	2.5
276	North-East Thames	0.91	0.76	−3.6	5.70	5.17	−1.9	4.35	4.47	0.5
277	South-East Thames	0.78	0.60	−5.0	5.66	5.71	0.2	5.04	5.12	0.3
278	South-West Thames	0.58	0.47	−4.0	4.78	4.13	−2.9	4.07	3.83	−1.2
279	Wessex	0.44	0.26	−10.2	5.35	5.12	−0.9	4.27	4.69	1.9
280	Oxford	0.46	0.42	−1.5	3.73	4.93	5.7	3.22	3.99	4.4
281	South-Western	0.52	0.35	−7.7	6.05	6.31	0.8	5.30	6.13	2.9
282	West Midlands	0.81	0.59	−6.1	6.97	6.15	−2.5	6.11	5.49	−2.1
283	Mersey	0.82	0.46	−10.8	10.13	9.20	−1.9	8.92	7.48	−3.5
284	North-Western	0.81	0.62	−5.0	8.44	7.73	−1.7	6.39	6.72	1.0
285	Wales	0.70	0.35	−12.7	7.40	7.77	1.0	5.99	6.78	2.5
UK: NORTHERN IRELAND		0.70	0.36	−12.7	5.57	4.31	−5.0	4.85	3.93	−4.2
286	Northern Ireland	0.70	0.36	−12.7	5.57	4.31	−5.0	4.85	3.93	−4.2
UK: SCOTLAND		1.10	0.66	−9.6	6.85	6.57	−0.8	5.49	5.68	0.7
287	Highlands and Islands	0.40	0.38	−0.9	7.04	5.51	−4.8	5.90	4.12	−7.0
288	Grampian	0.72	0.48	−7.8	5.22	5.38	0.6	3.48	6.13	12.0
289	Tayside	0.76	0.44	−10.3	4.41	5.76	5.5	4.03	3.99	−0.2
290	Fife	0.23	0.45	14.7	10.50	6.45	−9.3	9.05	6.35	−6.9
291	Lothian	0.45	0.59	5.7	6.58	6.11	−1.5	6.00	4.91	−3.9
292	Borders	0.24	0.48	14.7	4.14	7.00	11.1	3.84	5.85	8.8
293	Forth Valley	1.13	0.47	−16.2	6.28	7.72	4.2	3.55	5.57	9.4
294	Argyll and Clyde	1.77	0.81	−14.6	7.06	8.77	4.4	4.98	7.10	7.4
295	Greater Glasgow	2.27	1.22	−11.7	6.90	6.11	−2.4	5.76	5.83	0.2
296	Lanarkshire	0.79	0.50	−8.6	7.42	6.89	−1.5	5.68	5.76	0.3
297	Ayrshire and Arran	1.09	0.54	−13.0	8.83	8.13	−1.6	6.54	6.77	0.7
298	Dumfries and Galloway	1.17	0.49	−16.1	6.12	5.95	−0.6	5.67	5.50	−0.6
PORTUGAL		4.26	2.83	−7.9	3.04	2.91	−0.9	5.63	5.21	−1.5
299	Viana do Castelo	3.88	3.11	−4.3	2.57	3.23	4.6	7.52	5.31	−6.7
300	Braga	3.40	1.92	−10.8	1.90	1.74	−1.7	4.88	3.99	−3.9
301	Vila Real	3.70	4.00	1.6	2.01	2.87	7.4	4.10	5.45	5.8
302	Bragança	2.05	2.66	5.3	2.73	3.57	5.5	7.43	8.57	2.9
303	Guarda	2.53	2.22	−2.6	1.47	0.96	−8.1	5.44	4.35	−4.4
304	Viseu	5.91	3.82	−8.4	2.58	1.90	−5.9	4.60	5.71	4.4
305	Porto	5.88	3.08	−12.1	4.11	3.41	−3.6	7.60	6.36	−3.5
306	Aveiro	2.93	2.05	−6.9	2.35	2.86	4.0	7.06	5.13	−6.2
307	Coimbra	2.41	1.56	−8.3	1.73	3.50	15.2	5.22	4.92	−1.2
308	Castelo Branco	3.41	2.14	−8.9	0.98	2.10	16.6	3.21	3.26	0.3
309	Portalegre	2.18	1.47	−7.6	1.54	2.49	10.0	5.97	4.49	−5.5
310	Santarem	2.71	1.89	−6.9	2.12	2.97	7.0	5.69	5.08	−2.2
311	Leiria	3.04	1.63	−11.7	3.04	1.26	−16.2	5.54	3.97	−6.5
312	Lisboa	5.46	4.00	−6.0	3.74	3.50	−1.3	4.72	4.95	0.9
313	Setubal	3.80	2.17	−10.6	3.73	2.83	−5.4	4.74	4.41	−1.5
314	Evora	2.00	0.89	−14.9	1.82	1.89	0.7	4.48	3.28	−6.0
315	Beja	3.55	2.60	−6.0	1.87	2.37	4.9	4.76	4.49	−1.2
316	Faro	2.98	2.89	−0.6	3.58	2.09	−10.2	5.65	8.01	7.2
317	Madeira	5.54	3.60	−8.3	3.74	3.57	−0.9	5.26	5.59	1.2
318	Azores	7.20	3.20	−15.0	4.73	4.24	−2.1	8.74	7.21	−3.8
SPAIN		2.49	1.54	−8.4	1.55	1.95	4.3	3.86	3.10	−3.9
319	La Coruña	4.54	3.20	−6.2	1.90	3.41	11.2	4.71	5.01	1.1
320	Lugo	3.25	1.76	−10.6	1.35	1.39	0.5	5.19	3.66	−6.2
321	Orense	3.65	2.12	−9.4	0.92	1.33	6.9	3.86	2.88	−5.2
322	Pontevedra	3.33	2.51	−5.0	0.87	2.35	19.7	5.80	3.69	−7.9

Table 9.4(a)—*cont.*

Area		Age-standardized mortality rates (per 100000) and percentage changes TUB			CERV			UTER		
		1980–84	1985–89	Annual % change	1980–84	1985–89	Annual % change	1980–84	1985–89	Annual % change
323	Asturias	2.95	1.82	−8.4	2.10	2.16	0.6	4.31	2.68	−8.3
324	Cantabria	2.27	0.86	−16.2	2.24	2.86	4.6	4.72	2.88	−8.6
325	Alava	1.72	0.75	−13.9	0.54	1.20	15.5	1.77	0.97	−10.4
326	Guipuzcoa	1.96	1.21	−8.5	1.13	1.78	8.6	2.84	1.60	−9.9
327	Vizcaya	2.46	1.41	−9.6	1.67	1.99	3.3	3.68	2.94	−4.0
328	Navarra	2.15	0.81	−16.2	0.51	1.08	14.6	1.67	2.03	3.7
329	Rioja	1.98	1.19	−8.8	0.49	0.89	11.6	1.73	2.12	3.8
330	Huesca	0.53	0.92	10.7	0.82	1.04	4.5	4.22	3.29	−4.4
331	Teruel	0.75	2.20	21.5	0.00	0.54	5.9	3.87	2.61	−6.9
332	Zaragoza	1.82	1.68	−1.5	0.64	1.20	12.0	3.26	2.93	−1.9
333	Madrid Centro	1.97	1.17	−9.0	1.28	1.54	3.5	2.20	2.24	0.3
334	Avila	1.70	1.01	−9.1	0.67	1.31	13.0	2.14	2.89	5.6
335	Burgos	2.04	1.89	−1.4	0.87	1.94	15.7	1.70	0.81	−12.7
336	Leon	2.70	1.40	−11.2	1.12	1.27	2.3	4.01	3.07	−4.7
337	Palencia	1.99	2.02	0.3	0.66	0.85	4.9	5.21	1.56	−19.7
338	Salamanca	3.92	2.04	−11.2	0.85	2.39	20.7	4.12	2.10	−11.5
339	Segovia	1.16	0.21	−26.6	0.41	0.00	−100.0	1.99	1.95	−0.3
340	Soria	0.72	0.65	−1.8	0.00	0.84	6.0	3.74	1.03	−20.9
341	Valladolid	1.91	0.75	−15.6	1.26	0.98	−4.5	5.16	3.18	−8.4
342	Zamora	1.53	0.92	−8.7	0.51	1.68	24.4	4.35	4.49	0.6
343	Albacete	2.98	1.77	−9.0	1.37	0.98	−6.0	3.63	3.11	−2.8
344	Ciudad Real	2.55	1.30	−11.6	0.26	1.04	28.1	2.84	1.85	−7.5
345	Cuenca	1.48	0.46	−19.3	0.85	1.55	11.4	4.24	3.38	−4.0
346	Guadalajara	1.76	1.59	−1.8	0.45	3.53	45.6	1.13	4.52	28.7
347	Toledo	1.78	0.99	−10.1	0.67	1.01	7.8	2.89	3.47	3.4
348	Badajoz	2.79	1.25	−13.6	0.51	0.41	−4.2	3.40	2.23	−7.4
349	Caceres	2.78	0.98	−17.2	1.39	1.23	−2.2	3.82	2.13	−10.1
350	Barcelona	1.89	1.42	−5.0	1.78	2.41	5.7	4.01	3.66	−1.6
351	Gerona	1.66	1.27	−4.8	1.44	1.74	3.4	3.80	4.06	1.2
352	Lerida	1.60	1.38	−2.6	0.84	2.31	20.2	4.74	3.44	−5.7
353	Tarragona	2.27	0.76	−18.0	0.98	1.45	7.3	5.43	2.45	−13.5
354	Alicante	1.87	1.17	−8.2	1.38	1.50	1.6	4.18	3.57	−2.8
355	Castellon de la Plana	2.13	1.49	−6.3	1.00	1.92	12.5	4.51	3.79	−3.1
356	Valencia	2.17	1.82	−3.1	2.24	2.72	3.6	4.45	3.48	−4.4
357	Baleares	2.24	1.07	−12.6	3.56	3.60	0.2	5.48	5.08	−1.4
358	Almeria	3.69	0.94	−22.0	1.20	1.04	−2.6	4.05	1.59	−15.6
359	Cadiz	3.32	2.00	−8.8	2.16	2.29	1.1	4.97	3.15	−8.0
360	Cordoba	2.50	1.23	−12.1	1.19	2.09	10.7	3.22	3.26	0.2
361	Granada	2.54	1.44	−9.8	1.59	0.98	−8.5	2.86	2.51	−2.4
362	Huelva	4.00	2.64	−7.2	1.63	2.07	4.4	4.00	3.29	−3.5
363	Jaen	2.50	2.00	−4.0	1.05	0.53	−11.7	3.84	2.84	−5.3
364	Malaga	3.51	1.97	−10.0	1.73	1.45	−3.2	4.81	2.70	−9.9
365	Sevilla	5.78	2.69	−13.0	2.95	2.87	−0.5	5.97	4.15	−6.4
366	Murcia	1.80	1.51	−3.2	1.72	1.76	0.5	3.44	3.07	−2.0
367	Las Palmas	3.36	1.73	−11.4	2.79	4.18	7.7	4.26	4.68	1.7
368	Sta Cruz de Tenerife	1.83	1.49	−3.7	4.48	3.48	−4.5	5.16	3.60	−6.3
EC		1.37	0.79	−9.4	3.56	3.18	−1.9	4.36	3.67	−2.8

Table 9.4(b)

Area	Age-standardized mortality rates (per 100 000) and percentage changes HODG			CRHD			RESP		
	1980–84	1985–89	Annual % change	1980–84	1985–89	Annual % change	1980–84	1985–89	Annual % change
BELGIUM	1.09	0.67	–9.1	0.04	0.03	–7.6	1.77	1.47	–3.7
1 Antwerpen	1.45	0.68	–14.1	0.02	0.00	–100.0	1.49	1.39	–1.3
2 Brabant	0.79	0.48	–9.3	0.05	0.02	–20.9	2.02	1.01	–13.0
3 West-Vlaanderen	1.04	1.07	0.6	0.03	0.00	–100.0	1.29	1.45	2.3
4 Oost-Vlaanderen	1.54	0.68	–15.2	0.03	0.03	–1.4	2.39	2.13	–2.3
5 Hainaut	0.99	0.57	–10.4	0.09	0.03	–21.4	1.46	1.43	–0.3
6 Liege	0.92	0.60	–8.1	0.08	0.07	–1.6	2.41	2.22	–1.6
7 Limburg	1.06	1.18	2.2	0.00	0.09	13.3	1.31	1.26	–0.8
8 Luxembourg (province)	1.06	0.67	–8.8	0.00	0.16	–2.2	0.91	0.45	–13.2
9 Namur	0.81	0.24	–21.7	0.00	0.00	0.0	1.78	1.54	–2.9
LUXEMBOURG	0.68	0.89	5.5	0.46	0.09	–28.5	1.29	1.32	0.6
10 Luxembourg	0.68	0.89	5.5	0.46	0.09	–28.5	1.29	1.32	0.6
FEDERAL REPUBLIC OF GERMANY	1.06	0.73	–7.0	0.17	0.09	–11.7	1.76	1.18	–7.6
11 Schleswig-Holstein	1.03	0.62	–9.6	0.04	0.07	13.1	1.35	0.86	–8.8
12 Hamburg	0.61	0.91	8.2	0.19	0.13	–7.9	2.13	0.45	–26.8
13 Braunschweig	1.63	1.08	–7.8	0.08	0.07	–3.8	1.94	0.86	–15.0
14 Hannover	1.84	1.13	–9.3	0.14	0.07	–13.1	2.24	1.86	–3.7
15 Lüneburg	1.27	0.84	–7.9	0.02	0.14	45.5	1.69	0.86	–12.7
16 Weser-Ems	1.23	0.72	–10.2	0.13	0.12	–1.5	1.88	1.88	–0.0
17 Bremen	0.69	0.57	–3.6	0.10	0.10	1.9	1.30	1.77	6.4
18 Düsseldorf	0.91	0.59	–8.4	0.14	0.06	–15.4	1.62	1.10	–7.4
19 Köln	0.98	0.47	–13.5	0.17	0.06	–18.2	1.06	1.20	2.4
20 Munster	0.81	0.72	–2.3	0.25	0.10	–16.1	1.27	0.92	–6.4
21 Detmold	0.96	0.74	–5.1	0.19	0.04	–26.2	2.43	1.46	–9.7
22 Arnsberg	0.93	0.80	–2.9	0.21	0.10	–13.7	2.31	1.46	–8.7
23 Darmstadt	1.12	0.85	–5.3	0.31	0.12	–16.8	1.37	0.93	–7.5
24 Giessen	0.98	0.79	–4.1	0.31	0.11	–18.6	1.71	1.45	–3.3
25 Kassel	0.98	0.86	–2.4	0.32	0.09	–21.6	1.87	1.12	–9.8
26 Koblenz	1.60	0.76	–13.9	0.18	0.19	1.5	1.51	0.93	–9.2
27 Trier	1.46	0.66	–14.6	0.16	0.17	1.1	1.28	0.00	–100.0
28 Rheinhessen-Pfalz	1.24	0.68	–11.3	0.33	0.24	–6.6	1.82	1.56	–3.0
29 Stuttgart	0.97	0.69	–6.7	0.26	0.14	–12.1	1.46	1.38	–1.1
30 Karlsruhe	0.77	0.76	–0.3	0.29	0.07	–24.6	1.85	1.43	–5.0
31 Freiburg	0.79	0.52	–7.9	0.16	0.06	–18.7	1.65	1.76	1.2
32 Tübingen	0.85	0.55	–8.2	0.15	0.05	–21.2	2.50	0.97	–17.3
33 Oberbayern	0.91	0.74	–4.1	0.02	0.07	23.7	2.41	1.01	–15.9
34 Niederbayern	1.06	0.76	–6.3	0.00	0.00	0.0	1.44	0.72	–13.0
35 Oberpfalz	1.44	0.85	–10.1	0.04	0.00	–100.0	2.04	1.42	–6.9
36 Oberfranken	1.32	0.71	–11.6	0.10	0.04	–18.4	1.56	1.18	–5.4
37 Mittelfranken	1.47	0.71	–13.6	0.02	0.09	33.9	1.23	0.65	–11.9
38 Unterfranken	0.89	0.64	–6.4	0.03	0.03	1.1	1.59	0.63	–16.9
39 Schwaben	1.23	0.72	–10.0	0.06	0.00	–100.0	1.78	1.65	–1.6
40 Saarland	1.03	0.65	–8.6	0.41	0.10	–24.3	2.73	0.71	–23.7
41 Berlin (West)	1.02	1.04	0.4	0.13	0.11	–3.0	1.99	1.20	–9.6
DENMARK	0.82	0.58	–6.9	0.17	0.10	–10.2	1.34	1.11	–3.8
42 Kobenhavn and Frederiksberg (M)	0.91	0.82	–2.1	0.20	0.18	–2.2	0.63	0.34	–11.4
43 Kobenhavns County	1.12	0.66	–9.9	0.15	0.10	–8.2	1.30	1.27	–0.3
44 Frederiksborg County	0.76	0.43	–10.9	0.17	0.08	–14.3	0.30	0.69	17.9
45 Roskilde County	1.37	0.45	–19.8	0.14	0.00	–100.0	1.44	2.18	8.7
46 Vestsjællands County	1.39	0.72	–12.4	0.25	0.11	–14.9	1.17	1.28	1.8
47 Storstroms County	0.69	0.68	–0.2	0.28	0.00	–100.0	4.03	1.48	–18.2
48 Bornholms County	0.55	0.00	–100.0	0.00	0.00	0.0	0.00	2.49	1.4
49 Fyns County	0.57	0.78	6.4	0.08	0.07	–2.0	1.46	0.81	–11.1
50 Sonderjyllands County	0.63	0.51	–4.3	0.14	0.13	–1.2	2.88	0.45	–31.0
51 Ribe County	0.61	0.12	–28.1	0.65	0.00	–100.0	1.38	0.99	–6.4
52 Vejle County	0.80	0.62	–5.0	0.00	0.00	0.0	1.59	0.35	–26.0
53 Ringkobing County	0.70	0.29	–16.2	0.00	0.00	0.0	1.44	0.79	–11.2
54 Århus County	0.63	0.51	–3.9	0.17	0.10	–10.0	0.91	1.41	9.1

Table 9.4(b)—*cont.*

Area		HODG 1980–84	HODG 1985–89	HODG Annual % change	CRHD 1980–84	CRHD 1985–89	CRHD Annual % change	RESP 1980–84	RESP 1985–89	RESP Annual % change
55	Viborg County	0.57	0.45	–4.7	0.00	0.43	22.2	0.00	0.96	17.0
56	Nordjyllands County	0.75	0.58	–5.0	0.22	0.13	–9.5	1.54	1.94	4.7
FRANCE		0.71	0.54	–5.1	0.18	0.13	–6.5	1.20	1.05	–2.7
57	Ain	0.43	0.69	9.6	0.17	0.22	5.1	0.42	2.47	42.3
58	Aisne	0.55	0.53	–0.5	0.15	0.20	6.2	1.48	1.55	0.8
59	Allier	0.84	0.55	–8.1	0.00	0.00	0.0	1.82	0.67	–18.1
60	Alpes-de-Haute-Provence	0.43	0.79	13.0	0.31	0.00	–100.0	0.95	1.82	13.9
61	Hautes-Alpes	0.24	0.23	–1.0	0.00	0.00	0.0	0.00	0.97	–0.8
62	Alpes-Maritimes	0.84	0.73	–2.9	0.17	0.04	–26.1	1.03	1.13	1.9
63	Ardèche	0.97	0.37	–17.5	0.14	0.00	–100.0	1.15	1.19	0.7
64	Ardennes	0.62	0.69	2.3	0.13	0.12	–1.3	2.29	0.92	–16.6
65	Ariège	0.76	0.56	–6.0	0.00	0.57	12.4	0.90	0.00	–100.0
66	Aube	0.46	0.53	3.2	0.00	0.24	12.7	0.33	1.05	26.2
67	Aude	1.01	0.35	–19.1	0.00	0.00	0.0	1.71	3.03	12.1
68	Aveyron	0.75	0.37	–13.2	0.15	0.00	–100.0	2.03	0.89	–15.2
69	Bouches-du-Rhône	0.88	0.65	–5.9	0.24	0.27	1.8	0.82	0.62	–5.6
70	Calvados	0.94	0.34	–18.3	0.13	0.17	6.1	0.88	0.62	–6.7
71	Cantal	0.96	0.00	–100.0	0.25	0.48	13.6	1.96	1.44	–6.0
72	Charente	0.84	0.37	–15.0	0.12	0.11	–1.8	1.51	0.65	–15.6
73	Charente-Maritime	0.56	0.59	0.9	0.16	0.07	–14.8	0.80	1.28	9.8
74	Cher	0.57	0.96	10.8	0.25	0.22	–1.8	1.31	1.38	0.9
75	Corrèze	0.63	0.63	–0.2	0.00	0.00	0.0	0.98	1.59	10.1
76	Corse	0.52	0.20	–17.3	0.15	0.42	23.6	0.95	0.48	–12.8
77	Côte-d'Or	0.83	0.53	–8.6	0.23	0.14	–9.6	1.19	1.24	0.9
78	Côtes-du-Nord	0.43	0.38	–2.7	0.23	0.14	–9.3	1.09	0.40	–18.3
79	Creuse	1.70	0.56	–20.0	0.34	0.31	–1.7	0.00	4.27	34.7
80	Dordogne	0.47	0.58	4.4	0.00	0.20	12.4	1.86	1.64	–2.5
81	Doubs	0.33	0.59	12.3	0.37	0.07	–28.5	1.43	1.54	1.5
82	Drôme	0.74	0.31	–15.9	0.28	0.00	–100.0	1.21	1.45	3.6
83	Eure	0.58	0.59	0.4	0.16	0.00	–100.0	0.92	1.45	9.4
84	Eure-et-Loir	0.59	0.55	–1.3	0.00	0.09	–2.7	1.69	1.41	–3.5
85	Finistère	0.50	0.24	–13.4	0.15	0.13	–1.8	0.12	1.01	53.8
86	Gard	0.76	0.49	–8.5	0.22	0.37	11.4	0.20	0.97	37.3
87	Haute-Garonne	0.49	0.56	2.9	0.09	0.00	–100.0	1.34	0.66	–13.3
88	Gers	0.59	0.70	3.6	0.00	0.22	–1.2	3.50	4.56	5.4
89	Gironde	0.68	0.52	–5.3	0.13	0.09	–8.3	0.99	1.39	7.0
90	Hérault	0.72	0.40	–11.0	0.27	0.09	–19.3	1.06	1.21	2.6
91	Ille-et-Vilaine	0.46	0.53	3.2	0.05	0.05	–2.3	0.70	0.62	–2.3
92	Indre	0.87	0.74	–3.0	0.17	0.16	–1.4	0.46	2.05	34.9
93	Indre-et-Loire	0.89	0.70	–4.8	0.15	0.00	–100.0	1.16	0.60	–12.4
94	Isère	0.58	0.39	–7.6	0.11	0.17	8.5	1.07	0.69	–8.5
95	Jura	1.09	0.52	–13.6	0.64	0.15	–25.6	0.79	1.23	9.4
96	Landes	0.43	0.16	–17.8	0.14	0.00	–100.0	1.12	1.53	6.5
97	Loir-et-Cher	0.72	0.43	–9.9	0.14	0.12	–2.0	1.36	1.43	1.1
98	Loire	0.56	0.52	–1.7	0.20	0.10	–14.1	0.89	1.08	3.8
99	Haute-Loire	1.40	0.25	–29.4	0.40	0.00	–100.0	0.00	2.68	38.9
100	Loire-Atlantique	0.56	0.45	–4.1	0.04	0.07	12.1	1.63	0.81	–12.9
101	Loiret	0.74	0.65	–2.6	0.14	0.48	28.6	1.36	1.21	–2.3
102	Lot	0.17	0.48	23.7	0.00	0.25	–1.7	0.77	0.00	–100.0
103	Lot-et-Garonne	0.85	0.75	–2.5	0.13	0.00	–100.0	0.37	0.76	15.7
104	Lozère	0.71	0.70	–0.2	0.00	0.00	0.0	1.44	1.56	1.5
105	Maine-et-Loire	1.02	0.70	–7.3	0.06	0.05	–2.1	1.17	1.14	–0.7
106	Manche	0.73	0.33	–15.0	0.54	0.00	–100.0	0.58	0.82	7.1
107	Marne	0.78	0.99	4.9	0.27	0.06	–25.7	1.45	0.86	–9.9
108	Haute-Marne	1.53	0.76	–13.1	0.19	0.00	–100.0	1.67	0.93	–11.2
109	Mayenne	0.79	0.38	–13.5	0.15	0.27	12.8	1.25	1.01	–4.1
110	Meurthe-et-Moselle	0.58	0.28	–13.3	0.10	0.29	23.4	1.02	1.25	4.1
111	Meuse	0.93	0.65	–6.9	0.40	0.19	–14.0	0.46	0.00	–100.0
112	Morbihan	0.67	0.21	–20.6	0.27	0.00	–100.0	1.54	1.46	–1.1
113	Moselle	0.71	0.47	–8.0	0.25	0.07	–22.7	1.35	0.75	–11.0

Age-standardized mortality rates (per 100 000) and percentage changes

Table 9.4(b)—*cont.*

Area		HODG 1980–84	HODG 1985–89	HODG Annual % change	CRHD 1980–84	CRHD 1985–89	CRHD Annual % change	RESP 1980–84	RESP 1985–89	RESP Annual % change
		Age-standardized mortality rates (per 100000) and percentage changes								
114	Nièvre	0.56	0.76	6.5	0.00	0.16	−1.5	0.94	1.00	1.2
115	Nord	0.89	0.73	−3.8	0.22	0.08	−17.1	1.40	1.33	−0.9
116	Oise	0.56	0.30	−11.9	0.21	0.05	−26.3	0.88	2.25	20.7
117	Orne	1.07	0.79	−5.9	0.00	0.13	−1.3	0.92	1.32	7.5
118	Pas-de-Calais	0.96	0.83	−2.9	0.31	0.18	−10.5	1.17	1.21	0.5
119	Puy-de-dôme	1.02	0.67	−8.2	0.25	0.11	−14.5	0.68	0.56	−3.9
120	Pyrénées-Atlantiques	0.56	0.36	−8.7	0.07	0.06	−2.0	0.39	0.82	15.9
121	Hautes-Pyrénées	0.77	0.43	−10.9	0.00	0.00	0.0	2.00	2.22	2.1
122	Pyrénées-Orientales	0.38	0.65	11.1	0.13	0.33	21.4	1.71	1.74	0.3
123	Bas-Rhin	0.73	0.54	−6.0	0.23	0.11	−14.1	1.59	1.56	−0.5
124	Haut-Rhin	0.71	0.53	−5.7	0.27	0.10	−17.7	2.47	1.95	−4.6
125	Rhône	0.56	0.34	−9.4	0.24	0.20	−3.5	1.62	0.96	−10.0
126	Haute-Saône	0.70	0.34	−13.3	0.34	0.16	−14.3	1.53	2.07	6.2
127	Saône-et-Loire	0.83	0.50	−9.6	0.07	0.13	13.3	1.21	0.76	−8.9
128	Sarthe	0.64	0.87	6.4	0.08	0.07	−2.1	0.54	0.58	1.5
129	Savoie	0.55	0.37	−7.7	0.33	0.20	−10.1	0.59	1.83	25.3
130	Haute-Savoie	0.83	0.51	−9.1	0.27	0.11	−15.6	1.10	0.70	−8.5
131	Paris	0.65	0.62	−1.2	0.20	0.11	−10.5	1.08	0.95	−2.5
132	Seine-Maritime	1.17	0.47	−16.6	0.28	0.11	−16.5	1.84	1.06	−10.4
133	Seine-et-Marne	0.57	0.69	4.0	0.19	0.12	−7.9	2.18	1.13	−12.4
134	Yvelines	0.61	0.46	−5.6	0.08	0.12	8.5	1.40	0.93	−8.0
135	Deux-Sèvres	0.23	0.15	−8.5	0.12	0.00	−100.0	0.28	0.59	16.5
136	Somme	1.24	0.91	−5.9	0.22	0.13	−9.8	1.29	0.70	−11.6
137	Tarn	0.60	1.17	14.2	0.12	0.00	−100.0	1.29	0.34	−23.4
138	Tarn-et-Garonne	0.55	0.90	10.6	0.00	0.00	0.0	0.58	0.59	0.3
139	Var	0.43	0.58	6.5	0.27	0.23	−2.9	1.09	0.59	−11.5
140	Vaucluse	0.66	0.73	2.1	0.33	0.22	−7.6	0.47	0.46	−0.1
141	Vendée	0.67	0.62	−1.4	0.09	0.08	−2.4	1.78	0.76	−15.6
142	Vienne	0.79	0.48	−9.3	0.00	0.00	0.0	0.00	0.58	16.6
143	Haute-Vienne	0.51	0.42	−3.5	0.00	0.00	0.0	1.66	1.08	−8.2
144	Vosges	0.61	0.47	−5.2	0.10	0.00	−100.0	1.38	0.50	−18.3
145	Yonne	0.87	0.50	−10.6	0.13	0.00	−100.0	1.58	0.97	−9.3
146	Territoire-de-Belfort	0.59	0.57	−0.5	0.27	0.51	13.2	0.00	0.00	0.0
147	Essonne	0.52	0.65	4.8	0.25	0.12	−14.5	1.75	0.72	−16.3
148	Hauts-de-Seine	0.74	0.43	−10.2	0.15	0.11	−4.9	1.30	0.65	−12.9
149	Seine-Saint-Denis	0.62	0.42	−7.4	0.10	0.16	10.1	1.39	1.02	−6.0
150	Val-de-Marne	0.57	0.53	−1.7	0.14	0.18	5.7	1.22	0.70	−10.5
151	Val-d'Oise	0.81	0.57	−6.8	0.25	0.28	2.2	0.73	0.35	−13.7
GREECE		0.96	0.87	−1.6	0.31	0.09	−19.4	2.37	1.13	−11.6
152	Greater Athens	0.94	0.90	−0.7	0.13	0.10	−4.5	1.80	0.82	−12.3
153	Rest of Central Greece and Eubea	1.10	0.80	−5.2	0.23	0.06	−19.1	2.39	0.87	−15.5
154	Peloponnisos	0.77	0.83	1.4	0.27	0.04	−27.6	1.74	1.04	−8.2
155	Ionian Islands	0.73	0.71	−0.5	0.38	0.22	−8.5	0.86	1.55	10.4
156	Epirus	0.97	0.65	−6.5	0.00	0.00	0.0	3.50	0.79	−21.9
157	Thessaly	0.82	0.62	−4.4	0.08	0.05	−8.6	2.23	1.95	−2.2
158	Macedonia	0.90	0.83	−1.3	0.49	0.13	−20.3	1.91	1.39	−5.2
159	Thrace	1.69	1.03	−7.9	0.85	0.10	−29.6	10.14	1.79	−25.1
160	Aegean Islands	1.17	1.23	0.8	0.63	0.00	−100.0	2.81	0.84	−18.2
161	Crete	1.10	1.26	2.4	0.91	0.08	−34.1	2.71	1.29	−11.6
ITALY		1.29	0.84	−6.9	0.94	0.39	−13.4	2.55	1.53	−8.1
162	Torino	1.36	0.80	−8.4	0.84	0.37	−12.5	2.07	0.83	−14.1
163	Vercelli	1.87	0.67	−15.8	0.99	0.76	−4.3	1.02	1.72	9.0
164	Novara	1.63	0.47	−18.7	0.75	0.21	−19.0	2.37	1.17	−11.0
165	Cuneo	1.23	1.04	−2.7	0.84	0.46	−9.5	1.13	1.05	−1.1
166	Asti	1.06	0.68	−7.1	1.23	0.18	−27.6	4.47	0.00	−100.0
167	Alessandria	1.17	1.10	−1.1	0.87	0.00	−100.0	0.96	1.64	9.4
168	Aosta	1.07	0.61	−9.0	0.58	0.29	−10.8	3.19	1.29	−14.0
169	Imperia	2.19	1.37	−7.5	0.80	0.51	−7.4	0.63	1.60	16.7
170	Savona	1.38	1.27	−1.4	0.47	0.13	−19.6	2.90	0.64	−22.3

Table 9.4(b)—*cont.*

	Area	HODG 1980–84	HODG 1985–89	HODG Annual % change	CRHD 1980–84	CRHD 1985–89	CRHD Annual % change	RESP 1980–84	RESP 1985–89	RESP Annual % change
		Age-standardized mortality rates (per 100000) and percentage changes								
171	Genova	1.69	0.94	−9.3	0.61	0.40	−6.8	1.41	1.47	0.8
172	La Spezia	1.60	0.89	−9.2	0.60	0.47	−4.0	0.58	0.75	4.5
173	Varese	1.60	0.60	−15.1	0.86	0.29	−16.5	2.18	1.17	−9.8
174	Como/Sondrio	1.12	0.94	−2.9	0.70	0.28	−14.2	2.21	1.20	−9.7
175	Milano	1.39	0.91	−6.8	0.75	0.29	−14.5	1.89	1.01	−9.9
176	Bergamo	1.55	0.76	−11.2	0.84	0.36	−13.3	1.76	1.97	1.9
177	Brescia	1.58	0.96	−8.0	0.80	0.13	−26.4	1.82	0.73	−14.1
178	Pavia	2.24	0.92	−13.8	0.41	0.22	−10.1	1.62	0.00	−100.0
179	Cremona	1.03	0.98	−0.7	0.82	0.64	−4.2	0.74	0.45	−7.9
180	Mantova	1.77	1.01	−8.9	0.28	0.19	−6.3	1.94	1.24	−7.1
181	Bolzano	0.93	0.23	−20.8	0.40	0.08	−23.7	1.76	2.06	2.6
182	Trento	0.93	0.76	−3.3	1.11	0.53	−11.5	1.25	1.18	−0.9
183	Verona	1.24	0.64	−10.4	0.35	0.26	−4.9	0.97	0.17	−25.3
184	Vicenza	1.17	0.65	−9.3	0.56	0.18	−17.1	1.96	1.03	−10.2
185	Belluno	1.25	1.11	−2.0	0.48	0.16	−16.7	1.63	2.05	3.9
186	Treviso	1.55	0.66	−13.3	0.48	0.18	−14.7	1.02	1.07	0.8
187	Venezia	1.62	1.01	−7.6	0.32	0.24	−4.7	0.91	0.86	−0.9
188	Padova	1.64	1.37	−2.9	0.50	0.12	−20.9	3.34	1.29	−14.6
189	Rovigo	1.18	1.22	0.5	0.44	0.29	−6.9	0.45	0.57	4.0
190	Udine/Gorizia	0.99	0.78	−4.0	0.50	0.25	−10.8	0.93	1.65	10.1
191	Trieste	1.69	1.05	−7.7	0.87	0.82	−1.0	1.15	0.77	−6.5
192	Pordenone	0.93	0.79	−2.8	0.74	0.12	−26.0	0.00	2.06	31.1
193	Piacenza	1.30	1.02	−4.0	0.90	0.13	−27.1	0.51	0.00	−100.0
194	Parma	1.34	1.30	−0.5	0.36	0.37	0.5	1.75	1.32	−4.6
195	Reggio Emilia	2.18	0.96	−12.7	0.26	0.09	−16.7	0.91	1.12	3.4
196	Modena	1.62	1.24	−4.4	0.46	0.34	−4.8	1.05	0.79	−4.7
197	Bologna	1.08	0.62	−8.9	0.65	0.30	−12.1	1.59	1.45	−1.5
198	Ferrara	1.00	0.80	−3.7	0.28	0.19	−6.0	2.11	0.00	−100.0
199	Ravenna	0.68	0.72	1.0	0.29	0.10	−16.2	0.74	0.98	4.9
200	Forli	1.24	0.93	−4.7	0.23	0.11	−11.0	1.33	1.18	−2.0
201	Pesaro	0.60	1.00	8.9	0.43	0.32	−4.8	3.37	1.23	−15.5
202	Ancona	0.85	0.65	−4.4	0.41	0.00	−100.0	2.42	0.65	−19.6
203	Macerata	1.09	0.72	−6.6	0.37	0.51	5.4	1.25	0.48	−14.7
204	Ascoli Piceno	1.18	0.72	−7.9	0.50	0.41	−3.4	0.96	0.37	−14.8
205	Massa-Carrara	1.46	0.69	−11.7	1.07	0.18	−25.8	1.19	1.44	3.2
206	Lucca	1.23	0.87	−5.6	0.18	0.19	0.2	0.96	0.79	−3.1
207	Pistoia	1.40	0.81	−8.8	1.05	0.13	−29.2	1.39	1.14	−3.2
208	Firenze	1.40	0.95	−6.2	0.54	0.23	−13.2	1.72	0.27	−26.6
209	Livorno	0.99	1.44	6.5	0.40	0.20	−10.8	1.78	0.91	−10.6
210	Pisa	1.46	0.97	−6.5	0.45	0.09	−23.5	1.60	0.39	−21.0
211	Arezzo	0.93	0.68	−5.2	0.92	0.23	−20.7	1.21	0.95	−3.9
212	Siena	1.12	0.46	−13.8	0.58	0.15	−20.2	2.81	0.68	−21.1
213	Grosseto	0.54	0.42	−4.1	0.80	0.16	−23.4	0.00	0.00	0.0
214	Perugia	1.92	1.07	−9.2	0.92	0.31	−16.8	1.85	0.94	−10.6
215	Terni	1.05	1.54	6.6	1.72	0.64	−15.1	2.20	1.34	−7.9
216	Viterbo/Rieti	1.51	0.80	−10.1	1.00	0.35	−16.0	3.26	1.52	−12.0
217	Roma	1.34	0.79	−8.4	0.85	0.47	−9.3	2.12	1.38	−6.9
218	Latina	1.40	0.86	−7.7	1.50	0.44	−18.5	2.17	0.88	−14.0
219	Frosinone	1.13	1.10	−0.5	1.54	0.46	−18.4	0.41	0.89	13.7
220	Caserta	0.85	1.05	3.6	2.14	0.77	−15.7	3.36	1.38	−13.7
221	Benevento	1.19	0.51	−13.1	1.24	1.34	1.3	1.94	1.40	−5.4
222	Napoli	1.27	0.80	−7.4	1.71	0.76	−12.7	4.58	2.23	−11.3
223	Avellino	0.80	1.03	4.3	1.43	0.34	−21.2	4.26	3.23	−4.5
224	Salerno	1.24	0.87	−5.8	2.08	0.60	−18.6	3.22	2.10	−6.9
225	L'Aquila	0.69	0.74	1.3	1.60	0.76	−11.6	2.22	1.22	−9.5
226	Teramo	1.15	0.71	−7.8	0.54	0.40	−5.1	1.47	1.64	1.8
227	Pescara	0.80	0.33	−13.7	1.38	0.50	−15.6	2.84	2.07	−5.1
228	Chieti	1.23	1.22	−0.1	1.01	0.29	−18.8	1.67	1.25	−4.7
229	Isernia/Campobasso	1.35	1.12	−3.0	2.14	0.93	−13.0	2.79	1.74	−7.6
230	Foggia	0.95	0.65	−6.2	1.19	0.38	−17.4	4.15	2.36	−9.0
231	Bari	0.97	0.55	−9.0	1.64	0.72	−12.8	2.96	1.62	−9.6

Table 9.4(b)—*cont.*

Area		Age-standardized mortality rates (per 100000) and percentage changes HODG			CRHD			RESP		
		1980–84	1985–89	Annual % change	1980–84	1985–89	Annual % change	1980–84	1985–89	Annual % change
232	Taranto	1.15	0.52	−12.3	1.18	0.70	−8.4	3.40	2.17	−7.2
233	Brindisi	1.38	0.71	−10.6	2.15	0.53	−20.7	4.10	1.38	−16.6
234	Lecce	1.38	1.05	−4.5	1.21	0.45	−15.2	3.09	2.43	−3.9
235	Potenza/Matera	0.93	0.86	−1.2	1.33	0.50	−15.0	3.59	2.30	−7.2
236	Cosenza	0.66	0.50	−4.7	1.43	0.62	−13.1	3.69	1.01	−19.4
237	Catanzaro	1.21	0.48	−14.2	2.10	0.73	−16.2	3.54	1.18	−16.7
238	Reggio Calabria	1.29	1.08	−3.0	1.09	0.59	−9.8	2.54	1.95	−4.3
239	Trapani	1.28	0.59	−12.1	1.15	0.34	−18.3	2.34	1.17	−10.9
240	Palermo	1.32	0.66	−10.8	1.03	0.38	−15.5	4.84	2.70	−9.3
241	Messina	1.13	0.55	−11.3	1.15	0.66	−8.9	4.14	3.16	−4.4
242	Agrigento	1.40	1.01	−5.2	1.63	0.71	−12.9	4.09	2.55	−7.6
243	Caltanisetta	0.87	0.45	−10.4	1.07	0.91	−2.6	2.28	1.61	−5.7
244	Enna	1.25	0.93	−4.9	1.60	0.00	−100.0	3.18	4.42	5.6
245	Catania	1.29	0.85	−6.7	1.12	0.55	−11.2	4.39	3.05	−5.9
246	Ragusa	1.16	0.53	−12.2	1.77	0.39	−22.4	4.53	3.11	−6.1
247	Siracusa	0.96	0.69	−5.2	1.10	0.26	−21.4	1.71	1.19	−5.9
248	Sassari	1.33	0.97	−5.2	0.74	0.23	−17.8	3.20	2.18	−6.2
249	Nuoro	1.43	0.75	−10.1	0.96	0.13	−28.2	3.39	4.10	3.2
250	Cagliari/Oristano	0.75	0.95	4.1	0.82	0.22	−19.5	3.57	1.55	−13.0
IRELAND		1.30	0.80	−9.3	0.28	0.15	−12.2	2.63	1.81	−7.2
251	Eastern	0.97	0.46	−13.6	0.26	0.17	−7.5	1.96	1.93	−0.3
252	Midland	1.65	1.44	−2.7	0.21	0.00	−100.0	2.66	2.33	−2.6
253	Mid-Western	0.98	0.75	−5.1	0.54	0.00	−100.0	3.11	0.92	−21.7
254	North-Eastern	1.26	1.09	−2.9	0.14	0.25	11.5	3.88	1.58	−16.5
255	North-Western	2.21	0.72	−20.1	0.00	0.38	12.1	2.38	1.70	−6.5
256	South-Eastern	1.95	0.92	−13.9	0.22	0.20	−2.4	2.69	2.65	−0.3
257	Southern	1.54	1.10	−6.5	0.39	0.07	−29.0	2.97	1.65	−11.1
258	Western	0.98	0.87	−2.3	0.39	0.12	−21.6	2.96	1.48	−12.9
THE NETHERLANDS		0.77	0.69	−2.5	0.18	0.09	−13.5	1.28	1.12	−3.0
259	Groningen	0.84	0.57	−8.3	0.06	0.14	19.7	0.96	0.54	−11.9
260	Friesland	0.69	0.66	−1.1	0.18	0.07	−19.7	1.10	1.73	10.7
261	Drenthe	0.49	0.79	11.4	0.33	0.00	−100.0	0.94	0.32	−21.4
262	Overijssel	0.98	0.73	−6.3	0.27	0.00	−100.0	1.17	1.18	0.2
263	Gelderland	0.79	0.81	0.7	0.24	0.02	−41.1	1.21	1.41	3.4
264	Utrecht	0.70	0.68	−0.7	0.11	0.08	−7.0	1.12	0.87	−5.5
265	Noord Holland	0.88	0.54	−10.5	0.14	0.11	−5.4	0.89	1.26	8.1
266	Zuid Holland	0.79	0.71	−2.4	0.15	0.11	−7.1	1.51	0.99	−8.8
267	Zeeland	0.90	1.00	2.4	0.20	0.00	−100.0	1.42	0.78	−12.4
268	Noord Brabant	0.60	0.60	−0.2	0.20	0.12	−10.5	1.70	1.04	−10.3
269	Limburg	0.73	0.76	0.8	0.15	0.14	−1.8	1.33	1.40	1.2
270	Flevoland	0.68	1.22	13.7	0.07	0.38	45.6	0.85	1.02	4.1
UK: ENGLAND AND WALES		0.85	0.71	−3.6	0.29	0.15	−12.0	2.79	1.53	−11.3
271	Northern	0.98	0.75	−5.2	0.26	0.22	−3.1	2.73	1.47	−11.6
272	Yorkshire	1.07	0.68	−8.6	0.35	0.16	−14.2	3.07	1.75	−10.6
273	Trent	0.84	0.75	−2.3	0.38	0.17	−15.0	2.75	1.47	−11.7
274	East Anglian	0.68	0.67	−0.1	0.26	0.05	−27.9	2.56	1.37	−11.7
275	North-West Thames	0.83	0.57	−7.2	0.24	0.22	−2.2	2.54	1.51	−9.9
276	North-East Thames	0.76	0.69	−1.9	0.26	0.20	−4.7	2.98	1.62	−11.5
277	South-East Thames	0.86	0.71	−3.8	0.28	0.09	−21.1	2.61	1.47	−10.9
278	South-West Thames	0.78	0.64	−3.7	0.18	0.12	−7.3	2.48	1.36	−11.3
279	Wessex	0.79	0.63	−4.3	0.20	0.11	−11.4	3.55	1.20	−19.5
280	Oxford	0.73	0.92	4.7	0.13	0.09	−6.8	2.31	1.43	−9.0
281	South-Western	0.72	0.77	1.5	0.16	0.11	−6.9	2.71	1.29	−13.8
282	West Midlands	1.01	0.78	−5.0	0.34	0.14	−15.8	3.21	1.67	−12.3
283	Mersey	0.77	0.63	−3.8	0.21	0.14	−7.6	2.16	1.53	−6.7
284	North-Western	0.72	0.72	0.2	0.42	0.16	−18.2	2.74	1.99	−6.2
285	Wales	1.06	0.63	−9.8	0.45	0.21	−14.1	2.90	1.40	−13.6

Table 9.4(b)—*cont.*

Area	HODG 1980–84	HODG 1985–89	HODG Annual % change	CRHD 1980–84	CRHD 1985–89	CRHD Annual % change	RESP 1980–84	RESP 1985–89	RESP Annual % change
	Age-standardized mortality rates (per 100000) and percentage changes								
UK: NORTHERN IRELAND	1.23	0.97	−4.5	0.28	0.16	−9.9	3.07	1.95	−8.7
286 Northern Ireland	1.23	0.97	−4.5	0.28	0.16	−9.9	3.07	1.95	−8.7
UK: SCOTLAND	0.86	0.73	−3.1	0.35	0.18	−12.2	2.45	2.26	−1.7
287 Highlands and Islands	0.99	1.04	0.9	0.14	0.00	−100.0	1.77	3.02	11.2
288 Grampian	0.70	0.71	0.4	0.15	0.07	−15.0	1.49	1.31	−2.5
289 Tayside	0.92	1.10	3.7	0.19	0.27	7.1	3.37	1.47	−15.3
290 Fife	1.14	1.04	−1.8	0.11	0.20	12.9	2.99	1.58	−12.0
291 Lothian	0.72	0.54	−5.5	0.39	0.05	−34.9	2.43	2.10	−2.8
292 Borders	1.30	0.50	−17.2	0.00	0.35	−2.0	1.12	2.36	16.0
293 Forth Valley	0.85	1.02	3.7	0.27	0.00	−100.0	4.51	3.26	−6.3
294 Argyll and Clyde	1.03	0.69	−7.9	0.16	0.31	14.1	2.45	1.94	−4.6
295 Greater Glasgow	0.73	0.56	−5.1	0.72	0.43	−9.6	1.98	2.85	7.6
296 Lanarkshire	1.00	0.49	−13.2	0.56	0.12	−26.4	3.13	2.19	−6.9
297 Ayrshire and Arran	0.83	0.68	−3.9	0.39	0.18	−13.9	1.89	2.87	8.7
298 Dumfries and Galloway	0.53	1.37	20.8	0.00	0.00	0.0	2.24	2.35	1.0
PORTUGAL	0.72	0.52	−6.4	1.62	0.62	−17.6	6.25	3.82	−9.4
299 Viana do Castelo	0.22	0.31	7.2	1.04	0.64	−9.4	10.38	2.91	−22.5
300 Braga	0.46	0.52	2.5	2.57	0.65	−24.1	8.31	5.17	−9.1
301 Vila Real	0.32	0.42	5.4	1.89	0.50	−23.5	9.72	4.64	−13.8
302 Bragança	0.44	0.43	−0.5	1.22	0.72	−10.0	9.69	4.60	−13.9
303 Guarda	0.93	0.55	−10.0	2.03	0.23	−35.6	4.40	3.94	−2.2
304 Viseu	0.40	0.92	18.1	1.48	0.72	−13.5	9.96	4.99	−12.9
305 Porto	0.70	0.39	−10.7	2.15	0.66	−21.1	6.54	4.36	−7.8
306 Aveiro	0.44	0.28	−8.6	1.59	0.82	−12.4	6.05	3.19	−12.0
307 Coimbra	0.42	0.57	6.6	1.43	0.51	−18.7	5.89	2.65	−14.7
308 Castelo Branco	0.45	0.00	−100.0	2.71	1.54	−10.7	5.66	3.78	−7.7
309 Portalegre	0.53	0.55	0.7	1.55	1.27	−3.8	4.75	0.88	−28.6
310 Santarem	0.67	0.33	−13.3	1.04	0.08	−39.4	4.67	3.46	−5.8
311 Leiria	0.56	0.82	8.1	0.63	0.69	1.7	4.25	3.02	−6.6
312 Lisboa	1.13	0.62	−11.2	1.36	0.45	−20.1	5.11	4.25	−3.6
313 Setubal	0.81	0.53	−8.2	1.10	0.41	−18.0	3.68	2.64	−6.4
314 Evora	1.11	0.85	−5.1	1.37	0.00	−100.0	4.06	1.94	−13.7
315 Beja	0.69	0.86	4.7	2.55	1.46	−10.6	1.12	1.95	11.7
316 Faro	0.94	0.38	−16.7	1.32	0.67	−12.6	2.52	2.54	0.2
317 Madeira	0.70	0.32	−14.4	1.86	1.09	−10.2	6.66	2.57	−17.3
318 Azores	0.48	0.71	8.4	2.32	1.70	−6.0	11.04	4.63	−15.9
SPAIN	0.81	0.69	−2.8	1.03	0.43	−14.8	2.67	1.36	−11.6
319 La Coruña	1.23	0.86	−6.4	1.26	0.36	−20.4	4.35	0.90	−24.9
320 Lugo	0.68	0.72	1.0	0.62	0.57	−1.5	4.05	1.19	−20.0
321 Orense	0.29	0.30	0.4	0.62	0.24	−16.0	3.91	2.09	−10.7
322 Pontevedra	0.59	0.66	2.1	0.53	0.05	−33.8	2.81	1.36	−12.4
323 Asturias	0.92	0.81	−2.3	1.11	0.09	−36.1	2.18	0.97	−13.8
324 Cantabria	0.77	0.61	−4.1	0.95	0.20	−24.5	3.23	2.14	−7.2
325 Alava	0.93	0.57	−8.6	0.54	0.31	−9.7	3.05	0.36	−32.3
326 Guipuzcoa	1.10	0.40	−16.7	0.21	0.20	−1.1	2.55	1.40	−10.3
327 Vizcaya	0.83	0.78	−1.1	0.77	0.35	−13.3	2.16	0.74	−17.7
328 Navarra	0.93	0.87	−1.3	0.91	0.38	−14.7	2.62	1.56	−9.0
329 Rioja	0.81	0.61	−5.1	0.31	0.40	4.6	1.81	0.00	−100.0
330 Huesca	0.35	0.89	18.4	0.21	0.29	6.4	2.95	1.34	−13.4
331 Teruel	0.51	0.45	−2.1	0.30	1.35	31.5	3.01	3.27	1.5
332 Zaragoza	0.80	1.18	7.2	0.99	0.54	−10.3	1.85	1.61	−2.5
333 Madrid Centro	0.57	0.57	0.0	1.01	0.18	−26.8	2.36	0.97	−15.0
334 Avila	0.72	0.57	−4.1	1.71	0.00	−100.0	2.81	4.88	10.6
335 Burgos	0.65	0.71	1.6	0.57	0.15	−21.4	1.34	1.10	−3.5
336 Leon	0.59	0.75	4.5	1.96	1.19	−8.6	3.32	1.99	−8.9
337 Palencia	0.97	0.89	−1.7	0.23	0.32	6.3	1.60	1.50	−1.1
338 Salamanca	0.96	0.85	−2.2	1.68	0.83	−12.0	3.37	2.02	−8.9
339 Segovia	1.07	1.37	4.7	0.89	0.00	−100.0	5.36	0.00	−100.0

Table 9.4(b)—*cont.*

Area		HODG 1980–84	HODG 1985–89	HODG Annual % change	CRHD 1980–84	CRHD 1985–89	CRHD Annual % change	RESP 1980–84	RESP 1985–89	RESP Annual % change
		Age-standardized mortality rates (per 100000) and percentage changes								
340	Soria	1.57	0.00	−100.0	1.83	0.69	−16.2	4.53	1.74	−16.0
341	Valladolid	1.19	0.52	−14.0	0.87	0.47	−10.5	1.98	0.60	−19.5
342	Zamora	0.68	0.60	−2.2	0.79	0.58	−5.4	1.02	0.77	−5.0
343	Albacete	0.58	0.51	−2.1	1.12	0.51	−13.4	3.39	0.99	−20.1
344	Ciudad Real	1.03	0.59	−9.7	1.28	1.05	−3.5	3.93	2.17	−10.3
345	Cuenca	0.38	0.34	−1.9	1.26	0.95	−5.1	1.43	0.73	−11.6
346	Guadalajara	0.76	0.73	−0.7	0.64	1.34	14.3	2.67	0.89	−18.0
347	Toledo	0.51	0.35	−6.5	1.82	0.62	−17.7	2.81	2.49	−2.2
348	Badajoz	1.30	1.01	−4.4	1.83	1.06	−9.5	2.94	3.01	0.5
349	Caceres	0.98	0.60	−8.6	1.47	0.15	−33.8	3.32	1.94	−9.3
350	Barcelona	0.80	0.61	−4.6	0.66	0.42	−7.9	2.17	0.82	−16.3
351	Gerona	0.89	0.66	−5.3	0.52	0.11	−24.6	2.47	0.90	−16.7
352	Lerida	0.79	0.80	0.2	0.72	0.65	−1.8	1.97	1.86	−1.1
353	Tarragona	0.77	0.42	−10.6	0.78	0.85	1.7	2.64	0.38	−29.8
354	Alicante	0.59	0.51	−2.9	1.15	0.44	−16.1	3.01	1.24	−14.9
355	Castellon de la Plana	0.73	0.59	−4.0	1.20	0.23	−25.9	2.43	1.46	−8.9
356	Valencia	1.01	0.74	−5.5	1.56	0.66	−14.4	2.59	1.26	−12.3
357	Baleares	1.16	0.92	−4.2	0.47	0.41	−2.2	2.65	1.23	−13.1
358	Almeria	0.77	0.58	−4.9	0.69	0.63	−1.7	3.56	0.67	−26.3
359	Cadiz	0.78	0.98	4.4	1.21	0.45	−16.5	2.49	1.50	−8.8
360	Cordoba	0.62	1.11	11.2	1.23	0.72	−9.3	4.48	2.00	−13.6
361	Granada	1.04	1.13	1.6	0.83	0.30	−17.1	2.19	2.26	0.6
362	Huelva	0.61	0.85	6.2	1.20	0.53	−14.0	2.17	2.28	0.9
363	Jaen	0.66	0.67	0.1	1.93	0.65	−17.9	4.56	1.25	−20.9
364	Malaga	1.12	0.68	−8.6	1.70	0.63	−16.5	2.30	1.82	−4.1
365	Sevilla	1.00	0.81	−3.9	1.61	0.54	−18.1	2.74	2.49	−1.7
366	Murcia	0.50	0.55	1.7	0.80	0.53	−7.3	3.05	1.67	−10.4
367	Las Palmas	0.67	0.59	−2.1	1.12	0.42	−16.3	2.34	1.52	−7.5
368	Sta Cruz de Tenerife	1.01	0.72	−5.8	0.99	0.29	−20.3	2.87	2.17	−4.9
EC		0.95	0.71	−5.3	0.47	0.21	−12.9	2.27	1.43	−8.0

Table 9.4(c)

Area	Age-standardized mortality rates (per 100000) and percentage changes								
	ASTH			APP			HERN		
	1980–84	1985–89	Annual % change	1980–84	1985–89	Annual % change	1980–84	1985–89	Annual % change
BELGIUM	0.95	0.78	–4.0	0.07	0.03	–16.8	0.10	0.07	–7.8
1 Antwerpen	0.79	0.59	–5.7	0.03	0.00	–100.0	0.05	0.00	–100.0
2 Brabant	0.88	0.92	1.0	0.10	0.04	–15.5	0.13	0.07	–11.1
3 West-Vlaanderen	1.13	0.67	–9.9	0.02	0.02	–1.3	0.10	0.02	–25.6
4 Oost-Vlaanderen	0.62	0.37	–10.1	0.15	0.02	–34.6	0.10	0.13	5.6
5 Hainaut	1.50	1.23	–3.8	0.06	0.07	5.7	0.18	0.16	–2.6
6 Liege	1.15	0.78	–7.4	0.05	0.00	–100.0	0.07	0.02	–20.4
7 Limburg	0.45	0.48	1.3	0.04	0.00	–100.0	0.04	0.11	21.5
8 Luxembourg (province)	0.34	1.09	26.7	0.00	0.00	0.0	0.11	0.11	–1.3
9 Namur	1.79	1.34	–5.7	0.18	0.12	–8.5	0.12	0.00	–100.0
LUXEMBOURG	0.75	0.91	3.9	0.28	0.00	–100.0	0.15	0.13	–2.4
10 Luxembourg	0.75	0.91	3.9	0.28	0.00	–100.0	0.15	0.13	–2.4
FEDERAL REPUBLIC OF GERMANY	1.04	0.80	–5.1	0.19	0.09	–14.5	0.17	0.09	–11.3
11 Schleswig-Holstein	1.07	0.89	–3.7	0.21	0.10	–14.5	0.15	0.12	–4.4
12 Hamburg	1.06	0.68	–8.5	0.22	0.11	–13.2	0.12	0.11	–0.9
13 Braunschweig	1.18	0.94	–4.5	0.29	0.16	–10.9	0.17	0.13	–5.3
14 Hannover	1.22	0.82	–7.7	0.23	0.04	–31.4	0.15	0.07	–14.3
15 Lüneburg	1.21	0.83	–7.2	0.28	0.10	–18.6	0.21	0.02	–40.3
16 Weser-Ems	0.97	0.76	–4.8	0.26	0.12	–14.8	0.14	0.11	–6.0
17 Bremen	1.41	1.31	–1.5	0.26	0.33	5.1	0.14	0.07	–13.6
18 Düsseldorf	1.11	0.77	–7.1	0.14	0.05	–19.8	0.11	0.07	–8.5
19 Köln	1.05	0.81	–4.9	0.12	0.07	–10.3	0.10	0.05	–12.5
20 Munster	1.01	0.79	–4.8	0.19	0.07	–18.1	0.13	0.08	–9.7
21 Detmold	1.13	0.98	–2.8	0.15	0.05	–19.1	0.09	0.06	–5.3
22 Arnsberg	1.09	0.91	–3.5	0.25	0.09	–18.4	0.19	0.07	–17.0
23 Darmstadt	1.25	0.76	–9.5	0.17	0.08	–13.0	0.29	0.05	–30.3
24 Giessen	1.23	0.92	–5.7	0.29	0.08	–23.5	0.34	0.12	–18.7
25 Kassel	1.39	0.64	–14.5	0.29	0.10	–19.0	0.12	0.12	–1.2
26 Koblenz	1.10	1.04	–1.1	0.20	0.03	–29.5	0.21	0.10	–14.3
27 Trier	0.84	0.47	–10.9	0.05	0.20	30.7	0.26	0.10	–18.3
28 Rheinhessen-Pfalz	1.37	1.03	–5.6	0.25	0.08	–20.7	0.13	0.11	–2.0
29 Stuttgart	0.86	0.57	–8.0	0.14	0.05	–19.1	0.19	0.08	–16.9
30 Karlsruhe	0.79	0.76	–0.7	0.20	0.09	–14.8	0.15	0.15	–0.5
31 Freiburg	0.96	0.63	–7.9	0.14	0.01	–37.7	0.22	0.13	–9.7
32 Tübingen	0.79	0.43	–11.6	0.12	0.13	1.4	0.17	0.07	–16.8
33 Oberbayern	0.80	0.75	–1.2	0.12	0.11	–2.0	0.09	0.09	0.1
34 Niederbayern	0.88	0.90	0.5	0.28	0.12	–15.6	0.31	0.19	–9.5
35 Oberpfalz	0.86	0.70	–4.1	0.26	0.15	–10.6	0.32	0.10	–21.1
36 Oberfranken	1.07	1.00	–1.2	0.24	0.11	–13.6	0.33	0.24	–6.1
37 Mittelfranken	1.09	0.98	–2.2	0.20	0.08	–16.8	0.25	0.09	–18.0
38 Unterfranken	1.01	0.65	–8.4	0.15	0.10	–7.5	0.13	0.10	–5.4
39 Schwaben	0.79	0.92	3.3	0.27	0.14	–11.6	0.12	0.06	–11.9
40 Saarland	1.18	0.69	–10.2	0.11	0.07	–10.6	0.14	0.19	6.5
41 Berlin (West)	0.94	0.90	–0.9	0.21	0.13	–8.2	0.13	0.07	–12.9
DENMARK	0.42	0.47	2.6	0.15	0.15	–1.0	0.14	0.15	1.7
42 Kobenhavn and Frederiksberg (M)	0.59	0.37	–9.0	0.13	0.20	9.1	0.12	0.15	3.9
43 Kobenhavns County	0.27	0.71	21.7	0.12	0.20	11.4	0.08	0.04	–12.9
44 Frederiksborg County	0.28	0.09	–20.1	0.16	0.15	–1.1	0.09	0.08	–1.9
45 Roskilde County	0.15	0.42	23.3	0.13	0.00	–100.0	0.00	0.26	12.1
46 Vestsjællands County	0.00	0.48	30.6	0.09	0.36	31.9	0.09	0.09	–0.2
47 Storstroms County	0.14	0.27	14.1	0.28	0.10	–19.4	0.18	0.19	0.3
48 Bornholms County	0.00	0.00	0.0	0.00	0.00	0.0	0.00	0.00	0.0
49 Fyns County	0.62	0.30	–13.8	0.17	0.11	–7.6	0.17	0.17	0.1
50 Sonderjyllands County	0.70	0.28	–17.0	0.31	0.00	–100.0	0.43	0.20	–13.9
51 Ribe County	0.64	0.61	–0.8	0.00	0.24	14.6	0.13	0.00	–100.0
52 Vejle County	0.74	0.71	–0.8	0.24	0.24	0.0	0.24	0.40	10.5
53 Ringkobing County	0.39	0.62	9.9	0.20	0.00	–100.0	0.11	0.00	–100.0
54 Århus County	0.40	0.54	5.9	0.14	0.18	5.9	0.14	0.10	–7.8

Table 9.4(c)—*cont.*

	Area	Age-standardized mortality rates (per 100 000) and percentage changes ASTH			APP			HERN		
		1980–84	1985–89	Annual % change	1980–84	1985–89	Annual % change	1980–84	1985–89	Annual % change
55	Viborg County	0.47	0.91	14.0	0.11	0.11	0.3	0.22	0.23	0.2
56	Nordjyllands County	0.44	0.42	–0.8	0.16	0.05	–19.4	0.05	0.27	38.5
FRANCE		0.38	0.65	11.3	0.17	0.07	–16.6	0.27	0.20	–6.1
57	Ain	0.25	0.96	31.1	0.37	0.29	–4.9	0.52	0.24	–14.2
58	Aisne	0.48	1.18	19.8	0.34	0.05	–32.6	0.30	0.48	9.6
59	Allier	0.22	0.63	23.9	0.26	0.13	–13.4	0.26	0.31	3.6
60	Alpes-de-Haute-Provence	0.00	0.29	–1.2	0.21	0.00	–100.0	0.00	0.00	0.0
61	Hautes-Alpes	1.70	0.96	–10.8	0.24	0.00	–100.0	0.23	0.00	–100.0
62	Alpes-Maritimes	0.54	0.82	8.6	0.11	0.03	–25.3	0.13	0.10	–5.8
63	Ardèche	0.00	0.94	46.2	0.18	0.00	–100.0	0.46	0.09	–28.5
64	Ardennes	0.48	0.94	14.6	0.00	0.08	–0.7	0.74	0.26	–18.9
65	Ariège	1.23	0.00	–100.0	0.17	0.00	–100.0	0.00	0.48	23.8
66	Aube	0.12	0.48	30.8	0.27	0.00	–100.0	0.38	0.18	–13.7
67	Aude	0.29	0.54	13.0	0.00	0.08	–0.8	0.32	0.23	–6.6
68	Aveyron	0.58	0.72	4.3	0.00	0.08	–0.7	0.51	0.40	–4.8
69	Bouches-du-Rhône	0.24	0.63	21.0	0.13	0.01	–35.7	0.21	0.15	–7.0
70	Calvados	0.47	0.39	–3.8	0.18	0.00	–100.0	0.38	0.00	–100.0
71	Cantal	0.24	0.47	14.6	0.45	0.00	–100.0	0.30	0.14	–13.6
72	Charente	0.22	0.65	23.7	0.15	0.07	–13.6	0.30	0.21	–6.7
73	Charente-Maritime	0.23	0.86	30.7	0.10	0.14	7.5	0.09	0.18	13.3
74	Cher	0.47	0.45	–0.8	0.32	0.15	–13.5	0.40	0.15	–17.6
75	Corrèze	0.50	0.82	10.1	0.29	0.10	–20.0	0.47	0.00	–100.0
76	Corse	0.30	0.58	14.2	0.00	0.00	0.0	0.10	0.10	–1.0
77	Côte-d'Or	0.44	0.35	–4.8	0.17	0.00	–100.0	0.30	0.22	–5.3
78	Côtes-du-Nord	0.22	0.85	31.2	0.09	0.13	7.9	0.40	0.08	–26.7
79	Creuse	0.00	0.00	0.0	0.34	0.17	–13.5	0.32	0.30	–1.1
80	Dordogne	0.55	0.52	–1.1	0.31	0.06	–28.1	0.35	0.11	–20.6
81	Doubs	0.07	0.34	37.2	0.11	0.00	–100.0	0.18	0.12	–8.8
82	Drôme	0.28	1.02	29.7	0.39	0.12	–20.9	0.27	0.18	–7.4
83	Eure	0.60	1.10	12.7	0.12	0.16	7.0	0.25	0.17	–7.0
84	Eure-et-Loir	0.10	0.45	35.6	0.15	0.07	–14.1	0.00	0.00	0.0
85	Finistère	0.41	1.05	20.7	0.09	0.06	–8.3	0.27	0.29	1.2
86	Gard	0.21	0.51	19.3	0.41	0.04	–36.3	0.27	0.17	–8.9
87	Haute-Garonne	0.46	0.48	0.9	0.03	0.06	13.4	0.13	0.06	–14.1
88	Gers	0.46	0.23	–13.2	0.00	0.00	0.0	0.13	0.12	–1.9
89	Gironde	0.51	0.81	9.7	0.18	0.15	–3.5	0.18	0.11	–9.8
90	Hérault	0.41	0.41	0.1	0.14	0.13	–1.3	0.38	0.06	–29.9
91	Ille-et-Vilaine	0.42	0.61	7.6	0.17	0.07	–17.6	0.26	0.28	1.4
92	Indre	0.98	0.80	–4.0	0.21	0.20	–0.6	0.71	0.29	–16.6
93	Indre-et-Loire	0.43	0.27	–9.1	0.26	0.05	–28.2	0.27	0.10	–17.8
94	Isère	0.14	0.30	16.0	0.20	0.05	–23.1	0.18	0.36	14.8
95	Jura	0.61	0.73	3.5	0.10	0.00	–100.0	0.00	0.50	36.6
96	Landes	0.13	0.49	30.2	0.00	0.08	–1.5	0.00	0.07	–2.1
97	Loir-et-Cher	0.65	0.73	2.6	0.00	0.00	0.0	0.18	0.08	–14.3
98	Loire	0.44	0.43	–0.6	0.24	0.03	–32.7	0.39	0.17	–15.5
99	Haute-Loire	0.19	0.00	–100.0	0.24	0.12	–13.7	0.48	0.45	–1.3
100	Loire-Atlantique	0.43	0.76	12.2	0.21	0.05	–25.1	0.31	0.10	–19.6
101	Loiret	0.33	0.97	24.1	0.05	0.14	23.0	0.16	0.14	–1.5
102	Lot	0.00	0.51	14.2	0.00	0.00	0.0	0.29	0.27	–1.3
103	Lot-et-Garonne	0.26	0.25	–0.6	0.24	0.00	–100.0	0.00	0.37	36.9
104	Lozère	1.07	0.52	–13.5	0.33	0.00	–100.0	0.33	0.32	–0.4
105	Maine-et-Loire	0.43	0.80	13.5	0.16	0.04	–25.1	0.22	0.28	5.2
106	Manche	0.25	0.70	23.3	0.00	0.05	–0.9	0.22	0.00	–100.0
107	Marne	0.25	0.42	10.7	0.30	0.15	–13.6	0.27	0.57	15.8
108	Haute-Marne	0.17	0.52	24.6	0.25	0.12	–13.4	0.13	0.12	–1.1
109	Mayenne	0.28	0.79	23.3	0.48	0.09	–28.1	0.39	0.09	–25.1
110	Meurthe-et-Moselle	0.38	0.14	–18.1	0.04	0.14	31.0	0.39	0.22	–10.9
111	Meuse	0.19	0.55	24.3	0.52	0.12	–24.8	0.54	0.37	–7.1
112	Morbihan	0.45	0.84	13.4	0.13	0.12	–1.1	0.17	0.20	3.0
113	Moselle	0.47	0.63	6.1	0.23	0.17	–5.6	0.30	0.08	–24.0

Table 9.4(c)—*cont.*

Area		ASTH 1980–84	ASTH 1985–89	ASTH Annual % change	APP 1980–84	APP 1985–89	APP Annual % change	HERN 1980–84	HERN 1985–89	HERN Annual % change
114	Nièvre	0.34	0.66	14.3	0.42	0.10	–24.7	0.51	0.29	–10.6
115	Nord	0.59	1.40	18.9	0.35	0.12	–18.5	0.46	0.36	–4.8
116	Oise	0.41	0.83	15.5	0.13	0.00	–100.0	0.37	0.09	–25.5
117	Orne	0.00	0.25	14.5	0.17	0.00	–100.0	0.09	0.08	–1.1
118	Pas-de-Calais	0.78	1.19	8.8	0.20	0.07	–18.7	0.52	0.37	–6.6
119	Puy-de-dôme	0.42	0.69	10.5	0.13	0.12	–0.6	0.22	0.17	–5.4
120	Pyrénées-Atlantiques	0.62	1.03	10.9	0.00	0.09	13.6	0.22	0.17	–5.7
121	Hautes-Pyrénées	0.33	0.66	14.5	0.11	0.00	–100.0	0.41	0.29	–6.5
122	Pyrénées-Orientales	0.24	0.89	29.9	0.21	0.00	–100.0	0.13	0.12	–1.4
123	Bas-Rhin	0.22	0.35	9.7	0.00	0.03	–1.0	0.34	0.26	–5.2
124	Haut-Rhin	0.37	0.66	12.4	0.24	0.08	–20.6	0.26	0.24	–1.6
125	Rhône	0.19	0.38	15.3	0.09	0.09	–0.5	0.31	0.13	–16.0
126	Haute-Saône	0.32	0.77	19.7	0.45	0.00	–100.0	0.23	0.11	–13.7
127	Saône-et-Loire	0.20	0.46	18.1	0.31	0.04	–32.5	0.18	0.21	3.6
128	Sarthe	0.66	0.35	–12.0	0.31	0.05	–30.7	0.22	0.20	–1.3
129	Savoie	0.21	0.40	13.1	0.08	0.00	–100.0	0.49	0.15	–21.0
130	Haute-Savoie	0.26	0.29	2.1	0.16	0.05	–21.2	0.46	0.21	–14.8
131	Paris	0.34	0.42	4.0	0.10	0.08	–4.3	0.26	0.20	–5.1
132	Seine-Maritime	0.41	0.61	8.6	0.09	0.09	–0.5	0.33	0.34	0.5
133	Seine-et-Marne	0.33	0.54	10.2	0.22	0.00	–100.0	0.25	0.35	7.2
134	Yvelines	0.43	0.75	11.9	0.16	0.06	–16.5	0.18	0.16	–1.5
135	Deux-Sèvres	0.33	0.75	17.5	0.38	0.00	–100.0	0.38	0.14	–17.9
136	Somme	0.26	0.44	10.8	0.15	0.05	–20.2	0.21	0.20	–1.0
137	Tarn	0.58	0.67	2.8	0.07	0.00	–100.0	0.28	0.00	–100.0
138	Tarn-et-Garonne	0.21	0.19	–1.7	0.00	0.00	0.0	0.00	0.12	–1.4
139	Var	0.53	0.86	10.3	0.07	0.00	–100.0	0.20	0.18	–2.1
140	Vaucluse	0.41	0.62	8.4	0.12	0.00	–100.0	0.12	0.11	–1.5
141	Vendée	0.24	0.37	9.3	0.16	0.00	–100.0	0.22	0.00	–100.0
142	Vienne	0.50	0.47	–1.0	0.14	0.00	–100.0	0.22	0.00	–100.0
143	Haute-Vienne	0.55	0.31	–10.6	0.00	0.07	–0.7	0.14	0.19	7.3
144	Vosges	0.09	0.46	37.6	0.20	0.06	–20.0	0.41	0.07	–30.7
145	Yonne	0.75	0.70	–1.3	0.25	0.24	–1.0	0.33	0.23	–6.8
146	Territoire-de-Belfort	0.52	0.25	–13.6	0.20	0.00	–100.0	0.43	0.20	–14.2
147	Essonne	0.38	0.69	12.5	0.17	0.03	–31.0	0.19	0.17	–1.8
148	Hauts-de-Seine	0.22	0.59	21.8	0.13	0.07	–10.4	0.07	0.26	28.7
149	Seine-Saint-Denis	0.42	0.71	10.9	0.12	0.04	–20.0	0.30	0.27	–2.0
150	Val-de-Marne	0.25	0.43	11.4	0.15	0.04	–22.2	0.18	0.22	4.3
151	Val-d'Oise	0.39	0.63	10.4	0.06	0.06	–1.3	0.23	0.21	–1.4
GREECE		0.00	0.08	.	0.06	0.01	–33.9	0.09	0.03	–15.4
152	Greater Athens	0.00	0.05	.	0.06	0.02	–18.4	0.12	0.03	–18.4
153	Rest of Central Greece and Eubea	0.00	0.06	.	0.04	0.00	–100.0	0.08	0.02	–19.1
154	Peloponnisos	0.00	0.08	.	0.04	0.00	–100.0	0.04	0.02	–8.7
155	Ionian Islands	0.00	0.00	.	0.45	0.00	–100.0	0.22	0.00	–100.0
156	Epirus	0.00	0.35	.	0.00	0.00	0.0	0.00	0.16	2.7
157	Thessaly	0.00	0.00	.	0.12	0.00	–100.0	0.13	0.04	–18.6
158	Macedonia	0.00	0.13	.	0.06	0.00	–100.0	0.09	0.01	–27.6
159	Thrace	0.00	0.10	.	0.00	0.00	0.0	0.00	0.00	0.0
160	Aegean Islands	0.00	0.00	.	0.00	0.00	0.0	0.10	0.06	–8.7
161	Crete	0.00	0.15	.	0.09	0.00	–100.0	0.00	0.05	–8.8
ITALY		0.15	0.21	5.6	0.15	0.06	–14.0	0.26	0.15	–8.2
162	Torino	0.19	0.29	7.4	0.21	0.10	–11.9	0.40	0.23	–8.6
163	Vercelli	0.00	0.10	0.6	0.12	0.06	–11.9	0.06	0.26	28.3
164	Novara	0.29	0.14	–10.7	0.00	0.00	0.0	0.30	0.22	–5.0
165	Cuneo	0.34	0.27	–3.6	0.22	0.04	–24.5	0.66	0.31	–11.7
166	Asti	0.18	0.19	0.2	0.11	0.00	–100.0	0.11	0.20	10.3
167	Alessandria	0.26	0.53	12.9	0.31	0.00	–100.0	0.34	0.31	–1.3
168	Aosta	0.00	1.22	25.9	0.22	0.00	–100.0	0.22	0.38	10.0
169	Imperia	0.17	0.53	20.7	0.63	0.00	–100.0	0.20	0.46	14.5
170	Savona	0.00	0.13	0.7	0.08	0.15	11.5	0.15	0.07	–12.1

Age-standardized mortality rates (per 100000) and percentage changes

Table 9.4(c)—*cont.*

	Area	ASTH 1980–84	ASTH 1985–89	ASTH Annual % change	APP 1980–84	APP 1985–89	APP Annual % change	HERN 1980–84	HERN 1985–89	HERN Annual % change
171	Genova	0.29	0.35	2.9	0.13	0.09	–6.7	0.29	0.14	–11.7
172	La Spezia	0.00	0.33	12.7	0.00	0.00	0.0	0.36	0.00	–100.0
173	Varese	0.30	0.22	–5.4	0.07	0.03	–12.3	0.17	0.18	0.5
174	Como/Sondrio	0.25	0.14	–9.1	0.03	0.02	–1.6	0.14	0.17	3.1
175	Milano	0.10	0.09	–2.6	0.12	0.02	–28.0	0.22	0.15	–6.5
176	Bergamo	0.19	0.07	–14.5	0.12	0.05	–12.5	0.22	0.08	–15.6
177	Brescia	0.17	0.13	–3.9	0.18	0.11	–6.9	0.08	0.09	2.3
178	Pavia	0.15	0.46	20.7	0.14	0.13	–1.1	0.23	0.04	–25.0
179	Cremona	0.22	0.33	7.2	0.22	0.00	–100.0	0.22	0.32	6.6
180	Mantova	0.20	0.20	0.0	0.06	0.00	–100.0	0.25	0.23	–1.6
181	Bolzano	0.16	0.15	–0.3	0.25	0.06	–21.6	0.14	0.18	4.5
182	Trento	0.16	0.16	–0.4	0.00	0.16	18.4	0.24	0.16	–6.9
183	Verona	0.09	0.18	11.9	0.13	0.06	–12.1	0.03	0.03	–2.2
184	Vicenza	0.05	0.09	11.7	0.18	0.00	–100.0	0.23	0.23	0.1
185	Belluno	0.17	0.33	12.4	0.11	0.00	–100.0	0.11	0.00	–100.0
186	Treviso	0.14	0.14	–0.6	0.00	0.07	10.5	0.27	0.10	–15.4
187	Venezia	0.24	0.36	6.9	0.12	0.03	–21.6	0.16	0.00	–100.0
188	Padova	0.17	0.25	6.6	0.06	0.03	–12.1	0.23	0.09	–15.2
189	Rovigo	0.15	0.14	–0.2	0.10	0.18	10.9	0.48	0.09	–25.1
190	Udine/Gorizia	0.16	0.21	5.0	0.11	0.03	–17.3	0.25	0.07	–20.0
191	Trieste	0.28	0.30	1.2	0.24	0.00	–100.0	0.07	0.07	–0.0
192	Pordenone	0.00	0.00	0.0	0.09	0.00	–100.0	0.19	0.17	–2.0
193	Piacenza	0.00	0.00	0.0	0.17	0.08	–11.6	0.00	0.07	–1.5
194	Parma	0.29	0.19	–6.4	0.17	0.11	–7.2	0.22	0.31	5.6
195	Reggio Emilia	0.00	0.18	12.1	0.06	0.00	–100.0	0.00	0.00	0.0
196	Modena	0.06	0.06	–0.1	0.04	0.11	18.9	0.20	0.00	–100.0
197	Bologna	0.12	0.24	12.8	0.15	0.05	–17.2	0.19	0.11	–8.7
198	Ferrara	0.00	0.10	0.5	0.06	0.06	–0.6	0.12	0.00	–100.0
199	Ravenna	0.10	0.00	–100.0	0.07	0.06	–1.0	0.13	0.17	5.1
200	Forli	0.00	0.06	–0.2	0.00	0.04	–1.3	0.12	0.07	–8.5
201	Pesaro	0.11	0.00	–100.0	0.22	0.14	–7.5	0.14	0.00	–100.0
202	Ancona	0.09	0.17	12.1	0.05	0.00	–100.0	0.21	0.14	–6.3
203	Macerata	0.13	0.00	–100.0	0.16	0.00	–100.0	0.08	0.07	–1.7
204	Ascoli Piceno	0.00	0.10	0.0	0.07	0.13	10.8	0.20	0.12	–8.5
205	Massa-Carrara	0.19	0.00	–100.0	0.35	0.00	–100.0	0.23	0.20	–1.9
206	Lucca	0.39	0.10	–20.6	0.25	0.06	–21.4	0.18	0.06	–18.1
207	Pistoia	0.42	0.00	–100.0	0.09	0.00	–100.0	0.18	0.16	–1.6
208	Firenze	0.03	0.18	34.9	0.04	0.02	–11.7	0.14	0.12	–1.6
209	Livorno	0.11	0.53	30.6	0.54	0.20	–15.5	0.20	0.25	3.8
210	Pisa	0.29	0.57	12.0	0.06	0.18	19.0	0.06	0.05	–1.5
211	Arezzo	0.00	0.24	12.2	0.15	0.07	–11.7	0.07	0.13	10.5
212	Siena	0.31	0.63	12.5	0.44	0.00	–100.0	0.50	0.08	–26.8
213	Grosseto	0.17	0.69	26.1	0.00	0.20	11.3	0.10	0.00	–100.0
214	Perugia	0.06	0.13	11.9	0.00	0.00	0.0	0.31	0.18	–9.1
215	Terni	0.17	0.00	–100.0	0.00	0.10	–0.7	0.19	0.09	–12.1
216	Viterbo/Rieti	0.19	0.45	15.8	0.12	0.05	–12.0	0.34	0.00	–100.0
217	Roma	0.15	0.27	10.9	0.14	0.07	–11.4	0.27	0.14	–10.4
218	Latina	0.08	0.07	–1.2	0.06	0.05	–2.3	0.20	0.11	–9.5
219	Frosinone	0.08	0.22	19.0	0.06	0.00	–100.0	0.23	0.35	7.3
220	Caserta	0.19	0.08	–12.3	0.18	0.00	–100.0	0.85	0.21	–21.1
221	Benevento	0.13	0.13	–0.7	0.00	0.00	0.0	0.18	0.47	17.4
222	Napoli	0.23	0.30	4.3	0.24	0.05	–22.4	0.56	0.30	–9.9
223	Avellino	0.17	0.08	–11.6	0.06	0.05	–1.4	0.06	0.16	17.6
224	Salerno	0.14	0.17	2.9	0.29	0.12	–14.0	0.20	0.26	4.9
225	L'Aquila	0.26	0.00	–100.0	0.08	0.15	11.3	0.24	0.00	–100.0
226	Teramo	0.14	0.26	11.6	0.09	0.26	18.2	0.19	0.08	–12.9
227	Pescara	0.25	0.12	–11.2	0.26	0.00	–100.0	0.18	0.23	4.6
228	Chieti	0.10	0.29	19.1	0.26	0.00	–100.0	0.07	0.18	18.0
229	Isernia/Campobasso	0.12	0.00	–100.0	0.08	0.07	–1.2	0.31	0.14	–12.5
230	Foggia	0.00	0.25	29.6	0.04	0.07	10.6	0.35	0.19	–9.6
231	Bari	0.17	0.18	1.1	0.23	0.03	–27.0	0.21	0.24	2.0

Age-standardized mortality rates (per 100000) and percentage changes

Table 9.4(c)—*cont.*

Area		ASTH 1980–84	ASTH 1985–89	ASTH Annual % change	APP 1980–84	APP 1985–89	APP Annual % change	HERN 1980–84	HERN 1985–89	HERN Annual % change
		Age-standardized mortality rates (per 100000) and percentage changes								
232	Taranto	0.06	0.39	36.9	0.24	0.13	−9.8	0.43	0.18	−13.1
233	Brindisi	0.00	0.00	0.0	0.34	0.00	−100.0	0.15	0.19	4.8
234	Lecce	0.19	0.09	−12.0	0.10	0.03	−18.5	0.34	0.09	−19.2
235	Potenza/Matera	0.18	0.41	14.7	0.22	0.00	−100.0	0.32	0.16	−11.1
236	Cosenza	0.10	0.18	10.9	0.11	0.07	−8.4	0.36	0.20	−9.1
237	Catanzaro	0.19	0.05	−21.5	0.26	0.07	−20.1	0.17	0.11	−6.9
238	Reggio Calabria	0.13	0.49	25.1	0.09	0.09	−1.1	0.25	0.09	−15.7
239	Trapani	0.61	0.33	−9.7	0.00	0.06	−1.5	0.26	0.17	−6.7
240	Palermo	0.12	0.36	20.3	0.20	0.10	−10.8	0.34	0.13	−15.2
241	Messina	0.06	0.59	48.1	0.23	0.11	−12.0	0.35	0.14	−14.2
242	Agrigento	0.15	0.07	−11.6	0.11	0.05	−12.5	0.49	0.10	−22.7
243	Caltanisetta	0.38	0.12	−17.2	0.28	0.09	−17.8	0.40	0.18	−12.8
244	Enna	0.38	0.37	−0.2	0.13	0.13	−1.1	0.56	0.13	−22.1
245	Catania	0.04	0.13	24.3	0.27	0.14	−9.9	0.20	0.17	−2.6
246	Ragusa	0.27	0.12	−11.9	0.19	0.00	−100.0	0.20	0.26	4.7
247	Siracusa	0.00	0.17	11.3	0.00	0.12	10.7	0.44	0.32	−5.0
248	Sassari	0.00	0.52	36.7	0.00	0.06	−1.8	0.35	0.12	−16.3
249	Nuoro	0.39	0.00	−100.0	0.20	0.00	−100.0	0.33	0.00	−100.0
250	Cagliari/Oristano	0.23	0.18	−4.2	0.13	0.09	−6.3	0.35	0.15	−13.1
IRELAND		1.01	0.97	−0.9	0.14	0.07	−12.3	0.13	0.12	−1.7
251	Eastern	1.11	0.75	−7.7	0.13	0.07	−10.5	0.03	0.03	−1.1
252	Midland	0.76	1.93	20.4	0.00	0.14	−0.3	0.15	0.15	−0.0
253	Mid-Western	0.49	1.35	22.6	0.37	0.00	−100.0	0.20	0.10	−12.9
254	North-Eastern	1.04	1.41	6.3	0.20	0.19	−0.6	0.33	0.11	−19.9
255	North-Western	0.78	0.53	−7.3	0.27	0.00	−100.0	0.14	0.45	25.8
256	South-Eastern	1.11	0.84	−5.5	0.08	0.00	−100.0	0.17	0.08	−13.3
257	Southern	0.93	0.66	−6.5	0.05	0.11	14.7	0.06	0.00	−100.0
258	Western	1.40	1.40	0.0	0.16	0.08	−12.7	0.26	0.45	11.7
THE NETHERLANDS		0.35	0.25	−7.1	0.12	0.10	−4.4	0.15	0.12	−5.0
259	Groningen	0.12	0.07	−10.8	0.19	0.06	−22.6	0.05	0.13	22.6
260	Friesland	0.52	0.34	−8.8	0.14	0.17	4.8	0.20	0.06	−23.3
261	Drenthe	0.00	0.28	32.4	0.06	0.30	42.1	0.06	0.23	32.7
262	Overijssel	0.23	0.24	1.4	0.18	0.20	1.9	0.22	0.28	4.8
263	Gelderland	0.34	0.27	−5.3	0.11	0.09	−3.5	0.12	0.12	−0.2
264	Utrecht	0.32	0.24	−5.8	0.03	0.07	21.3	0.16	0.04	−27.6
265	Noord Holland	0.44	0.29	−9.2	0.10	0.07	−7.7	0.18	0.12	−8.8
266	Zuid Holland	0.40	0.30	−5.7	0.10	0.11	2.9	0.14	0.12	−3.7
267	Zeeland	0.10	0.00	−100.0	0.30	0.19	−9.9	0.08	0.19	22.2
268	Noord Brabant	0.30	0.14	−15.2	0.13	0.03	−27.5	0.23	0.11	−14.5
269	Limburg	0.48	0.33	−8.0	0.19	0.11	−10.6	0.10	0.06	−11.4
270	Flevoland	0.29	0.20	−8.3	0.28	0.00	−100.0	0.08	0.22	26.9
UK: ENGLAND AND WALES		0.95	1.00	1.1	0.10	0.09	−2.4	0.21	0.18	−2.7
271	Northern	1.07	0.92	−2.9	0.15	0.11	−6.5	0.16	0.10	−9.8
272	Yorkshire	0.75	1.04	6.7	0.09	0.05	−11.2	0.18	0.18	0.6
273	Trent	0.88	1.14	5.3	0.10	0.14	7.3	0.20	0.15	−6.1
274	East Anglian	1.12	1.14	0.4	0.08	0.09	2.8	0.31	0.15	−13.2
275	North-West Thames	1.03	0.95	−1.8	0.06	0.04	−8.4	0.24	0.17	−6.2
276	North-East Thames	1.02	1.00	−0.4	0.11	0.10	−1.9	0.15	0.18	3.4
277	South-East Thames	0.89	1.01	2.5	0.13	0.10	−5.4	0.18	0.16	−2.6
278	South-West Thames	0.95	1.06	2.0	0.10	0.11	2.2	0.13	0.13	−0.6
279	Wessex	0.95	1.05	2.2	0.08	0.05	−7.9	0.21	0.20	−1.8
280	Oxford	0.76	1.00	5.6	0.09	0.12	6.2	0.11	0.22	14.5
281	South-Western	1.07	0.83	−5.0	0.10	0.07	−7.1	0.28	0.22	−4.8
282	West Midlands	1.10	0.90	−4.0	0.11	0.08	−5.3	0.28	0.26	−1.5
283	Mersey	0.83	1.05	4.9	0.08	0.04	−12.3	0.16	0.14	−3.3
284	North-Western	0.85	1.03	3.9	0.12	0.13	1.8	0.28	0.23	−4.4
285	Wales	0.90	0.96	1.3	0.09	0.08	−1.6	0.19	0.19	0.5

Table 9.4(c)—*cont.*

Area		ASTH 1980–84	ASTH 1985–89	ASTH Annual % change	APP 1980–84	APP 1985–89	APP Annual % change	HERN 1980–84	HERN 1985–89	HERN Annual % change
		Age-standardized mortality rates (per 100000) and percentage changes								
UK: NORTHERN IRELAND		1.05	0.96	−1.8	0.14	0.11	−5.6	0.25	0.09	−17.4
286	Northern Ireland	1.05	0.96	−1.8	0.14	0.11	−5.6	0.25	0.09	−17.4
UK: SCOTLAND		0.83	0.93	2.3	0.12	0.08	−6.3	0.20	0.13	−8.5
287	Highlands and Islands	1.21	1.54	4.9	0.19	0.09	−13.4	0.10	0.29	23.5
288	Grampian	0.58	0.74	5.1	0.11	0.05	−13.4	0.17	0.11	−8.3
289	Tayside	0.56	1.47	21.2	0.06	0.19	24.9	0.38	0.06	−30.1
290	Fife	0.42	1.01	19.2	0.00	0.07	0.2	0.00	0.00	0.0
291	Lothian	0.80	0.91	2.7	0.07	0.00	−100.0	0.10	0.07	−7.5
292	Borders	0.38	0.36	−1.1	0.24	0.00	−100.0	0.24	0.24	0.1
293	Forth Valley	0.78	1.40	12.4	0.09	0.09	0.2	0.47	0.37	−4.5
294	Argyll and Clyde	0.47	0.47	0.1	0.22	0.00	−100.0	0.28	0.23	−4.1
295	Greater Glasgow	1.27	0.83	−8.1	0.07	0.13	12.4	0.17	0.16	−1.7
296	Lanarkshire	0.72	0.96	5.9	0.18	0.18	0.2	0.23	0.09	−16.9
297	Ayrshire and Arran	1.34	0.75	−10.9	0.20	0.07	−19.5	0.34	0.07	−27.5
298	Dumfries and Galloway	0.52	0.75	7.8	0.17	0.00	−100.0	0.00	0.00	0.0
PORTUGAL		0.00	0.50	.	0.20	0.07	−19.0	0.19	0.12	−8.8
299	Viana do Castelo	0.00	0.84	.	0.00	0.10	−0.3	0.20	0.20	−0.2
300	Braga	0.00	0.56	.	0.20	0.08	−17.9	0.09	0.22	18.2
301	Vila Real	0.00	0.69	.	0.10	0.00	−100.0	0.10	0.10	0.5
302	Bragança	0.00	0.00	.	0.13	0.13	0.4	0.26	0.00	−100.0
303	Guarda	0.00	0.41	.	0.12	0.13	1.5	0.12	0.25	16.7
304	Viseu	0.00	0.00	.	0.18	0.00	−100.0	0.25	0.13	−12.3
305	Porto	0.00	0.37	.	0.21	0.07	−21.0	0.16	0.12	−4.6
306	Aveiro	0.00	0.51	.	0.13	0.24	13.3	0.19	0.09	−14.4
307	Coimbra	0.00	0.58	.	0.17	0.11	−8.3	0.11	0.05	−13.6
308	Castelo Branco	0.00	0.18	.	0.30	0.11	−18.8	0.29	0.00	−100.0
309	Portalegre	0.00	0.00	.	0.16	0.00	−100.0	0.60	0.00	−100.0
310	Santarem	0.00	0.17	.	0.10	0.10	−0.3	0.20	0.30	7.9
311	Leiria	0.00	0.58	.	0.35	0.00	−100.0	0.24	0.11	−13.8
312	Lisboa	0.00	0.69	.	0.24	0.04	−28.5	0.20	0.08	−16.8
313	Setubal	0.00	0.52	.	0.26	0.03	−34.9	0.16	0.09	−9.8
314	Evora	0.00	0.23	.	0.13	0.00	−100.0	0.24	0.12	−12.9
315	Beja	0.00	0.69	.	0.50	0.13	−23.4	0.36	0.00	−100.0
316	Faro	0.00	0.45	.	0.15	0.07	−13.5	0.00	0.21	23.8
317	Madeira	0.00	0.53	.	0.22	0.11	−13.7	0.12	0.12	−1.3
318	Azores	0.00	0.92	.	0.22	0.11	−12.6	0.35	0.24	−7.3
SPAIN		0.23	0.29	4.4	0.16	0.06	−17.3	0.21	0.11	−11.3
319	La Coruña	0.07	0.34	34.3	0.14	0.09	−8.7	0.17	0.21	3.5
320	Lugo	0.41	0.14	−17.9	0.00	0.00	0.0	0.27	0.14	−11.5
321	Orense	0.27	0.24	−2.1	0.28	0.07	−22.1	0.11	0.20	12.1
322	Pontevedra	0.38	0.35	−1.1	0.18	0.07	−15.5	0.29	0.00	−100.0
323	Asturias	0.17	0.17	0.2	0.24	0.03	−33.3	0.17	0.00	−100.0
324	Cantabria	0.29	0.63	14.9	0.20	0.06	−19.7	0.10	0.18	11.1
325	Alava	0.00	0.29	15.6	0.43	0.12	−21.0	0.12	0.13	1.7
326	Guipuzcoa	0.15	0.24	9.2	0.08	0.00	−100.0	0.16	0.14	−2.5
327	Vizcaya	0.24	0.50	14.6	0.11	0.07	−6.8	0.16	0.08	−12.5
328	Navarra	0.29	0.35	3.6	0.20	0.06	−19.7	0.26	0.00	−100.0
329	Rioja	0.15	0.37	17.9	0.10	0.00	−100.0	0.10	0.00	−100.0
330	Huesca	0.00	0.77	28.5	0.00	0.13	4.1	0.21	0.00	−100.0
331	Teruel	0.00	0.00	0.0	0.15	0.00	−100.0	0.00	0.20	5.3
332	Zaragoza	0.00	0.28	39.3	0.18	0.07	−15.7	0.24	0.17	−5.6
333	Madrid Centro	0.16	0.09	−8.9	0.05	0.03	−6.4	0.11	0.05	−13.2
334	Avila	0.00	0.64	21.0	0.00	0.00	0.0	0.13	0.00	−100.0
335	Burgos	0.10	0.13	4.6	0.14	0.08	−8.4	0.07	0.00	−100.0
336	Leon	0.38	0.21	−10.1	0.37	0.06	−28.6	0.09	0.06	−8.6
337	Palencia	0.42	0.00	−100.0	0.13	0.17	4.6	0.13	0.00	−100.0
338	Salamanca	0.11	0.73	41.2	0.21	0.00	−100.0	0.00	0.09	4.4
339	Segovia	0.27	0.00	−100.0	0.16	0.00	−100.0	0.00	0.00	0.0

Table 9.4(c)—*cont.*

Area		Age-standardized mortality rates (per 100000) and percentage changes ASTH			APP			HERN		
		1980–84	1985–89	Annual % change	1980–84	1985–89	Annual % change	1980–84	1985–89	Annual % change
340	Soria	0.00	0.61	6.9	0.24	0.00	−100.0	0.00	0.00	0.0
341	Valladolid	0.07	0.09	2.9	0.17	0.06	−16.0	0.18	0.21	2.6
342	Zamora	0.00	0.00	0.0	0.00	0.00	0.0	0.10	0.13	4.8
343	Albacete	0.00	0.44	27.9	0.15	0.09	−8.5	0.32	0.20	−8.6
344	Ciudad Real	0.17	0.34	13.7	0.11	0.00	−100.0	0.43	0.00	−100.0
345	Cuenca	0.39	0.28	−6.0	0.45	0.00	−100.0	0.11	0.30	19.4
346	Guadalajara	0.00	0.00	0.0	0.17	0.00	−100.0	0.17	0.00	−100.0
347	Toledo	0.34	0.11	−18.4	0.11	0.00	−100.0	0.27	0.00	−100.0
348	Badajoz	0.49	0.41	−3.0	0.20	0.11	−11.3	0.25	0.27	1.3
349	Caceres	0.00	0.13	6.0	0.12	0.00	−100.0	0.31	0.08	−21.7
350	Barcelona	0.22	0.36	8.8	0.10	0.04	−16.1	0.09	0.08	−2.8
351	Gerona	0.58	0.90	8.4	0.37	0.06	−27.7	0.37	0.25	−7.0
352	Lerida	0.00	0.44	27.8	0.27	0.08	−19.3	0.00	0.08	3.6
353	Tarragona	0.67	0.17	−21.8	0.20	0.11	−9.5	0.15	0.06	−15.9
354	Alicante	0.19	0.25	5.2	0.12	0.05	−13.7	0.17	0.05	−18.8
355	Castellon de la Plana	0.27	0.32	3.5	0.23	0.14	−9.0	0.00	0.42	43.2
356	Valencia	0.27	0.19	−6.2	0.25	0.16	−7.8	0.41	0.23	−9.8
357	Baleares	0.57	0.19	−17.8	0.16	0.09	−9.6	0.08	0.05	−9.4
358	Almeria	0.27	0.45	9.4	0.07	0.00	−100.0	0.37	0.09	−23.0
359	Cadiz	0.25	0.56	15.6	0.18	0.14	−4.4	0.51	0.32	−8.2
360	Cordoba	0.16	0.07	−14.2	0.26	0.00	−100.0	0.12	0.19	9.4
361	Granada	0.10	0.06	−7.9	0.32	0.00	−100.0	0.56	0.18	−18.7
362	Huelva	0.19	0.23	4.3	0.13	0.00	−100.0	0.41	0.17	−14.5
363	Jaen	0.18	0.32	10.9	0.29	0.10	−17.1	0.31	0.22	−6.2
364	Malaga	0.42	0.49	2.6	0.13	0.06	−13.4	0.41	0.03	−36.7
365	Sevilla	0.32	0.45	6.3	0.24	0.07	−21.1	0.49	0.17	−17.7
366	Murcia	0.00	0.23	38.4	0.34	0.03	−34.7	0.22	0.07	−18.3
367	Las Palmas	0.58	0.32	−10.3	0.25	0.05	−26.5	0.36	0.06	−28.3
368	Sta Cruz de Tenerife	0.32	0.38	3.2	0.04	0.10	16.9	0.20	0.06	−19.8
EC		0.54	0.59	1.6	0.15	0.07	−11.6	0.21	0.14	−7.0

Table 9.4(d)

Area	CHOLY 1980–84	CHOLY 1985–89	CHOLY Annual % change	HYP/S 1980–84	HYP/S 1985–89	HYP/S Annual % change	MAT 1980–84	MAT 1985–89	MAT Annual % change
	Age-standardized mortality rates (per 100000) and percentage changes								
BELGIUM	0.35	0.11	−20.2	35.74	30.61	−3.0	7.27	4.55	−8.9
1 Antwerpen	0.25	0.09	−18.9	35.72	29.13	−4.0	9.21	4.26	−14.3
2 Brabant	0.36	0.09	−23.7	33.24	27.88	−3.5	8.28	6.68	−4.2
3 West-Vlaanderen	0.38	0.13	−19.4	26.99	21.35	−4.6	4.44	3.09	−7.0
4 Oost-Vlaanderen	0.17	0.16	−1.4	31.68	26.46	−3.5	3.80	4.09	1.5
5 Hainaut	0.51	0.18	−19.1	43.06	35.84	−3.6	3.91	2.59	−7.9
6 Liege	0.36	0.00	−100.0	40.72	44.86	2.0	8.54	8.28	−0.6
7 Limburg	0.32	0.18	−11.3	33.42	27.18	−4.0	11.65	2.19	−28.4
8 Luxembourg (province)	0.92	0.00	−100.0	43.88	32.41	−5.9	13.46	0.00	−100.0
9 Namur	0.37	0.17	−14.0	47.07	40.97	−2.7	7.51	3.71	−13.2
LUXEMBOURG	0.51	0.32	−8.8	52.22	46.54	−2.3	0.00	4.54	−0.6
10 Luxembourg	0.51	0.32	−8.8	52.22	46.54	−2.3	0.00	4.54	−0.6
FEDERAL REPUBLIC OF GERMANY	0.45	0.23	−12.2	40.28	31.26	−4.9	15.97	8.19	−12.5
11 Schleswig-Holstein	0.46	0.32	−7.0	34.12	28.14	−3.8	12.43	11.63	−1.3
12 Hamburg	0.36	0.16	−15.2	36.99	27.43	−5.8	13.67	7.01	−12.5
13 Braunschweig	0.49	0.13	−23.6	41.58	30.82	−5.8	12.00	5.21	−15.4
14 Hannover	0.57	0.17	−21.7	39.59	28.62	−6.3	6.61	4.33	−8.1
15 Lüneburg	0.47	0.18	−17.5	37.37	27.91	−5.7	4.28	5.45	4.9
16 Weser-Ems	0.38	0.29	−5.1	38.69	29.77	−5.1	13.73	4.06	−21.6
17 Bremen	0.43	0.07	−30.7	45.25	28.02	−9.1	3.46	10.04	23.7
18 Düsseldorf	0.30	0.18	−9.8	39.62	32.94	−3.6	21.23	8.92	−15.9
19 Köln	0.35	0.22	−8.5	39.39	29.10	−5.9	18.94	6.35	−19.6
20 Munster	0.48	0.24	−12.6	43.45	32.39	−5.7	19.84	7.24	−18.3
21 Detmold	0.43	0.21	−13.5	37.67	31.32	−3.6	14.38	3.11	−26.4
22 Arnsberg	0.48	0.26	−11.4	45.05	35.04	−4.9	20.41	9.60	−14.0
23 Darmstadt	0.48	0.19	−17.0	38.35	30.82	−4.3	19.98	8.97	−14.8
24 Giessen	0.45	0.24	−11.5	38.66	31.08	−4.3	16.21	9.91	−9.4
25 Kassel	0.62	0.29	−14.0	37.35	30.75	−3.8	14.51	3.51	−24.7
26 Koblenz	0.25	0.23	−1.7	48.18	33.56	−7.0	14.68	9.93	−7.5
27 Trier	0.26	0.14	−11.5	48.64	35.05	−6.3	15.65	3.96	−24.0
28 Rheinhessen-Pfalz	0.36	0.11	−20.8	49.71	38.11	−5.2	24.47	10.61	−15.4
29 Stuttgart	0.43	0.29	−7.5	34.57	26.33	−5.3	14.00	4.06	−21.9
30 Karlsruhe	0.51	0.28	−11.3	41.44	29.89	−6.3	14.15	6.29	−15.0
31 Freiburg	0.56	0.39	−7.1	34.68	30.30	−2.7	14.58	1.88	−33.6
32 Tübingen	0.33	0.28	−3.3	36.15	26.13	−6.3	10.27	1.07	−36.4
33 Oberbayern	0.25	0.24	−1.5	32.76	26.03	−4.5	10.21	13.03	5.0
34 Niederbayern	0.70	0.21	−21.3	44.18	34.94	−4.6	25.88	10.26	−16.9
35 Oberpfalz	0.62	0.27	−15.3	47.57	37.21	−4.8	23.63	17.95	−5.4
36 Oberfranken	0.82	0.28	−19.2	47.65	39.24	−3.8	16.68	14.52	−2.7
37 Mittelfranken	0.60	0.21	−18.5	39.47	31.51	−4.4	15.60	15.81	0.3
38 Unterfranken	0.83	0.18	−26.5	34.15	31.13	−1.8	14.50	8.44	−10.3
39 Schwaben	0.24	0.31	5.8	37.28	30.53	−3.9	25.80	11.03	−15.6
40 Saarland	0.55	0.43	−4.5	53.95	41.57	−5.1	9.77	15.25	9.3
41 Berlin (West)	0.74	0.24	−20.4	55.75	40.13	−6.4	13.01	12.16	−1.3
DENMARK	0.26	0.32	4.1	33.44	31.28	−1.3	5.62	5.23	−1.4
42 Kobenhavn and Frederiksberg (M)	0.24	0.48	15.1	42.05	42.11	0.0	7.65	6.74	−2.5
43 Kobenhavns County	0.23	0.27	3.2	31.46	31.56	0.1	6.78	0.00	−100.0
44 Frederiksborg County	0.26	0.31	3.9	30.49	27.44	−2.1	12.06	0.00	−100.0
45 Roskilde County	0.00	0.00	0.0	31.44	29.34	−1.4	0.00	17.37	11.6
46 Vestsjællands County	0.18	0.27	8.2	30.85	33.71	1.8	14.26	6.45	−14.7
47 Storstroms County	0.28	0.56	15.1	33.32	29.16	−2.6	0.00	7.67	−1.3
48 Bornholms County	0.00	0.00	0.0	27.56	35.33	5.1	0.00	0.00	0.0
49 Fyns County	0.51	0.34	−7.7	29.38	23.61	−4.3	0.00	8.09	13.3
50 Sonderjyllands County	0.22	0.31	7.2	32.92	31.29	−1.0	0.00	6.82	−0.5
51 Ribe County	0.25	0.50	14.4	32.85	27.69	−3.4	0.00	14.83	14.0
52 Vejle County	0.32	0.24	−5.8	34.97	32.76	−1.3	0.00	5.36	−0.7
53 Ringkobing County	0.63	0.10	−30.4	38.82	30.86	−4.5	6.24	0.00	−100.0
54 Århus County	0.19	0.24	4.5	30.28	30.01	−0.2	3.13	5.76	13.0

Table 9.4(d)—*cont.*

Area		CHOLY 1980–84	CHOLY 1985–89	CHOLY Annual % change	HYP/S 1980–84	HYP/S 1985–89	HYP/S Annual % change	MAT 1980–84	MAT 1985–89	MAT Annual % change
55	Viborg County	0.22	0.34	8.6	36.15	27.86	−5.1	7.59	7.30	−0.8
56	Nordjyllands County	0.16	0.43	22.1	32.25	32.76	0.3	15.17	0.00	−100.0
FRANCE		0.36	0.20	−11.3	34.14	27.31	−4.4	13.85	9.82	−6.6
57	Ain	0.39	0.18	−14.3	29.69	24.55	−3.7	19.90	6.50	−20.1
58	Aisne	0.41	0.38	−1.2	40.15	29.35	−6.1	19.07	7.50	−17.0
59	Allier	0.19	0.24	4.8	37.60	28.10	−5.7	14.78	10.94	−5.8
60	Alpes-de-Haute-Provence	0.20	0.00	−100.0	31.55	24.61	−4.9	14.46	0.00	−100.0
61	Hautes-Alpes	0.23	0.44	13.7	28.53	23.69	−3.7	14.09	13.95	−0.2
62	Alpes-Maritimes	0.37	0.12	−19.9	24.20	21.15	−2.7	10.13	11.19	2.0
63	Ardèche	0.28	0.17	−9.1	35.31	29.13	−3.8	18.30	18.62	0.4
64	Ardennes	0.75	0.26	−19.1	39.41	30.26	−5.1	12.89	8.98	−7.0
65	Ariège	0.00	0.00	0.0	25.19	25.74	0.4	0.00	0.00	0.0
66	Aube	0.95	0.09	−37.5	35.32	30.22	−3.1	14.91	10.26	−7.2
67	Aude	0.40	0.15	−17.7	26.58	23.83	−2.2	13.12	18.76	7.4
68	Aveyron	0.34	0.24	−6.9	28.28	25.88	−1.8	19.65	0.00	−100.0
69	Bouches-du-Rhône	0.29	0.10	−18.6	31.89	25.09	−4.7	19.81	10.18	−12.5
70	Calvados	0.19	0.09	−14.2	37.58	28.62	−5.3	8.56	4.51	−12.0
71	Cantal	0.30	0.43	7.5	43.63	35.56	−4.0	10.42	23.91	18.1
72	Charente	0.45	0.21	−14.0	29.53	31.11	1.0	18.38	14.79	−4.3
73	Charente-Maritime	0.24	0.44	13.2	28.93	25.09	−2.8	6.25	3.32	−11.9
74	Cher	0.48	0.23	−13.9	34.33	29.73	−2.8	10.28	5.28	−12.5
75	Corrèze	0.28	0.36	5.1	34.92	28.51	−4.0	0.00	0.00	0.0
76	Corse	0.10	0.48	36.5	33.07	29.73	−2.1	6.91	6.71	−0.6
77	Côte-d'Or	0.42	0.17	−16.6	29.68	22.25	−5.6	16.69	11.84	−6.6
78	Côtes-du-Nord	0.18	0.21	3.5	45.64	31.70	−7.0	8.66	6.22	−6.4
79	Creuse	0.48	0.15	−20.7	48.32	23.70	−13.3	2.88	0.00	−100.0
80	Dordogne	0.35	0.28	−4.8	38.33	24.26	−8.7	48.27	15.40	−20.4
81	Doubs	0.25	0.12	−14.0	33.44	27.98	−3.5	20.00	11.54	−10.4
82	Drôme	0.54	0.24	−14.7	27.45	23.47	−3.1	2.55	0.00	−100.0
83	Eure	0.44	0.34	−4.7	34.95	30.58	−2.6	14.29	8.05	−10.8
84	Eure-et-Loir	0.08	0.14	12.9	30.38	21.09	−7.0	7.20	7.20	0.0
85	Finistère	0.39	0.23	−10.2	44.32	31.58	−6.6	14.12	9.39	−7.8
86	Gard	0.41	0.21	−12.3	26.71	26.61	−0.1	20.48	19.56	−0.9
87	Haute-Garonne	0.26	0.06	−25.3	26.12	20.97	−4.3	13.63	3.65	−23.2
88	Gers	0.40	0.00	−100.0	29.04	23.08	−4.5	11.74	11.97	0.4
89	Gironde	0.30	0.22	−6.1	31.98	25.10	−4.7	9.32	4.08	−15.2
90	Hérault	0.45	0.23	−12.9	29.24	20.22	−7.1	17.90	16.85	−1.2
91	Ille-et-Vilaine	0.41	0.03	−39.0	41.68	30.25	−6.2	10.54	12.96	4.2
92	Indre	0.61	0.09	−31.0	36.03	24.91	−7.1	0.00	0.00	0.0
93	Indre-et-Loire	0.22	0.15	−6.9	22.61	21.28	−1.2	8.69	8.85	0.4
94	Isère	0.67	0.14	−26.9	28.14	21.87	−4.9	10.10	5.64	−11.0
95	Jura	0.11	0.10	−1.1	37.19	21.47	−10.4	12.13	0.00	−100.0
96	Landes	0.24	0.29	3.6	32.47	27.47	−3.3	0.00	6.07	0.4
97	Loir-et-Cher	0.35	0.08	−25.5	38.20	25.19	−8.0	5.33	0.00	−100.0
98	Loire	0.25	0.33	6.1	31.94	26.05	−4.0	9.52	4.16	−15.2
99	Haute-Loire	0.72	0.33	−14.2	37.60	30.42	−4.2	16.22	34.48	16.3
100	Loire-Atlantique	0.26	0.26	0.4	37.57	29.59	−4.7	7.73	4.15	−11.7
101	Loiret	0.26	0.29	2.0	29.06	23.41	−4.2	2.50	17.68	47.8
102	Lot	0.15	0.00	−100.0	35.30	28.69	−4.1	0.00	13.11	1.7
103	Lot-et-Garonne	0.00	0.07	−0.9	31.72	22.72	−6.5	11.23	5.81	−12.3
104	Lozère	0.00	0.00	0.0	37.58	28.84	−5.2	21.65	0.00	−100.0
105	Maine-et-Loire	0.18	0.24	6.4	31.02	26.38	−3.2	5.28	7.81	8.1
106	Manche	0.44	0.05	−34.9	36.73	28.98	−4.6	8.72	5.92	−7.4
107	Marne	0.17	0.31	13.4	32.31	31.89	−0.3	18.41	9.63	−12.2
108	Haute-Marne	0.53	0.37	−6.8	34.01	30.42	−2.2	43.41	20.82	−13.7
109	Mayenne	0.30	0.19	−9.0	34.85	24.91	−6.5	4.83	21.17	34.4
110	Meurthe-et-Moselle	0.39	0.11	−22.5	38.22	27.16	−6.6	11.03	13.67	4.4
111	Meuse	0.41	0.25	−9.4	42.82	30.91	−6.3	33.54	28.82	−3.0
112	Morbihan	0.22	0.20	−1.7	53.09	42.12	−4.5	9.35	19.68	16.1
113	Moselle	0.86	0.38	−14.9	44.10	36.98	−3.5	34.83	6.74	−28.0

Age-standardized mortality rates (per 100 000) and percentage changes

Table 9.4(d)—*cont.*

Area		CHOLY 1980–84	CHOLY 1985–89	CHOLY Annual % change	HYP/S 1980–84	HYP/S 1985–89	HYP/S Annual % change	MAT 1980–84	MAT 1985–89	MAT Annual % change
114	Nièvre	0.20	0.39	13.6	39.27	32.52	−3.7	14.34	15.41	1.4
115	Nord	0.54	0.34	−9.0	47.62	39.09	−3.9	11.75	9.99	−3.2
116	Oise	0.23	0.13	−11.3	35.21	31.45	−2.2	7.62	5.53	−6.2
117	Orne	0.26	0.00	−100.0	35.12	28.68	−4.0	9.36	0.00	−100.0
118	Pas-de-Calais	0.54	0.31	−10.4	49.17	39.71	−4.2	14.39	9.68	−7.6
119	Puy-de-dôme	0.40	0.33	−3.5	37.16	28.57	−5.1	10.41	23.00	17.2
120	Pyrénées-Atlantiques	0.14	0.08	−9.2	29.42	28.30	−0.8	21.04	6.24	−21.6
121	Hautes-Pyrénées	0.00	0.39	30.5	35.71	26.10	−6.1	8.01	0.00	−100.0
122	Pyrénées-Orientales	0.40	0.19	−14.2	28.59	24.25	−3.2	46.67	9.99	−26.5
123	Bas-Rhin	0.44	0.29	−7.9	41.37	30.62	−5.8	6.05	7.61	4.7
124	Haut-Rhin	0.52	0.32	−9.4	42.01	33.35	−4.5	18.54	10.39	−10.9
125	Rhône	0.35	0.13	−18.0	27.74	22.59	−4.0	14.87	8.96	−9.6
126	Haute-Saône	0.24	0.33	7.3	41.79	29.71	−6.6	23.92	32.74	6.5
127	Saône-et-Loire	0.53	0.08	−30.9	34.57	26.19	−5.4	16.10	5.89	−18.2
128	Sarthe	0.49	0.10	−27.1	25.48	21.52	−3.3	19.63	11.82	−9.6
129	Savoie	0.17	0.15	−1.7	33.08	24.19	−6.1	4.47	0.00	−100.0
130	Haute-Savoie	0.35	0.00	−100.0	30.51	25.71	−3.4	10.81	12.96	3.7
131	Paris	0.22	0.12	−11.4	28.53	22.67	−4.5	18.51	13.10	−6.7
132	Seine-Maritime	0.55	0.16	−21.9	36.94	31.27	−3.3	9.11	4.22	−14.3
133	Seine-et-Marne	0.39	0.13	−20.1	29.36	28.84	−0.4	14.76	9.01	−9.4
134	Yvelines	0.30	0.23	−5.1	27.39	22.25	−4.1	22.71	8.98	−16.9
135	Deux-Sèvres	1.00	0.07	−41.0	29.58	20.20	−7.3	17.52	0.00	−100.0
136	Somme	0.73	0.24	−19.5	35.71	31.38	−2.5	16.96	20.13	3.5
137	Tarn	0.41	0.13	−20.8	28.09	21.37	−5.3	10.11	16.18	9.8
138	Tarn-et-Garonne	0.13	0.23	13.2	32.32	21.48	−7.8	0.00	0.00	0.0
139	Var	0.76	0.15	−27.9	29.99	23.34	−4.9	8.75	10.09	2.9
140	Vaucluse	0.42	0.17	−16.9	29.52	25.17	−3.1	10.30	15.95	9.1
141	Vendée	0.22	0.10	−15.0	35.68	28.14	−4.6	0.00	12.44	35.1
142	Vienne	0.22	0.20	−1.4	27.84	19.47	−6.9	8.25	9.03	1.8
143	Haute-Vienne	0.34	0.32	−1.2	34.01	25.28	−5.8	15.74	5.68	−18.5
144	Vosges	0.28	0.13	−13.8	42.21	29.55	−6.9	34.38	22.55	−8.1
145	Yonne	0.33	0.08	−25.3	37.00	30.24	−4.0	9.51	0.00	−100.0
146	Territoire-de-Belfort	0.43	0.20	−14.3	38.12	24.08	−8.8	9.62	21.11	17.0
147	Essonne	0.41	0.14	−18.9	30.95	23.96	−5.0	19.89	6.21	−20.8
148	Hauts-de-Seine	0.11	0.20	13.0	28.93	22.31	−5.1	15.69	5.51	−18.9
149	Seine-Saint-Denis	0.20	0.13	−8.4	32.96	28.73	−2.7	15.48	15.75	0.4
150	Val-de-Marne	0.14	0.22	10.4	28.75	24.32	−3.3	17.52	15.06	−3.0
151	Val-d'Oise	0.27	0.18	−7.0	29.01	23.78	−3.9	11.84	11.91	0.1
GREECE		0.19	0.10	−9.8	47.04	41.56	−2.0	8.40	5.83	−5.9
152	Greater Athens	0.18	0.13	−4.9	47.90	42.54	−2.0	4.81	5.24	1.4
153	Rest of Central Greece and Eubea	0.25	0.05	−24.4	49.11	39.56	−3.5	12.42	6.60	−10.0
154	Peloponnisos	0.13	0.12	−0.6	43.96	34.14	−4.1	4.48	3.64	−3.4
155	Ionian Islands	0.00	0.00	0.0	47.07	38.75	−3.2	9.04	0.00	−100.0
156	Epirus	0.14	0.00	−100.0	40.44	34.88	−2.4	18.07	6.05	−16.7
157	Thessaly	0.38	0.07	−23.9	48.78	40.47	−3.1	0.00	4.95	16.4
158	Macedonia	0.16	0.11	−6.7	46.11	46.66	0.2	6.79	4.22	−7.6
159	Thrace	0.00	0.09	−7.9	62.88	67.05	1.1	42.23	19.34	−12.2
160	Aegean Islands	0.21	0.00	−100.0	43.85	38.75	−2.0	21.06	8.10	−14.7
161	Crete	0.27	0.21	−4.3	42.19	30.44	−5.3	8.00	9.52	2.9
ITALY		0.69	0.36	−10.2	51.55	38.40	−4.8	11.39	6.08	−9.9
162	Torino	1.11	0.43	−14.6	53.48	38.37	−5.4	13.70	4.43	−17.2
163	Vercelli	0.72	0.32	−12.7	67.17	50.50	−4.6	6.68	7.55	2.1
164	Novara	0.50	0.31	−7.8	63.11	45.05	−5.5	9.12	5.23	−8.8
165	Cuneo	0.80	0.43	−9.8	55.99	45.21	−3.5	12.02	8.69	−5.3
166	Asti	0.76	0.68	−1.9	56.29	40.35	−5.4	37.95	13.74	−15.6
167	Alessandria	0.78	0.45	−8.9	51.91	39.71	−4.4	6.51	14.77	14.6
168	Aosta	0.65	0.77	2.7	46.59	39.74	−2.6	0.00	21.38	0.4
169	Imperia	0.71	0.46	−7.1	43.66	31.84	−5.1	0.00	0.00	0.0
170	Savona	0.44	0.34	−4.4	46.61	37.17	−3.7	0.00	0.00	0.0

Age-standardized mortality rates (per 100 000) and percentage changes

Table 9.4(d)—*cont.*

	Area	CHOLY 1980–84	CHOLY 1985–89	CHOLY Annual % change	HYP/S 1980–84	HYP/S 1985–89	HYP/S Annual % change	MAT 1980–84	MAT 1985–89	MAT Annual % change
171	Genova	1.00	0.53	−10.0	44.72	33.07	−4.9	12.03	15.99	4.9
172	La Spezia	0.62	0.42	−6.3	44.03	30.05	−6.2	12.27	0.00	−100.0
173	Varese	0.82	0.47	−8.9	54.47	37.20	−6.2	7.90	8.72	1.7
174	Como/Sondrio	0.78	0.30	−14.9	58.29	39.65	−6.2	2.05	4.55	14.2
175	Milano	0.51	0.24	−11.7	53.15	35.63	−6.5	7.33	4.36	−8.3
176	Bergamo	0.71	0.32	−12.3	65.71	37.95	−8.7	8.02	2.22	−19.3
177	Brescia	0.48	0.30	−7.7	62.72	39.65	−7.4	5.60	0.00	−100.0
178	Pavia	0.54	0.24	−12.7	69.42	49.95	−5.3	11.01	0.00	−100.0
179	Cremona	0.65	0.38	−8.6	70.61	51.25	−5.2	14.20	7.91	−9.3
180	Mantova	0.31	0.28	−1.7	62.62	40.41	−7.0	6.68	0.00	−100.0
181	Bolzano	0.82	0.12	−27.6	45.76	29.07	−7.3	18.73	0.00	−100.0
182	Trento	1.03	0.41	−14.0	45.97	36.67	−3.7	4.55	0.00	−100.0
183	Verona	0.74	0.21	−19.3	57.88	34.66	−8.2	13.04	2.85	−22.4
184	Vicenza	0.88	0.26	−18.2	59.23	37.94	−7.2	10.72	0.00	−100.0
185	Belluno	0.66	0.31	−12.1	63.00	40.57	−7.1	20.99	12.18	−8.7
186	Treviso	0.61	0.32	−10.1	46.13	33.36	−5.3	5.58	3.13	−9.2
187	Venezia	0.54	0.14	−20.4	43.79	32.18	−5.0	0.00	6.23	14.4
188	Padova	0.40	0.20	−10.8	48.05	31.19	−6.9	7.56	5.57	−5.0
189	Rovigo	0.77	0.17	−22.3	51.41	38.14	−4.9	17.48	10.03	−8.8
190	Udine/Gorizia	0.75	0.29	−14.5	53.38	38.66	−5.2	7.58	12.74	9.1
191	Trieste	0.89	0.66	−4.8	39.40	31.86	−3.5	12.58	0.00	−100.0
192	Pordenone	0.67	0.34	−10.9	45.33	37.43	−3.1	8.15	0.00	−100.0
193	Piacenza	0.80	0.51	−7.2	54.12	42.23	−4.0	10.45	12.02	2.4
194	Parma	0.78	0.26	−17.0	47.66	34.13	−5.4	14.35	7.84	−9.6
195	Reggio Emilia	0.45	0.25	−9.0	42.99	29.75	−6.0	0.00	0.00	0.0
196	Modena	0.63	0.25	−14.4	42.50	37.50	−2.1	8.47	0.00	−100.0
197	Bologna	0.68	0.24	−16.1	43.33	31.09	−5.4	17.36	7.36	−13.3
198	Ferrara	0.46	0.53	2.4	45.13	37.90	−2.9	15.90	18.82	2.9
199	Ravenna	0.52	0.12	−22.1	37.25	27.45	−5.0	0.00	0.00	0.0
200	Forli	0.33	0.29	−2.2	36.71	24.81	−6.3	18.78	4.30	−21.8
201	Pesaro	0.72	0.26	−15.8	40.74	26.89	−6.7	18.93	0.00	−100.0
202	Ancona	0.48	0.19	−14.3	41.93	30.09	−5.4	5.06	0.00	−100.0
203	Macerata	0.71	0.21	−18.2	42.43	35.12	−3.1	15.41	0.00	−100.0
204	Ascoli Piceno	0.54	0.30	−9.5	44.44	32.29	−5.2	5.54	0.00	−100.0
205	Massa-Carrara	0.69	0.31	−12.7	49.70	34.31	−6.0	11.31	0.00	−100.0
206	Lucca	0.43	0.06	−29.0	44.16	37.42	−2.7	6.20	0.00	−100.0
207	Pistoia	0.45	0.16	−15.6	35.75	28.42	−3.8	0.00	0.00	0.0
208	Firenze	0.53	0.42	−3.6	38.20	29.21	−4.4	4.37	4.60	0.9
209	Livorno	0.79	0.18	−21.5	42.22	32.35	−4.3	22.34	0.00	−100.0
210	Pisa	0.97	0.44	−12.4	33.63	28.87	−2.5	18.59	0.00	−100.0
211	Arezzo	0.73	0.26	−15.6	40.92	31.21	−4.4	7.51	7.93	0.9
212	Siena	0.66	0.46	−6.0	41.18	31.66	−4.3	0.00	0.00	0.0
213	Grosseto	0.60	0.63	1.0	47.63	30.24	−7.3	48.47	0.00	−100.0
214	Perugia	0.47	0.49	0.7	45.51	31.76	−5.8	7.19	3.99	−9.3
215	Terni	0.38	0.53	5.4	41.12	32.94	−3.6	0.00	0.00	0.0
216	Viterbo/Rieti	0.85	0.25	−18.3	50.48	36.47	−5.3	13.80	10.20	−4.9
217	Roma	0.64	0.45	−5.9	42.36	35.38	−3.0	10.65	6.32	−8.3
218	Latina	0.88	0.39	−12.7	52.31	39.49	−4.6	6.82	10.90	8.1
219	Frosinone	0.52	0.15	−18.7	59.79	42.43	−5.6	12.95	3.66	−19.0
220	Caserta	0.70	0.59	−2.9	80.45	56.13	−5.8	16.78	6.50	−14.6
221	Benevento	0.36	0.31	−2.4	55.49	45.72	−3.2	29.78	10.49	−16.0
222	Napoli	0.95	0.42	−12.6	69.96	57.10	−3.3	10.60	6.88	−7.0
223	Avellino	0.75	0.60	−3.6	49.70	44.51	−1.8	6.66	3.75	−9.1
224	Salerno	0.65	0.48	−5.1	57.93	49.30	−2.7	18.17	2.82	−26.7
225	L'Aquila	0.65	0.15	−21.9	51.20	40.03	−4.0	11.89	0.00	−100.0
226	Teramo	0.68	0.25	−15.2	47.44	33.25	−5.8	12.01	0.00	−100.0
227	Pescara	0.54	0.31	−8.8	47.33	37.80	−3.7	25.40	13.78	−9.7
228	Chieti	0.99	0.53	−9.9	41.60	33.33	−3.6	4.74	5.34	2.0
229	Isernia/Campobasso	0.85	0.48	−9.1	57.19	42.79	−4.7	15.47	0.00	−100.0
230	Foggia	0.31	0.47	6.8	50.61	41.44	−3.3	9.46	2.11	−22.1
231	Bari	0.60	0.44	−4.9	49.09	34.22	−5.8	5.49	7.02	4.2

Age-standardized mortality rates (per 100000) and percentage changes

Table 9.4(d)—*cont.*

Area		CHOLY 1980–84	CHOLY 1985–89	CHOLY Annual % change	HYP/S 1980–84	HYP/S 1985–89	HYP/S Annual % change	MAT 1980–84	MAT 1985–89	MAT Annual % change
		Age-standardized mortality rates (per 100000) and percentage changes								
232	Taranto	0.75	0.28	−15.4	45.69	37.79	−3.1	24.97	12.89	−10.4
233	Brindisi	0.44	0.26	−8.6	51.20	41.52	−3.4	9.15	7.86	−2.5
234	Lecce	0.53	0.54	0.1	46.73	35.46	−4.5	8.69	6.60	−4.5
235	Potenza/Matera	0.65	0.16	−20.9	55.89	42.36	−4.5	7.10	16.13	14.7
236	Cosenza	1.08	0.30	−19.1	59.76	44.52	−4.8	9.19	6.43	−5.8
237	Catanzaro	0.54	0.22	−14.3	49.45	43.25	−2.2	16.88	7.67	−12.3
238	Reggio Calabria	0.45	0.44	−0.1	49.84	40.65	−3.3	2.26	7.38	21.8
239	Trapani	0.52	0.17	−17.0	63.31	36.57	−8.7	10.20	0.00	−100.0
240	Palermo	0.49	0.48	−0.1	58.49	41.28	−5.6	17.57	3.39	−24.0
241	Messina	0.82	0.38	−11.9	48.87	43.24	−2.0	16.38	14.94	−1.5
242	Agrigento	0.37	0.47	4.0	52.45	39.93	−4.4	5.57	19.50	23.2
243	Caltanisetta	0.51	0.71	5.7	55.58	50.73	−1.5	18.20	15.29	−2.9
244	Enna	0.71	0.25	−15.9	66.46	52.63	−3.8	20.44	33.53	8.6
245	Catania	1.01	0.32	−17.5	60.85	51.46	−2.8	19.83	9.35	−11.8
246	Ragusa	0.79	0.52	−6.8	57.04	42.80	−4.7	50.81	10.82	−22.7
247	Siracusa	0.59	0.45	−4.3	53.91	48.98	−1.6	17.62	11.51	−6.9
248	Sassari	0.70	0.60	−2.6	50.14	38.57	−4.3	15.18	4.35	−18.8
249	Nuoro	0.90	0.97	1.3	51.04	34.85	−6.2	21.80	0.00	−100.0
250	Cagliari/Oristano	1.32	0.36	−19.3	47.06	33.92	−5.3	11.57	10.75	−1.2
IRELAND		0.37	0.21	−10.3	50.78	35.82	−6.7	6.83	4.12	−9.6
251	Eastern	0.33	0.11	−19.3	52.81	35.46	−7.7	4.08	2.90	−6.6
252	Midland	0.31	0.15	−13.0	44.59	39.86	−2.2	13.87	17.29	4.5
253	Mid-Western	0.10	0.10	−0.0	56.34	36.87	−8.1	6.28	11.69	13.2
254	North-Eastern	0.56	0.55	−0.3	55.14	42.10	−5.3	9.65	0.00	−100.0
255	North-Western	0.43	0.00	−100.0	52.95	30.32	−10.6	4.90	0.00	−100.0
256	South-Eastern	0.43	0.08	−27.9	50.30	37.70	−5.6	10.30	0.00	−100.0
257	Southern	0.53	0.42	−4.8	49.56	34.96	−6.7	3.86	4.72	4.1
258	Western	0.26	0.36	6.8	41.37	31.10	−5.5	12.05	3.61	−21.4
THE NETHERLANDS		0.43	0.29	−8.3	28.75	24.76	−3.3	7.60	7.43	−0.5
259	Groningen	0.15	0.13	−4.0	29.27	23.77	−4.5	3.00	3.83	5.6
260	Friesland	0.30	0.30	0.1	29.47	23.35	−5.0	9.91	3.23	−22.1
261	Drenthe	0.51	0.30	−11.0	27.38	24.20	−2.7	11.74	0.00	−100.0
262	Overijssel	0.42	0.52	4.7	30.83	25.45	−4.2	8.50	14.63	12.8
263	Gelderland	0.39	0.43	2.2	30.05	27.41	−2.0	2.81	8.95	29.4
264	Utrecht	0.22	0.22	−0.1	29.99	26.76	−2.5	8.64	9.95	3.2
265	Noord Holland	0.54	0.30	−12.0	24.83	21.38	−3.3	9.88	4.41	−16.4
266	Zuid Holland	0.43	0.23	−13.4	28.35	23.95	−3.7	9.25	9.08	−0.4
267	Zeeland	0.31	0.19	−10.3	25.02	20.38	−4.5	0.00	0.00	0.0
268	Noord Brabant	0.59	0.34	−11.6	30.70	27.12	−2.7	8.53	5.59	−9.0
269	Limburg	0.45	0.17	−19.1	31.41	26.56	−3.7	4.97	11.70	20.9
270	Flevoland	0.14	0.22	10.2	26.34	20.70	−5.2	1.82	0.00	−100.0
UK: ENGLAND AND WALES		0.25	0.21	−2.7	44.37	36.57	−3.8	8.52	6.80	−4.4
271	Northern	0.27	0.25	−2.1	54.90	45.53	−3.7	10.07	6.44	−8.5
272	Yorkshire	0.19	0.19	0.6	48.84	39.75	−4.0	10.29	7.30	−6.6
273	Trent	0.21	0.20	−1.5	47.01	37.99	−4.2	8.94	6.58	−5.9
274	East Anglian	0.21	0.21	−0.3	33.68	28.79	−3.1	11.86	9.37	−4.6
275	North-West Thames	0.19	0.11	−9.7	36.76	31.98	−2.7	6.95	8.51	4.1
276	North-East Thames	0.29	0.17	−10.6	37.74	34.53	−1.8	8.39	6.20	−5.9
277	South-East Thames	0.26	0.23	−2.6	40.13	34.13	−3.2	7.19	6.04	−3.4
278	South-West Thames	0.16	0.18	2.7	34.69	28.03	−4.2	6.44	5.78	−2.1
279	Wessex	0.13	0.13	−0.0	33.00	30.38	−1.6	5.99	4.33	−6.3
280	Oxford	0.18	0.22	4.2	35.74	28.64	−4.3	5.67	6.93	4.1
281	South-Western	0.26	0.24	−1.8	40.79	30.35	−5.7	7.90	6.06	−5.2
282	West Midlands	0.32	0.28	−2.9	49.98	40.57	−4.1	9.61	8.30	−2.9
283	Mersey	0.36	0.24	−7.9	52.19	41.74	−4.4	10.69	4.83	−14.7
284	North-Western	0.30	0.27	−2.2	54.83	45.75	−3.6	8.98	7.41	−3.8
285	Wales	0.28	0.27	−0.7	52.60	40.84	−4.9	8.32	6.86	−3.8

Table 9.4(d)—*cont.*

Area		Age-standardized mortality rates (per 100000) and percentage changes CHOLY			HYP/S			MAT		
		1980–84	1985–89	Annual % change	1980–84	1985–89	Annual % change	1980–84	1985–89	Annual % change
UK: NORTHERN IRELAND		0.38	0.13	−19.0	54.30	43.63	−4.3	8.64	0.72	−39.1
286	Northern Ireland	0.38	0.13	−19.0	54.30	43.63	−4.3	8.64	0.72	−39.1
UK: SCOTLAND		0.30	0.21	−6.3	62.55	50.81	−4.1	13.38	9.09	−7.4
287	Highlands and Islands	0.40	0.19	−13.7	57.69	47.90	−3.7	10.81	5.68	−12.1
288	Grampian	0.22	0.05	−24.7	50.06	40.11	−4.3	18.51	15.32	−3.7
289	Tayside	0.31	0.25	−4.4	54.93	43.19	−4.7	12.42	12.61	0.3
290	Fife	0.37	0.07	−27.5	65.85	49.26	−5.6	8.76	8.84	0.2
291	Lothian	0.28	0.21	−5.3	54.85	50.32	−1.7	15.36	8.40	−11.4
292	Borders	0.47	0.00	−100.0	63.83	35.67	−11.0	0.00	17.63	−0.3
293	Forth Valley	0.75	0.37	−13.1	60.49	52.18	−2.9	23.07	6.01	−23.6
294	Argyll and Clyde	0.34	0.29	−3.3	67.12	52.70	−4.7	9.83	10.16	0.7
295	Greater Glasgow	0.34	0.21	−9.4	70.16	59.03	−3.4	13.79	7.78	−10.8
296	Lanarkshire	0.09	0.18	14.5	66.16	56.51	−3.1	14.81	5.41	−18.2
297	Ayrshire and Arran	0.07	0.47	47.5	74.63	48.54	−8.2	12.05	4.16	−19.2
298	Dumfries and Galloway	0.16	0.16	−0.6	52.96	50.40	−1.0	0.00	22.74	14.8
PORTUGAL		0.33	0.27	−4.0	86.72	67.92	−4.8	17.71	9.25	−12.2
299	Viana do Castelo	0.10	0.10	−0.2	90.26	76.11	−3.4	14.77	0.00	−100.0
300	Braga	0.24	0.22	−1.7	93.03	75.62	−4.1	19.90	14.82	−5.7
301	Vila Real	0.30	0.10	−19.4	104.66	89.98	−3.0	23.36	0.00	−100.0
302	Bragança	0.00	0.00	0.0	95.38	72.86	−5.2	7.47	19.91	21.7
303	Guarda	0.12	0.13	1.6	98.40	80.46	−3.9	21.93	0.00	−100.0
304	Viseu	0.37	0.32	−2.9	103.95	87.83	−3.3	14.15	3.59	−24.0
305	Porto	0.52	0.27	−12.4	87.76	73.58	−3.5	15.60	9.41	−9.6
306	Aveiro	0.38	0.17	−14.5	89.55	60.79	−7.5	21.05	2.29	−35.8
307	Coimbra	0.28	0.05	−28.1	93.44	67.96	−6.2	12.96	8.31	−8.5
308	Castelo Branco	0.39	0.00	−100.0	84.77	59.11	−7.0	42.31	8.74	−27.0
309	Portalegre	0.15	0.78	39.0	76.29	74.99	−0.3	23.33	14.04	−9.7
310	Santarem	0.51	0.05	−37.3	84.66	65.18	−5.1	20.23	4.27	−26.7
311	Leiria	0.18	0.23	4.9	99.74	78.95	−4.6	25.47	11.65	−14.5
312	Lisboa	0.27	0.37	6.4	75.68	55.48	−6.0	15.06	7.13	−13.9
313	Setubal	0.28	0.38	6.3	70.78	54.35	−5.1	18.90	12.46	−8.0
314	Evora	0.61	0.61	0.0	86.92	64.77	−5.7	25.59	0.00	−100.0
315	Beja	0.36	0.25	−6.9	70.25	67.34	−0.8	16.67	10.74	−8.4
316	Faro	0.36	0.41	3.0	68.87	62.69	−1.9	4.55	25.07	40.7
317	Madeira	0.87	0.35	−16.7	128.23	101.98	−4.5	8.94	15.27	11.3
318	Azores	0.12	0.37	25.2	118.28	94.97	−4.3	27.75	18.08	−8.2
SPAIN		0.38	0.17	−13.7	43.55	34.27	−4.3	10.64	4.76	−13.6
319	La Coruña	0.37	0.15	−15.2	51.91	38.39	−5.3	18.53	2.37	−31.2
320	Lugo	0.11	0.14	4.5	35.20	33.50	−0.9	14.13	0.00	−100.0
321	Orense	0.32	0.07	−24.8	44.99	34.69	−4.6	16.47	8.63	−11.1
322	Pontevedra	0.16	0.12	−6.0	48.29	39.54	−3.6	4.79	7.83	9.4
323	Asturias	0.43	0.20	−12.8	41.14	30.15	−5.5	18.92	2.56	−30.5
324	Cantabria	0.31	0.00	−100.0	43.58	31.67	−5.6	17.25	4.70	−21.1
325	Alava	0.24	0.00	−100.0	31.19	24.25	−4.5	5.70	0.00	−100.0
326	Guipuzcoa	0.25	0.10	−15.9	34.28	30.21	−2.3	10.29	4.06	−15.6
327	Vizcaya	0.43	0.11	−22.3	41.13	31.17	−4.9	11.17	2.33	−24.8
328	Navarra	0.42	0.13	−19.8	37.49	23.05	−8.5	3.18	0.00	−100.0
329	Rioja	0.30	0.48	9.0	39.31	36.08	−1.5	32.17	0.00	−100.0
330	Huesca	0.52	0.26	−12.0	33.94	28.60	−3.1	8.72	0.00	−100.0
331	Teruel	0.74	0.20	−21.3	36.54	28.02	−4.7	12.36	0.00	−100.0
332	Zaragoza	0.57	0.28	−12.1	39.28	30.71	−4.4	10.59	12.74	3.4
333	Madrid Centro	0.18	0.08	−13.1	31.55	24.14	−4.8	6.11	2.76	−13.5
334	Avila	0.13	0.00	−100.0	32.50	27.88	−2.8	19.98	0.00	−100.0
335	Burgos	0.49	0.34	−6.3	34.41	28.61	−3.3	0.00	0.00	0.0
336	Leon	0.46	0.11	−22.6	39.97	31.82	−4.1	22.25	4.94	−23.9
337	Palencia	0.40	0.00	−100.0	43.80	26.16	−8.9	8.60	0.00	−100.0
338	Salamanca	0.42	0.09	−24.6	37.11	28.80	−4.5	18.51	0.00	−100.0
339	Segovia	0.00	0.00	0.0	35.99	28.43	−4.2	23.02	0.00	−100.0

Table 9.4(d)—*cont.*

Area		CHOLY 1980–84	CHOLY 1985–89	CHOLY Annual % change	HYP/S 1980–84	HYP/S 1985–89	HYP/S Annual % change	MAT 1980–84	MAT 1985–89	MAT Annual % change
340	Soria	0.00	0.00	0.0	35.56	23.16	−7.5	0.00	0.00	0.0
341	Valladolid	0.87	0.07	−36.5	31.15	24.15	−4.5	19.00	5.26	−20.8
342	Zamora	0.00	0.13	4.9	31.89	32.56	0.4	33.69	0.00	−100.0
343	Albacete	0.98	0.40	−15.1	48.87	43.99	−1.9	3.99	5.69	6.7
344	Ciudad Real	0.32	0.20	−8.2	52.15	38.72	−5.3	26.84	4.03	−29.2
345	Cuenca	0.34	0.00	−100.0	41.50	40.13	−0.6	16.18	0.00	−100.0
346	Guadalajara	0.35	0.22	−7.6	31.94	22.24	−6.4	0.00	0.00	0.0
347	Toledo	0.48	0.00	−100.0	38.56	33.49	−2.5	9.02	0.00	−100.0
348	Badajoz	0.51	0.11	−24.4	60.43	49.65	−3.5	16.44	5.60	−17.8
349	Caceres	0.13	0.17	5.0	54.51	40.84	−5.1	31.31	9.60	−19.3
350	Barcelona	0.27	0.18	−7.0	39.42	28.52	−5.7	5.84	5.37	−1.5
351	Gerona	0.16	0.25	8.6	33.50	27.72	−3.4	0.00	14.52	30.6
352	Lerida	0.39	0.24	−8.6	41.57	33.11	−4.1	10.07	0.00	−100.0
353	Tarragona	0.15	0.53	25.5	42.12	30.04	−6.0	11.60	13.04	2.2
354	Alicante	0.32	0.20	−8.8	54.38	41.43	−4.8	12.49	3.26	−21.7
355	Castellon de la Plana	0.47	0.29	−8.8	44.42	38.01	−2.8	21.19	5.31	−22.2
356	Valencia	0.64	0.27	−14.8	59.02	44.16	−5.1	7.02	7.71	1.7
357	Baleares	0.40	0.33	−3.6	47.46	36.01	−4.9	6.50	11.38	10.7
358	Almeria	0.15	0.00	−100.0	46.84	39.76	−2.9	16.58	0.00	−100.0
359	Cadiz	0.58	0.16	−20.9	56.52	50.64	−2.0	13.67	10.76	−4.3
360	Cordoba	0.47	0.10	−25.0	46.80	44.13	−1.1	12.43	2.45	−25.6
361	Granada	0.49	0.32	−7.6	40.65	35.65	−2.4	16.94	11.65	−6.6
362	Huelva	0.62	0.00	−100.0	55.22	52.00	−1.1	5.76	0.00	−100.0
363	Jaen	0.13	0.11	−3.5	45.05	43.16	−0.8	8.12	8.30	0.4
364	Malaga	0.82	0.40	−12.3	50.54	43.41	−2.7	7.22	3.40	−12.8
365	Sevilla	0.47	0.15	−19.3	54.74	40.02	−5.5	11.64	1.15	−34.4
366	Murcia	0.50	0.11	−24.3	46.25	39.37	−2.9	8.56	3.52	−14.9
367	Las Palmas	0.52	0.12	−23.8	63.22	48.47	−4.7	11.36	4.52	−15.4
368	Sta Cruz de Tenerife	0.30	0.12	−15.4	47.13	38.42	−3.6	1.89	7.83	29.4
EC		0.42	0.24	−9.4	43.67	34.72	−4.3	11.71	7.30	−8.2

Age-standardized mortality rates (per 100000) and percentage changes

Table 9.4(e)

Area		Age-standardized mortality rates (per 100000) and percentage changes								
		PER			BREAST			ISHD		
		1980–84	1985–89	Annual % change	1980–84	1985–89	Annual % change	1980–84	1985–89	Annual % change
BELGIUM		12.74	10.23	–4.3	40.24	40.22	–0.0	96.57	73.62	–5.3
1	Antwerpen	13.00	9.64	–5.8	41.99	40.21	–0.9	81.84	68.91	–3.4
2	Brabant	12.37	11.55	–1.4	40.63	43.04	1.2	82.25	64.73	–4.7
3	West-Vlaanderen	13.59	9.74	–6.4	48.60	44.77	–1.6	84.08	60.39	–6.4
4	Oost-Vlaanderen	12.84	10.68	–3.6	42.57	43.49	0.4	103.28	74.87	–6.2
5	Hainaut	12.10	9.98	–3.8	38.72	38.01	–0.4	111.24	84.43	–5.4
6	Liege	11.71	10.00	–3.1	33.34	33.90	0.3	113.65	85.26	–5.6
7	Limburg	13.98	9.28	–7.9	34.94	34.86	–0.0	104.26	81.56	–4.8
8	Luxembourg (province)	13.05	9.22	–6.7	38.72	34.65	–2.2	107.83	81.90	–5.4
9	Namur	12.66	9.17	–6.3	33.75	36.41	1.5	133.63	90.82	–7.4
LUXEMBOURG		11.04	8.40	–5.3	39.66	41.01	0.7	133.07	95.08	–6.5
10	Luxembourg	11.04	8.40	–5.3	39.66	41.01	0.7	133.07	95.08	–6.5
FEDERAL REPUBLIC OF GERMANY		9.94	7.10	–6.5	32.79	34.92	1.3	108.33	93.98	–2.8
11	Schleswig-Holstein	9.42	6.99	–5.8	34.75	38.74	2.2	118.58	102.87	–2.8
12	Hamburg	8.76	7.25	–3.7	35.07	38.32	1.8	93.59	78.25	–3.5
13	Braunschweig	10.31	6.29	–9.4	30.46	33.54	1.9	111.32	100.00	–2.1
14	Hannover	9.46	6.73	–6.6	32.29	35.71	2.0	111.74	97.13	–2.8
15	Lüneburg	9.22	6.48	–6.8	31.25	35.05	2.3	106.24	93.93	–2.4
16	Weser-Ems	10.95	7.73	–6.7	34.02	34.94	0.5	119.63	99.18	–3.7
17	Bremen	9.24	7.33	–4.5	34.52	34.87	0.2	102.27	93.81	–1.7
18	Düsseldorf	11.62	7.80	–7.7	34.53	36.52	1.1	125.46	103.27	–3.8
19	Köln	9.84	7.09	–6.4	33.49	35.71	1.3	110.97	96.82	–2.7
20	Munster	12.36	8.04	–8.2	34.87	36.53	0.9	121.53	102.78	–3.3
21	Detmold	10.50	7.64	–6.1	32.49	33.74	0.8	105.69	92.37	–2.7
22	Arnsberg	11.46	8.14	–6.6	34.19	34.96	0.4	128.28	110.73	–2.9
23	Darmstadt	9.20	6.53	–6.6	33.60	35.64	1.2	100.81	86.75	–3.0
24	Giessen	9.34	7.49	–4.3	28.70	33.89	3.4	103.43	93.04	–2.1
25	Kassel	10.14	7.59	–5.6	31.60	32.01	0.3	103.07	87.50	–3.2
26	Koblenz	9.82	7.32	–5.7	35.38	36.13	0.4	112.74	100.04	–2.4
27	Trier	9.08	7.44	–3.9	35.71	31.88	–2.2	114.54	92.29	–4.2
28	Rheinhessen-Pfalz	10.45	7.04	–7.6	34.50	34.82	0.2	116.33	95.79	–3.8
29	Stuttgart	8.74	6.40	–6.0	31.36	33.67	1.4	92.46	80.57	–2.7
30	Karlsruhe	9.14	6.85	–5.6	31.21	30.61	–0.4	104.93	93.96	–2.2
31	Freiburg	8.21	5.87	–6.5	30.77	32.69	1.2	86.46	77.04	–2.3
32	Tübingen	8.33	6.20	–5.7	30.91	31.43	0.3	88.75	78.96	–2.3
33	Oberbayern	8.79	6.91	–4.7	31.43	34.08	1.6	81.29	73.91	–1.9
34	Niederbayern	9.23	6.36	–7.2	26.61	30.91	3.0	103.76	94.12	–1.9
35	Oberpfalz	10.42	7.23	–7.0	28.18	33.10	3.3	116.41	102.88	–2.4
36	Oberfranken	9.25	6.75	–6.1	30.94	32.45	1.0	113.74	106.09	–1.4
37	Mittelfranken	9.40	6.59	–6.9	30.40	34.92	2.8	106.78	99.35	–1.4
38	Unterfranken	9.80	6.81	–7.0	30.92	31.34	0.3	94.68	83.46	–2.5
39	Schwaben	9.52	6.55	–7.2	30.09	35.11	3.1	91.11	84.85	–1.4
40	Saarland	11.35	8.52	–5.6	35.34	35.94	0.3	139.40	111.82	–4.3
41	Berlin (West)	10.93	7.72	–6.7	36.33	40.89	2.4	109.79	93.79	–3.1
DENMARK		8.83	8.61	–0.5	38.33	42.59	2.1	146.34	124.50	–3.2
42	Kobenhavn and Frederiksberg (M)	8.49	7.95	–1.3	47.48	49.06	0.7	154.27	135.19	–2.6
43	Kobenhavns County	6.54	7.25	2.1	40.00	45.20	2.5	128.55	106.52	–3.7
44	Frederiksborg County	7.90	8.04	0.4	39.95	49.35	4.3	132.01	112.95	–3.1
45	Roskilde County	8.53	9.73	2.7	44.80	44.24	–0.3	158.04	124.40	–4.7
46	Vestsjællands County	9.84	9.22	–1.3	32.92	42.86	5.4	167.24	135.50	–4.1
47	Storstroms County	7.53	7.98	1.2	35.69	42.48	3.5	163.30	143.18	–2.6
48	Bornholms County	10.29	9.80	–1.0	32.96	31.03	–1.2	156.29	159.87	0.5
49	Fyns County	8.18	7.80	–0.9	32.63	36.51	2.3	137.26	121.34	–2.4
50	Sonderjyllands County	9.80	7.97	–4.0	32.82	36.62	2.2	151.02	134.61	–2.3
51	Ribe County	8.25	9.86	3.6	30.89	30.91	0.0	144.92	135.84	–1.3
52	Vejle County	7.74	8.74	2.5	41.52	40.93	–0.3	142.54	109.37	–5.2
53	Ringkobing County	9.80	9.99	0.4	32.63	42.61	5.5	151.43	133.24	–2.5
54	Århus County	10.69	8.46	–4.6	41.21	43.12	0.9	148.13	116.37	–4.7

Table 9.4(e)—*cont.*

	Area	PER 1980–84	PER 1985–89	PER Annual % change	BREAST 1980–84	BREAST 1985–89	BREAST Annual % change	ISHD 1980–84	ISHD 1985–89	ISHD Annual % change
171	Genova	13.17	9.63	–5.1	34.02	37.86	2.2	86.54	59.69	–7.2
172	La Spezia	12.76	12.79	0.0	42.29	31.70	–5.6	70.47	59.00	–3.5
173	Varese	14.91	9.62	–7.0	34.32	37.21	1.6	91.06	67.72	–5.8
174	Como/Sondrio	12.01	8.66	–5.3	36.99	36.44	–0.3	97.31	80.50	–3.7
175	Milano	13.27	9.44	–5.5	37.50	38.31	0.4	94.42	69.86	–5.8
176	Bergamo	13.95	10.22	–5.1	39.29	36.02	–1.7	94.20	75.61	–4.3
177	Brescia	12.66	8.70	–6.1	32.77	36.36	2.1	107.44	75.20	–6.9
178	Pavia	13.49	10.07	–4.8	33.98	34.20	0.1	110.77	77.72	–6.8
179	Cremona	13.49	8.94	–6.6	41.85	32.26	–5.1	112.98	83.69	–5.8
180	Mantova	12.62	9.89	–4.0	31.93	30.08	–1.2	98.16	79.58	–4.1
181	Bolzano	12.36	7.99	–7.0	25.58	33.74	5.7	84.21	66.42	–4.6
182	Trento	12.85	9.52	–4.9	35.96	34.86	–0.6	92.82	67.35	–6.2
183	Verona	14.89	11.00	–4.9	35.74	36.25	0.3	97.68	67.92	–7.0
184	Vicenza	12.06	9.71	–3.5	33.52	30.17	–2.1	93.81	71.68	–5.2
185	Belluno	11.96	9.50	–3.8	34.03	37.94	2.2	102.54	75.12	–6.0
186	Treviso	11.73	7.63	–6.9	32.56	32.72	0.1	79.03	58.85	–5.7
187	Venezia	14.07	8.88	–7.4	35.45	34.83	–0.3	81.05	57.42	–6.7
188	Padova	13.51	9.05	–6.4	33.18	33.83	0.4	89.15	66.11	–5.8
189	Rovigo	12.15	9.73	–3.6	29.71	33.43	2.4	91.93	66.60	–6.2
190	Udine/Gorizia	13.18	7.94	–8.1	33.53	33.21	–0.2	93.36	71.24	–5.3
191	Trieste	8.43	6.63	–3.9	40.66	31.71	–4.9	82.45	56.83	–7.2
192	Pordenone	11.90	7.25	–7.9	30.21	32.61	1.5	81.84	56.19	–7.2
193	Piacenza	13.38	15.63	2.6	38.07	32.98	–2.8	92.36	75.30	–4.0
194	Parma	16.35	9.96	–7.9	37.63	34.69	–1.6	88.63	72.46	–3.9
195	Reggio Emilia	13.59	8.33	–7.8	31.75	39.36	4.4	76.91	61.08	–4.5
196	Modena	13.72	10.96	–3.7	36.56	29.48	–4.2	79.53	70.96	–2.3
197	Bologna	13.86	9.50	–6.1	40.71	36.02	–2.4	85.25	66.47	–4.9
198	Ferrara	13.75	9.79	–5.5	32.53	34.36	1.1	84.66	72.65	–3.0
199	Ravenna	13.24	11.01	–3.0	31.82	31.17	–0.4	68.44	52.70	–5.1
200	Forli	12.20	11.88	–0.5	31.29	27.99	–2.2	63.70	53.05	–3.6
201	Pesaro	13.00	10.59	–3.4	30.62	29.31	–0.9	66.50	52.13	–4.8
202	Ancona	12.75	11.12	–2.3	30.76	30.00	–0.5	61.09	53.18	–2.7
203	Macerata	16.18	10.34	–7.2	32.07	26.81	–3.5	62.49	52.59	–3.4
204	Ascoli Piceno	14.95	11.02	–5.0	28.21	24.95	–2.4	68.04	51.83	–5.3
205	Massa-Carrara	15.04	10.20	–6.3	32.93	28.60	–2.8	71.95	64.20	–2.3
206	Lucca	13.70	10.50	–4.3	30.63	34.44	2.4	76.73	55.74	–6.2
207	Pistoia	12.37	12.86	0.7	31.39	26.03	–3.7	74.19	60.35	–4.0
208	Firenze	14.41	9.98	–5.9	29.11	30.53	1.0	65.64	53.84	–3.9
209	Livorno	14.90	9.95	–6.5	33.59	37.43	2.2	73.04	55.73	–5.3
210	Pisa	13.88	13.89	0.0	30.90	32.43	1.0	70.62	57.54	–4.0
211	Arezzo	14.79	9.44	–7.2	22.85	27.61	3.9	57.28	51.66	–2.0
212	Siena	16.09	11.16	–5.9	25.71	29.55	2.8	68.40	48.25	–6.7
213	Grosseto	14.54	10.07	–5.9	29.86	29.06	–0.5	69.26	56.79	–3.9
214	Perugia	11.26	11.46	0.3	25.86	27.41	1.2	74.74	62.39	–3.5
215	Terni	17.90	12.32	–6.0	26.25	26.22	–0.0	65.26	56.70	–2.8
216	Viterbo/Rieti	14.99	11.07	–4.9	25.53	29.92	3.2	79.01	67.41	–3.1
217	Roma	14.73	10.65	–5.3	34.55	33.54	–0.6	82.89	66.15	–4.4
218	Latina	15.86	10.72	–6.3	28.48	27.85	–0.4	71.29	57.79	–4.1
219	Frosinone	15.61	12.56	–3.6	20.37	22.40	1.9	80.32	60.70	–5.4
220	Caserta	18.43	14.36	–4.1	24.47	23.62	–0.7	95.42	82.98	–2.8
221	Benevento	16.48	14.64	–2.0	21.20	21.64	0.4	81.32	66.80	–3.9
222	Napoli	18.63	14.68	–3.9	29.44	28.22	–0.8	112.30	89.70	–4.4
223	Avellino	15.22	14.00	–1.4	19.07	19.93	0.9	74.69	65.94	–2.5
224	Salerno	17.54	15.11	–2.5	23.23	24.22	0.8	89.11	66.54	–5.7
225	L'Aquila	16.11	13.89	–2.4	22.85	21.31	–1.4	79.25	59.54	–5.6
226	Teramo	13.03	11.24	–2.4	23.27	24.09	0.7	73.70	51.41	–7.0
227	Pescara	14.60	14.75	0.2	24.48	26.90	1.9	62.81	59.54	–1.1
228	Chieti	16.29	10.25	–7.4	21.72	18.45	–3.2	64.27	55.14	–3.0
229	Isernia/Campobasso	16.09	13.32	–3.1	20.92	22.41	1.4	70.65	62.31	–2.5
230	Foggia	18.10	13.57	–4.7	25.20	28.37	2.4	76.83	61.52	–4.3
231	Bari	18.12	12.69	–5.8	32.98	30.69	–1.4	70.59	52.96	–5.6

Age-standardized mortality rates (per 100000) and percentage changes

Table 9.4(e)—*cont.*

Area		Age-standardized mortality rates (per 100000) and percentage changes PER			BREAST			ISHD		
		1980–84	1985–89	Annual % change	1980–84	1985–89	Annual % change	1980–84	1985–89	Annual % change
232	Taranto	18.09	14.33	−3.8	29.95	26.12	−2.7	72.24	54.14	−5.6
233	Brindisi	17.70	14.03	−3.8	33.75	30.80	−1.8	71.94	56.07	−4.9
234	Lecce	17.16	15.45	−1.7	29.49	31.35	1.2	65.64	44.93	−7.3
235	Potenza/Matera	16.83	13.49	−3.6	20.31	24.95	4.2	73.09	59.63	−4.0
236	Cosenza	17.36	14.43	−3.0	20.39	22.07	1.6	76.99	59.44	−5.0
237	Catanzaro	16.88	14.34	−2.7	16.41	18.54	2.5	70.67	60.36	−3.1
238	Reggio Calabria	19.28	15.33	−3.7	24.82	28.93	3.1	66.83	54.33	−4.1
239	Trapani	14.72	12.21	−3.1	28.49	31.43	2.0	76.51	63.10	−3.8
240	Palermo	22.14	13.86	−7.5	24.80	26.32	1.2	73.78	58.63	−4.5
241	Messina	19.21	17.18	−1.8	29.22	24.78	−3.2	66.88	57.20	−3.1
242	Agrigento	15.79	13.22	−2.9	23.65	24.31	0.6	73.51	62.30	−3.3
243	Caltanisetta	20.57	17.07	−3.1	23.90	24.35	0.4	71.06	58.70	−3.7
244	Enna	16.69	17.60	0.9	22.66	21.81	−0.8	79.24	67.57	−3.1
245	Catania	19.15	16.13	−2.8	31.85	31.22	−0.4	78.92	66.35	−3.4
246	Ragusa	16.82	15.15	−1.7	31.66	37.33	3.3	77.53	50.75	−8.1
247	Siracusa	18.04	15.27	−2.7	29.99	28.90	−0.7	72.66	66.72	−1.7
248	Sassari	16.88	13.84	−3.3	31.90	35.76	2.3	74.04	63.59	−3.0
249	Nuoro	16.35	14.57	−1.9	24.12	24.43	0.3	80.01	66.90	−3.5
250	Cagliari/Oristano	19.30	15.06	−4.0	31.73	33.83	1.3	66.17	55.32	−3.5
IRELAND		13.83	11.28	−4.0	43.42	44.30	0.4	209.26	180.85	−2.9
251	Eastern	14.43	11.41	−4.6	46.49	45.84	−0.3	214.43	178.96	−3.6
252	Midland	11.42	12.51	1.8	44.35	39.73	−2.2	218.11	186.42	−3.1
253	Mid-Western	13.45	10.95	−4.0	44.90	47.58	1.2	213.50	188.20	−2.5
254	North-Eastern	14.29	10.77	−5.5	42.48	41.06	−0.7	220.50	176.30	−4.4
255	North-Western	14.07	11.56	−3.8	37.67	45.36	3.8	193.08	173.44	−2.1
256	South-Eastern	14.91	12.03	−4.2	38.48	38.33	−0.1	212.26	193.04	−1.9
257	Southern	14.05	12.72	−2.0	46.07	42.58	−1.6	218.38	188.69	−2.9
258	Western	11.36	7.51	−7.9	36.48	49.97	6.5	170.59	160.34	−1.2
THE NETHERLANDS		10.39	9.53	−1.9	38.93	39.34	0.2	119.56	104.11	−3.0
259	Groningen	10.09	11.08	2.1	34.00	38.35	2.7	154.23	137.08	−2.6
260	Friesland	10.28	8.74	−3.5	37.79	36.16	−1.0	135.11	119.53	−2.7
261	Drenthe	10.25	9.22	−2.3	34.71	37.30	1.6	138.08	126.99	−1.8
262	Overijssel	10.02	10.30	0.6	41.16	41.71	0.3	127.28	113.23	−2.6
263	Gelderland	10.48	9.89	−1.3	37.49	39.32	1.1	124.68	103.28	−4.1
264	Utrecht	10.66	9.11	−3.4	37.15	41.92	2.7	111.36	90.44	−4.5
265	Noord Holland	10.61	10.08	−1.1	42.19	40.25	−1.0	107.34	96.53	−2.3
266	Zuid Holland	10.11	8.91	−2.8	38.75	40.53	1.0	109.23	96.55	−2.7
267	Zeeland	10.86	8.76	−4.7	34.91	40.94	3.6	92.08	80.32	−3.0
268	Noord Brabant	10.51	9.47	−2.3	39.27	36.65	−1.5	119.04	101.59	−3.5
269	Limburg	10.99	9.50	−3.2	39.88	39.02	−0.5	144.30	125.45	−3.1
270	Flevoland	8.32	9.33	2.6	34.74	27.61	−5.0	123.58	94.07	−5.9
UK: ENGLAND AND WALES		11.45	9.05	−4.6	44.51	44.30	−0.1	180.62	161.91	−2.7
271	Northern	12.48	9.31	−5.7	41.89	42.45	0.3	228.56	210.62	−2.0
272	Yorkshire	13.05	9.59	−6.0	44.95	41.01	−2.3	210.90	191.28	−2.4
273	Trent	11.32	9.32	−3.8	45.34	45.65	0.2	193.70	175.82	−2.4
274	East Anglian	10.10	7.75	−5.2	44.31	41.46	−1.6	136.52	120.10	−3.2
275	North-West Thames	9.83	8.53	−2.8	41.66	44.09	1.4	150.15	132.24	−3.1
276	North-East Thames	11.30	9.15	−4.1	45.16	46.75	0.9	161.77	143.59	−2.9
277	South-East Thames	11.21	8.81	−4.7	44.99	43.62	−0.8	151.78	132.46	−3.3
278	South-West Thames	10.16	7.96	−4.8	43.79	43.81	0.0	137.96	118.08	−3.8
279	Wessex	9.86	8.77	−2.3	43.15	43.72	0.3	149.61	130.98	−3.3
280	Oxford	9.97	7.88	−4.6	46.61	43.13	−1.9	146.61	125.34	−3.8
281	South-Western	10.49	8.10	−5.0	43.64	44.05	0.2	158.38	139.90	−3.1
282	West Midlands	13.40	10.49	−4.8	45.78	46.15	0.2	189.02	174.36	−2.0
283	Mersey	11.14	8.78	−4.6	45.39	45.33	−0.0	216.47	203.69	−1.5
284	North-Western	12.45	9.73	−4.8	43.52	44.33	0.5	231.07	206.05	−2.8
285	Wales	12.07	9.32	−5.0	47.47	46.26	−0.6	201.52	183.47	−2.3

Table 9.4(e)—*cont.*

Area		Age-standardized mortality rates (per 100 000) and percentage changes PER			BREAST			ISHD		
		1980–84	1985–89	Annual % change	1980–84	1985–89	Annual % change	1980–84	1985–89	Annual % change
UK: NORTHERN IRELAND		13.64	9.58	–6.8	43.68	43.70	0.0	250.45	206.85	–3.8
286	Northern Ireland	13.64	9.58	–6.8	43.68	43.70	0.0	250.45	206.85	–3.8
UK: SCOTLAND		11.59	9.29	–4.3	44.72	42.68	–0.9	246.93	219.00	–2.4
287	Highlands and Islands	11.30	8.23	–6.1	50.24	54.30	1.6	246.21	209.43	–3.2
288	Grampian	10.21	9.19	–2.1	39.95	35.27	–2.5	193.52	172.08	–2.3
289	Tayside	8.86	7.57	–3.1	42.91	44.99	1.0	213.17	199.90	–1.3
290	Fife	11.57	10.30	–2.3	42.39	39.11	–1.6	246.06	211.96	–2.9
291	Lothian	11.78	8.61	–6.1	42.75	37.84	–2.4	213.29	186.32	–2.7
292	Borders	11.65	6.17	–11.9	37.09	37.03	–0.0	200.07	183.92	–1.7
293	Forth Valley	13.03	9.98	–5.2	47.05	50.67	1.5	231.87	209.09	–2.0
294	Argyll and Clyde	11.89	9.89	–3.6	48.97	42.63	–2.7	281.05	242.67	–2.9
295	Greater Glasgow	11.22	9.50	–3.3	46.63	42.65	–1.8	263.57	244.30	–1.5
296	Lanarkshire	12.34	10.12	–3.9	48.44	45.06	–1.4	298.32	254.90	–3.1
297	Ayrshire and Arran	14.30	10.23	–6.5	41.47	45.50	1.9	274.23	245.29	–2.2
298	Dumfries and Galloway	11.38	8.64	–5.4	39.66	45.03	2.6	258.05	219.81	–3.2
PORTUGAL		21.70	18.38	–3.3	26.07	27.60	1.2	60.48	54.77	–2.0
299	Viana do Castelo	23.44	20.25	–2.9	17.49	20.94	3.7	50.97	51.31	0.1
300	Braga	23.18	19.35	–3.5	12.07	19.51	10.1	58.96	54.73	–1.5
301	Vila Real	30.14	21.94	–6.2	15.16	14.27	–1.2	37.07	38.28	0.6
302	Bragança	23.82	21.21	–2.3	17.83	22.42	4.7	51.99	43.83	–3.4
303	Guarda	20.68	17.94	–2.8	14.17	20.96	8.1	43.68	45.30	0.7
304	Viseu	25.08	17.43	–7.0	20.47	22.88	2.2	44.67	44.18	–0.2
305	Porto	23.92	19.62	–3.9	20.18	25.30	4.6	72.35	55.62	–5.1
306	Aveiro	21.97	17.39	–4.6	20.42	21.84	1.4	56.20	45.26	–4.2
307	Coimbra	19.80	16.30	–3.8	27.13	25.61	–1.1	49.08	40.12	–4.0
308	Castelo Branco	25.04	21.16	–3.3	20.19	24.95	4.3	44.26	42.89	–0.6
309	Portalegre	24.97	18.25	–6.1	24.30	26.71	1.9	56.20	52.49	–1.4
310	Santarem	20.77	16.25	–4.8	24.72	29.92	3.9	39.09	41.98	1.4
311	Leiria	16.74	14.53	–2.8	26.44	27.24	0.6	43.98	45.64	0.7
312	Lisboa	17.65	17.53	–0.1	35.60	32.72	–1.7	79.42	65.45	–3.8
313	Setubal	19.05	15.70	–3.8	34.61	33.37	–0.7	46.54	53.33	2.8
314	Evora	19.19	18.94	–0.3	28.13	27.56	–0.4	49.64	55.02	2.1
315	Beja	21.42	14.07	–8.1	30.94	31.25	0.2	57.59	65.55	2.6
316	Faro	20.96	18.70	–2.2	32.73	32.72	–0.0	63.78	51.57	–4.2
317	Madeira	24.85	20.71	–3.6	30.27	26.82	–2.4	68.59	51.01	–5.7
318	Azores	24.54	23.28	–1.0	30.44	38.41	4.8	87.91	125.92	7.5
SPAIN		13.16	9.99	–4.9	23.73	25.99	2.0	58.11	52.98	–2.0
319	La Coruña	12.37	10.22	–3.4	27.01	24.16	–2.5	55.16	52.66	–1.0
320	Lugo	16.62	12.91	–4.5	18.10	25.71	8.1	45.46	47.74	1.1
321	Orense	23.17	13.64	–9.2	13.56	21.82	11.1	36.95	35.21	–1.1
322	Pontevedra	12.06	8.17	–6.8	25.23	25.23	–0.0	47.85	44.17	–1.8
323	Asturias	13.83	11.11	–3.9	22.39	25.52	2.9	68.18	58.40	–3.4
324	Cantabria	13.34	10.10	–4.9	20.93	23.31	2.4	53.62	50.38	–1.4
325	Alava	12.31	9.97	–3.8	25.23	26.26	0.9	45.53	37.82	–4.0
326	Guipuzcoa	13.63	10.03	–5.4	23.66	25.07	1.3	59.45	55.42	–1.5
327	Vizcaya	14.21	12.21	–2.7	24.64	29.83	4.3	45.80	38.27	–3.9
328	Navarra	12.01	7.84	–7.5	27.79	28.52	0.6	62.46	50.38	–4.7
329	Rioja	16.41	14.38	–2.4	23.02	24.49	1.4	48.00	46.95	–0.5
330	Huesca	12.21	8.90	–5.6	22.63	32.26	8.2	41.23	41.75	0.3
331	Teruel	10.51	6.28	–8.9	26.04	27.40	1.1	45.45	45.82	0.2
332	Zaragoza	13.30	8.79	–7.3	25.86	31.03	4.1	56.84	48.59	–3.4
333	Madrid Centro	11.49	7.81	–6.8	19.01	24.01	5.3	48.49	41.82	–3.2
334	Avila	13.28	9.77	–5.4	19.48	20.72	1.4	51.35	39.48	–5.7
335	Burgos	9.03	6.40	–6.1	22.53	22.76	0.2	41.25	40.64	–0.3
336	Leon	17.89	16.63	–1.3	24.84	26.97	1.8	42.37	46.23	2.0
337	Palencia	15.22	7.75	–11.5	24.55	33.61	7.2	50.86	47.21	–1.6
338	Salamanca	15.04	13.04	–2.6	16.23	27.22	12.2	46.23	46.04	–0.1
339	Segovia	10.71	9.16	–2.8	17.43	26.94	10.2	48.12	34.32	–7.2

Table 9.4(e)—*cont.*

Area		Age-standardized mortality rates (per 100000) and percentage changes PER			BREAST			ISHD		
		1980–84	1985–89	Annual % change	1980–84	1985–89	Annual % change	1980–84	1985–89	Annual % change
340	Soria	10.86	8.74	−3.9	23.93	18.31	−5.8	43.33	38.66	−2.5
341	Valladolid	7.00	2.16	−19.3	26.28	30.59	3.4	42.42	40.48	−1.0
342	Zamora	14.49	10.57	−5.6	18.98	19.50	0.6	39.13	38.49	−0.4
343	Albacete	17.09	11.10	−7.5	24.71	19.56	−5.1	50.33	48.87	−0.7
344	Ciudad Real	13.33	11.65	−2.4	22.83	26.24	3.1	49.38	53.18	1.7
345	Cuenca	15.77	11.16	−6.1	23.27	23.57	0.3	44.53	48.27	1.8
346	Guadalajara	10.77	3.49	−18.5	23.95	20.35	−3.5	48.20	35.12	−6.8
347	Toledo	13.53	10.20	−5.0	19.73	21.75	2.2	49.94	46.54	−1.6
348	Badajoz	13.63	11.29	−3.4	28.84	27.47	−1.1	76.22	72.10	−1.2
349	Caceres	13.98	10.95	−4.4	18.62	23.51	5.3	62.35	65.73	1.2
350	Barcelona	8.44	7.90	−1.2	27.96	27.44	−0.4	48.99	46.51	−1.1
351	Gerona	11.43	8.57	−5.1	25.81	30.82	4.0	77.40	52.99	−8.1
352	Lerida	12.99	10.11	−4.4	21.35	26.62	5.0	43.95	42.57	−0.7
353	Tarragona	11.48	8.95	−4.4	21.04	23.65	2.6	51.46	43.07	−3.9
354	Alicante	11.66	8.39	−5.8	26.04	26.17	0.1	78.28	69.64	−2.6
355	Castellon de la Plana	14.09	10.63	−5.0	24.24	22.85	−1.3	55.21	54.50	−0.3
356	Valencia	11.47	8.16	−6.0	27.02	27.79	0.6	65.78	58.57	−2.5
357	Baleares	14.33	9.34	−7.5	24.89	27.79	2.5	100.82	82.60	−4.3
358	Almeria	16.25	11.83	−5.6	23.88	16.56	−7.8	64.01	60.78	−1.1
359	Cadiz	17.71	15.18	−2.8	22.90	26.28	3.1	84.57	81.18	−0.9
360	Cordoba	14.10	10.81	−4.7	21.58	22.03	0.5	54.62	56.29	0.7
361	Granada	14.41	12.28	−2.9	22.77	23.62	0.8	58.39	53.87	−1.8
362	Huelva	18.44	12.38	−7.0	22.12	26.61	4.2	69.03	67.29	−0.6
363	Jaen	16.37	12.87	−4.3	18.68	19.97	1.5	46.02	43.57	−1.2
364	Malaga	16.22	12.30	−4.9	21.31	27.50	5.8	86.33	72.22	−3.9
365	Sevilla	17.39	12.80	−5.4	26.00	27.91	1.6	72.07	69.79	−0.7
366	Murcia	11.06	9.56	−2.6	24.62	27.47	2.5	64.91	59.65	−1.9
367	Las Palmas	16.85	9.72	−9.5	30.13	33.27	2.2	106.56	88.00	−4.2
368	Sta Cruz de Tenerife	12.22	10.25	−3.1	24.58	24.81	0.2	77.44	72.96	−1.3
EC		12.85	9.98	−4.4	32.57	34.10	0.4	97.24	88.51	−2.8

Table 9.4(f)

Area	Age-standardized mortality rates (per 100 000) and percentage changes PEPTIC			ALL (age 5–64)			ALL (all ages)		
	1980–84	1985–89	Annual % change	1980–84	1985–89	Annual % change	1980–84	1985–89	Annual % change
BELGIUM	1.30	0.89	−7.3	312.51	279.03	−2.2	1148.57	1049.22	−1.8
1 Antwerpen	0.65	0.42	−8.3	279.55	250.38	−2.2	1099.77	995.88	−2.0
2 Brabant	1.64	1.05	−8.6	294.75	265.15	−2.1	1089.33	1004.93	−1.6
3 West-Vlaanderen	0.82	0.54	−7.9	285.86	252.38	−2.5	1071.95	974.92	−1.9
4 Oost-Vlaanderen	1.08	0.68	−9.0	298.48	269.30	−2.0	1141.04	1041.38	−1.8
5 Hainaut	2.02	1.46	−6.3	370.71	336.62	−1.9	1255.82	1165.83	−1.5
6 Liege	1.20	1.18	−0.3	356.77	314.55	−2.5	1267.53	1141.98	−2.1
7 Limburg	1.14	0.50	−15.1	280.61	245.92	−2.6	1099.04	1001.17	−1.8
8 Luxembourg (province)	0.91	1.19	5.6	357.08	310.03	−2.8	1191.27	1101.64	−1.6
9 Namur	2.12	1.28	−9.7	376.10	335.63	−2.3	1279.88	1158.40	−2.0
LUXEMBOURG	2.85	1.11	−17.1	363.16	309.45	−3.2	1250.91	1115.93	−2.3
10 Luxembourg	2.85	1.11	−17.1	363.16	309.45	−3.2	1250.91	1115.93	−2.3
FEDERAL REPUBLIC OF GERMANY	2.31	1.49	−8.4	308.76	276.77	−2.2	1121.41	1021.27	−1.9
11 Schleswig-Holstein	2.32	1.54	−7.9	305.90	277.55	−1.9	1110.62	1034.16	−1.4
12 Hamburg	2.10	2.28	1.7	333.03	306.55	−1.6	1132.02	1031.29	−1.8
13 Braunschweig	2.84	1.46	−12.5	303.45	275.05	−1.9	1110.68	1020.17	−1.7
14 Hannover	2.50	1.19	−13.8	315.32	282.96	−2.1	1092.81	1022.65	−1.3
15 Lüneburg	2.43	1.07	−15.2	308.55	274.13	−2.3	1121.33	1037.60	−1.5
16 Weser-Ems	2.13	1.21	−10.6	311.93	274.27	−2.5	1125.52	1016.41	−2.0
17 Bremen	3.45	2.17	−8.8	338.25	317.29	−1.3	1114.90	1031.20	−1.5
18 Düsseldorf	2.29	1.44	−8.9	327.30	292.25	−2.2	1157.18	1050.00	−1.9
19 Köln	1.94	1.12	−10.4	295.56	265.57	−2.1	1140.05	1029.45	−2.0
20 Munster	1.89	1.57	−3.6	322.13	287.74	−2.2	1173.07	1054.40	−2.1
21 Detmold	1.82	1.18	−8.3	301.03	267.86	−2.3	1079.93	974.36	−2.0
22 Arnsberg	2.34	1.57	−7.7	330.38	297.10	−2.1	1172.71	1066.30	−1.9
23 Darmstadt	2.10	1.58	−5.5	295.26	267.49	−2.0	1083.92	997.99	−1.6
24 Giessen	2.28	1.42	−9.0	285.77	264.16	−1.6	1108.42	1035.07	−1.4
25 Kassel	1.45	1.13	−4.9	286.11	260.77	−1.8	1084.71	1012.33	−1.4
26 Koblenz	1.82	1.24	−7.4	302.11	273.05	−2.0	1135.62	1033.01	−1.9
27 Trier	1.81	0.98	−11.6	320.62	281.84	−2.5	1151.81	1038.53	−2.0
28 Rheinhessen-Pfalz	2.63	1.53	−10.2	322.77	280.75	−2.8	1162.88	1044.07	−2.1
29 Stuttgart	2.25	1.49	−7.9	270.89	241.63	−2.3	1025.28	930.58	−1.9
30 Karlsruhe	3.48	2.07	−9.9	295.79	265.59	−2.1	1092.82	998.98	−1.8
31 Freiburg	2.29	1.30	−10.7	274.59	248.75	−2.0	1025.83	925.60	−2.0
32 Tübingen	2.42	1.48	−9.4	269.00	237.66	−2.4	1017.81	921.20	−2.0
33 Oberbayern	1.95	1.47	−5.5	270.61	249.07	−1.6	1015.86	941.84	−1.5
34 Niederbayern	2.68	1.45	−11.6	327.84	290.36	−2.4	1196.47	1070.56	−2.2
35 Oberpfalz	2.84	1.95	−7.2	340.75	301.71	−2.4	1220.81	1093.63	−2.2
36 Oberfranken	2.81	2.11	−5.6	343.51	300.83	−2.6	1192.99	1069.91	−2.2
37 Mittelfranken	1.86	1.65	−2.3	312.43	282.37	−2.0	1139.20	1037.69	−1.8
38 Unterfranken	2.04	1.34	−8.1	291.71	259.75	−2.3	1134.55	1018.31	−2.1
39 Schwaben	1.47	1.10	−5.6	290.94	264.47	−1.9	1108.57	1003.34	−2.0
40 Saarland	2.45	1.62	−7.9	346.13	303.51	−2.6	1230.62	1110.88	−2.0
41 Berlin (West)	4.05	1.84	−14.6	417.28	357.58	−3.0	1273.10	1150.18	−2.0
DENMARK	2.06	2.42	3.3	326.40	320.05	−0.4	1101.17	1072.87	−0.5
42 Kobenhavn and Frederiksberg (M)	2.54	3.74	8.1	452.30	450.49	−0.1	1195.53	1172.87	−0.4
43 Kobenhavns County	2.36	2.06	−2.7	315.17	309.88	−0.3	1081.07	1055.93	−0.5
44 Frederiksborg County	2.16	1.95	−2.0	302.03	296.66	−0.4	1092.17	1048.46	−0.8
45 Roskilde County	1.15	3.45	24.5	301.13	305.92	0.3	1107.75	1097.56	−0.2
46 Vestsjællands County	1.74	1.43	−3.9	324.71	319.29	−0.3	1112.21	1107.99	−0.1
47 Storstroms County	2.76	3.81	6.7	333.95	343.26	0.6	1141.42	1120.09	−0.4
48 Bornholms County	2.46	1.68	−7.4	299.37	277.06	−1.5	1112.67	1044.38	−1.3
49 Fyns County	2.23	1.87	−3.4	303.32	301.04	−0.2	1082.43	1034.13	−0.9
50 Sonderjyllands County	1.69	2.24	5.8	292.31	297.07	0.3	1051.64	1051.50	−0.0
51 Ribe County	1.40	1.57	2.2	303.53	285.84	−1.2	1049.36	990.82	−1.1
52 Vejle County	1.91	3.14	10.4	312.18	304.10	−0.5	1068.91	1043.31	−0.5
53 Ringkobing County	1.50	1.63	1.7	297.97	296.66	−0.1	1058.97	1022.86	−0.7
54 Århus County	1.81	1.95	1.4	314.51	297.86	−1.1	1084.71	1043.56	−0.8

Table 9.4(f)—*cont.*

Area		PEPTIC			ALL (age 5–64)			ALL (all ages)		
		Age-standardized mortality rates (per 100000) and percentage changes								
		1980–84	1985–89	Annual % change	1980–84	1985–89	Annual % change	1980–84	1985–89	Annual % change
55	Viborg County	2.66	2.50	−1.3	288.95	291.23	0.2	1046.37	1017.56	−0.6
56	Nordjyllands County	1.67	2.62	9.4	308.06	310.81	0.2	1069.94	1071.78	0.0
FRANCE		1.64	1.18	−6.3	307.14	283.01	−1.6	983.39	960.12	−0.5
57	Ain	1.33	1.05	−4.7	284.98	257.76	−2.0	953.60	925.78	−0.6
58	Aisne	2.00	1.52	−5.3	358.44	335.24	−1.3	1111.41	1094.12	−0.3
59	Allier	1.01	1.84	12.6	313.23	286.88	−1.7	1002.45	978.25	−0.5
60	Alpes-de-Haute-Provence	1.29	0.87	−7.6	288.24	250.98	−2.7	786.40	880.22	2.3
61	Hautes-Alpes	1.11	1.76	9.7	278.47	257.68	−1.5	939.91	892.75	−1.0
62	Alpes-Maritimes	0.95	0.96	0.2	265.04	252.39	−1.0	847.19	844.42	−0.1
63	Ardèche	1.16	0.41	−18.9	285.79	252.78	−2.4	964.30	926.06	−0.8
64	Ardennes	2.64	1.10	−16.1	362.47	334.54	−1.6	1089.13	1068.65	−0.4
65	Ariège	0.26	1.00	31.2	253.39	227.73	−2.1	923.48	907.92	−0.3
66	Aube	2.97	1.57	−12.0	317.47	292.52	−1.6	970.72	959.98	−0.2
67	Aude	0.76	1.09	7.4	248.47	228.91	−1.6	895.03	901.77	0.2
68	Aveyron	0.67	0.89	5.7	235.27	209.93	−2.3	892.68	881.81	−0.2
69	Bouches-du-Rhône	1.20	0.83	−7.3	288.62	268.92	−1.4	978.06	959.01	−0.4
70	Calvados	1.67	0.92	−11.2	326.37	294.77	−2.0	1011.95	982.26	−0.6
71	Cantal	1.40	1.36	−0.7	308.18	281.71	−1.8	1034.96	979.97	−1.1
72	Charente	1.29	1.00	−5.0	272.55	266.52	−0.4	933.53	925.64	−0.2
73	Charente-Maritime	1.13	0.98	−2.7	277.12	256.05	−1.6	921.35	897.45	−0.5
74	Cher	1.63	0.84	−12.5	311.59	289.23	−1.5	975.28	977.28	0.0
75	Corrèze	1.33	0.57	−15.5	277.58	254.30	−1.7	970.49	941.77	−0.6
76	Corse	1.10	0.60	−11.4	294.66	272.46	−1.6	960.96	978.95	0.4
77	Côte-d'Or	1.96	2.04	0.8	293.96	274.05	−1.4	935.05	907.44	−0.6
78	Côtes-du-Nord	1.46	0.80	−11.4	355.26	320.86	−2.0	1080.36	1022.49	−1.1
79	Creuse	1.51	0.72	−13.9	312.57	279.01	−2.2	970.07	981.94	0.2
80	Dordogne	0.93	0.70	−5.4	277.47	256.80	−1.5	955.38	928.35	−0.6
81	Doubs	1.55	0.91	−10.0	289.53	264.08	−1.8	965.13	938.78	−0.6
82	Drôme	0.96	0.87	−1.9	277.79	245.69	−2.4	930.61	889.81	−0.9
83	Eure	2.73	1.44	−12.0	340.04	321.75	−1.1	1026.96	1033.14	0.1
84	Eure-et-Loir	1.23	0.91	−5.9	290.58	280.54	−0.7	942.03	918.33	−0.5
85	Finistère	2.24	1.27	−10.6	368.52	334.12	−1.9	1086.23	1048.65	−0.7
86	Gard	1.28	1.21	−1.2	279.81	259.90	−1.5	946.44	949.55	0.1
87	Haute-Garonne	0.86	0.52	−9.6	248.07	220.84	−2.3	900.70	870.28	−0.7
88	Gers	1.68	1.15	−7.3	258.10	220.12	−3.1	912.77	873.25	−0.9
89	Gironde	1.05	0.83	−4.6	283.47	262.21	−1.5	965.51	935.96	−0.6
90	Hérault	1.15	0.66	−10.4	256.68	237.32	−1.6	921.60	896.57	−0.5
91	Ille-et-Vilaine	1.69	0.76	−14.7	315.47	277.81	−2.5	1064.13	979.98	−1.6
92	Indre	0.64	1.35	16.2	293.30	268.82	−1.7	962.07	946.35	−0.3
93	Indre-et-Loire	0.94	0.56	−9.8	268.97	249.82	−1.5	887.11	863.81	−0.5
94	Isère	1.04	1.36	5.4	282.04	254.63	−2.0	958.67	917.69	−0.9
95	Jura	1.50	0.79	−12.0	283.68	263.28	−1.5	963.60	927.50	−0.8
96	Landes	1.66	1.27	−5.2	273.37	255.27	−1.4	949.69	934.40	−0.3
97	Loir-et-Cher	0.97	0.90	−1.6	287.31	260.80	−1.9	900.24	888.42	−0.3
98	Loire	2.22	1.47	−7.9	308.30	264.99	−3.0	1003.19	942.83	−1.2
99	Haute-Loire	2.25	1.94	−2.9	307.13	285.79	−1.4	987.92	999.87	0.2
100	Loire-Atlantique	1.51	0.95	−8.9	342.53	305.49	−2.3	1033.90	985.61	−1.0
101	Loiret	1.63	1.13	−7.0	282.29	268.31	−1.0	928.62	916.84	−0.3
102	Lot	1.15	0.43	−17.8	242.00	226.73	−1.3	927.73	902.41	−0.6
103	Lot-et-Garonne	0.85	0.47	−11.3	250.25	229.31	−1.7	931.19	893.86	−0.8
104	Lozère	3.10	1.01	−20.1	278.57	256.26	−1.7	986.75	928.11	−1.2
105	Maine-et-Loire	1.31	0.70	−11.9	286.43	254.03	−2.4	941.16	887.83	−1.2
106	Manche	0.95	0.81	−3.1	303.75	279.03	−1.7	1013.77	994.62	−0.4
107	Marne	1.98	1.55	−4.8	328.49	311.74	−1.0	995.84	1006.49	0.2
108	Haute-Marne	1.04	0.99	−1.1	331.95	298.89	−2.1	1029.15	981.79	−0.9
109	Mayenne	1.09	0.73	−7.5	286.66	253.87	−2.4	967.37	905.28	−1.3
110	Meurthe-et-Moselle	2.16	1.97	−1.8	342.63	301.32	−2.5	1064.43	1012.76	−1.0
111	Meuse	3.20	1.78	−11.1	360.10	307.17	−3.1	1073.10	1013.82	−1.1
112	Morbihan	1.91	0.89	−14.3	400.63	346.92	−2.8	1162.97	1088.01	−1.3
113	Moselle	3.46	1.94	−10.9	346.15	309.70	−2.2	1149.67	1093.44	−1.0

Table 9.4(f)—*cont.*

Area		PEPTIC			ALL (age 5–64)			ALL (all ages)		
		Age-standardized mortality rates (per 100000) and percentage changes								
		1980–84	1985–89	Annual % change	1980–84	1985–89	Annual % change	1980–84	1985–89	Annual % change
114	Nièvre	2.09	1.22	−10.1	333.05	325.61	−0.5	1008.51	996.00	−0.2
115	Nord	3.24	2.13	−8.0	404.14	372.22	−1.6	1185.62	1145.92	−0.7
116	Oise	2.11	1.33	−8.7	325.81	312.89	−0.8	1037.41	1041.55	0.1
117	Orne	1.38	0.39	−22.2	312.23	280.91	−2.1	1001.48	960.28	−0.8
118	Pas-de-Calais	2.58	2.63	0.3	408.25	378.36	−1.5	1181.87	1164.09	−0.3
119	Puy-de-dôme	1.65	1.44	−2.8	319.78	297.09	−1.5	1023.87	1007.36	−0.3
120	Pyrénées-Atlantiques	1.34	0.99	−6.0	274.36	251.05	−1.8	940.87	925.00	−0.3
121	Hautes-Pyrénées	1.14	1.08	−0.9	272.39	245.86	−2.0	959.66	920.27	−0.8
122	Pyrénées-Orientales	1.38	1.38	0.1	265.06	236.95	−2.2	930.38	898.65	−0.7
123	Bas-Rhin	2.75	1.56	−10.7	331.94	296.34	−2.2	1082.99	1045.01	−0.7
124	Haut-Rhin	1.96	2.06	1.1	332.59	303.62	−1.8	1104.41	1057.77	−0.9
125	Rhône	1.68	1.33	−4.7	282.56	258.99	−1.7	936.91	911.14	−0.6
126	Haute-Saône	2.04	1.24	−9.5	312.26	286.92	−1.7	1029.06	984.68	−0.9
127	Saône-et-Loire	1.47	1.47	−0.0	302.48	269.46	−2.3	968.43	957.14	−0.2
128	Sarthe	0.86	1.12	5.5	271.34	258.37	−1.0	912.00	884.83	−0.6
129	Savoie	1.82	0.96	−12.0	300.67	277.73	−1.6	978.08	946.59	−0.7
130	Haute-Savoie	1.72	1.22	−6.6	301.70	277.02	−1.7	977.16	941.47	−0.7
131	Paris	1.43	0.84	−10.2	302.14	291.54	−0.7	860.72	868.23	0.2
132	Seine-Maritime	2.03	1.62	−4.4	353.42	323.41	−1.8	1042.77	1018.09	−0.5
133	Seine-et-Marne	1.21	1.04	−3.0	302.56	295.91	−0.4	1013.55	1008.84	−0.1
134	Yvelines	1.69	0.87	−12.3	262.06	251.22	−0.8	914.57	901.59	−0.3
135	Deux-Sèvres	0.72	0.90	4.5	242.89	220.92	−1.9	904.03	877.09	−0.6
136	Somme	1.63	2.25	6.6	353.44	332.10	−1.2	1104.82	1087.96	−0.3
137	Tarn	0.76	0.62	−4.1	241.71	212.46	−2.5	907.62	866.67	−0.9
138	Tarn-et-Garonne	1.19	0.74	−9.0	252.56	227.09	−2.1	907.72	887.19	−0.5
139	Var	1.04	0.89	−3.1	281.12	256.33	−1.8	937.27	911.31	−0.6
140	Vaucluse	1.41	0.96	−7.4	283.08	262.34	−1.5	963.87	925.44	−0.8
141	Vendée	1.40	0.55	−17.1	274.56	255.34	−1.4	956.28	923.85	−0.7
142	Vienne	0.68	0.75	1.8	256.85	234.09	−1.8	859.37	868.04	0.2
143	Haute-Vienne	0.76	0.31	−16.5	262.91	251.05	−0.9	903.35	914.88	0.3
144	Vosges	2.61	1.67	−8.6	347.30	313.92	−2.0	1048.28	1024.28	−0.5
145	Yonne	1.96	1.35	−7.2	337.32	314.05	−1.4	990.99	999.71	0.2
146	Territoire-de-Belfort	2.36	1.89	−4.3	323.28	283.52	−2.6	1052.39	1004.17	−0.9
147	Essonne	1.13	0.85	−5.5	275.69	260.51	−1.1	920.60	913.84	−0.1
148	Hauts-de-Seine	1.53	0.92	−9.7	280.79	271.17	−0.7	906.31	895.37	−0.2
149	Seine-Saint-Denis	1.52	1.25	−3.8	326.15	313.38	−0.8	992.72	992.55	−0.0
150	Val-de-Marne	1.45	1.15	−4.4	289.17	270.68	−1.3	944.47	934.12	−0.2
151	Val-d'Oise	2.11	1.01	−13.8	290.99	276.30	−1.0	988.29	975.92	−0.3
GREECE		0.92	0.41	−12.8	236.21	247.59	0.8	1032.19	1075.77	0.7
152	Greater Athens	1.01	0.55	−9.8	238.58	260.61	1.5	1058.96	1166.32	1.6
153	Rest of Central Greece and Eubea	0.58	0.50	−2.3	229.67	226.21	−0.3	988.41	993.03	0.1
154	Peloponnisos	0.94	0.19	−23.1	217.43	220.81	0.3	963.31	987.00	0.4
155	Ionian Islands	2.04	0.20	−32.2	230.07	216.86	−1.0	1112.78	1036.57	−1.2
156	Epirus	0.64	0.00	−100.0	236.35	218.68	−1.3	978.75	974.67	−0.1
157	Thessaly	0.79	0.29	−15.5	249.91	245.20	−0.3	1057.00	1082.45	0.4
158	Macedonia	0.89	0.37	−13.6	241.25	266.09	1.6	1071.65	1116.26	0.7
159	Thrace	1.35	0.55	−13.9	291.75	315.51	1.3	1165.57	1259.50	1.3
160	Aegean Islands	0.97	0.56	−8.7	224.55	223.16	−0.1	1035.23	1017.19	−0.3
161	Crete	0.84	0.24	−18.7	211.31	211.51	0.0	910.78	934.90	0.4
ITALY		1.96	1.25	−8.6	284.89	247.22	−2.3	1101.92	950.67	−2.4
162	Torino	2.20	1.57	−6.6	293.49	251.34	−2.6	1158.35	954.38	−3.2
163	Vercelli	2.22	1.25	−10.9	322.70	285.72	−2.0	1143.36	1033.24	−1.7
164	Novara	1.86	1.31	−6.8	326.13	291.28	−1.9	1171.58	1006.23	−2.5
165	Cuneo	1.58	1.60	0.2	313.32	271.82	−2.3	1163.09	1008.23	−2.4
166	Asti	2.55	0.62	−24.7	274.84	239.81	−2.2	1133.76	981.17	−2.4
167	Alessandria	1.44	0.70	−13.4	286.00	263.08	−1.4	1090.77	960.08	−2.1
168	Aosta	1.70	2.11	4.5	363.40	322.47	−2.0	1138.32	1029.74	−1.7
169	Imperia	2.22	1.15	−12.3	286.48	245.97	−2.5	1078.93	942.28	−2.2
170	Savona	1.96	0.85	−15.3	276.75	244.35	−2.1	1097.79	945.40	−2.5

Table 9.4(f)—*cont.*

	Area	PEPTIC 1980–84	PEPTIC 1985–89	PEPTIC Annual % change	ALL (age 5–64) 1980–84	ALL (age 5–64) 1985–89	ALL (age 5–64) Annual % change	ALL (all ages) 1980–84	ALL (all ages) 1985–89	ALL (all ages) Annual % change
171	Genova	1.88	0.84	−14.9	292.36	252.50	−2.4	1121.90	965.54	−2.5
172	La Spezia	0.84	0.53	−8.6	264.39	228.42	−2.4	1055.17	915.55	−2.3
173	Varese	1.60	1.47	−1.6	291.87	248.32	−2.7	1141.96	941.27	−3.2
174	Como/Sondrio	1.48	1.04	−6.7	322.40	277.32	−2.5	1184.94	988.23	−3.0
175	Milano	2.00	1.00	−12.9	308.70	261.36	−2.7	1157.94	946.74	−3.3
176	Bergamo	1.89	0.80	−15.8	360.05	298.35	−3.1	1165.39	1032.25	−2.0
177	Brescia	2.07	1.39	−7.6	368.70	303.95	−3.2	1268.93	1026.55	−3.5
178	Pavia	2.32	0.89	−17.5	349.46	302.14	−2.4	1218.72	1045.55	−2.5
179	Cremona	1.57	1.10	−6.9	373.65	316.66	−2.7	1254.17	1092.24	−2.3
180	Mantova	1.17	1.25	1.3	309.86	263.25	−2.7	1175.38	988.07	−2.9
181	Bolzano	1.27	1.29	0.3	314.54	262.17	−3.0	1117.31	917.89	−3.2
182	Trento	1.60	1.55	−0.6	335.08	288.83	−2.4	1136.87	967.56	−2.7
183	Verona	2.15	1.11	−12.4	315.48	267.38	−2.7	1140.84	949.54	−3.0
184	Vicenza	2.73	1.29	−14.0	325.86	272.74	−2.9	1171.28	965.85	−3.2
185	Belluno	3.96	1.61	−16.5	391.89	328.38	−2.9	1181.19	1020.71	−2.4
186	Treviso	2.50	0.92	−18.2	310.19	254.73	−3.2	1084.41	899.51	−3.1
187	Venezia	1.61	1.29	−4.4	324.42	269.54	−3.0	1099.61	951.01	−2.4
188	Padova	1.62	1.51	−1.5	318.19	263.10	−3.1	1116.34	958.89	−2.5
189	Rovigo	3.16	2.01	−8.6	323.85	274.80	−2.7	1156.68	979.92	−2.7
190	Udine/Gorizia	2.90	1.64	−10.8	367.06	299.43	−3.3	1189.34	1007.44	−2.7
191	Trieste	4.77	1.86	−17.1	332.13	281.70	−2.7	1121.66	987.77	−2.1
192	Pordenone	1.95	1.59	−3.9	345.43	280.78	−3.4	1117.28	956.05	−2.6
193	Piacenza	1.74	0.80	−14.4	324.46	276.23	−2.6	1097.49	962.43	−2.2
194	Parma	2.52	1.69	−7.6	279.37	249.98	−1.8	1067.17	911.70	−2.6
195	Reggio Emilia	1.39	0.96	−7.2	266.96	239.99	−1.8	1035.02	886.47	−2.5
196	Modena	1.23	1.23	−0.0	277.58	243.46	−2.2	1056.27	907.24	−2.5
197	Bologna	1.27	1.26	−0.3	267.23	235.68	−2.1	1041.92	884.18	−2.7
198	Ferrara	2.08	1.77	−3.2	295.61	263.55	−1.9	1068.03	953.74	−1.9
199	Ravenna	0.81	0.82	0.3	248.11	220.27	−2.0	975.74	816.30	−2.9
200	Forli	1.28	0.57	−15.0	250.69	222.73	−2.0	1011.53	863.28	−2.6
201	Pesaro	1.02	0.82	−4.3	245.87	214.17	−2.3	999.53	868.20	−2.3
202	Ancona	1.18	0.99	−3.4	232.94	205.93	−2.0	991.75	850.60	−2.5
203	Macerata	0.86	0.34	−17.2	232.90	202.95	−2.3	1002.20	843.25	−2.8
204	Ascoli Piceno	1.90	0.85	−15.0	226.60	198.25	−2.2	1005.44	864.77	−2.5
205	Massa-Carrara	1.62	0.64	−16.8	289.53	260.80	−1.7	1076.34	954.22	−2.0
206	Lucca	2.11	0.70	−19.8	285.22	252.67	−2.0	1078.02	964.88	−1.8
207	Pistoia	0.56	1.15	15.5	257.24	218.46	−2.7	1034.88	872.74	−2.8
208	Firenze	1.43	0.69	−13.5	241.47	212.70	−2.1	984.39	875.24	−1.9
209	Livorno	1.54	0.68	−15.2	264.03	231.24	−2.2	1042.70	924.54	−2.0
210	Pisa	1.22	0.69	−10.8	249.16	224.54	−1.7	1043.72	914.98	−2.2
211	Arezzo	0.45	0.42	−1.7	245.46	217.62	−2.0	1012.70	878.06	−2.3
212	Siena	2.20	1.21	−11.3	235.16	211.24	−1.8	992.01	873.06	−2.1
213	Grosseto	1.09	1.15	1.0	269.65	223.24	−3.1	1047.25	923.61	−2.1
214	Perugia	1.40	1.05	−5.6	250.64	217.86	−2.3	1015.03	883.68	−2.3
215	Terni	1.80	1.39	−5.0	231.17	203.79	−2.1	1048.46	899.56	−2.5
216	Viterbo/Rieti	1.94	0.80	−16.3	275.15	236.65	−2.5	1108.39	971.61	−2.2
217	Roma	1.83	1.24	−7.6	262.62	236.34	−1.7	1091.28	949.73	−2.3
218	Latina	1.59	0.61	−17.3	260.02	227.74	−2.2	1081.74	923.09	−2.6
219	Frosinone	2.43	1.02	−15.8	257.10	230.95	−1.8	1051.25	938.94	−1.9
220	Caserta	2.95	2.18	−5.9	306.77	278.94	−1.6	1214.54	1082.54	−1.9
221	Benevento	1.26	1.97	9.4	244.15	220.18	−1.7	1054.94	911.04	−2.4
222	Napoli	3.02	1.69	−10.9	333.58	285.53	−2.6	1318.93	1146.34	−2.3
223	Avellino	2.52	1.63	−8.3	290.58	210.80	−5.2	1188.48	869.38	−5.1
224	Salerno	2.03	1.24	−9.4	261.71	224.49	−2.5	1029.70	923.59	−1.8
225	L'Aquila	2.40	1.98	−3.7	276.68	242.67	−2.2	1080.41	933.45	−2.4
226	Teramo	1.20	1.06	−2.6	243.86	203.55	−3.0	1027.71	856.04	−3.0
227	Pescara	1.81	1.47	−4.1	225.55	216.62	−0.7	987.94	885.69	−1.8
228	Chieti	2.68	1.02	−17.5	232.49	199.26	−2.5	994.47	858.58	−2.4
229	Isernia/Campobasso	2.54	1.31	−12.4	251.48	221.03	−2.1	1022.47	870.71	−2.6
230	Foggia	1.75	1.23	−6.8	248.41	227.56	−1.5	1022.90	938.25	−1.4
231	Bari	1.90	1.04	−11.3	249.99	217.02	−2.3	1032.46	932.58	−1.7

Age-standardized mortality rates (per 100000) and percentage changes

Table 9.4(f)—*cont.*

Area		Age-standardized mortality rates (per 100000) and percentage changes PEPTIC			ALL (age 5–64)			ALL (all ages)		
		1980–84	1985–89	Annual % change	1980–84	1985–89	Annual % change	1980–84	1985–89	Annual % change
232	Taranto	1.17	1.16	−0.3	249.04	229.04	−1.4	1077.09	953.29	−2.0
233	Brindisi	2.42	1.94	−4.3	261.78	231.31	−2.0	1116.01	963.12	−2.4
234	Lecce	1.95	1.19	−9.4	244.99	210.12	−2.5	1079.98	906.38	−2.9
235	Potenza/Matera	2.53	1.70	−7.6	242.55	217.20	−1.8	1027.34	903.98	−2.1
236	Cosenza	2.44	2.02	−3.7	245.68	204.48	−3.0	1005.14	875.59	−2.3
237	Catanzaro	2.35	1.93	−3.9	246.77	226.01	−1.5	1005.07	913.00	−1.6
238	Reggio Calabria	2.40	1.33	−11.1	258.18	249.80	−0.5	1001.76	952.74	−0.8
239	Trapani	1.84	0.81	−15.1	248.48	203.43	−3.3	1066.51	955.58	−1.8
240	Palermo	2.17	1.49	−7.2	262.64	236.89	−1.7	1098.53	1011.72	−1.4
241	Messina	3.10	2.08	−7.7	228.52	212.38	−1.2	1034.91	896.62	−2.4
242	Agrigento	2.21	0.91	−16.3	236.07	211.61	−1.8	1051.33	926.51	−2.1
243	Caltanisetta	2.38	2.52	1.1	261.85	242.28	−1.3	1127.19	1012.37	−1.8
244	Enna	1.78	2.40	6.1	253.15	224.39	−2.0	1120.31	990.25	−2.0
245	Catania	2.20	1.27	−10.4	262.50	236.23	−1.7	1141.88	1032.01	−1.7
246	Ragusa	0.77	0.95	4.4	239.85	211.02	−2.1	1162.43	959.27	−3.2
247	Siracusa	1.60	1.21	−5.4	243.80	230.51	−0.9	1086.07	995.55	−1.4
248	Sassari	1.74	1.59	−1.8	270.05	242.98	−1.7	1045.12	952.61	−1.5
249	Nuoro	1.58	1.22	−5.0	291.55	250.82	−2.5	1036.72	923.82	−1.9
250	Cagliari/Oristano	1.67	1.39	−3.6	273.66	238.06	−2.3	1043.65	930.75	−1.9
IRELAND		2.73	1.97	−6.3	340.70	299.07	−2.6	1321.11	1235.37	−1.3
251	Eastern	1.97	2.03	0.7	343.77	293.43	−3.1	1275.20	1191.03	−1.4
252	Midland	4.11	2.17	−12.0	341.12	313.02	−1.7	1376.79	1309.33	−1.0
253	Mid-Western	2.44	2.28	−1.4	355.56	310.84	−2.7	1411.40	1304.83	−1.6
254	North-Eastern	2.47	1.91	−5.0	347.03	301.70	−2.8	1346.19	1248.31	−1.5
255	North-Western	4.99	2.37	−13.8	328.10	299.52	−1.8	1298.75	1228.67	−1.1
256	South-Eastern	2.43	1.72	−6.7	339.93	300.35	−2.4	1356.48	1247.73	−1.7
257	Southern	3.28	2.08	−8.8	351.87	302.57	−3.0	1358.91	1264.92	−1.4
258	Western	2.76	1.29	−14.1	304.66	290.05	−1.0	1251.33	1200.69	−0.8
THE NETHERLANDS		1.17	0.84	−7.2	252.90	239.08	−1.2	988.19	955.70	−0.7
259	Groningen	1.44	1.20	−4.1	262.54	251.42	−1.0	982.34	981.70	−0.0
260	Friesland	1.58	1.23	−5.4	251.71	236.10	−1.4	983.67	960.75	−0.5
261	Drenthe	1.10	0.83	−6.1	255.65	256.31	0.1	981.92	962.79	−0.4
262	Overijssel	1.23	0.81	−8.8	258.79	245.27	−1.2	999.65	986.72	−0.3
263	Gelderland	1.30	0.76	−11.1	256.51	238.18	−1.6	999.09	966.58	−0.7
264	Utrecht	1.00	0.70	−7.7	242.65	230.18	−1.2	973.72	936.11	−0.9
265	Noord Holland	1.04	0.71	−8.2	253.79	242.82	−1.0	986.19	958.74	−0.6
266	Zuid Holland	1.11	1.00	−2.4	248.68	236.59	−1.1	965.15	932.13	−0.8
267	Zeeland	0.97	0.74	−5.8	234.93	222.75	−1.2	937.72	903.85	−0.8
268	Noord Brabant	1.01	0.75	−6.2	249.53	233.16	−1.5	1010.88	957.08	−1.2
269	Limburg	1.53	0.82	−13.0	269.62	252.78	−1.4	1055.63	1017.07	−0.8
270	Flevoland	1.25	0.00	−100.0	227.89	193.40	−3.6	914.79	751.61	−4.3
UK: ENGLAND AND WALES		2.62	2.31	−3.1	302.22	277.19	−1.7	1117.99	1066.42	−0.9
271	Northern	3.54	2.90	−4.9	355.43	327.69	−1.6	1242.25	1191.46	−0.8
272	Yorkshire	2.96	2.28	−6.3	323.16	296.75	−1.7	1175.90	1112.84	−1.1
273	Trent	2.60	2.44	−1.6	309.53	284.16	−1.7	1147.48	1095.82	−0.9
274	East Anglian	1.59	1.73	2.1	250.85	234.18	−1.4	1020.23	986.41	−0.7
275	North-West Thames	2.58	2.15	−4.5	274.40	254.42	−1.5	1041.67	990.92	−1.0
276	North-East Thames	2.55	2.56	0.0	287.84	269.89	−1.3	1064.11	1021.89	−0.8
277	South-East Thames	2.44	2.40	−0.4	284.14	263.68	−1.5	1068.71	1026.92	−0.8
278	South-West Thames	2.02	1.47	−7.7	260.02	235.65	−1.9	1025.38	984.12	−0.8
279	Wessex	1.92	1.59	−4.5	257.09	241.14	−1.3	980.82	982.23	0.0
280	Oxford	2.01	1.67	−4.5	257.63	236.77	−1.7	1042.39	1001.71	−0.8
281	South-Western	1.82	1.46	−5.4	286.66	248.04	−2.9	1099.59	996.08	−2.0
282	West Midlands	3.12	2.27	−7.6	312.98	287.52	−1.7	1166.09	1110.00	−1.0
283	Mersey	3.18	2.93	−2.0	346.56	319.11	−1.6	1213.03	1150.46	−1.1
284	North-Western	3.22	3.34	0.9	351.33	322.85	−1.7	1235.15	1184.62	−0.8
285	Wales	2.67	2.87	1.8	326.67	296.47	−1.9	1170.19	1104.66	−1.1

Table 9.4(f)—*cont.*

Area		PEPTIC 1980–84	PEPTIC 1985–89	PEPTIC Annual % change	ALL (age 5–64) 1980–84	ALL (age 5–64) 1985–89	ALL (age 5–64) Annual % change	ALL (all ages) 1980–84	ALL (all ages) 1985–89	ALL (all ages) Annual % change
		Age-standardized mortality rates (per 100000) and percentage changes								
UK: NORTHERN IRELAND		2.70	2.42	−2.2	362.43	321.49	−2.4	1285.29	1189.67	−1.5
286	Northern Ireland	2.70	2.42	−2.2	362.43	321.49	−2.4	1285.29	1189.67	−1.5
UK: SCOTLAND		3.68	2.99	−4.1	382.67	352.26	−1.6	1285.72	1224.23	−1.0
287	Highlands and Islands	3.62	1.96	−11.6	390.69	356.31	−1.8	1278.67	1193.42	−1.4
288	Grampian	2.43	2.60	1.4	324.15	307.39	−1.1	1184.96	1143.50	−0.7
289	Tayside	2.67	2.07	−4.9	335.07	324.14	−0.7	1202.11	1169.84	−0.5
290	Fife	2.72	1.77	−8.2	353.01	319.58	−2.0	1238.38	1178.62	−1.0
291	Lothian	3.37	2.65	−4.7	343.96	316.13	−1.7	1203.83	1162.03	−0.7
292	Borders	1.50	2.25	8.5	322.82	290.21	−2.1	1188.22	1110.94	−1.3
293	Forth Valley	3.70	2.35	−8.7	367.62	342.48	−1.4	1277.81	1228.59	−0.8
294	Argyll and Clyde	4.40	3.36	−5.2	417.98	375.34	−2.1	1371.68	1283.50	−1.3
295	Greater Glasgow	4.32	4.49	0.8	442.23	415.35	−1.2	1363.03	1309.77	−0.8
296	Lanarkshire	4.63	3.26	−6.8	405.42	358.19	−2.4	1378.29	1290.26	−1.3
297	Ayrshire and Arran	4.66	3.38	−6.2	397.55	352.39	−2.4	1365.43	1252.87	−1.7
298	Dumfries and Galloway	3.12	1.77	−10.7	369.87	377.46	0.4	1246.43	1212.91	−0.5
PORTUGAL		2.53	1.67	−7.9	334.96	305.43	−1.8	1196.53	1066.59	−2.3
299	Viana do Castelo	2.44	2.58	1.2	335.94	323.02	−0.8	1179.51	1089.05	−1.6
300	Braga	2.18	1.11	−12.7	334.16	316.31	−1.1	1237.15	1136.73	−1.7
301	Vila Real	3.82	1.64	−15.6	382.33	358.08	−1.3	1335.63	1232.02	−1.6
302	Bragança	4.21	1.51	−18.6	321.35	310.67	−0.7	1185.96	1081.63	−1.8
303	Guarda	2.93	1.40	−13.8	347.60	327.78	−1.2	1137.67	1062.97	−1.3
304	Viseu	3.14	1.74	−11.2	344.30	328.62	−0.9	1206.73	1129.34	−1.3
305	Porto	2.75	1.21	−15.2	346.84	309.82	−2.2	1259.88	1130.79	−2.1
306	Aveiro	1.86	1.09	−10.1	352.03	298.87	−3.2	1239.31	1079.60	−2.7
307	Coimbra	2.68	0.95	−18.7	322.85	277.23	−3.0	1165.09	1032.24	−2.4
308	Castelo Branco	2.13	2.27	1.3	321.57	313.95	−0.5	1088.15	1016.68	−1.3
309	Portalegre	2.12	1.72	−4.1	283.06	277.61	−0.4	1090.42	1014.34	−1.4
310	Santarem	1.13	0.79	−6.9	320.37	291.30	−1.9	1147.38	1012.45	−2.5
311	Leiria	1.52	1.55	0.3	358.57	322.84	−2.1	1257.30	1125.14	−2.2
312	Lisboa	2.96	2.09	−6.7	321.83	289.44	−2.1	1184.17	1069.20	−2.0
313	Setubal	1.23	1.28	0.7	313.61	266.29	−3.2	1161.25	984.77	−3.2
314	Evora	3.07	2.32	−5.4	278.60	280.77	0.2	1125.97	1090.20	−0.6
315	Beja	3.18	3.56	2.3	309.95	324.71	0.9	1129.96	1098.37	−0.6
316	Faro	3.13	1.84	−10.1	314.81	319.80	0.3	1116.78	1006.95	−2.0
317	Madeira	2.36	2.96	4.6	421.11	391.62	−1.4	1230.06	883.95	−6.4
318	Azores	2.82	3.48	4.3	429.33	391.73	−1.8	1341.98	942.57	−6.8
SPAIN		1.71	1.00	−11.3	259.52	247.81	−0.8	969.14	924.34	−0.9
319	La Coruña	1.15	0.79	−8.1	291.37	274.92	−1.1	985.05	923.89	−1.2
320	Lugo	0.84	0.21	−26.2	243.66	246.67	0.2	960.78	899.11	−1.2
321	Orense	1.18	0.42	−20.5	221.05	215.81	−0.4	871.85	808.03	−1.4
322	Pontevedra	0.92	0.91	−0.3	277.52	269.53	−0.5	1006.41	943.53	−1.2
323	Asturias	1.77	1.12	−9.7	285.88	262.38	−1.5	989.47	933.09	−1.1
324	Cantabria	0.98	1.55	10.8	275.68	250.10	−1.8	961.79	902.58	−1.1
325	Alava	0.94	1.03	2.1	265.07	215.75	−3.7	970.31	852.19	−2.3
326	Guipuzcoa	2.33	1.12	−15.0	250.40	258.44	0.6	903.06	928.51	0.5
327	Vizcaya	1.40	0.58	−17.9	282.97	252.05	−2.1	1010.38	937.06	−1.4
328	Navarra	1.08	1.18	2.1	264.82	224.74	−2.9	982.36	866.00	−2.3
329	Rioja	2.17	0.56	−26.0	233.47	240.62	0.5	959.14	937.44	−0.4
330	Huesca	0.81	1.21	9.2	207.38	222.52	1.3	795.94	854.43	1.3
331	Teruel	1.39	0.62	−16.5	222.71	209.82	−1.1	860.32	814.93	−1.0
332	Zaragoza	2.24	1.74	−5.4	235.75	221.63	−1.1	901.36	890.54	−0.2
333	Madrid Centro	0.81	0.51	−9.7	245.34	228.60	−1.3	891.59	837.83	−1.1
334	Avila	2.01	0.26	−36.7	219.34	203.18	−1.4	804.02	788.17	−0.4
335	Burgos	2.65	1.08	−18.1	248.71	239.14	−0.7	805.37	819.30	0.3
336	Leon	1.71	0.78	−15.9	271.02	258.50	−0.9	967.86	881.48	−1.7
337	Palencia	1.86	1.05	−12.0	284.85	275.73	−0.6	955.72	880.56	−1.5
338	Salamanca	0.87	1.24	8.1	225.68	220.43	−0.4	821.21	794.79	−0.6
339	Segovia	0.77	0.00	−100.0	236.14	217.98	−1.4	900.80	833.19	−1.4

Table 9.4(f)—*cont.*

Area		Age-standardized mortality rates (per 100 000) and percentage changes PEPTIC			ALL (age 5–64)			ALL (all ages)		
		1980–84	1985–89	Annual % change	1980–84	1985–89	Annual % change	1980–84	1985–89	Annual % change
340	Soria	1.47	0.00	−100.0	225.76	209.67	−1.3	790.90	732.89	−1.4
341	Valladolid	1.06	1.33	5.1	224.69	214.10	−0.9	819.55	811.13	−0.2
342	Zamora	0.78	0.20	−25.9	225.69	218.28	−0.6	859.81	823.79	−0.8
343	Albacete	3.05	1.39	−16.0	241.57	226.28	−1.2	1015.90	933.54	−1.5
344	Ciudad Real	2.54	1.48	−11.3	257.96	246.87	−0.8	1028.22	971.41	−1.0
345	Cuenca	1.93	0.70	−20.2	243.69	226.76	−1.3	945.78	847.18	−2.0
346	Guadalajara	0.54	0.70	5.9	217.79	220.36	0.2	778.87	824.93	1.1
347	Toledo	1.09	0.72	−8.9	229.03	214.32	−1.2	945.37	894.57	−1.0
348	Badajoz	2.53	2.40	−1.2	283.23	281.56	−0.1	1052.18	1003.96	−0.8
349	Caceres	2.38	1.55	−9.1	258.49	259.43	0.1	971.47	916.28	−1.1
350	Barcelona	1.39	0.96	−7.8	232.94	228.77	−0.3	880.11	883.55	0.1
351	Gerona	1.68	1.19	−7.4	255.35	240.42	−1.1	1009.85	938.29	−1.3
352	Lerida	1.85	1.13	−10.4	229.39	224.23	−0.4	897.40	890.45	−0.1
353	Tarragona	1.66	0.55	−21.7	249.13	221.21	−2.1	974.95	934.47	−0.8
354	Alicante	2.29	0.91	−18.5	261.34	246.60	−1.1	1048.14	961.18	−1.6
355	Castellon de la Plana	2.04	1.11	−12.6	228.01	231.73	0.3	977.18	954.97	−0.4
356	Valencia	1.76	1.03	−11.2	282.28	259.66	−1.5	1096.40	1021.36	−1.3
357	Baleares	2.71	0.74	−25.2	277.69	276.37	−0.1	997.94	987.75	−0.2
358	Almeria	1.86	0.97	−13.5	260.41	262.44	0.1	1035.80	1000.80	−0.6
359	Cadiz	3.32	1.44	−16.9	308.51	307.15	−0.1	1127.74	1092.76	−0.6
360	Cordoba	2.13	0.60	−24.6	245.06	248.80	0.3	988.35	968.23	−0.4
361	Granada	3.08	1.85	−10.7	258.54	250.63	−0.6	1028.98	983.16	−0.8
362	Huelva	1.82	1.35	−6.4	280.67	274.76	−0.4	1076.67	1019.80	−1.0
363	Jaen	1.81	1.28	−7.3	231.64	242.40	0.8	960.39	964.56	0.1
364	Malaga	2.06	1.14	−12.3	306.28	292.56	−0.8	1122.73	1044.77	−1.3
365	Sevilla	3.49	1.86	−13.0	289.76	277.53	−0.8	1100.47	1045.61	−0.9
366	Murcia	2.16	0.90	−17.6	268.06	247.38	−1.4	1056.59	977.72	−1.4
367	Las Palmas	1.94	1.54	−5.0	341.84	309.70	−1.8	1143.42	1055.06	−1.5
368	Sta Cruz de Tenerife	1.49	0.65	−16.7	293.99	300.00	0.4	1032.29	988.65	−0.8
EC		2.00	1.45	−5.9	296.83	270.58	−1.7	1077.74	1005.63	−1.3

APPENDIX A SELECTION OF DISEASES

Disease Tuberculosis	Age group: 5–64 years	ICD codes from 8th and 9th revisions

Interventions

Screening, early detection of cases, immunization
Contact tracing
Antibiotics

Health care providers

Public health programme*
Primary care
Hospital

Other potential contributory factors to excess mortality

Incidence —social class
—ethnic group
Non-compliance with treatment

ICD8: 010–019

010 Silicotuberculosis
011 Pulmonary tuberculosis
012 Other respiratory tuberculosis
013 Tuberculosis of meninges and central nervous system
014 Tuberculosis of intestines, peritoneum, and mesenteric glands
015 Tuberculosis of bones and joints
016 Tuberculosis of genito-urinary system
017 Tuberculosis of other organs
018 Disseminated tuberculosis
019 Late effects of tuberculosis

ICD9: 010–018, 137

010 Primary tuberculouis infection
011 Pulmonary tuberculosis
012 Other respiratory tuberculosis
013 Tuberculosis of meninges and central nervous system
014 Tuberculosis of intestines, peritoneum, and mesenteric glands
015 Tuberculosis of bones and joints
016 Tuberculosis of genito-urinary system
017 Tuberculosis of other organs
018 Miliary tuberculosis
137 Late effects of tuberculosis

*Most important provider(s)

References
British Thoracic and Tuberculosis Association (1971). A survey of tuberculosis mortality in England and Wales in 1968. *Tubercle*, **52**, 1–18.
Johnston, R.F. and Wildnick, K.H. (1974). State of the art. Review of the impact of chemotherapy on the care of patients with tuberculosis. *American Review of Respiratory Disease*, **109**, 636–64.

Disease Malignant neoplasm of cervix uteri	Age group: 15–64 years	ICD code from 8th and 9th revisions

Interventions

Screening, cytology
Surgery
Radiation therapy

Health care providers

Community health services*
Primary care
Hospital

Other potential contributory factors to excess mortality

Incidence —social class
—sexual habits

180 Malignant neoplasm of cervix uteri

*Most important provider(s)

References
Clark, B.A. and Anderson, T.W. (1979) Does screening by 'PAP' smears help prevent cervical cancer? *Lancet*, **ii**, 1–4.
Editorial (whole issue on cancer of the cervix) (1976). Screening for carcinoma of the cervix. *Canadian Medical Association Journal*, **114**, 1013–26.
Macgregor, J.E. and Teper, S. (1978). Mortality from carcinoma of the cervix uteri in Britain. *Lancet*, **ii**, 774–6.

Disease Malignant neoplasm of cervix uteri and body of the uterus | Age group: 15–54 years | ICD codes from 8th and 9th revisions

Interventions

Screening, cytology
Surgery
Radiation therapy

Health care providers

Community health services*
Primary care
Hospital

Other potential contributory factors to excess mortality

Incidence —social class
—sexual habits

Due to variation in coding practices between countries and possible inclusion of malignant neoplasm of the body of the uterus with that of the cervix uteri, the two have been combined for between country comparisons. (Age limit 54 years for combined SMR, to exclude the bulk of malignant neoplasm body uterus deaths which are not avoidable.)

ICD8: 180, 182

180 Malignant neoplasm of cervix uteri
182 Other malignant neoplasm of uterus

ICD9: 179, 180, 182

179 Malignant neoplasm of uterus, part unspecified
180 Malignant neoplasm of cervix uteri
182 Other malignant neoplasm of uterus

*Most important provider(s)

References
Clark, B.A. and Anderson, T.W. (1979) Does screening by 'PAP' smears help prevent cervical cancer? *Lancet*, **ii**, 1–4.
Editorial (whole issue on cancer of the cervix) (1976). Screening for carcinoma of the cervix. *Canadian Medical Association Journal*, **114**, 1013–26.
Macgregor, J.E. and Teper, S. (1978). Mortality from carcinoma of the cervix uteri in Britain. *Lancet*, **ii**, 774–6.

Disease Hodgkin's disease | Age group: 5–64 years | ICD code from 8th and 9th revisions

Interventions

Case detection
Chemotherapy
Radiation therapy

Health care providers

Hospital*
Primary care
Pathology services

Other potential contributory factors to excess mortality

Social class
Radiation therapy services may be not available in each small area. Excess mortality may reflect non referral or delayed referral of cases to regional treatment centres.

201 Hodgkin's disease

*Most important provider(s)

References
Aisenberg, A.C. (1978). The staging and treatment of Hodgkin's disease. *New England Journal of Medicine*, **299**, 1228–32.
Kaplan, H.S. (1980) *Hodgkin's disease* (2nd edn). Havard University Press, Cambridge, Massachusetts.

Disease Chronic rheumatic heart disease	Age group: 5–44 years	ICD codes from 8th and 9th revisions

Interventions

Case detection of streptococci
Antibiotics
Prophylaxis
Valve replacement surgery

Health care providers

Hospital*
Primary care

Other potential contributory factors to excess mortality

Social class

Long lag period between acute rheumatic fever and mortality. Cardiothoracic surgery services may not be available at small area level in all areas.

393 Chronic rheumatic pericarditis
394 Diseases of mitral valve
395 Diseases of aortic valve
396 Diseases of mitral and aortic valves
397 Diseases of other endocardial structures
398 Other rheumatic heart disease

*Most important provider(s)

References
Feinstein, A.R., Stern, E.K. and Spagnuola, M. (1966). The prognosis of acute rheumatic fever. *American Heart Journal*, **68**, 817–34.
Gordis, L. (1973). Effectiveness of comprehensive-care programs in preventing rheumatic fever. *New England Journal of Medicine*, **289**, 331–5.
Rammelkamp, C.H. (1952). Studies in the epidemiology of rheumatic fever in the armed services. In *Rheumatic fever*, (ed L. Thomas). University of Minneapolis Press, Minneapolis.

Disease All respiratory diseases	Age group: 1–14 years	ICD codes from 8th and 9th revisions

Interventions

Early detection of complications

Health care providers

Primary care
Hospital

Other potential contributory factors to excess mortality

Social class
Urban pollution

ICD8: 460–519

Acute respiratory infection (460–466)
Influenza (470–474)
Pneumonia (480–486)
Bronchitis, emphysema and asthma (490-493)
Other diseases of upper respiratory tract (500–508)
Other diseases of respiratory system (510–519)

ICD9: 460-519

Acute respiratory infections (460–466)
Other diseases of upper respiratory tract (470–478)
Pneumonia and influenza (480–487)
Chronic obstructive pulmonary disease and allied conditions (490–496)
Pneumoconiosis and other lung diseases due to external agents (500–508)
Other diseases of respiratory system (510–519)

References
Editorial (1985). Acute respiratory infections in under-fives: 15 million deaths a year. *Lancet*, **ii**, 699–701.

Disease Asthma	Age group: 5–44 years	ICD codes from 8th and 9th revisions
Interventions Casualty department care Treatment Early referral of status asthmaticus **Health care providers** Primary care* Hospital **Other potential contributory factors to excess mortality** Social class Prevalence Inappropriate drug treatment There is potential coding error with chronic obstructive airways disease. Not all asthma deaths are avoidable and therefore variation in prevalence between areas is an important consideration.		493 Asthma

*Most important provider(s)

References

Johnston, A.J., Nunn, A.J., Somner, A.R., Stableforth, D.E. and Stewart, C.J. (1984). Circumstances of death from asthma., *British Medical Journal*, **288**, 1870–2.
Speizer, F.E., Doll, R. and Heaf, P. (1968). Observations on recent increase in mortality from asthma, *British Medical Journal*, **1**, 335–9.
Stableforth, D.E. (1983). Death from asthma (editorial). *Thorax*, **38**, 801–5.

Disease Appendicitis	Age group: 5–64 years	ICD codes from 8th and 9th revisions
Interventions Case detection Surgery **Health care providers** Hospital* Primary care **Other potential contributory factors to excess mortality** Coding error—acute abdominal pain with no positive diagnosis		540 Acute appendicitis 541 Appendicitis, unqualified 542 Other appendicitis 543 Other diseases of appendix

*Most important provider(s)

Reference

Editorial (1985). Perioperative deaths, *Lancet*, **ii**, 1049.

Disease Abdominal hernia	Age group: 5–64 years	ICD codes from 8th and 9th revisions
Interventions Case detection Surgery prior to complications **Health care providers** Hospital* Primary care **Other potential contributory factors to excess mortality** Coding error—acute abdominal pain with no positive diagnosis Incidence of strangulated abdominal hernia		**ICD8: 550–553** 550 Inguinal hernia without mention of obstruction 551 Other hernia of abdominal cavity without mention of obstruction 552 Inguinal hernia with obstruction 553 Other hernia of abdominal cavity with obstruction **IDC9: 550-553** 550 Inguinal hernia 551 Other hernia of abdominal cavity, with gangrene 552 Other hernia of abdominal cavity with obstruction, without mention of gangrene 553 Other hernia of abdominal cavity without mention of obstruction or gangrene

*Most important provider(s)

Reference

Editorial (1985). Perioperative deaths. *Lancet*, **ii**, 1049.

Disease Cholelithiasis and cholecystitis	Age group: 5–64 years	ICD codes from 8th and 9th revisions

Interventions

Case detection
Surgery prior to complications

Health care providers

Hospital*
Primary care

Other potential contributory factors to excess mortality

Coding error—acute abdominal pain with no positive diagnosis

ICD8: 574–575

574 Cholelithiasis
575 Other disorders of the gallbladder

ICD9: 574–575.1, 576.1

574 Cholelithiasis
575.0 Acute cholecystitis
575.1 Other cholecystitis
576.1 Cholangitis

*Most important provider(s)

References

Editorial (1985). Perioperative deaths. *Lancet*, **ii**, 1049

Fitzpatrick, G., Neutra, R., and Gilbert, J.P. (1977). Cost benefits of cholecystectomy for silent gallstones. In *Cost, risks and effectiveness of surgery*, (ed J.P. Bunker, B.A. Barnes and F. Mosteller), pp. 246–76. Oxford University Press, New York.

Ransohoff, D.F., Gracie, W.A., Wolfenson, L B., and Neuhauser, D. (1983). Prophylactic cholecystectomy or expectant management for silent gallstones. A decision analysis to assess survival. *Annals of Internal Medicine*, **99**, 199–204.

Disease Hypertensive and cerebrovascular diseases	Age group: 35–64 years	ICD codes from 8th and 9th revisions

Interventions

Case detection
Antihypertensive medication
Treatment of complications of cerebrovascular disease

Health care providers

Primary care*
Hospital

Other potential contributory factors to excess mortality

Coding error—ischaematic heart disease
Lack of screening/case finding
Social factors
Non-compliance with treatment
Nutrition
Weight
Smoking (cerebrovascular disease)
Malignant hypertension

Due to potential case transfer (coding) between hypertension and cerebrovascular disease, the two diseases have been combined. The lower age limit has been raised to 35 years to exclude cerebrovascular disease which is not considered avoidable, for example, Berry aneurysms.

ICD8: 400–404, 430–438

400 Malignant hypertension
401 Essential benign hypertension
402 Hypertensive heart disease
403 Hypertensive renal disease
404 Hypertensive heart and renal disease

430 Subarachnoid haemorrhage
431 Cerebral haemorrhage
432 Occlusion of precerebral arteries
433 Cerebral thrombosis
434 Cerebral embolism
435 Transient cerebral ischaemia
436 Acute but ill-defined cerebrovascular disease
437 Generalized ischaemic cerebrovascular disease
438 Other and ill-defined cerebrovascular disease

ICD9: 401–405, 430–438

401 Essential hypertension
402 Hypertensive heart disease
403 Hypertensive renal disease
404 Hypertensive heart and renal disease
405 Secondary hypertension

430 Subarachnoid haemorrhage
431 Intracerebral haemorrhage
432 Other and unspecified intracranial haemorrhage
433 Occlusion and stenosis of precerebral arteries
434 Occlusion of cerebral arteries
435 Transient cerebral ischaemia
436 Acute but ill-defined cerebrovascular disease
437 Other and ill-defined cerebrovascular disease
438 Late effects of cerebrovascular disease

*Most important provider(s)

References

Hypertension Detection and Follow-Up Program Cooperative Group (1979). Five year findings of the hypertension detection and follow-up program. I. Reduction in mortality in persons with high blood pressure, including mild hypertension. *Journal of the American Medical Association*, **242**, 2562–71.

Hypertension Detection and Follow-Up Program Cooperative Group (1982). Five year findings of the hypertension detection and follow-up program. II. Reduction in stroke incidence among persons with high blood pressure. *Journal of the American Medical Association*, **247**, 633–8.

Veteran's Adminstration Cooperative Study Group on Antihypertensive Agents (1972). Effects of treatment on morbidity in hypertension. *Circulation*, **45**, 991–1004.

Disease Maternal deaths (all causes) Age group: all years ICD codes from 8th and 9th revisions

Interventions

Antenatal care
Obstetric care

Health care providers

Hospital*
Primary care

Other potential contributory factors to excess mortality

None

ICD8: 630–678

630–634 Complications of pregnancy
635–639 Urinary infections and toxaemias of pregnancy and the puerperium
640–645 Abortion
650–662 Delivery
670–678 Complications of the puerperium

ICD9: 630–676

630–639 Pregnancy with abortive outcome
640–648 Complications mainly related to pregnancy
650–659 Normal delivery and other indications for care in pregnancy, labour and delivery
660–669 Complications occuring mainly in the course of labour and delivery
670–676 Complications of the puerperium

*Most important provider(s)

References

Department of Health and Social Security (1982). Report on confidential enquiries into maternal deaths in England and Wales 1976–8. *Report on Health and Social Subjects, 26.* HMSO, London.
Dambrosio, F. and Buscaglia, M. (1976). La mortalilita in Lombardia e le sue cause. Risultati di un'indagine condotta nelgi ospedali della Lombardia per gli anni 1966–73. *Annali di Ostetricia, Ginecologia, Medicina Perinatale*, **97**, 302–25
Rumeau-Rouquette, C., du Mazaubrun, C., and Rabarison, Y. (1984). *Naître en France. Dix ans d'évolution.* INSERM-Doin, Paris.

Disease Perinatal mortality All causes, aged under 1 week, plus stillbirths

Interventions

Antnatal care
Obstetric care
Paediatric neonatal care

Health care providers

Hospital*
Primary care

Other potential contributory factors to excess mortality

Incidence —low birth weight
—social class

*Most important provider(s).

References

Alberman, E. (1982). Perinatal audit (editorial). *Community Medicine*, **4**, 95–6.
Mersey Regional Health Authority (1982). Report of Working Party. Confidential Enquiry into perinatal deaths in the Mersey Region. *Lancet*, **i**, 491–4.
Donzelli, G. and Assenza, G. (1984). L'audit perinatale. *Salute e Territorio*, **34–35**, 71–4.
Rumeau-Rouquette, C., de Mazaubrun, C., and Rabarison, Y. (1984). *Naître en France. Dix ans d'évolution.* INSERM-Doin, Paris.

Disease Cancer of the breast	Age group: 25–64 years	ICD codes for 8th and 9th revisions
Interventions Case finding Screening Surgery Radiotherapy Chemotherapy **Health care providers** Public health programmes: screening in ages 50–64* Primary health care Hospital **Other potential contributory factors to excess mortality** Incidence Risk factors: obesity, family history		174 Malignant neoplasm of female breast

*Most important provider(s)

References

Forrest, P. (1990). *Breast cancer: the decision to screen.* Nuffield Provincial Hospital Trust.

Disease Ischaemic heart disease	Age group: 35–64 years	ICD codes from 8th and 9th revisions
Interventions Primary prevention **Health care providers** Primary health care* Hospital Health education **Other potential contributory factors to excess mortality** Coding error Social factors		**ICD8: 410–414** 410 Acute myocardial infarction 411 Other acute and sub-acute forms of ischaemic heart disease 412 Chronic ischaemic heart disease 413 Angina pectoris 414 Asymptomatic ischaemic heart disease **ICD9: 410–414, 429.2** 410 Acute myocardial infarction 411 Other acute and sub-acute forms of ischaemic heart disease 412 Old myocardial infarctions 413 Angina pectoris 414 Other forms of chronic ischaemic heart disease 429.2 Cardiovascular disease, unspecified

*Most important provider(s)

References

Hypertension Detection and Follow-Up Program Cooperative Group (1979). Five year findings of the hypertension detection and follow-up program. I. Reduction in mortality in persons with high blood pressure, including mild hypertension. *Journal of the American Medical Association*, **242**, 2562–71.

Hjermann, I., Byrne, K.V., Holme, J., *et al* (1981). Effect of diet and smoking intervention on the incidence of coronary heart disease: report from the Oslo Study Group of randomised trials in healthy men. *Lancet* **ii**, 1303–9.

Puska, P., Nissenen, A., Tuomilehto, J. *et al.* (1985). The community based strategy to prevent coronary heart disease: conclusions from the ten years of the North Karelia Project. *Annual Review of Public Health*, **6**, 177–93

Disease Peptic ulcers	Age group: 25–64 years	ICD codes from 8th and 9th revisions
Interventions Anti-ulcer drugs Surgery for complications **Health care providers** Primary health care Hospital* **Other potential contributory factors to excess mortality** Alcohol Smoking		531 Gastric ulcer 532 Duodenal ulcer 533 Peptic ulcer, site unspecified 534 Gastrojejunal ulcer

*Most important provider(s)

Reference

Boyd, E. and Wormsley, K.G. (1985). Etiology and pathogenesis of peptic ulcer disease. In *Bockus gastroenterology* (4th edn) (ed J.E. Berk), Vol II. W.E. Saunders.

APPENDIX B DATA SOURCES

Belgium

The National Institute for Statistics and the Ministry of Economic Affairs.

Luxembourg

Statistiques des causes de deces 1980–84/1985–89
Direction de la Sante
Service des Statistiques Sanitaires
22, rue Goethe
1637 Luxembourg.

Federal Republic of Germany

Bevölkerung nach Alter und Familienstand (1980), Statistisches Bundesamt.

Fachserie 1, Bevölkerung und Erwebstätigkeit, Reihe 1–3.

Fachserie 1, Bevölkerung und Erwerbstätigkeit, Reihe 1. Gebiet und Bevölkerung (1981,...1989).

Fachserie 12, Gesundheitswesen–Reihe 4. 'Todesursachen' (1980,...1989), Statistisches Bundesamt.

Gestorbene nach Todesursachen–Bericht A IV/3 (1980,...1989). Berichte der Statistischen Landesämter.

Denmark

Mortality data

The National Board of Health and the Danish Institute for Clinical Epidemiology.

Population data

The Central Bureau of Statistics.

France

Service d'Information sur les causes médicales de décès–SC8
Institut National de la Santé et de la Recherche Médicale
44 Chemin de Ronde
78110 Le Vesinet
Paris.

Greece

Published and unpublished material (census, vital registration) compiled and offered by the National Statistical Service of Greece.

Italy

Mortality records were made available to the Istituto Superiore di Sanita by the ISTAT in the original form.

1. Capocaccia, R., *et al.* La mortalità in Italia nel periodo 1970–79 ... 1989. *Rapporti ISTISAN,* (84/10, 85/10, 89/6, 90/17, 90/18, 91/37, 92/22).

2. Capocaccia, R., Caselli G. *Popolazione residente per età e sesso nelle provincia italiane anni 1972–81.* Università degli Studi di Roma 'La Sapienza' Dip. Sc. Demografiche, Fonti e Strumenti, 2, 1990.

Ireland

Central Statistics Office
Ardee Road
Dublin 6.

The Netherlands

Mortality data

Data from the Central Bureau of Statistics, processed by the Department of Public Health and Social Medicine, Erasmus University, Rotterdam.

Population data

Central Bureau of Statistics.

United Kingdom: England and Wales

Mortality data

Mortality statistics series VS3 (augmented) 1980–84/1985–89
Office of Population Censuses and Surveys
St Catherine's House
10 Kingsway
London WC2B 6JP.

Population data

Population Estimates Unit, Office of Population Censuses and Surveys.

United Kingdom: Scotland

Registrar General for Scotland
Ladywell House
Ladywell Road
Edinburgh EH12 7TF.

United Kingdom: Northern Ireland

General Register Office
Department of Health and Social Services
Oxford House
49–55 Chichester Street
Belfast BT1 4HL.

Portugal

Instituto Nacional de Estatística, Lisboa.

'Estatísticas da Saúde'
Departamento de Estudos e Planeamento da Saúde
Ministério da Saúde
Lisboa.

'Risco de Morrer em Portugal'
Serviço de Informaçäo de Saúde
Direcção-Geral da Saúde
Lisboa.

Spain

All data were supplied by the National Statistics Institute and were collected and prepared by the 'Subdirección General de Información Sanitaria y Epidemiologia' of the Spanish Ministry of Health.

Mortality data

'Movimiento Natural de la Población Española'
Instituto Nacional de Estadística
Paseo de la Castellana, 176
28071 Madrid.

Population data

1981 Census of the Spanish population
Instituto Nacional de Estatística.

APPENDIX C FURTHER READING

References to related work in participant countries

Belgium

Belgian Group on Avoidable Mortality (submitted for publication). *Atlas de la mortalité évitable en Belgique, 1980–84—Atlas van de vermijdbare sterfe in België* (Collaboratorsi R. Lagasse, P.C. Humblet, G.F.G. Moens, H. van de Voorde and E. Wollast). Archives of Public Health.

Berghmans, L., Gilbert, M., Aelvoet, W., and Lagasse, R. (1990*a*). Evaluation of death certificates' quality. Report of the feasibility study. Document polycopié. Bruxelles.

Berghams, L., Gilbert, M., Aelvort, W., and Lagasse, R. (1990*b*). Collaborative project on variations in certification and coding of the causes of death in the EC, Workshop, Brussels, 10–11 September 1990. Document polycopié.

Gruppo di lavoro Italiano per lo studio della qualità della certificazione e codifica, Berghmans, L. and Lagasse, R. (1990). Lo studio sulla qualità della certificione e codifica della cause di morte nei paesi della comunitá Europea (CEE). In Atti preliminari, 5° Convego Nazionale sugli Studi di Mortalita, Firenze, 24–26 ottobre 1990, p. 179.

Hooft, P. (1987). Relatieve risicogebbieden in het arrondissement Leuven: een geografische analyse van gezondheid. Unpublished thesis. Katholeike Universiteit, Leuven.

Hooft, P., and van den Voorde, H. (1989). Relatieve risicogebieden in het arrondissement Leuven. Een ordinale geografische analyse van de gezondheidstoetand en de spreiding van de gezondheidszorg. *Archives, Belges de Médecine Sociale, Hygiène, Médecine Travail et Médecine Légale,* **47** (1–4) 157.

Humblet, P., Lagasse, R., Moens, G.F.G., van de Voorde, H., and Wollast, E. (ed.) (1986). Atlas de la mortalité évitable en Belgique, 1974–1978—*Atlas van de vermijdbare sterfte in Belgie*. Ecole de Santé Publique, Université Libre de Bruxelles/School voor Maatschappelijke Gezondheidszorg, Katholeike Universiteit, Leuven.

Humblet, P.C., Lagasse, R., and Moens, G.F.G. (1988). Fiabilité du processus de codage des causes de décès en Belgique. *Archives, Belges de Médecine Sociale, Hygiène, Médecine Travail et Médecine Légale,* **46** (1–2), 42.

Humblet, P.C., Lagasse, R., Moens, G.F.G., Wollast, E., and van de Voorde, H. (1987). La mortalité évitable en Belgique. *Social Science and Medicine,* **25** (5), 485.

Humblet, P.C., Wollast, E., Vandenbussche, P., Leleux, P., and Buekens, P. (1989). Organization of prenatal care in Belgium. *Biology of the Neonate,* **55,** 55.

Lagasse, R., Humblet, P.C., Hooft, P., Van de Voorde, H., and Wollast, E. (1991). The concept of avoidable death, its representation in atlases and use in public health. CBGS Monografie n°1, Brussels, p37–48.

Lagasse, R., Kittel, F., Dramaix, M., Gheyssens, H., De Backer, G., and Kornitzer, M. (1986). Ischemic heart disease and regional variations of sociocultural characteristics in Belgium. *Social Science and Medicine* **22** (9), 901.

Lagasse, R., Devlieger, H., de Wals, P., Casaer, P., Eggermont, E., and Lechat, M. (1989). Perinatal morbidity in Belgium. *Biology of the Neonate,* **55,** 19.

Lagasse, R., Gilbert, M., Humblet, P.C., Aelvort, W., and Berghmans, L. (1990*a*). Mortality statistics comparability in the European Community: first results of a feasibility study on death certification and coding practices. Actes de la IInd European Conference on Health Services Research and Primary Health Care, Köln, 14–15 December 1990.

Lagasse, R., Humblet, P.C., Lenaerts, A., Godin, I., and Moens, G.F.G. (1990). Health and social inequalities in Belgium. *Social Science and Medicine* **31,** 3, 237.

Mackenbach, J.P., Moens, G.F.G., and Lagasse, R. (1985). Verschillen in door gezondheidszorg vermijdbare sterfte tussen Nederland en Belgie. *Gezondheid en Samenleving* **6** (4), 265.

Moens, G.F.G. (1987). Evaluation of the effect of a health service using an ecological method. *Tijdschrift voor Sociale Gezondheidszorg* **65,** 764.

Moens, G.F.G., Van de voorde, H., Humblet, P.C., Lagasse, R., and Wollast, E. (1985*a*). Vermijde sterfte door tuberculose: een evaluatie instrument van de effectiviteit van tuberculosebestrijdingsprogramma's in België. *Tijdschrift voor Soziale Gezondheidszorg* **63**(21), 880.

Moens, G., Lagasse, R., Humblet, P., van de Voorde, M., and Wollast, E. (1985*b*). Evaluatie van de medische zorg in Belgie via monitoring van vermijdbare sterfte. *Tijdschrift voor Sociale Gezonheidszorg* **63,** 880.

Moens, G.F.G., Lagasse, R., Humblet, P., van de Voorde, M., and Wollast, E. (1986). 'Vermijdbare sterfte': een evaluatie instrument van de gezondheidszorg in Belgie? *Tijdschrift voor Geneeskunde* **42** (13), 921.

Moens, G.F.G., Haenen, W., and van de Voorde, H. (1988*a*). Epidemiological aspects of suicide among the young in selected European countries. *Journal Epidemiology and Community Health,* **42,** 279.

Moens, G.F.G., Loysch, M.J.M., and van de Voorde, H. (1988*b*). The geographical patterns of methods of suicide in Belgium: implications for prevention. *Acta Psychiatrica Scandinavica,* **77,** 320.

van de Voorde, H., Haenen, W., van Wonterghem, G., and Hooft, P. (1991). Gezondheidniuews in dagbladpers en Mattheuseffect. *Archives of Public Health* **48** (1–2), 32.

Van den Bussche, P., Dujardin, B., Wollast, E., Lagasse, R., Humblet, P.C., *et al.* (1987). *Atlas de la santé périnatale et infantile en Belgique–Atlas van périnatale en infantiele gezondheid in Belgie.* Sociéte Royale Belge de Gynécologie et d'Obstétrique, Bruxelles.

Federal Republic of Germany

Becker, N., Frentzel-Beyme, R., and Wagner, G. (1984). *Krebsatlas der Bundesrepublik Deutschland.* (2nd edn). Springer-Verlag, Berlin.

Borgers, D. (1989). Mortalitätsanalysen zur Beuteilung von Krankheitsrisiken und Gesundheitszustand der Bevölkerung. In *Epidemiologie und Gesundheitswissenschaft* (ed. D. Borgers). Argument-Verlag, Hamburg.

Gatzweiler, H.P., and Steins, G. (1982). Regionale Mortalitätsunterschiede in der Bundesrepublik Deutschland. Daten und Hypothesen. In *Jahrbuch für Regionalwissenschaft*, Vol 3, p. 36. Gesellschaft für Regionalforschung, Göttingen.

Giersdorf, P., and Lorenz, R. (1986). Zu regionalen Unterschieden der Mortalität in der DDR im Zeitraum 1980/1983. *Zeitschrift für Ärztliche Fortbildung*, **80**, 947.

Häussler, B., and Rescke, P. (1991). Vermeidbare Todesfälle in Rheinland-Pflaz. Ministerium für Arbeit, Soziales Familie, und Gesundheit Rheinland-Pflaz. Mainz.

Hölzel, D., and Altwein, J.E. (1991). Hodentumoren. Ist der Rückgang der Mortalität in der Bundesrepublik Deutschland zu langsam erfolgt? *Deutches Ärzteblatt,* **C88** (47), 2282.

Kern, K.D., and Braun, W. (1985). Einflufl wichtiger Todersursachen auf die Sterblichkeit und die Lebenserwartung. *Wirtschaft und Statistik*, **3**: 233.

Neuberger, G., and Frommholz, C. (1986). Kleinräumliche Sterblichkeitsdifferenzen und deren mögliche Ursachen—dargestellt am Beispiel Bayern. In *Öffentliche Gesundheitswesen*, **48**, 97.

Robra, B.P., Brecht, J.G., and Dralle, H. (1983). Appendizitis-Mortalität in der Bundesrepublik Deutschland 1952–1979. Trendanalyse und Alterskonturen. *Deutsche Medizinische Wochenschrift*, **125** (13), 485.

Denmark

Bjerregaard, P. (1988). Alchohol related death in Greenland. *Arctic Medical Research*, **47**, Supplement 1, 596.

Bjerregaard, P. (1988). Causes of death in Greenland 1968-85. *Arctic Medical Research*, **47** (3), 105.

Bjerregaard, P., and Juel, K. (1990). Avoidable deaths in Greenland 1968–85: variations by region and period. *Arctic Medical Research,* **49**, 119.

Bjerregaard, P., and Juel, K. (1993). Middellevetid og dødelighed i Danmark [Life expectancy and mortality in Denmark]. *Ugeskr Laeger*, **155**, 4097.

Bjerregaard, P., and Juel, K. (1993). *Middellevetid og dødelighed* [Life expectancy and mortality]. København: Sundhedsministeriet.

Johansen, L.G., and Bjerregaard, P. (1988). Lost years of life in Greenland in the period 1968 to 1983. *Arctic Medical Research,* **47** Supplement 1, 596.

Juel, K. (1984). Dodelighedsindeks for kommuner og amter 1971–80. Dansk Institut for Klinisk Epidemiologi. Sundhedsstyrelsen. *Vitalstatistik*, **1** (7), 1.

Juel, K., and Bjerregaard, P. (1994). Alkoholrelateret dødelighed i Danmark 1951–1992 [Alcohol related mortality in Denmark 1951–1992]. In *Alkohol-og narkotikamisbruget 1993* (ed. H. Strunge). København: Sundhedsstryrelsen.

Juel, K., and Kamper-Jorgensen, F. (1986). Avoidable deaths in Denmark during the period 1970-1983. Variations with hospital district and periods. *Ugeskrift for Laeger*, **148**, 1981.

Juel, K., and Pedersen, P.A. (1992). Increasing asthma mortality in Denmark 1969-1988 not a result of a changed coding practice. *Annals of Allergy*, **69**, 180.

Juel, K., and Sjøl, A. (1995). Decline in mortality from heart disease in Denmark: some methodological problems. *Journal of Clinical Epidemiology*, **48**, 467.

Knudsen, L. (1988). Fodsler og sociale forhold 1982–1983. Dansk Institut for Klinisk Epidemiologi. Sundhedsstyrelsen. *Vitalstatistik*, **1** (22), 141.

Life Expectancy Committee. (1994). *Life time in Denmark.* Ministry of Health, Denmark.

Madsen, M., Anderson, T.F., Roepstorff, C., Jørgensen, S., Keskimäki, I., Johnsson, M., Paulson, E,. and Nielsen, H.B. (1994). Rates of surgery in the Nordic countries - variation between and within nations. Dike & Nomesko, København.

France

Annuaire des Statistiques Sanitaires et Sociales SESI. (1989). Ministère des Affaires Sociales et de la Solidarité Nationale, Paris.

Arveiler, D., Bingham, A., Escudero, I., *et al.* (1988). Evaluation des conditions d'accès aux soins d'urgence des sujets atteints d'infarctus du myocarde. *Revue d'Epidémiologie et de Santé Publique*, **4–5**, 350.

Audirac, P.A. *Recensement général de la Population 1982: principaux résultats*. Les Collections de l'Insee, Paris, Series D, no. 97.

Bouvier-Colle, M.H. (1987). *Géographie de la mortalité en France*, Données Sociales, Paris INSEE, no. 445.

Bouvier-Colle, M.H., Varnoux, N., Costes, P., and Hatton, F. (1991). Reasons for the under-reporting of maternal mortality in France, as indicated by a survey of all deaths among women of childbearing age. *International Journal of Epidemiology*, **20**, 717.

Faur, B. *La situation démographique en 1982*. Les Collections de l'Insee, Paris, Series D, no. 106.

Garros, B., and Bouvier-Colle, M.H. (1990). Les variations géographiques de la mortalité. In *Mortalité en France*, (ed. M.H. Bouvier-Colle and F. Hatton). INSERM-Doin, Paris.

Giroud, M., Beuriat, P., Vion Ph., *et al.* (1988). Incidence des accidents vasculaires cérébraux dans une ville française moyenne. *Revue d'Epidémiologie et de Santé Publique*, **4–5**, 360.

Hatton, F., Tiret, L., Maujol, L., *et al.* (1983). Protocole de l'enquête épidémiologique sur les anesthésies. *Annales Françaises d'Anésthesie et de Réanimation*, **2**, 335.

L'Huillier, M-Ch., Steschenko, D., Olive, D., *et al.* (1988). Les registres des cancers de l'enfant en France. *Revue d' Epidémiologie et de Santé Publique*, **4-5**, 301.

Jougla, E. (1987). Analyse géographique de la relation entre le niveau du système de soins et le niveau de la mortalité en France, Université de Paris-Sud, DERBH.

Jougla, E., Ducimetiere, P., Bouvier-Colle, M.H., and Hatton, F. (1987). Relation entre le niveau de développement du système de soins et le niveau de la mortalité 'évitable' selon les départements français. *Revue d' Epidémiologie et de Santé Publique*, **35**, 365.

Jougla, E., Goldberg, M., and Hatton, F. (1988). Relation entre l'evolution de l'état de santé et l'activité du système de santé dans les pays développés. *Revue d' Epidémiologie et de Santé Publique*, **36**, 464.

Jougla, E., Bouvier-Colle, M.H., and Hatton, F. (1990). Relation entre le niveau de l'état de santé et le niveau des densités médicales. *Revue du Praticien*, **95**, 67.

Joulga, E., Papoz, L., Balkau, B., Maguin, P., Hatton, F., and The Eurodiab Sub-area C Study Goup (1992). Death certificate coding practices related to diabetes in European countries—The Eurodiab Sub-area C Study. *International Journal of Epidemiology,* 21, 343–51.

Jougla, E., Papoz, L., Balkau, B., Simon, D., Vauzelle-Kervroedan, F., and Hatton, F. (1991). Analyse de la mortalité liée au diabete en France à partir des causes multiples de décès (1970–1987). *Diabetes Metabolism,* **17** (3), 337.

Larroque, B., Bouvie-Colle, M.H., and Hatton, F. (1991). Agrégation temporospatiale de mort subite du nourripon en France de 1981 à 1986. (Space-time clustering of sudden infant death in France from 1981 to 1986). *Revue d'Epidémiologie et de Santé Publique*, **39** (1), 45.

Mallaret, M.R., Turquand, O., Blatier, J-F., *et al.* (1990). Salmonelloses humaines en rapport avec les tortues aquatiques dans le département de l'Isère. *Revue d'Epidemiologie et de Santé Publique*, **1**, 71.

Moatti, J-P., Le Gales, C., Julian, C., Lanoe, J-L., and Aymé, S. (1990). Analyse coût-bénéfice du diagnostic prénatal des anomalies chromosomiques par amniocentèse. *Revue d'Epidémiologie et de Santé Publique*, **4**, 309.

Noin, D., Thumerelle, P.J., and Kostrubiec, B. (1986). Analyse géographique des causes de décès en France. *Espace, Population, et Sociétés*, 269.

Nuttens, M-C., Arveiler, D., Zafra-Lopez, S., *et al.* (1988). L'infarctus du myocarde dans trois régions françaises: comparaison de l'incidence et de la mortalité en 1985. *Revue d'Epidémiologie et de Santé Publique*, **4–5**, 335.

Rumeau-Rouquette, C., Breart, G., and Padieu, R. (1985). Méthodes en épidémiologie. Flammarion Médecine Sciences, Paris.

Tiret, L., Desmonts, J.M., Hatton, F., and Vourc'h, G. (1986). Complications associated with anaesthesia: a prospective survey in France. *Canadian Anaesthetists' Society Journal*, **33**, 336–44.

Zanetti, R., Rosso, S., Faggiano, F., *et al.* (1988). Etudes cas-témoins sur le mélanome de la peau dans la province de Turin, Italie. *Revue d'Epidémiologie et de Santé Publique*, **4–5**, 309.

Greece

Papavangelou, G., Roumeliotou, A., Stergioy, G., Nestoridou, A., Trichopoulou, E., Kallinkos, G., Rizos, G. and Kornarou, E. (1991). HIV infection in Greek intravenous drug users. *European Journal of Epidemiology,* **7** (1), 88.

Italy

Baldi, P., and Morosini, P.L. (1984). *I dati di mortalitá per la programmazione sanitaria.* Atti del 2° Convegno Nazionale sugli Studi di Mortalitá Regione Toscana - CSPO, Firenze.

Buiatti, E., Barchielli, A., and Vannucchi, G. (1988). Eventi sentinella: esperienze, problemi aperti e prospettive. 4° Convegno Nazionale sugli Studi di Mortalitá, Firenze.

Lauriola, P., and Goldoni, C.A. (1989). Osservazioni, commenti e proposte su una indagine condotta nella Regione Emilia Romagna nel 1987, su alcuni eventi sentinella. *Epidemiologia e Prevenzione*, **39**, 22.

Marco, R., and Zanolin, E. (1990). Mortalitá per alcune cause riconducibili all'intervento medico nelle U.s.l. Lombarde (1980-1985). *Epidemiologia e Prevenzione*, **45**, 24.

Morosini, P., Lauriola, P., Magliola, E., Feola, G., and Paul, E.M. (1990). Le morti evitabili nella valutazione della attività del servizio sanitario nazionale. *Epidemiologia e Prevenzione*, **12** (45), 48.

Morosini, P.L., and Taroni, F. (1986). Valutazione di qualità dei servizi sanitari. *Salute e Territorio*, **49**, 48.

Parazzini, F., Grilli, R., Bruzzi, P., and Liberati, A. (1990). *La mortalità prevenibile con la terapia in ambito oncologico: il caso del tumore della mammella, dell'ovaio e del grosso intestino.* Atti 5° Convegno Nazionale sugli Studi di Mortalitá - Firenze, 24–26 Ottobre 1990.

Repetto, F., and Morosini, P.L. (1986). Sistema informativo, ricerca epidemiologica e valutazione dei servizi in Italia. *Epidemiologia e Prevenzione*, **26**, 1.

Taroni, F. (1985). *Il sistema informativo e la valutazione di qualità.* Atti del Convegno Internazionale di studio sulla Verifica e Revisione della Qualita' della Assistenza Sanitaria e delle Cure Mediche, June, Firenze.

The Netherlands

Beeck, E.F. van, Mackenbach, J.P., Kunst, A.E., and Looman, C.W.N. (1991). Determinants of traffic accident mortality patterns in the Netherlands: a geographic analysis. *International Journal of Epidemiology*, **20**, 698.

Kunst, A.E., Looman, C.W.N., and Mackenbach, J.P. (1988). Medical care and regional mortality differences within the countries of the European community. *European Journal of Population*, **4**, 223.

Kunst, A.E., Looman, C.W.N., and Mackenbach, J.P. (1991). Are regional mortality patterns in the Netherlands culturally determined? *Espaces, Populations et Sociétés*, **1**, 85.

Mackenbach, J.P. (1984). Gezondheidszorg en vermijdbare sterfte. *Tijdschrift voor Sociale Gezondheidszorg*, **62**, 433.

Mackenbach, J.P. (1985). Het effect van antibiotica op de sterfte aan infectieziekten in Nederland. *Tijdschrift voor Sociale Gezondheidszorg,* **63**, 518.

Mackenbach, J.P. (1987*a*). Internationale en regionale verschillen in sterfte aan enkele door medische zorg (gedeeltelijk) voorkoombare of behandelbare aandoeningen. *Nederlands Tijdschrift voor Geneeskunde*, **131** (37), 1612.

Mackenbach, J.P. (1987*b*). Verbeteringen in de overleving van kankerpatienten sinds de jaren 1950. *Tijdschrift voor Sociale Gezondheidszorg*, **65** (2), 30.

Mackenbach, J.P. (1987*c*). Health care policy and regional epidemiology; International comparisons and a case-study from the Netherlands. *Social Science and Medicine*, **23** (3), 247.

Mackenbach, J.P. (1991). Health care expenditure and mortality from amenable conditions in the European Community. *Health Policy,* **19**, 245.

Mackenbach, J.P., and Looman, C.W.N. (1988). Secular trends of infectious disease mortality in the Netherlands 1911–1978: quantitative estimates of changes coinciding with the introduction of antibiotics. *International Journal of Epidemiology*, **17** (3), 618.

Mackenbach, J.P., and Looman, C.W.N. (1994). Living standards and mortality in the European Community. *Journal of Epidemiology and Community Health,* **48**, 140.

Mackenbach, J.P., and Kunst, A.E. (1995). Socio-economic and cultural determinants of regional mortality patterns in the Netherlands. In *Adult mortality in developed countries. From description to explanation* (ed. A. Lopez, G. Caselli and T. Valkonen). Oxford University Press, Oxford.

Mackenbach, J.P., Moens, G., and Lagasse, R. (1985). Verschillen tussen Nederland en Belgie in door gezondheidszorg vermijdbare sterfte. *Gezondheid en Samenleving*, **6** (4), 265.

Mackenbach, J.P., Van Duyne, W.M.J., and Kelson, M.C. (1987). Certification and coding of two underlying causes of death in the Netherlands and other countries of the European Community. *Journal of Epidemiology and Community Health*, **41**, 156.

Mackenbach, J.P., Looman, C.W.N., and Kunst, A.E. (1988*a*). De ontwikkeling van de sterfte aan aandoeningen die (gedeeltelijk) door medische zorg voorkoombaar of behandelbaar zijn geworden, 1950-1984. *Nederlands Tijdschrift voor Geneeskunde*, **132** (36), 1665.

Mackenbach, J.P., Kunst, A.E., Looman, C.W.N., Habbema, J.D.F., and van der Maas, P.J. (1988*b*). Regional differences in mortality from conditions amenable to medical intervention in the Netherlands: a comparison of four time periods. *Journal of Epidemiology and Community Health*, **42** (4), 325.

Mackenbach, J.P., Looman, C.W.N., Kunst, A.E., Habbema, J.D.F., and van der Maas, P.J. (1988*c*). Post-1950 mortality trends and medical care: gains in life expectancy due to declines in mortality from conditions amenable to medical intervention in the Netherlands. *Social Science and Medicine*, **27** (9), 889.

Mackenbach, J.P., Looman, C.W.N., Kunst, A.E., Habbema, J.D.F., and van der Maas, P.J. (1988*d*). Regional differences in decline of mortality from conditions amenable to medical intervention in the Netherlands. *International Journal of Epidemiology*, **17** (4), 821.

Mackenbach, J.P., Stronks, K., and Kunst, A.E. (1989). The contribution of medical care to inequalities in health: differences between socio-economic groups in decline of mortality from conditions amenable to medical intervention. *Social Science and Medicine*, **29** (3), 369.

Mackenback, J.P., Bouvier-Colle, M.H., and Jougla, E. (1990). Avoidable mortality and health services—a review of aggregate data studies. *Journal of Epidemiology & Community Health*, **44**, 106.

Mackenbach, J.P., Kunst, A. E. and Looman, C.W.N. (1991). Cultural and economic determinants of regional mortality patterns in the Netherlands. *Journal of Epidemiology and Community Health,* **45**, 231.

United Kingdom—England and Wales

Bauer, R.L., and Charlton, J.R.H. (1986). Area variation in mortality from diseases amenable to medical intervention: the contribution of differences in morbidity. *International Journal of Epidemiology*, **15**, 408.

Buck N., Devlin, H.B., and Lunn, J.N. (1987). Report of the confidential enquiry into perioperative deaths. Nuffield Provincial Hospitals Trust and the King's Fund for Hospitals, London.

Charlton, J.R.H., and Lakhani, A. (1985). Is the Jarman underprivileged area score valid? *British Medical Journal*, **290**, 1714.

Charlton, J.R.H. and Velez, R. (1986). Some international comparisons of mortality amenable to medical intervention. *British Medical Journal*, **292**.

Charlton, J.R.H., Hartley, R.M., Silver, R., and Holland, W.W. (1983). Geographical variation in mortality from conditions amenable to medical intervention in England and Wales. *Lancet*, **i**, 691.

Charlton, J.R.H., Bauer, R., and Lakhani, A. (1984). Outcomes measures for district and regional health care planners. *Community Medicine*, **6**, 306.

Charlton, J.R.H., Lakhani, A., and Aristidou, M. (1986). How have 'avoidable death' indices for England and Wales changed? 1974–78 compared with 1979–83. *Community Medicine*, **8**, 304.

Charlton, J.R.H., Holland, W.W., Lakhani, A., and Paul, E.A. (1987). Variations in avoidable mortality and variations in health care. *Lancet*, **i**, 858.

Committee of Public accounts. (1989). *Quality of clinical care in National Health Service Hospitals*. HMSO, London.

Devlin, H.B., and Lunn, J.N. (1986). Confidential enquiry into perioperative deaths. *British Medical Journal*, **292**, 1622.

Holland, W.W. (1986). The 'avoidable death' guide to Europe. *Health Policy,* **6**, 115.

Holland, W.W. (1988). *European Community Atlas of 'Avoidable Death'*. CEC Health Services Research Series, no. 3. Published by Oxford University Press for the Council of the European Communities.

Holland, W.W. (1990*a*). Avoidable death in Europe. Guest editorial. *Archives of Public Health*, Belgium.

Holland, W.W. (1990*b*). Avoidable death as a measure of quality. *Quality Assurance in Health Care*, **2**, 227.

Holland, W.W. (1991). European Community Atlas of 'Avoidable Death'. Vol. 1, (2nd edn), CEC Health Services Research Series, no. 6. Published by Oxford University Press for the Council of the European Communities.

Holland, W.W., and Breeze, E. (1988). The performance of health services. In *The political economy of health and welfare* (ed. M. Keynes, D.A. Coleman, and N.H. Dimsdale). Macmillan, Basingstoke.

Holland, W.W., and Fitzsimmons, B. (1990). Avoidable Mortality - its use in developing countries. *Bridge* (Newsletter of health systems research and development), 5, 8, WHO Publications, Geneva.

Lunn, J.N., and Devlin, H.B. (1987). Lessons from the confidential enquiry into perioperative deaths in three NHS regions. *Lancet*, **ii**, 1384.

Mason, J.O., Koplan, J.P., and Layde, P.M. (1987). The prevention and control of chronic diseases: reducing unnecessary deaths and disability—a conference report. *Public Health Reports*, **102**, 17.

Moore, A. (1986). Preventable childhood deaths in Wolverhampton. *British Medical Journal*, **293**, 656.

O'Mahoney, M., and Holland, W.W. (1983). Review of the services for the control of Authority. In Annual Report (1983) of the Department of Community Medicine, UMDS, St Thomas's Campus, London SE1, p. 35.

Paul, E.A., Evans, J., Barry, J., *et al.* (1989). Variations géographiques de la mortalite due a des maladies justiciables d'unes communautés européennes: Atlas des décès 'évitables'. *World Health Statistics Quarterly*, **42**, 42.

Reynolds, F. (1986). Editorial: Obstetric anaesthetic services. *British Medical Journal*, **293**, 403.

Scrivens, E., and Charlton, J.R.H. (1983). Performance indicators: warning lights? *Health and Social Services Journal*, **15**, 1501.

Singal, G.M., Stilwell, P.J., Chambers, J, and Clews, B. (1985). A confidential enquiry into premature preventable deaths. Report to Walsall Health Authority, Walsall, England.

Smith, B.A. (1984). *Cost containment in health care: a study of twelve European countries 1977-83*. Bedford Square Press of the National Council for Voluntary Organisations, London. (Occasional Papers on Social Administration no. 73/ Social Administration Research Trust, London School of Economics.)

Smith, B.A., and Maynard, A. (1979). *The organisation, financing and cost of health care in the European Community*. Collection Studies, Social Policy Series no. 36. Office for Official Publications of the European Community, Luxembourg.

Valman, B. (1985). Preventing infant deaths. *British Medical Journal*, **290**, 339.

United Kingdom—Scotland

Carstairs, V. (1981). Multiple deprivation and health state. *Community Medicine*, **3**, 4.

Carstairs, V. (1989). Avoidable mortality in European countries—1974–1978. *Scottish Medical Journal*, Feb., 391.

Carstairs, V. (1991). Dying away from home: the influence on mortality statistics. *Population Trends*, no. 66.

Carstairs, V. (1993). Avoidable deaths in countries of the European Community and in Scotland. *Health Bulletin*, May (51), 3.

Carstairs, V., and Morris, R. (1989). Deprivation: explaining differences in mortality between Scotland and England and Wales. *British Medical Journal*, **299**, 886.

Carstairs, V., and Morris, R. (1990). Deprivation and health in Scotland. *Health Bulletin, Edinburgh*, **48** (4), 162.

Carstairs, V., and Morris, R. (1991). *Deprivation and health in Scotland*. Aberdeen University Press.

Cole, S.K. (1989). Accuracy of death certificates in neonatal deaths. *Community Medicine*, **11**, 1.

Crombie, I.K., Kenicer, M.B., Smith, W.C.S., and Tunstall-Pedoe, H. (1989). Unemployment, socioenviromental factors and coronary heart disease in Scotland. *British Heart Journal*, **61**, 172.

Crombie, I.K., Smith, W.C.S., Tavendale, R., and Tunstall-Pedoe, H. (1990). Geographical clustering of risk factors and lifestyle for coronary heart disease in the Scottish Heart Health Study. *British Heart Journal*, **64**, 199.

Smith, W.C.S., Tunstall-Pedoe, H., Crombie, I.K., and Tavendale, R. (1989). Concomitants of excess coronary deaths—major risk factor and lifestyle findings from 10,359 men and women in the Scottish Heart Health Study. *Scottish Medical Journal*, **34**, 550.

Tunstall-Pedoe, H., Smith, W.C.S., Crombie, I.K., and Tavendale, R. (1989). Coronary risk factor and lifestyle variation across Scotland: results from the Scottish Heart Health Study. *Scottish Medical Journal 34*, 556.

Woodward, M., Shewry, M.C., Smith, W.C.S., and Tunstall-Pedoe, H. (1992). Social status and coronary heart disease: results from the Scottish Heart Health Study. Preventive Medicine, **21**, 136.

Portugal

Araújo, M.P. (1990). *Evolução da mortalidade materna em Portugal: 1979–1987*. Saúde em Números, Direcção-Geral Cuidados de Saúde Primários 5 (1), Lisbon.

Cayolla da Motta, L. (1988). *Mortes evitáveis na Europa: diferenças nacionais e regionais*. Saúde em Números, Direcção-Geral Cuidados de Saúde Primários 4 (2), Lisbon.

Cayolla da Motta, L. (1990). Epidemiologia na década dos 90—prospectivas e futuro. *Temas de Reflexão, Revista Portuguesa de Saúde Pública*, **9** (1) 46.

Cayolla da Motta, L. (1990). Health levels in Portugal and Spain measured by years of potential life lost. *Abstracts of the Regional European Meeting of International Epidemiological Association*, Granada, p. 14.

Cayolla da Motta, L., and Marinho Falcão, J. (1987). *Atlas do Cancro em Portugal 1980-82*. Ministério da Saúde, Lisbon.

Cayolla da Motta, L., Sequeira, M.L., and Castanheira, J.L. (1989). *Anos de vida potenciais perdidos: mortalidade prematura (1-69 anos) por causas e distritos em Portugal e sua evolucao de 1976 a 1986 (Nota Prévia)*. Saúde em Números, Direcção-Geral dos Cuidados de Saúde Primários 4 (2).

Cayolla da Motta, L., Botelho, J. S., and Dias, A. (1992). Premature deaths by causes and their evolution in Portugal from 1980 to 1989.

Spain

Cerdá, T., and González, J. (1989). Distribución geográfica de la mortalidad evitable en España, período 1975–1983. *VIII Reunión Científica de la Sociedad Española de Epidemiología. Libro de Comunicaciones*. Abstract no. 113. Santiago de Compostela.

García Benavides, F., Pérez, S., Cayuela, A., *et al.* (1990). Razón de años de vida perdidos evitables: un indicator para identificar exceso de mortalidad en Areas de Salud. *Gaceta Sanitaria*, **3**, 12.

Gispert, R., and Segura, A. (1990). La indentificación de la mortalidad evitable y sus aplicaciones prácticas. *Gaceta Sanitaria*, **3**, 12.

González, J., and Cerda, T. (1989). Evolución temporal de la mortalidad evitable en España. VIII Reunión Científica de la Sociedad Española de Epidemiología. Libro de Comunicaciones. Abstract no. 113. Santiago de Compostela.

González, J., Cerda, T., Regidor, E., and Medrano, M.J. (1989). *Atlas de mortalidad evitable en España*. Ministerio de Sanidad y Consumo, Madrid.

Gil, L.M.B., and Rathwell, T. (1989). The effect of health services on mortality: amenable and non-amenable causes in Spain. *International Journal of Epidemiology*, **18** (3), 652.

Ortún, V. (1987). Criterios para la distribución de recursos sanitarios en España. *Gaceta Sanitaria*, **1**, 69.

Ortún Rubio, V., and Gispert Magarolas, R. (1988). Exploración de la mortalidad prematura como guía de la política sanitaria e indicator de calidad asistencia. *Medicina Clínica*, **90**, 399.

Regidor, E. (1991). Acerca de la mortalidad evitable. *Gaceta Sanitaria*, **5**, 139.

Portugal and Spain

Cayolla da Motta, L., and Rodriguez, L.A.G. (1988). Anos potenciais de vida perdidos: estudio comparativo de ‘mortalidade evitável’ por causas entre Portugal e Espanha. *Revista Portuguesa de Saúde Pública*, **3** (4), 39.

Cayolla da Motta, L., and Rodriguez, L.A. (1989). Years of potential life lost: Application of an indicator for assessing premature mortality in Spain and Portugal. *WHO Quarterly Rapport Trimestriel de Statistiques Sanitaires Mondiales*, **42**, 1.

Further references

Bouvier-Colle, M.H., Magescas, J.B., and Hatton, F. (1985). Causes de décès et jeunes étrangers en France. *Revue d’Epidémiologie et de Santé Publique*, **33**, 409.

Bouvier-Colle, M.H., Vallin, J., and Hatton, F. (1990). *Mortalité et causes de décès en France*. INSERM - Doin, Paris.

Dambrosio, F., and Buscaglia, M. (1976). La mortalità in Lombardia e le sue cause. Risultati di un'indagine e condotta negli ospedali della Lombardia per gli anni 1966-73. *Annali di Ostetricia, Ginecologia, Medicina Perinatale*, **97**, 302.

Editorial. (1985). Perioperative deaths. *Lancet*, **ii**, 1049.

Makenbach, J.P., Bouvier-Colle, M.H., and Jougla, E. (1990). Avoidable mortality and health services: a review of aggregate data studies. *Journal Epidemiology & Community Health*, **44**, 106.

Poikolainen, K., and Eskola, J. (1986). Mortality from causes amenable to health services intervention (letter). *Lancet*, **i**, 1387.

Rumeau-Rouquette, C., du Mazaubrun, C., and Rabarison, Y. (1984*a*). *Naître en France. Dix ans d'évolution*. INSERM-Doin, Paris.

Rutstein, D.D., Berenberg, W., Chalmers, T.C., *et al.* (1980). Measuring the quality of medical care: second revision of tables of indexes. *New England Journal of Medicine*, **302**, 1146.

Wigle, D.T., *et al.* (1987). Declining risk of death in Canada: achievement and a challenge. *Journal of Chronic Diseases, Canada*, **8**, 4.

Woolsey, T.D. (1981). *Toward an index of 'preventable' mortality*. United States Department of Health and Human Services, Hyattsville, Maryland.

World Health Organization MONICA Project. (1988). Geographical variation in the major risk factors of coronary heart disease in men and women aged 35–64 years. *World Health Statistics Quarterly*, **41**, 115.